12-Lead ECG

The Art of Interpretation

Lead I

Lead II   Lead III

Tomas B. Garcia, MD, FACEP

Neil E. Holtz, BS, EMT-P

JONES AND BARTLETT PUBLISHERS

Sudbury, Massachusetts

BOSTON   LONDON   TORONTO   SINGAPORE

Jones and Bartlett Publishers

World Headquarters
Jones and Bartlett Publishers
40 Tall Pine Drive
Sudbury, MA 01776
978-443-5000
info@jbpub.com
www.jbpub.com
www.12LeadECG.com

Jones and Bartlett Publishers Canada
2406 Nikanna Rd.
Mississauga, ON L5C 2W6
CANADA

Jones and Bartlett Publishers International
Barb House, Barb Mews
London W6 7PA
UK

ISBN: 0-7637-1284-1

Library of Congress Cataloging-in-Publication Data
Garcia, Tomas B., 1952-
   12-lead ECG: The art of interpretation/Tomas B. Garcia, Neil E. Holtz.
     p.cm.
   Includes index and bibliographical references.
   ISBN 0-7637-1284-1 (alk.paper)
   1. Electrocardiography. I. Holtz, Neil E. II. Title.

RC683.5.E5 G26 2000
616.1'207547--dc21   00-055359

Production Credits

Chief Executive Officer: Clayton Jones
Chief Operating Officer: Don W. Jones, Jr.
President: Robert W. Holland, Jr.
V.P. Production and Design: Anne Spencer
V.P. Manufacturing and Inventory Control: Therese Bräuer
V.P. Sales and Marketing: William Kane
Publisher, Public Safety Group: Kim Brophy
Associate Managing Editor: Carol E. Brewer
Design and Composition: Nesbitt Graphics, Inc.
Cover Design: Night & Day Design
Printing and Binding: Courier Corporation
Cover Printer: Lehigh Corporation

Cover and Illustration Credits: pp. v, 1, and 71 Proportions of the human figure, c. 1492 (Vitruvian Man) (pen & ink on paper) by Leonardo da Vinci (1452–1519) Galleria dell' Accademia, Venice, Italy/Bridgeman Art Library.

Printed in the United States of America
04

12-Lead ECG: The Art of Interpretation

Welcome to the comprehensive resource on 12-lead ECG! This text is the result of collaboration between a physician, a paramedic, and Jones and Bartlett Publishers. The result is an all-encompassing text designed to bring you from having little or no electrocardiographic knowledge to the level of a fully advanced interpreter of ECGs. Whether you are an EMT, nurse, medical student, or physician wanting to learn or brush up on your knowledge of electrocardiography, this book will meet your needs.

This text contains over 200 full-size ECG strips. Each chapter introduces background information that is followed by ECG strips, analyses and interpretations. The final chapter allows you to put together everything you have learned.

Unlike other texts, this book is set up to be accessed by three different levels of readers:

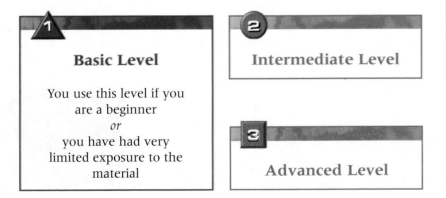

- **Level 1,** indicated in blue, provides basic information for the beginning student who has had minimal experience interpreting ECGs. This level addresses basic information that you will need to understand ECGs. They are the foundation concepts upon which we will build.

- **Level 2,** indicated in green, provides intermediate information applicable to those with a basic understanding of the principles of electrocardiography, but who want to solidify and begin to expand that knowledge. If you have completed Level 1 of this book or have read some basic books on rhythms or 12-leads, then you are probably at this level. If you are already at this level, you can skip Part 1 and start at Part 2.

- **Level 3,** indicated in red, provides advanced information. This is a level for those who have some mastery of electrocardiography, such as advanced practitioners. This level requires a solid understanding of the ECG and the disease complexes that can cause the changes shown on the ECG.

12-Lead ECG: The Art of Interpretation is designed to grow with you as your knowledge of electrocardiography progresses. Your journey into electrocardiography begins when you establish your level (see *How to Pick Your Starting Level*, p. iii). As a Level 1 or Level 2 student, read the text that pertains only to your level. Once you have mastered this material, return to the beginning of the book and read the text in the next level. You always have the previous levels' information available for reference, only a few pages away. The entire text, regardless of the level, is written in a friendly, easy-to-read tone that is clear and understandable, maximizing your comfort.

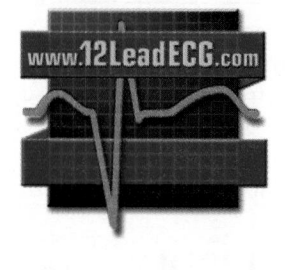

To enhance the knowledge you gain in this book, access this text's corresponding web site at www.12leadECG.com! At this site, you will find an online glossary and related web links. To learn more about the topic of a certain chapter, simply click on that chapter and view the link.

Read on to learn how to pick your starting level and to begin learning how to read an ECG. Before long, with the help of this multimedia learning system, you will become an advanced ECG interpreter and better equipped to save lives.

How to Use This Book

General Overview

Most electrocardiography textbooks were created for either beginners or advanced students, but leave the intermediate student, or person with some knowledge of 12-lead and arrhythmia recognition, out of the picture. This text was written for beginner, intermediate, and advanced students alike.

The format allows you to move at your own speed by providing information in bite-sized chunks. It is written in an easy-to-read, friendly, tone so that you can feel comfortable while you are reading.

There are plenty of jokes and humor throughout, because life is short and you have to have fun. We hope this approach enhances your reading experience and facilitates learning.

The book is broken down into two parts:

- **Part 1** presents basic information about the complexes, waves, and intervals, as well as the ECG and calibration. You will learn about the basic beat or complex and review the basic anatomy of the heart and the electrical conduction system. You will also learn how to use some tools that can be very helpful in interpreting the ECG.

- **Part 2** focuses on each wave and interval of the complex, the axis, and the 12-lead presentation of some rhythm disturbances. This book is not intended to cover all of the rhythms and you are referred to the reference section for some suggested reading on this material. Part 2 will cover the electrocardiographic criteria for the various types of acute myocardial infarctions and provides examples of each. Finally, Part 2 includes a chapter on putting it all together. This extremely useful chapter synthesizes all of the information you have learned to this point. You should plan on spending some time in this chapter and understanding the concepts thoroughly before you move on.

The book has been created to be continuously useful during your development and is intended to be read and reread as you advance in your knowledge and comfort level with the material. By rereading the material at increasingly advanced levels, you will get more out of the material and retain it with greater use.

How to Pick Your Starting Level

The first and most important thing you need to do as you begin the process of using this book is to establish your level of understanding. There are three levels of understanding represented by Levels 1, 2, and 3.

Level 1: As a beginner, start in Chapter 1 by reading the Level 1 material. When you get to Part 2, continue reading the Level 1 material and then look at the ECG examples to see if you can pick up the information that relates to what you have just read. **Look only at the information on the ECG that pertains to the Level 1 material.** Do not focus on interpretation at this time; that will come later. You can look at the rest of the waves and complexes, but only concentrate on learning the small amount of information for that section. Afterward, move on to the next section or chapter. When you have finished all of the book's Level 1 material and analyzed all of the ECGs for that pertinent information, restart the book in Part 2 using the Level 2 material.

Level 2: As an intermediate reader, you can either start with a review of the Level 1 material to refresh yourself, and then move on to Level 2, or simply start with the Level 2 material. Use the Quick Review questions to test your knowledge of the basic concepts. If you get them wrong, go back to the corresponding Level 1 material and review it. When you get to the ECGs, try to evaluate them without reading the corresponding text. Once you have done this, read the text that corresponds with each ECG and see if you had the concepts right. When you are done with all of the Level 2 material, go back and reread the book using the Level 3 material. To prevent gaps in knowledge, do not try to read the Level 3 text until you have completed Level 2.

Level 3: The Level 3 material is advanced. This information can be quite complex, but if you have finished all of the Level 2 material, you should be ready for this level. Review the sections you do not understand and use other reference books to supplement your knowledge at this level. Do not think that you need to have mastered the information upon completion of this book; it takes quite a few years and quite a few thousand ECGs to truly become a master.

Ready to start? If you are a beginner, begin at Chapter 1. If you are unsure of your level, try going back to Chapter 9 or 10 and see if you understand the material in Level 2. If you feel it is too elementary, then move up. If you feel it is too advanced, move back. Be truthful with yourself or you will become frustrated. Remember—use this book until you have gotten everything out of it that you can.

How to Read an ECG

The majority of this book is geared toward breaking down the various sections of the ECG and its complexes. The chapters teach you what each part of the ECG represents and the respective abnormalities. Each section covers the pathology associated with a wave or interval of the ECG by using a problems-oriented approach that consists of examining the list of possible causes for a pathological wave or interval and determining how these relate to the other complexes. This list of possible causes is called the *differential diagnosis*.

As you review the ECG, look at each wave and interval and create lists of abnormalities that you find in them. You will then have several lists. Find out what diseases or syndromes are common to all of those lists; that disease or syndrome will be, with almost complete certainty, the diagnosis.

Before you start the book, we would like to offer the following steps to guide you in ECG interpretation. These steps will become second nature after review and use. Don't worry if you are unfamiliar with some of the terminology—you will become familiar with it when you read the chapters. The most important task now is to develop a logical approach to examining and interpreting the ECG. You can adjust this system, as you need to, to match your particular style.

1. **Get a general impression of what is going on and keep it foremost in your mind.**

Look at the ECG for a few seconds and see what strikes you as the most important detail. Is it ischemia, arrhythmia, electrolyte problems, pacer problems, or something else? Don't let the details overwhelm you—instead, form the big picture first and keep it in your mind as you move on to interpret the ECG. Eventually, you will learn how to break down the ECG and methodically derive an interpretation.

2. Look at the ECG sequentially and in minute detail.

This is the second concept that involves all of the steps below. When starting out, try to use an ECG that contains a rhythm strip at the bottom that correlates with the leads above—it will make your life much easier. Look at the beats. If they look different, break them down and figure out which are the normal beats and which are the abnormal beats. Look at the normal beats first to determine your intervals, axis, blocks, etc. Then look at the abnormal beats and figure out what is causing them. Are they APCs, VPCs, aberrant conduction, paced beats, or something else?

3. What is the rate?

- Is it fast or slow?
- If it is irregular, what is the range?
- What are the intervals: PR, QRS, QTc, PP, RR?
- Are there irregularities in any of the intervals, for example, PR depression?

4. What is the rhythm?

- Is it fast or slow?
- Regular or irregular?
- Grouped or ungrouped?
- Can you see P waves? Are they all the same?
- Is there one-to-one conduction of the P waves to the QRS complexes?
- Wide or narrow?

5. What is the axis?

- What quadrant does it fall into?
- What is the isoelectric limb lead?
- Where is the transition zone in the precordials?
- Calculate the exact axis. (Advanced clinicians should also calculate the P, T, and ST axes.)
- Does the exact axis tell you anything?

6. Is there any evidence of hypertrophy?

- Left atrial?
- Right atrial?
- Biatrial?
- Left ventricular?
- Right ventricular?
- Biventricular?
- Left or right strain pattern?

7. Is there any evidence of ischemia or infarction?

- Are there regional T wave abnormalities?
- Are there regional ST segment abnormalities?
- Are there regional Q waves?

8. How can I put it all together?

Think of all the findings and try to come up with a common theme to the differential diagnosis that you have developed. Think of everything and overlook nothing. Be sure to consider the rate, rhythm, axis, hypertrophy, interval abnormalities, blocks, and ST and T wave abnormalities.

9. Can I put it all together with my patient's signs and symptoms?

Do the diagnosis and findings on the ECG make sense with the patient's presenting signs and symptoms? Can the ECG be a presentation of a problem or the cause of some pre-existing condition? Ask yourself, "How can I use the information to adequately treat the patient?"

10. What is my final diagnosis?

List your final single diagnosis or your abbreviated list of differential diagnoses.

In closing, don't forget that it takes time to learn to interpret ECGs. Some of the concepts we mention in the list above may be above your level now, but not for long! The more you use the book, the better you will become. Lastly, have fun! Life is short.

Contents

Acknowledgments

Author Acknowledgments:

We would like to begin by thanking all of those educators and clinicians who spent countless hours teaching us the specifics of Medicine. It was through your hard work and perseverance that we have learned how to treat patients. You have allowed us the privilege of becoming healers. Be secure in the knowledge that, just as ripples flow across a pond, so the ripples of knowledge that you have imparted on us shall continue on their journey to light the way for future clinicians. We hope that we have lived up to your expectations and have not let you down.

We would also like to thank all of the countless students, residents, paramedics, nurses, EMTs, physician assistants, and technicians that have asked us countless questions and continually questioned our authority. It is by answering your questions that we have been able to hone our knowledge and expand our abilities to teach. You have allowed us to pass on the knowledge that we have learned and this has been, in our opinion, our greatest honor. Always continue to question everyone and challenge the "standard" thinking of the time, because stagnation is the worst thing that could happen to Medicine.

We would like to thank Jones and Bartlett Publishers for having the foresight to publish a book that does not conform to the "norm." We would especially like to express our appreciation and our heartfelt gratitude to our editors: Tracy Foss, Carol Brewer, and Loren Marshall. Tracy, thanks for believing in our proposal and for your support throughout the project. Carol, thanks for putting up with the daily phone calls and the occasional tantrum. Your input, day by day, has molded this book into a reality. Loren, your insights and suggestions are appreciated and invaluable. Special thanks also goes to our Production Editor, Cynthia Maciel Knowles, whose hard work and guidance transformed the manuscript into a book. We thank all of Jones and Bartlett Publishers for your hard work and for the blood, sweat, and tears that you have poured into this project.

Finally, we would like to thank our families and friends who have sacrificed time away from us so that we could achieve our objectives. We know that it is time that will never be replaced. Some of the prices we have had to pay have been high. Hopefully, the lives saved because of the information we have passed on will be some consolation for our mutual loss. We thank you, we love you, and we will be forever in your debt.

Tomas B. Garcia, MD, FACEP
Neil E. Holtz, EMT-P

Publisher's Acknowledgments:

Jones and Bartlett Publishers and the authors would like to thank the following people for reviewing this text.

William A. Black
Alamo EMS
Vassar College
Ulster Community College
Wappinger Falls, NY

G. Richard Braen, MD
Buffalo General Hospital
Professor and Chairman, Department of
    Emergency Medicine
State University of New York at Buffalo,
School of Medicine
Buffalo, NY

Samuel F. Gates, EMT-P, EMS-I
Emergency Medical Services Institute
The Stamford Hospital
Stamford, CT

Carol Gupton, BSMES, NREMT-P
EMS Faculty
Training Division
Omaha Fire Department
Omaha, NE

Daniel G. Judkins, RN, MS, MPH
University of Arizona
Tuscon, AZ

Kathryn Lewis, RN, PhD
Department Chair
Phoenix College EMT/FSC
Phoenix, AZ

James Loflin, MD, FACEP
Texas Tech University Health Sciences Center
Department of Emergency Medicine
El Paso, TX

Jeff McDonald
EMS Coordinator
Tarrant County Junior College
Hurst, TX

John L. Morrissey, NREMT-P
New York State Instructor Coordinator,
    Regional Facility
AHA BCLS Instructor Trainer/ACLS/PALS
    Instructor
Senior Emergency Medical Care Representa-
    tive, New York State Department of Health,
    Bureau of Emergency Medical Services
Liverpool, NY

Gerard Oncale, RN, BSN, CEN, REMT-P
Louisiana Organ Procurement Agency
Metairie, LA

Kenneth Pardoe, MS, PA-C, NREMT-P
Captain, Anne Arundel County Fire
    Department
Physician Assistant, Department of Emergency
    Medicine
    North Arundel Hospital
Lieutenant, U.S. Naval Reserve, Medical Service
    Corps
Severn, MD

Douglas A. Rund, MD, FACEP
Professor and Chairman
Department of Emergency Medicine
The Ohio State University
Columbus, OH

John Saito, EMT-P, MPH
Dean, Allied Health Division
Mt. Hood Community College
Gresham, Oregon
Assistant Professor of Emergency Medicine
Oregon Health Sciences University
Portland, Oregon

Samuel J. Stratton, MD, MPH
Department of Emergency Medicine
Harbor-UCLA Medical Center
Torrance, CA

Paul A. Werfel, NREMT-P
Director, Paramedic Program
State University of New York
Stony Brook, NY

Frank G. Yanowitz, MD
Associate Professor of Medicine
University of Utah School of Medicine
Medical Director, ECG Department
Medical Director, The Fitness Institute
Chief, Geriatrics Division
LDS Hospital
Salt Lake City, UT

Dedications and Biographies

I dedicate this book to the two most wonderful and amazing people I know, my Mom and Dad. Thank you for the love, understanding, support, and tolerance you have given me throughout the years. You have been my inspiration and my foundation in life. Also to the light of my life, my son Daniel. You have added a depth to my life that goes beyond mere words. I love you and I am proud to be your dad. Finally, to my sister Sonia, who, from the time I was born, was always there for me.

Tomas B. Garcia, MD, FACEP

Dr. Tomas B. Garcia received his undergraduate degree from Florida International University. While applying to medical school, Dr. Garcia was licensed and practiced as an EMT in the state of Florida. Dr. Garcia received his medical degree from the University of Miami. He completed his internship and residency at Jackson Memorial Hospital in Miami, Florida and subsequently received board certification in both Internal Medicine and Emergency Medicine. Dr. Garcia taught and practiced in the Emergency Departments of the Brigham and Women's Hospital/Harvard Medical School in Boston, Massachusetts and Grady Memorial Hospital/Emory Medical School in Atlanta, Georgia. His main area of interest is emergency cardiac care and he lectures nationally on topics related to these issues. Presently, he is the president of *heartstuff.com*, an Internet site devoted to medical education and emergency cardiac care issues.

This book is dedicated first and foremost to my children Abbagail Lillian and Alec Irving Holtz. They are truly the future and the light in my life.

Secondly, to my brothers, Mark and Stephen Holtz, for their unwavering support from the beginning of time that I can remember.

Thirdly, to my Uncle and Aunt, the Doctors Noel and Carol Holtz, for their help, counseling, and support in the good times and bad.

Finally, to all the paramedics, nurses, clinic assistants, and docs at Grady, in the ECC and EMS departments, for their friendship and their patience listening to me talk about ECG and ACLS endlessly.

Neil E. Holtz, BS, EMT-P

Mr. Neil Holtz has been providing emergency care for the last twenty-two years. He started in the US Navy as a Hospital Corpsman assigned to the Second Marine Division. After an honorable discharge from the military, he went on to work for NYC*EMS as an EMS Specialist 1. He moved to Metro Atlanta in 1985 to attend Paramedic school at Dekalb Technical School and was employed by Grady Memorial Hospital in 1986, spending eight years in Grady EMS and the last six in the Emergency Care Center. Mr. Holtz has a BS degree from Georgia State University in Atlanta. He is currently the Director of the Emergency Medical Training Academy in Loganville, Georgia. He teaches ACLS, basic arrhythmia recognition, and 12-lead ECG interpretation.

Electrocardiography: The Art of Interpretation

Is medicine an art or a science? That question has been asked thousands of times in the past and continues to be asked to this day. I think the answer lies somewhere in the middle. It is both an art *and* a science. We use science to give us some objective answers, drugs, tools, and to prove facts. The science of medicine can be learned by anyone and requires only hard work and perseverance. It is the art of medicine, however, which has to be felt, loved, nurtured, and finally accepted if we are to become good clinicians.

When I teach medical students physical diagnosis, they spend the first couple of weeks merely observing patients from afar. They are not to talk to the patients or to examine them. Their only duty is to answer one simple question: Is the patient sick or not sick? They only have about 10 to 15 seconds to make up their minds so they cannot rationalize too much. Their decision has to be made from the gut, based on information that they gained through observation either consciously or unconsciously. It sounds complicated and yet students amaze me with how quickly they learn this task and how effectively they can put these lessons to use. This internal decision maker is an innate part of us all and will never steer you wrong. All we have to do is to develop it.

So what does this have to do with ECGs? Simple—we are going to use the same approach to learn electrocardiography. *The only way to learn electrocardiography is to look at thousands of ECGs and answer the question, "sick or not sick."* Most books about ECGs forget this one simple fact and instead go on for pages and pages writing about the ECGs and variations that can be seen, followed by one example. ECG findings are not as unique as fingerprints, but they do vary from person to person. If you only see one sample ECG for each pathology but never see the picture perfect example again in your life, you will never be able to diagnose it.

The complex language that is used in electrocardiography can be confusing and overwhelming. Most people buy an advanced textbook on electrocardiography, begin to read it, and then quickly give up. Sound familiar? You have to be very competent at electrocardiography to be able to understand the written word describing the possible variations. The simple way to learn about ECGs and one that has been largely underutilized is to see various examples and to develop a feel for what you are looking at. After a while, you will begin to feel your gut telling you whether the patient is "sick or not sick." The process of learning to interpret ECGs is not unlike learning to throw a ball. You can read about the throw, the trajectories, the spin, and the accuracy, but unless you see a few balls thrown and throw hundreds or thousands yourself, you will never really learn know how to throw a ball. In the same way, you need to see hundreds of ECGs before you become comfortable. By the time you finish this book, you will feel like you are beginning to understand the terminology and the concepts. After you reread this book, you will feel very comfortable.

You need to remember that specific findings can represent various disease processes. From that list of potential diseases, you will develop a list of differential diagnoses for each problem found on the ECG. We will teach you how to diagnose biatrial enlargement, right ventricular hypertrophy, and right-sided strain. We will give you the background necessary to diagnose severe mitral stenosis, but it will be up to you to talk to the patient and to examine them to determine if this is an accurate diagnosis. This is because you need real-time interpretation and a real live patient to be completely correct when you interpret an ECG. For example, it is difficult sometimes to interpret mild ST segment elevation in V_1 and V_2 in a patient with hypertension. Is it left ventricular hypertrophy (LVH) with strain or is it an injury? There are certain criteria for LVH with strain, but occasionally this is not as clear-cut as it may seem. Well, the answer is made simpler if you have the patient in front of you. If the patient is visiting you because they stubbed their toe, it's probably LVH with strain. If the patient is diaphoretic and clutching his chest, the diagnosis most likely would be ischemia and injury. This can also work in reverse, i.e., an ECG can guide your exam and diagnosis. There have been many times when I have been shown an ECG and I have told the clinician to go back and pick up some interesting finding on physical examination. A good example is a ventricular aneurysm. The ECG will inform you of the presence of the aneurysm and the aneurysmal heave on physical evidence will confirm diagnosis.

When you interpret ECGs, you have to be able to put the knowledge that you have gained from interpretation of the ECG and translate it to your patient. All of the ECGs in this book were obtained from real patients. The interpretations that we will offer are the interpretations we made by the patients' bedsides. You can disagree with some of them and that's okay. There are a lot of hard and fast rules in electrocardiography, but how you interpret an ECG will depend on how you were taught and your mood at the time you interpret the ECG. You can ask 20 cardiologists their opinions on an ECG and you would probably get a lot of different answers. If you show them the same ECG the next day, you would probably get more different interpretations from the same group. When it comes to interpretation, people just don't seem to agree on much. The key is to *understand* the concepts we are trying to offer you so that you can use them in your everyday practice. An ECG will offer you a wealth of knowledge about a patient. It can tell you about their past and their future (prognosis). It can tell you about their electrolyte problems, systemic illnesses, and their anatomy. Not bad for a simple bedside test.

I have been asked by a few hundred students to teach them what they *really* need to know. I can sum up the answer in one short, concise statement: You need to know the changes that your specific patient presented you on their ECG! You never know what will be important at any one point in your career; any one fact can cost the patient their life and will cost you countless hours of guilt, and possibly millions of dollars! Electrocardiographic interpretation is the same whether an EMT, paramedic, nurse, resident, attending physician, or cardiologist performs it. You cannot learn just enough to get by. Does a paramedic or a nurse need to know the changes of hyperkalemia that can lead to a lethal arrhythmia? Does a resident need to know that an axis shift can be a significant sign of cardiac disease or of a heart attack? To whom is it more important to know that an acute bifascicular block breaks down into complete heart block and possibly asystole in the setting of ischemia? It is important to you!

We are going to help you understand the basics of electrocardiography, the science. We are going to teach you using a programmed learning system that, we feel, will make it easy for you to learn at your own pace. Don't try to do everything at once, because it will overwhelm you. When you are first starting out, stick to the Level 1 (blue) material, which contains the basic teaching points written for beginners (see Introduction: How to Use This Book). As you advance, you can go back and read the more intermediate and advanced teaching points at your own pace. This is a book that is meant to be used over and over again until you have progressed through all three levels. Each time you use it you will find some additional pearls.

In closing, I would like to state that you need to look at everything at your disposal and trust yourself when you are interpreting an ECG. *Don't let anyone talk you out of something that you know is true.* Just smile at them and do what is best for the patient. You will not go wrong. Remember that an expert is someone who knows one more fact than you do. However, that one fact may not be relevant to your case so you may be the true expert!

Tomas B. Garcia, MD, FACEP

ECG: A Paramedic's Perspective

I remember staring at a 12-lead ECG with wonderment. I had just transferred from the ambulance department and off the streets to the emergency care center and inside the hospital. It struck me as curious, for I had seen the 12-lead before but only at a time when life was about running 9-1-1 calls. It seemed irrelevant to me. We were initially using LifePack 4s and then 5s, but nobody ever removed the lead selector from lead 2 with the notable exception of confirming asystole. Now, in the hospital as part of my job description, I was now doing 12-lead ECGs. I knew immediately that life was taking a strange twist. I stared at the thing and recognized the waves: the P, the QRS, the T, and the U. I noticed that the intervals I was used to peering at were there too: the PR, the R-R, the TP, the QRS duration. What did not make sense was why the deflections of the complexes were different. Moreover, how did the doctors reading these things get so much information out of them?

I grabbed a resident for whom I had done an ECG and asked him how he discerned all of the information out of that piece of paper. The harried doctor mumbled something under his breath and literally ran off. I went to another one and got some mumbo-jumbo about axis, QTc, and R wave progression. Before he would explain to my satisfaction, he too ran off. Before long, residents would see me coming with an ECG in my hand, immediately make an about-face, and walk off muttering something about having to look at an X-ray. I figured that this 12-lead ECG stuff was doctor knowledge that they were not allowed to divulge.

I finally cornered a medical attending and asked her to give me the down and dirty way that she interpreted an ECG. I scratched my head a lot and now I too was mumbling. I found a copy of a book on ECGs lying about the asthma room in the ER, and I started to read. It was difficult to read and I felt like I had to learn another language. Reading was making things significantly worse! Now the residents did not need to see me with an ECG in my hand, they just ran when they saw me. The charge nurses complained that I was "wasting" too much time on ECGs and not doing my work. One of the assistant clinical managers pulled me aside to voice his complaint too. I had to do something quick.

I purchased a programmed textbook to study 12-lead ECGs. It was awesome but incomplete. The author gave me a great piece of advice in her book; she said that the way to become good at reading ECGs was to practice, practice, practice. I then went back to my first book that made a bit more sense now. I was still missing information related to the practical application of my newfound knowledge and did not know where to get it. The hospital offered a 12-lead course six months from then. I signed up, but needed more information now. I read and read and read, and took the information I had read at face value. Unfortunately, as I later found out, some was incomplete and some outright wrong. I was not about to give up though. I had to know.

I soon realized that all this information would be of great use in the prehospital environment and that the world of 9-1-1 would be shifting to the use of 12-leads in the field. The EMS I had been affiliated with had no one who was familiar with 12-leads in the operations or training departments. I also began to realize that I was seeing a lot of poor prehospital care. Cognizably, I made the shift: I went from being a provider of EMS to a customer of the prehospital provider. I wanted to make an impact on the provision of prehospital care in the community, and what better way than to teach the medics 12-lead ECGs? Why should they have to learn in the same helter-skelter way that I had learned? They should have an easier time of it than I did. I envisioned a book that was complete, and with a bunch of examples that would make sense. It would have to be written in such a way that anybody—nurse, doctor, paramedic, or clinic assistants (who do the vast majority of ECGs in our clinic)—could read and "get" 12-lead ECG interpretation.

I believe that we have such a system. With this book, we developed a system that will transform the medical professional from a novice at 12-lead ECG to a knowledgeable interpreter. Readers will get the basics of 12-leads and then in the same book proceed to the intermediate and advanced levels. This system was developed for medical students, residents, practicing physicians, *and* for nurses, paramedics, and clinical assistants. Both I and Dr. Garcia, who was an EMT at one point, know the trials and tribulations of what it takes to be a non-physician struggling through the material.

I hope that you enjoy this book and are enthused by 12-lead ECGs as much as I am. A 12-lead ECG in many ways is like a piece of art. In time, you will develop a visceral feeling about them. A couple of years ago, I was teaching a basic arrhythmia course and was asked for the umpteenth time how to differentiate between atrial fibrillation and atrial flutter. After going through the criteria for again the umpteenth time, I stepped back from the screen and asked the students how the flutter made them feel. Did they feel the soothing symmetry of the undulating baseline? Did they feel the peace of looking at the regular rise and fall of the flutter waves, like staring out at the ocean? I then flashed up a slide of atrial fibrillation and asked if they could feel the chaos of the irregularly irregular pattern. I asked if they could feel the spasms of the fibrillating baseline undulated out of control. The vast majority understood this very right-brained perspective of ECG. An ECG is art; it is a right-brained exercise in feeling, sensing, perspective, and ultimately interpretation. I draw a correlation between interpreting a painting by Dali and interpreting an ECG. There are objective criteria for both, but it is the eye of the beholder that will be able to define both art and an ECG. When you are done with this book, you will appreciate the artistry that is the electrical conduction through the heart. It is that art that makes our hearts beat true.

Neil E. Holtz, BS, EMT-P

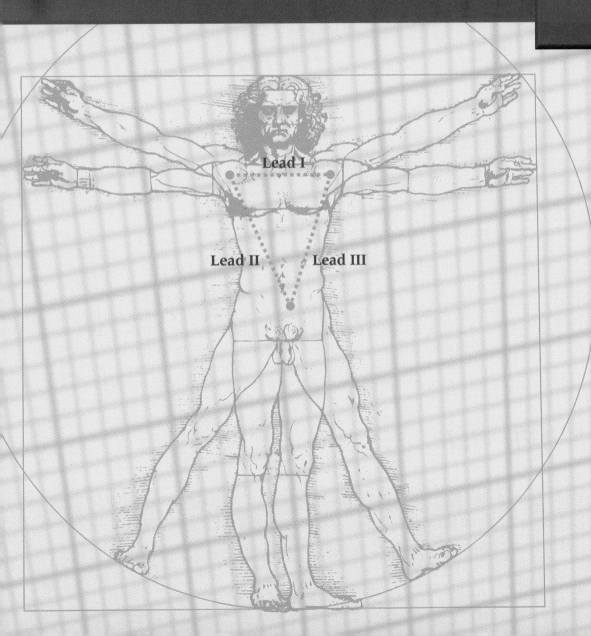

Lead I

Lead II   Lead III

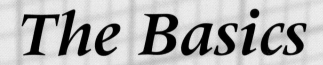
The Basics

The Basics

Part I covers ECG basics. Most of the boxes are presented as Level 1 material. Anyone dealing with ECGs should be extremely familiar with the information in this part. If you are an experienced clinician, you can skim over the information but should not skip over it completely. Make sure that you understand the material thoroughly before going on to Part II.

CHAPTER 1

Gross Anatomy

Since you are reading a book on electrocardiography, we assume that you have some basic knowledge of anatomy. However, a review is never a bad thing, so we are going to cover the basic anatomy of the heart and then concentrate on the electrical conduction system.

The heart sits in the middle of the chest at a slight angle pointing downward, to the left, and slightly anterior. Take a look at Figure 1-1.

Now, let's look at the heart itself. First, from an anterior view, and then in cross-section.

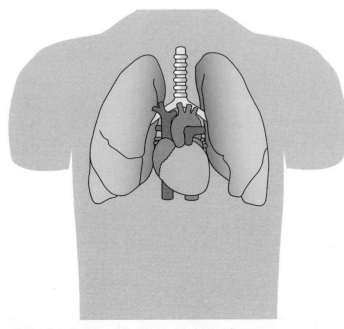

Figure 1-1: Location of the heart in the chest cavity.

Anterior View

The right ventricle (RV) dominates the anterior view. Most of the anterior surface of the ventricles consists of the RV surface. A key point to remember is that, though the RV dominates this visual view, the left ventricle (LV) dominates the electrical view. We will review this in more detail in Chapter 3 when we discuss vectors.

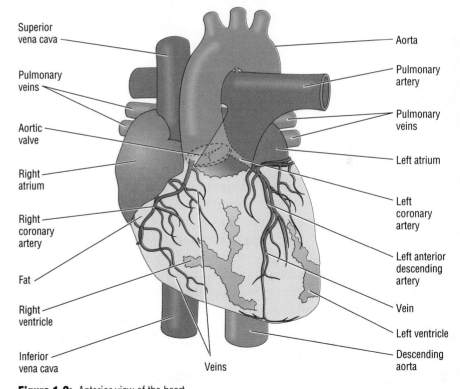

Figure 1-2: Anterior view of the heart.

The Heart in Cross Section

Here is a cross-sectional view of the heart (Figure 1-3). In the following sections, we will cover the function of the heart as a pump and review the electrical conduction system in greater detail.

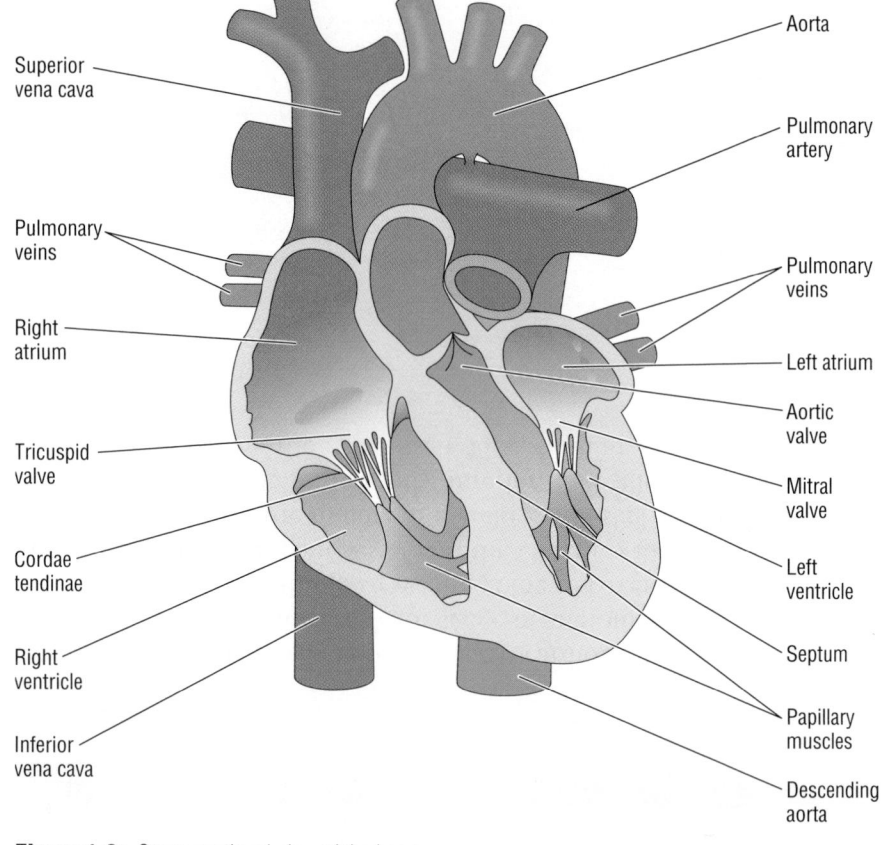

Figure 1-3: Cross-sectional view of the heart.

The Heart as a Pump

The heart consists of four main chambers: the two atria and the two ventricles. The atria empty into their corresponding ventricles. The left ventricle empties into the peripheral circulatory system, and the right ventricle empties into the pulmonary system. Veins bring blood to the heart, while arteries take blood away from the heart. As Figure 1-4 shows, this is a closed system. Blood circulates inside this closed system over and over, taking up oxygen in the lungs and giving it up to the peripheral tissues. This is a simplistic explanation of a very complicated system, but it will suffice for our purposes at this time.

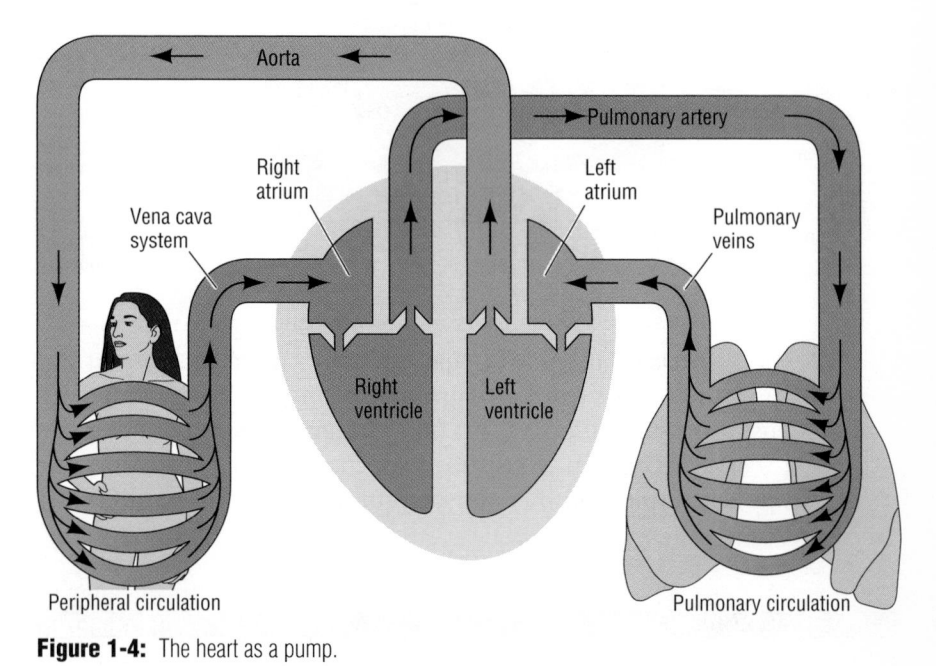

Figure 1-4: The heart as a pump.

Pump Function Simplified

It is simplest to think of the circulatory system as an engineer would: a system of interconnected pumps and pipes.

Take a look at Figure 1-5.

We see that there are four pumps in sequence. The two small primer pumps are the atria, whose sole purpose is to push a small amount of blood into the two larger ones, the ventricles. The ventricles differ in size and in the amount of pressure that they can generate. Because of the one-way valves found in the venous system, blood can only flow forward.

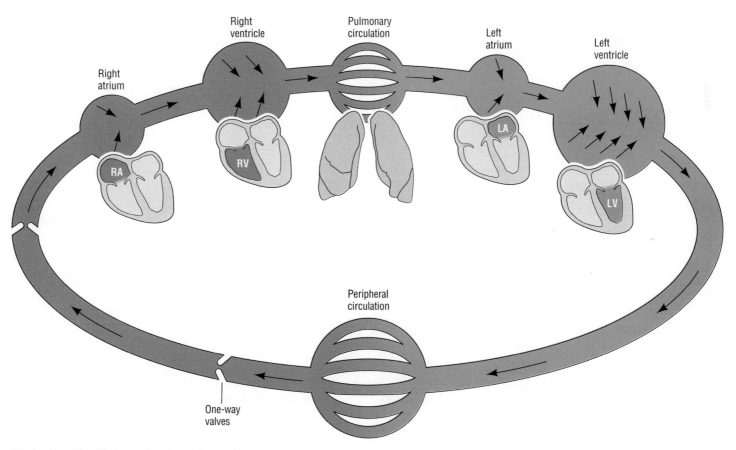

Figure 1-5: Simplified pump function of the circulatory system.

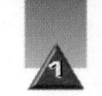
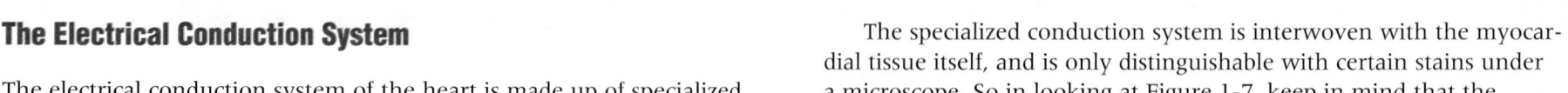

The Electrical Conduction System

The electrical conduction system of the heart is made up of specialized cells. Some of these are specialized for pacemaking functions and some for the transmission of the impulses that travel through them. We will break down the system in the following paragraphs and describe the functions of each of the parts in greater detail.

The main function of the system is to create an electrical impulse and transmit it in an organized manner to the rest of the myocardium. This is an electrochemical process that creates electrical energy that is picked up by the electrodes when we perform an electrocardiogram (ECG). (More on this in Chapter 3.)

The specialized conduction system is interwoven with the myocardial tissue itself, and is only distinguishable with certain stains under a microscope. So in looking at Figure 1-7, keep in mind that the system is actually in the heart walls. The atrial myocytes are innervated by direct contact from one cell to another; the first cell innervates the second, the second innervates the third, and so on. The internodal pathways transmit the impulse from the sino-atrial (SA) node to the AV node. The Purkinje system encircles the entire ventricles, just under the endocardium, and is the final component of the conduction system. The Purkinje cells innervate the myocardial cells themselves.

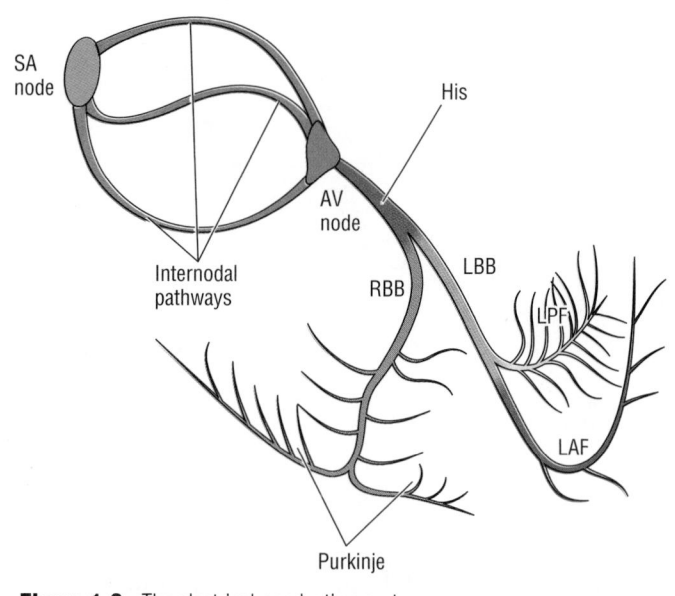

Figure 1-6: The electrical conduction system.

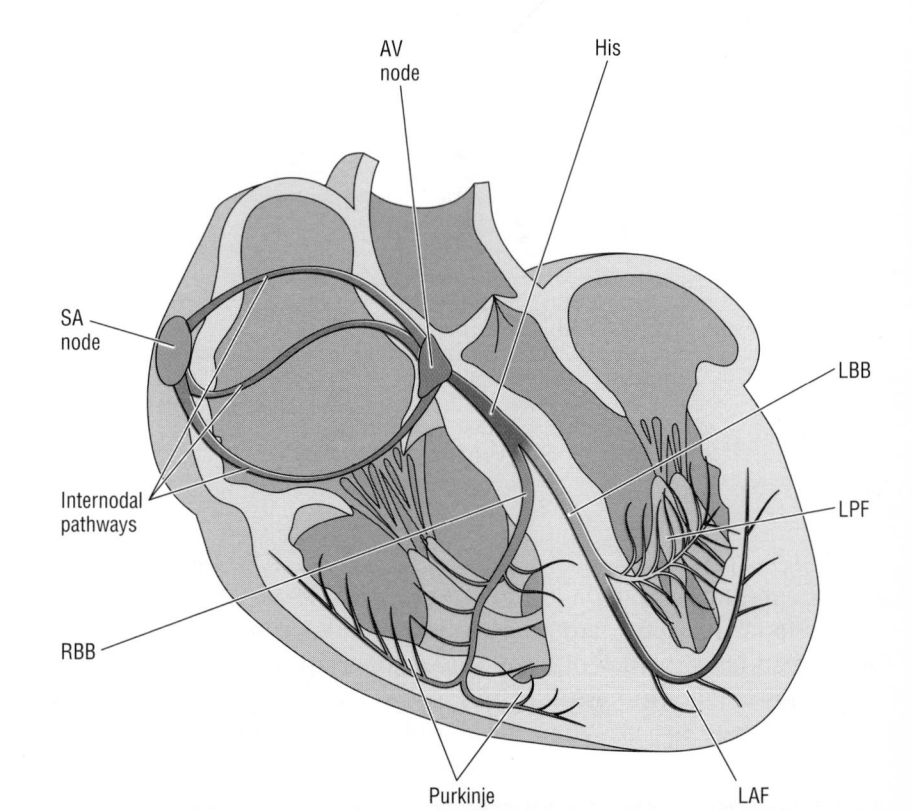

Figure 1-7: The electrical conduction system of the heart.

Pacemaker Function

What is the pacemaker function of the heart, and why do we need it? The pacemaker dictates the rate at which the heart will cycle through its pumping action to circulate the blood. The pacemaker creates an organized beating of all of the cardiac cells, in a specialized sequence, to produce effective pumping action. It sets the pace that all of the other cells will follow. Let's look at an analogy.

Imagine that each cell of the heart represents a single musician. When we have a few dozen of these musicians, we have an orchestra — the heart. Now, if each musician decides to play whenever he or she wants to, they would make an unrecognizable jumble of sound. The musicians need a beat or signal to cue them when to start to play, direct them when to come into the piece and when to leave, and coordinate their actions to create a beautiful melody. In music, that pacemaker is the underlying beat kept by the drummer or the conductor. In sections that are swift, the beat increases. In sections that are slow and soft, the beat decreases. The same thing happens in the heart; during exercise the pace speeds up, and during rest it slows.

As we have mentioned, there are specialized cells whose function is to create an electrical impulse and act as the heart's pacemaker. The main area that fills this important function is the SA node, found in the muscle of the right atrium. This area responds to the needs of the body, controlling the beat based on information it receives from the nervous, circulatory, and endocrine systems. The main pacemaker paces at a rate of 60 to 100 beats per minute (BPM), with an average of 70.

Pacemaker Settings

One thing we know about the body is that everything has a backup. Every cell in the conduction system is capable of setting the pace. However, the intrinsic rate of each type of cell is slower than the cells that precede it. This means that the fastest pacer is the SA node, the next fastest is the AV node, and so on. The fastest pacer sets the pace because it causes all the ones that come after it to reset after each beat. In this way, the slower pacers will never fire. If the faster pacer doesn't fire for some reason, the next fastest will be there as a backup to ensure function that is as close to normal as possible.

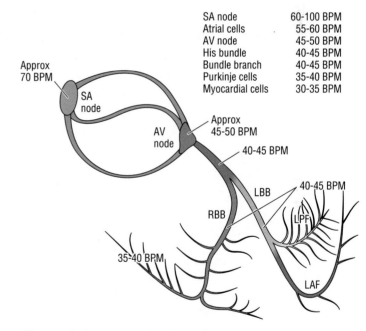

SA node	60-100 BPM
Atrial cells	55-60 BPM
AV node	45-50 BPM
His bundle	40-45 BPM
Bundle branch	40-45 BPM
Purkinje cells	35-40 BPM
Myocardial cells	30-35 BPM

Figure 1-8: Intrinsic rates of pacing cells.

The Sinoatrial (SA) Node

The SA node, the heart's main pacemaker, is found in the wall of the right atrium at its junction with the superior vena cava. Its blood supply comes from the right coronary artery in 59% of cases. In 38%, the blood supply originates from the left coronary artery, and in the last 3%, it arises from both.

The Internodal Pathways

There are three internodal pathways: anterior, middle, and posterior. Their main purpose is to transmit the pacing impulse from the SA node to the AV node. In addition, there is a small tract of specialized cells known as the Bachmann Bundle that transmits the impulses through the inter-atrial septum. All of these pathways are found in the walls of the right atrium and the inter-atrial septum.

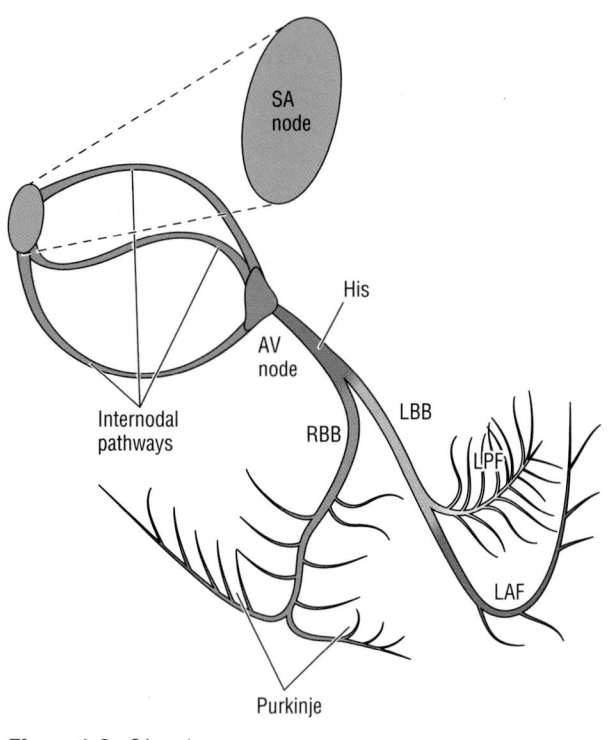

Figure 1-9: SA node.

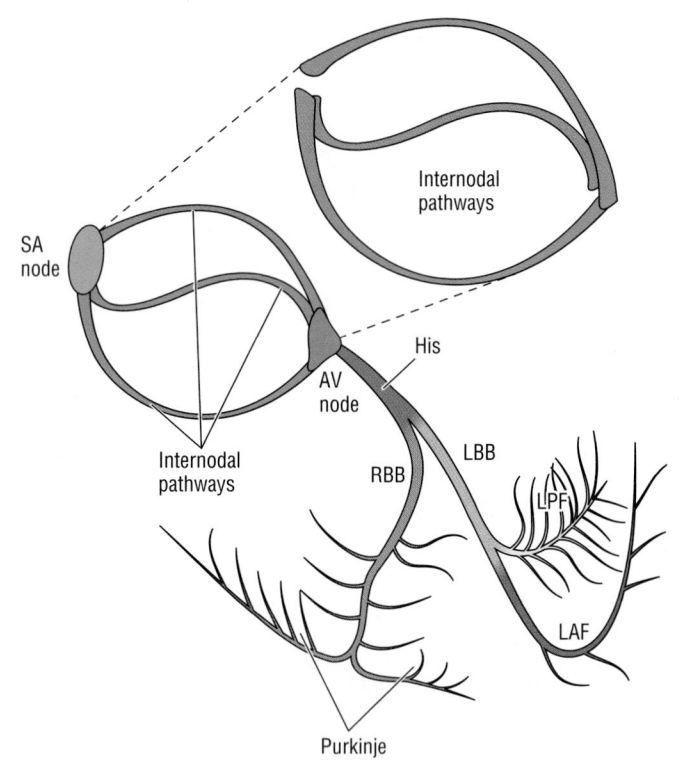

Figure 1-10: Internodal pathways.

The Atrioventricular (AV) Node

The AV node is located in the wall of the right atrium just next to the opening of the coronary sinus, the largest vein of the heart, and the septal leaflet of the tricuspid valve. It is responsible for slowing down conduction from the atria to the ventricles just long enough for atrial contraction to occur. This slowing allows the atria to "overfill" the ventricles and helps maintain the output of the heart at a maximum level. The AV node is always supplied by the right coronary artery.

The Bundle of His

The Bundle of His starts at the AV node and eventually gives rise to both the right and left bundle branches. It is found partially in the walls of the right atrium, and in the interventricular septum. The His bundle is the only route of communication between the atria and the ventricles.

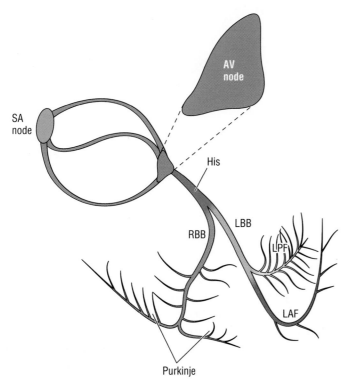

Figure 1-11: AV node.

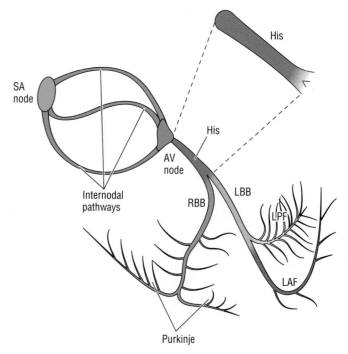

Figure 1-12: Bundle of His.

The Left Bundle Branch (LBB)

The left bundle begins at the end of the His bundle and travels through the interventricular septum. The left bundle gives rise to the fibers that will innervate the LV and the left face of the interventricular septum. It first connects to a small set of fibers that innervate the upper segment of the interventricular septum. This will be the first area to depolarize, meaning that the heart's cells fire. The left bundle ends at the beginning of the left anterior (LAF) and left posterior fascicles (LPF).

The Right Bundle Branch (RBB)

The right bundle, which also starts at the His bundle, gives rise to the fibers that will innervate the RV and the right face of the interventricular septum. It terminates in the Purkinje fibers associated with it.

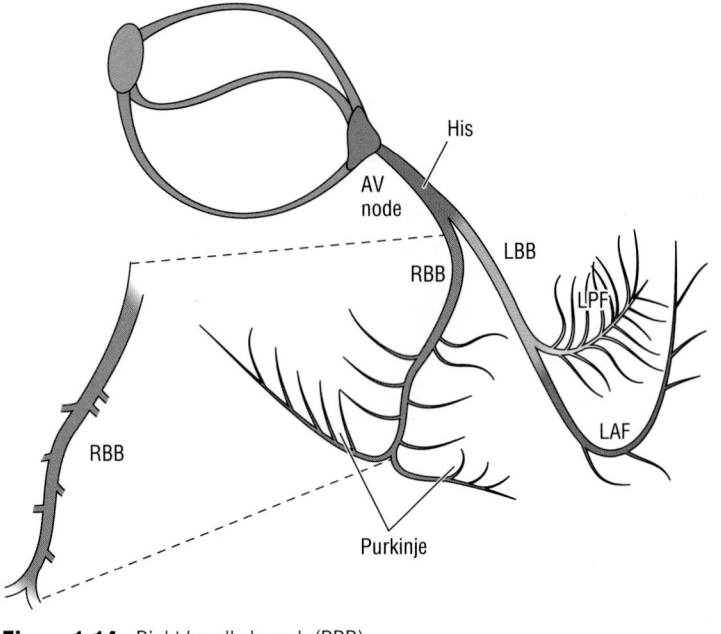

Figure 1-14: Right bundle branch (RBB).

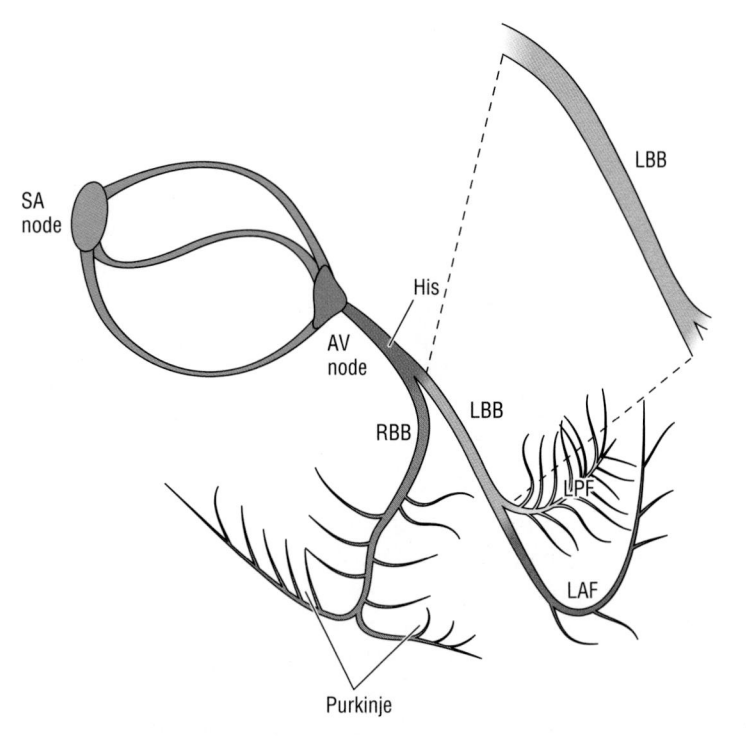

Figure 1-13: Left bundle branch (LBB).

The Left Anterior Fascicle (LAF)

The LAF, also known as the left anterior superior fascicle, travels through the left ventricle to the Purkinje cells that innervate the anterior and superior aspects of the left ventricle. It is a single-stranded fascicle, in comparison to the LPF.

The Left Posterior Fascicle (LPF)

The LPF is a fan-like structure leading to the Purkinje cells that will innervate the posterior and inferior aspects of the left ventricle. It is very difficult to block this fascicle because it is so widely distributed, rather than being just one strand.

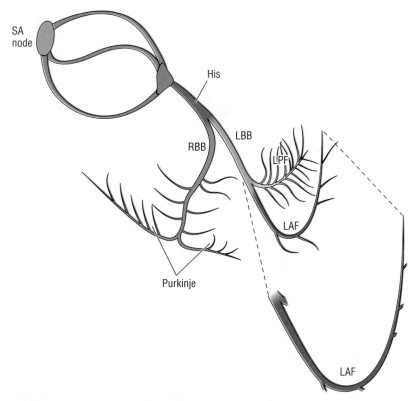

Figure 1-15: Left anterior fascicle (LAF).

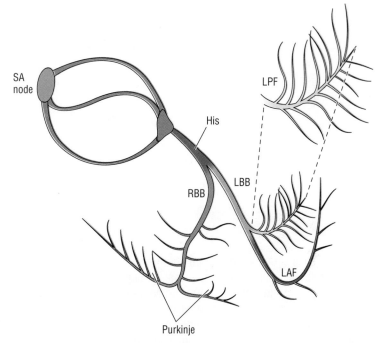

Figure 1-16: Left posterior fascicle (LPF).

The Purkinje System

The Purkinje system is made up of individual cells just beneath the endocardium. They are the cells that directly innervate the myocardial cells and initiate the ventricular depolarization cycle.

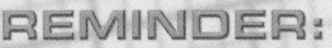

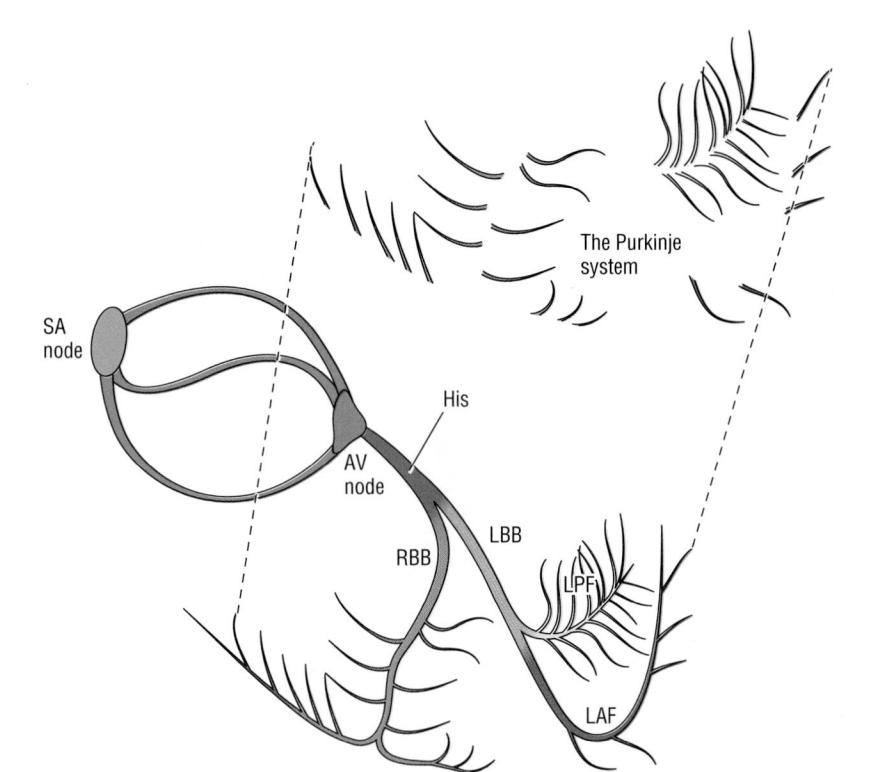

Figure 1-17: Purkinje system.

REMINDER:

So that the pathology that we will present in the rest of the book can be understood, it is critical to understand the heart's electrical conduction system. This pathology covers aberrantly transmitted beats, bundle blocks, fascicular blocks, AV blocks, and rhythm disturbances. We suggest at this point that you go back over the system a few times until you are familiar with its components and the way that the paced electrical impulse travels through the heart.

This is meant to be a cursory review of cardiac and conduction system anatomy. We will spend more time on various aspects of the system as we discuss the individual pathologic states. For a more extensive review of the subject, try the books mentioned in the Additional Readings section.

1. Visually, the right ventricle dominates the anterior view of the heart. True or False.

2. The right ventricle pumps the blood through the peripheral circulation. True or False.

3. Which of the statements below is incorrect:
   A. The electrical conduction system of the heart is made up of specialized cells.
   B. The conduction system is interwoven into the myocardial tissue.
   C. The conduction system is visible under the microscope without special stains.
   D. The internodal pathways transmit the impulse between the SA node and the AV node.

Match the following correctly:

4. ____ SA node   A. 40–45 BPM

5. ____ Atrial cells   B. 30–35 BPM

6. ____ AV node   C. 60–100 BPM

7. ____ His bundle   D. 35–40 BPM

8. ____ Purkinje cells   E. 55–60 BPM

9. ____ Myocardial cells   F. 45–50 BPM

10. The AV node is always supplied by:
    A. The left anterior descending artery
    B. The posterior descending artery
    C. The right coronary artery
    D. The left circumflex artery
    E. The first diagonal artery

1. True 2. False 3. C 4. C 5. E 6. F 7. A 8. D 9. B 10. C

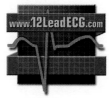

To enhance the knowledge you gain in this book, access this text's website at www.12leadECG.com! This valuable resource provides an online glossary and related web links. To learn more about the chapter topics, simply click on the chapter and view the link.

CHAPTER 2

W hy do you need to know about the generation of electrical activity in a cell and the effect of electrolytes on the electrocardiogram (ECG)? Because before you can understand what an ECG does, you need to know how it gets its information. Electrolytes are the means by which the cell develops "electricity." You also need to know about electrolytes because imbalances can cause life-threatening problems. For example, if you knew that peaked, sharp T waves were a sign of hyperkalemia (elevated potassium), or that a prolonged QT interval could be a sign of hypocalcemia or hypomagnesemia, you might avert a serious arrhythmia. It takes only minutes in some cases to go from peaked T waves to asystole. (By the way, pacers do not work in hyperkalemia!) A little knowledge about electrolytes and their effects on the ECG patterns can save the patient — and you.

To understand why the ECG is altered by an electrolyte abnormality, we will review the way in which the myocardial cell becomes polarized and depolarized, and the biochemical mechanisms that allow the cell to contract. We will try to make the concepts as painless as possible, so bear with us. This is intended to be only a very basic discussion of the topic, which you can supplement with a good physiology textbook as needed.

Mechanics of Contraction

Imagine that the heart is made up of a series of small barrels or cells (Figure 2-1). Each of these barrels is made up of two halves that slide over each other and are held together by interlocking pieces (actin and myosin proteins). The actin molecules are attached to the outside edges of the barrel wall, and the myosin molecules are interspersed between the actin molecules.

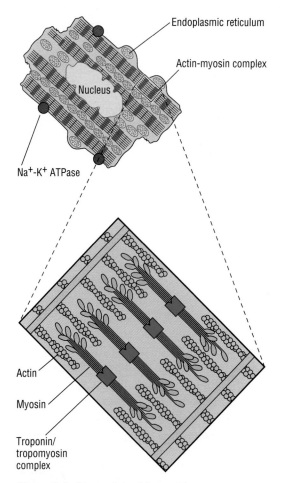

Figure 2-1: Myocardial cell (myocyte).

The outsides of the barrels (cells) are fused together to form long bands, or myofibrils (Figure 2-2). These bands, in turn, are held together side-to-side by wire (connective tissue) to form sheets, which are covered with fluid (extracellular fluid). The main function of the bands is to contract and expand. When one of the barrels contracts, the whole sheet shortens by a small amount. When all of the barrels contract, the whole sheet shortens significantly. The sheet returns to its starting size as all of the barrels relax. The sheets are arranged to form the four sacs that constitute the heart: two small, thin ones on top (the atria) and two large, thick ones on bottom (the ventricles).

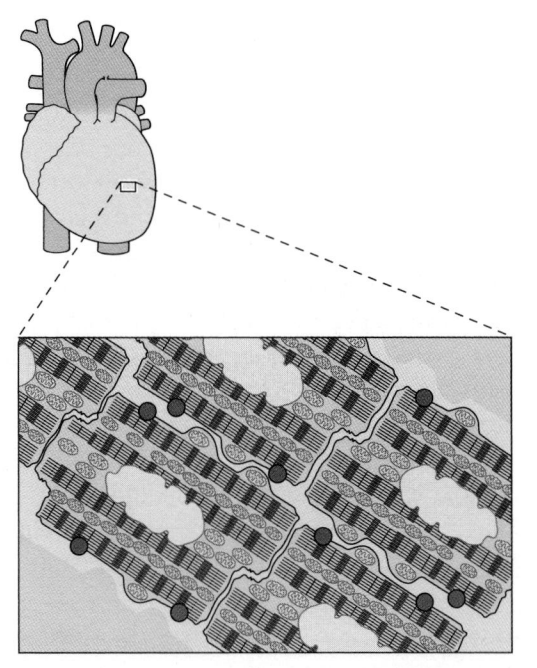

Figure 2-2: Barrels are held together, forming myofibrils and sheets.

Ion Movement and Polarity

The fluid inside and outside of the barrel contains water, salts, and proteins. The fluids are not the same, however; the concentrations of salt molecules and proteins are different in each one. In liquids, salts break down into positively and negatively charged particles known as ions (Figure 2-3). In other words, an ion is a positively or negatively charged particle in a solution. In the body, the main positively charged ions are sodium (Na+), potassium (K+), and calcium (Ca++). Chloride (Cl−) is the main negatively charged ion.

NaCl

Figure 2-3: Salts in a liquid medium turn into positively and negatively charged ions.

If the cell were not alive, the concentrations of all of the ions and charges would be the same on both sides of the barrel wall (the cell membrane). However, a live cell maintains differences in these concentrations across the cell membrane (Figure 2-4). The inside of the cell has a higher potassium concentration, whereas the outside has a higher concentration of sodium. The higher positive charge outside the cell thus causes relatively more negative charge inside the cell. The outside of the cell wall also has more calcium, which adds to the greater positive charge outside the cell. This difference between the charges outside and inside of the cell wall is known as its electrical potential.

Charges and ions naturally want to cancel themselves out and maintain neutrality. The cell wall is not a completely impermeable membrane. It is semi-permeable, because it contains small leaks that let some of the ions into and out of the cell. The natural tendency is for sodium to enter and potassium to exit. To maintain an electrical

potential, the cell must have some way of pushing the ions around against their wishes. Enter the sodium-potassium ATPase pumps (blue dots in figures). The pumps actively move ions around to maintain the resting concentration and charge of the cell. Now, how does the pump do that? The pump uses ATP, the body's fuel pellet, to push out two sodium ions (two positive charges) and bring in one potassium ion (one positive charge). The result is a greater number of positive charges outside the barrel than inside. In other words, the outside solution has a positive charge, while the inner solution has a more negative charge. Because of this pumping action, the electrical potential of the resting myocyte is approximately −70 to −90 mV.

As time passes, the number of ions entering into the cell starts to offset the effect of the pump, and the inside of the cell becomes less negative (increasing numbers of positively charged sodium ions are leaking in). This pattern of slowly increasing the cell's electrical potential is referred to as phase 4 of the action potential (Figure 2-5).

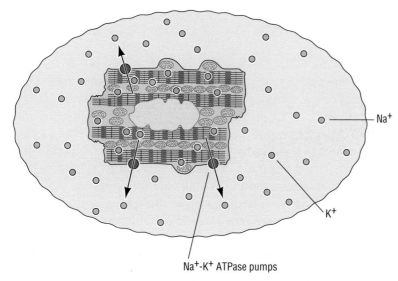

Figure 2-4: Solutions inside and outside the barrel are different. The pump (blue dots) maintains the right number of ions on both sides of the wall.

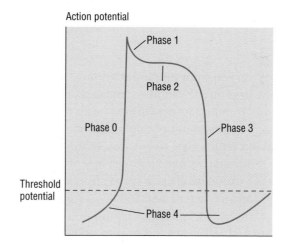

Figure 2-5: Phases of myocyte stimulation.

Membrane Channels and Action Potential Phases

Eventually, the cell becomes so positive that a new set of channels opens. The point at which the channels open is called the threshold potential, and the channels are the fast sodium channels. Think of this as a one-way valve at the end of a tube. When the positive charges inside the cell reach a certain point, the valve opens. Because it is a one-way valve, ions can only enter the cell, and what is the most common ion outside the cell? Sodium! This influx of sodium makes the cell even more positive, and the cycle continues. The rapid increase in sodium ions causes the cell to "spike," or fire. This is called phase 0

(Figure 2-5). The impulse is transmitted down the cell, which begins to influence the cell next to it, and so on, until they are all stimulated. At this point, the cell is no longer polarized, or negatively charged; it is now depolarized, and just as positive as the outside solution.

The next phase, when the cell is at its peak positive charge, is phase 1. At this point, some negatively charged chloride ions enter the cell and cause the influx of sodium to slow down. This initial slowdown slams shut the one-way valve on the rapid sodium channels. Two more types of channels now open: the slow sodium channels and the calcium channels, and a slow "plateau" phase begins — phase 2. The slow sodium channels are responsible for a slow influx of sodium ions, but not to the degree of

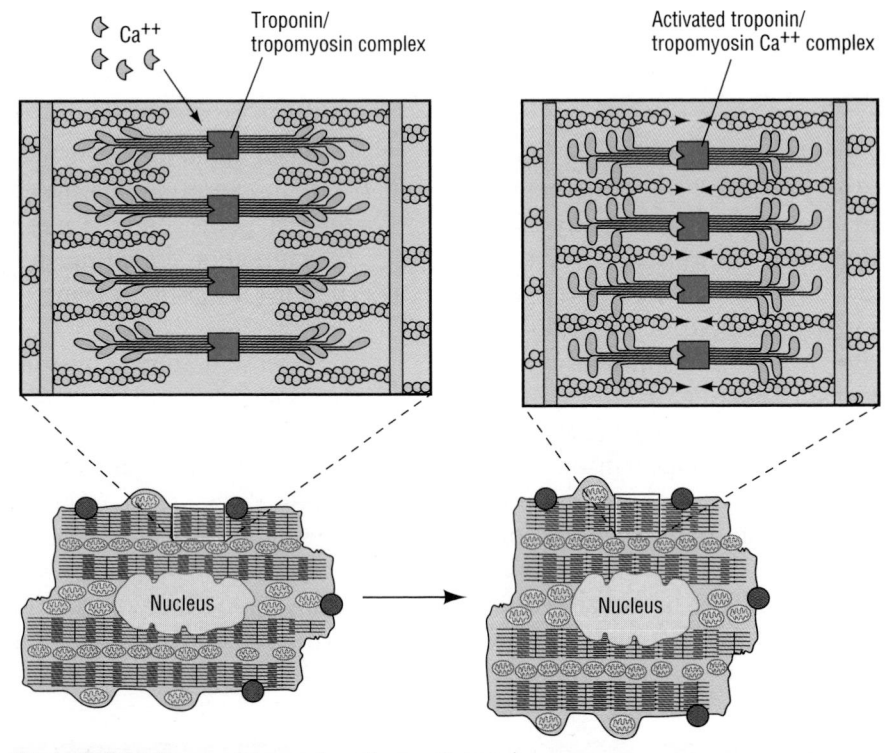

Figure 2-6: Action of calcium on the actin-myosin complex.

the fast sodium channels. The calcium channels open and begin to allow calcium to enter the cell. Calcium is a double positive ion; it has two positive charges instead of one. The influx of calcium and the slow influx of sodium help maintain the cell in the depolarized state.

This is where the fun starts: calcium is needed for the cell to contract. Calcium acts like a key, activating a clamp composed of the proteins troponin and tropomyosin. The clamp brings together the two ratcheting proteins, actin and myosin, and allows them to move along each other and cause the cell to contract (Figure 2-6). Without calcium, the right key configuration is not present to unlock and free the clamping proteins, and the actin and myosin do not come close enough together to engage their "teeth" with each other. The more calcium, the faster the clamping action, and the longer the contraction is maintained.

Next is phase 3. In this phase, some potassium channels open and allow potassium to escape the inside of the cell. During this phase of rapid repolarization, the exit of positive ions imparts a relatively negative charge to the inside of the cell (repolarizes it).

After the cell reaches resting potential, the whole process begins again. The Na-K ATPase pump begins to move sodium out and potassium in, the cell leaks, and it slowly creeps back up to the threshold potential to fire again. One critical point to understand about phase 4 is that different myocytes reach the threshold potential at different rates. Which ones reach it first? The ones that maintain the pacemaking function of the heart, the sinoatrial (SA) nodal cells. In sequence, the next ones are the atrial cells, the atrioventricular (AV) nodal cells, the bundle cells, the Purkinje cells, and finally the ventricular myocytes. Isn't it interesting that the independent rates for each of these systems is slower than the ones before? This is the body's protective mechanism, rather than having just one set of cells responsible for the pacing function. If all of the cells in the SA node die, then the next fastest phase 4 belongs to the atrial myocytes; they will fire before the other cells, and will set the pace. This continues down the line, as needed.

Moving On

As a closing thought, imagine that there are millions of action potentials occurring throughout the heart. Each individual cell is polarizing and depolarizing about 70 to 100 times each minute, and there are quite a few million myocytes in the heart. This translates to millions or billions of action potentials occurring each minute. Miraculously, they will all act in unison, thanks to the electrical conduction system we reviewed in Chapter 1. The sum of these collective electrical discharges will create one large electrical current — the electric axis of the heart. In the next few chapters, we will see how the ECG machine measures these electrical potentials and changes them into the patterns that we will learn to recognize on an ECG tracing. We will see how the normal heart gives off some characteristic waves and complexes and how these complexes are altered in pathologic states.

Laying down the foundation for electrocardiography may appear tedious. It is important, however, if we really want to understand and interpret the ECG correctly. Remember, it isn't enough just to read the ECG; you must understand what causes the tracings, and the pathology it represents, in order to translate that information into a diagnosis. That diagnosis will be, in turn, used to guide therapy — therapy that could save your patient's life.

CHAPTER IN REVIEW

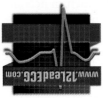

1. Which of the following is incorrect:
- **A.** Na+
- **B.** K−
- **C.** Ca++
- **D.** Cl−
- **E.** K+

2. There is a high concentration of sodium inside of the cell. True or False.

3. There is a high concentration of potassium outside the cell. True or False.

4. The electrical potential of the resting myocytes is:
- **A.** +70 to +90 mV
- **B.** +100 to +120 mV
- **C.** Approximately zero
- **D.** −70 to −90 mV
- **E.** −100 to −120 mV

5. The sodium-potassium ATPase pumps use ATP to push two sodium ions out and bring one potassium ion into the cell. This creates a net negative charge inside the cell. True or False.

6. Actin and myosin are the protein chains that shorten the myocytes. Which *ion* acts like a key that allows the troponin/tropomyosin complex to clamp these two together so they can interact?
- **A.** Sodium
- **B.** Potassium
- **C.** Calcium
- **D.** Magnesium
- **E.** Chloride

7. The cell is polarized in the normal resting state prior to firing. True or False.

8. The cell fires when the action potential is reached. The cell is polarized during this process. True or False.

9. Which one of the following has the fastest pacemaking function:
- **A.** SA node
- **B.** Atrial myocytes
- **C.** AV node
- **D.** Bundle branches
- **E.** Ventricular myocytes

10. The electrochemical activity of polarization-depolarization is measurable by the ECG. True or False.

1. B **2.** False **3.** False **4.** D **5.** True **6.** C **7.** True **8.** False **9.** A **10.** True

C H A P T E R **3**

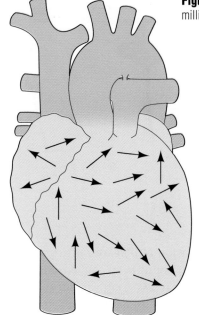

Figure 3-2: The heart contains millions of vectors.

Imagine each cell giving rise to its own electrical impulse. These impulses vary in intensity and direction. We use the term vector to describe these electrical impulses. A vector is a diagrammatic way to show the strength and the direction of the electrical impulse. For example, suppose the amount of electrical activity generated by a cell is worth $1.00 and is directed to the top of the page. We'll call that line Vector A (Figure 3-1). Now, another cell has an electrical discharge that is worth $2.00 and faces the upper right corner. The latter, Vector B, will be twice as big as Vector A. Well, as you can imagine, the heart has a few million of these individual vectors (Figure 3-2).

Adding and Subtracting Vectors

Vectors represent amounts of energy and direction. They add up when they are going in the same direction, and cancel each other out if they point in opposite directions. If they are at an angle to each other, they add or subtract energy and change directions when they meet (Figure 3-3). This is a brief introduction to vector mathematics. A good physics book will give you additional information.

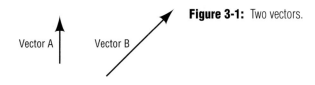

Figure 3-1: Two vectors.

Vector A   Vector B

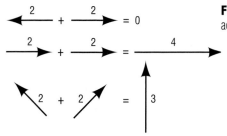

Figure 3-3: Examples of adding vectors.

The Electrical Axis of the Heart

Now, take the sum of all of the millions of vectors found in the ventricles of the heart. We'll wait a few minutes while you add them up. That final vector, after all of the addition, subtraction, and direction changes, is known as the electrical axis of the ventricle (Figure 3-4). In the same way, each wave and segment has its own respective vector. There is a P-wave vector, a T-wave vector, an ST segment vector, and a QRS vector. The ECG is a measurement of these vectors as they pass under an electrode. That's it! It is an electronic representation of the electrical movement of the main vectors passing under an electrode, or a lead. In the next pages, we are only going to discuss the QRS vector.

Electrodes and Waves

The electrodes are sensing devices that pick up the electrical activity occurring beneath them. When a positive electrical impulse is moving away from the electrode (Figure 3-5, A), the ECG machine converts it into a negative (downward) wave. When a positive wave moves toward an electrode, the ECG records a positive (upward) wave (Figure 3-5, C). When the electrode is somewhere in the middle (Figure 3-5, B), the ECG shows a positive deflection for the amount of energy that is coming toward it and a negative wave for the amount going away from it. This is similar to the Doppler effect. We are all familiar with this effect when an ambulance approaches us with its siren on. As it moves closer, it gets louder; as it gets further away, the noise diminishes.

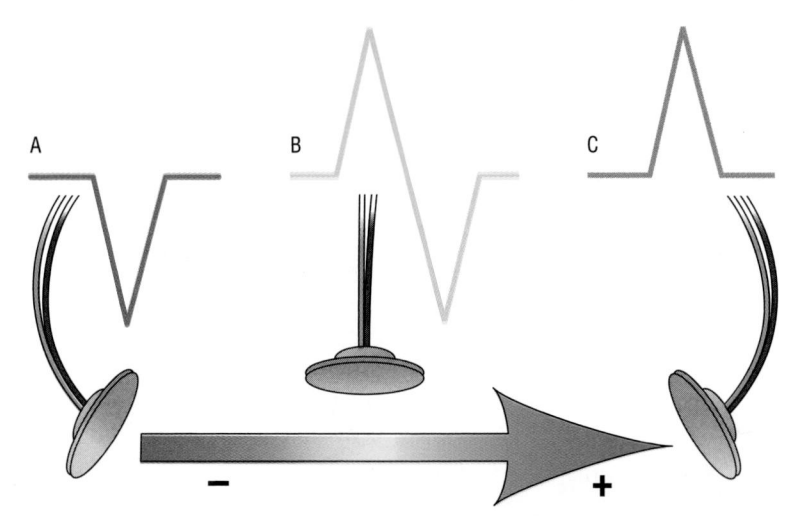

Figure 3-5: Three different ECGs resulting from the same vector, due to different lead placements.

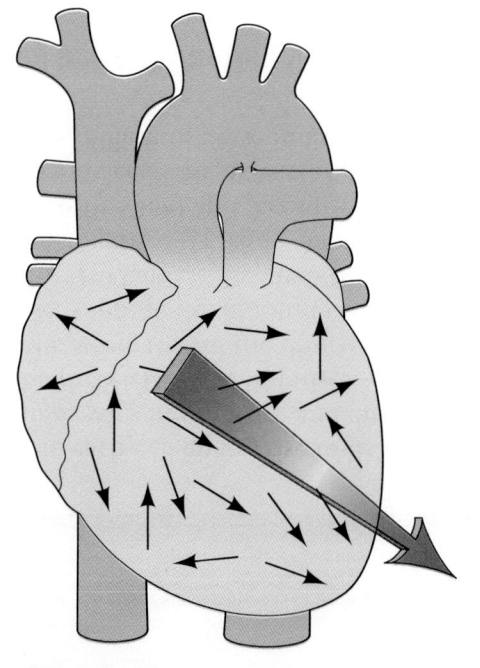

Figure 3-4: Sum of all ventricular vectors = electrical axis.

Leads Are Like Pictures of the Heart

So, the electrodes (leads) pick up the electrical activity of the vectors, and the ECG machine converts them to waves. Think of each set of waves as a picture. Now, imagine that we place various electrodes — or cameras, for this analogy — at certain angles to the main axis (Figure 3-6). We would get multiple pictures of the heart from a three-dimensional perspective. Think of an ECG as a picture album, and it will be easy. To make matters more interesting, suppose we gave you multiple photographs of a toy elephant, including some reference for scale. Would you be able to put them together three-dimensionally in your mind's eye? Of course you would! This is all an ECG is meant to give us: a three-dimensional picture of the heart's electrical axes. From this picture, we can get all sorts of information about where pathologic processes — such as infarcts, hypertrophy, and blocks — are occurring.

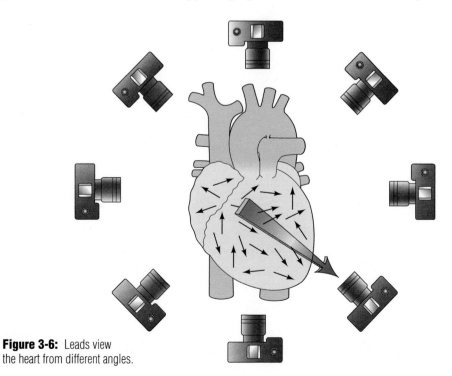

Figure 3-6: Leads view the heart from different angles.

Lead Placement (Where to Put the "Cameras")

All right, so where do you place the cameras, or electrodes? You place them over the areas shown in Figure 3-7. The limb leads (extremity leads) — the right arm (RA), left arm (LA), right leg (RL), and left leg (LL) — are placed at least 10 cm from the heart. It doesn't matter if you place the arm leads on the shoulders or the arms, as long as they're 10 cm from the heart. The precordial leads (chest leads), however, have to be placed exactly. Position V_1 and V_2 on each side of the sternum at the fourth intercostal space. To find the space, first isolate the Angle of Louis. This is a hump located near the top third of the sternum. Start feeling down your sternum from the top, and you'll feel it. It is located next to the second rib. The space directly beneath it is the second intercostal space. Count down two more spaces and you're there. V_4 is at the fifth intercostal space in the mid-clavicular line. Follow the diagram for the remaining positions.

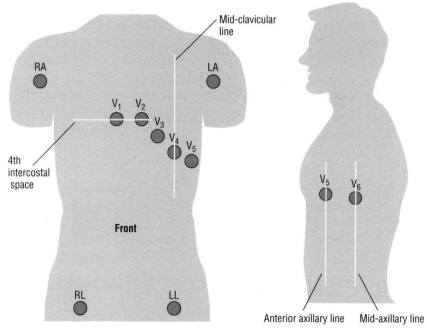

Figure 3-7: Lead placement.

How the Machine Manipulates the Leads

The ECG machine reads the positive and negative poles of the limb electrodes to produce leads I, II, and III on the ECG (Figure 3-8). In other words, the camera is placed at the positive pole and aimed down the lead in question. In physics, two vectors (or in this case leads) are equal as long as they are parallel and of the same intensity and polarity. Therefore, we can move the leads from the locations shown in Figure 3-8 to a point passing through the center of the heart, and they will be the same (Figure 3-9, A). By doing some complicated vector manipulation, the machine comes up with three additional leads (Figure 3-9, B).

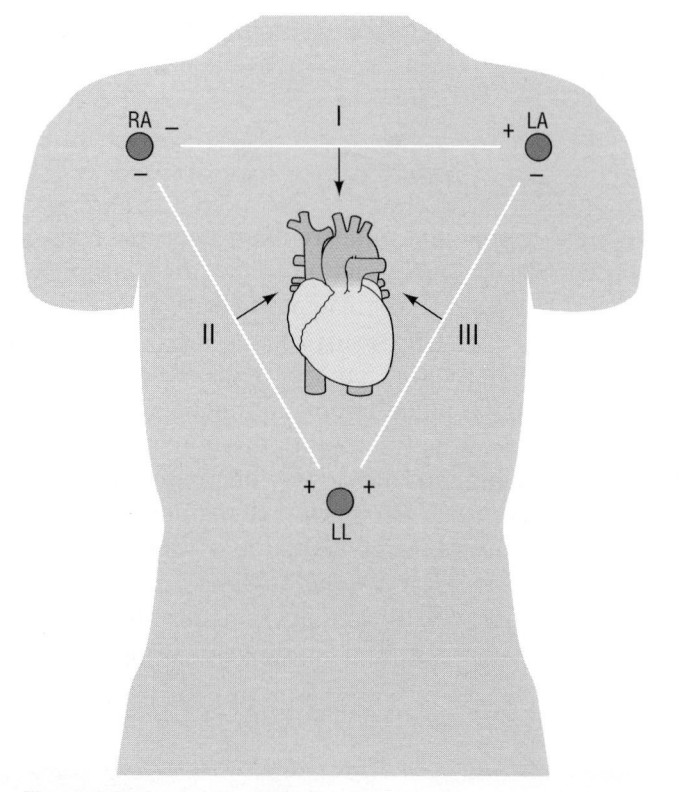

Figure 3-8: Leads I, II, and III.

The Two Lead Systems

The Hexaxial System

Now, let's combine A and B from Figure 3-9. Using the same principle as before — that leads can be moved as long as the resultant lead is parallel and of the same polarity — we can produce the hexaxial system (Figure 3-10). Think of this as a system of analyzing vectors that cuts the center of the heart along a plane, creating a front half and a back half. It would be as if there were a glass sheet dividing the body from ear to ear. In anatomical terminology, this is called a coronal cut. Keep in mind as you proceed that what you are evaluating is how the vector would project on the two dimensional glass sheet and not on the three dimensional anterior or posterior parts of the heart.

The hexaxial system gives rise to the six limb leads: I, II, III, aVR, aVL, and aVF. Traditionally, the side of the lead that has the positive electrode, or pole, is the one that has the lead name at its end (Figure 3-9). Hence, the positive pole of lead I is at the right side of the circle, the positive pole of aVF is down, and so on. Also, note that the leads are 30 degrees apart. This will be very useful when we talk about axis.

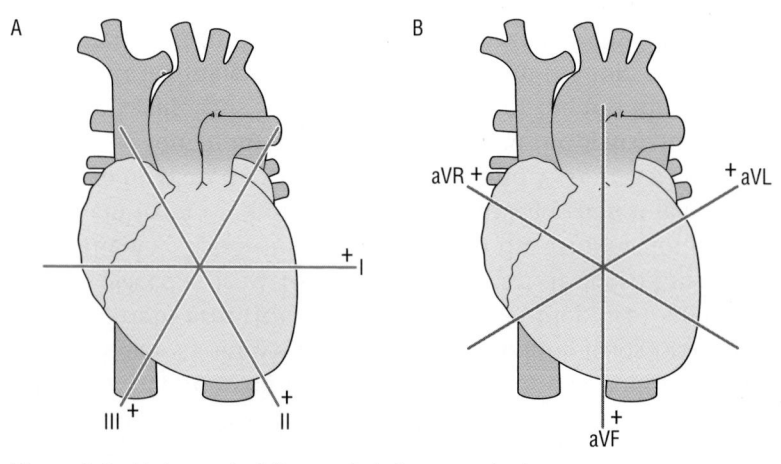

Figure 3-9: Vector manipulation results in three more leads.

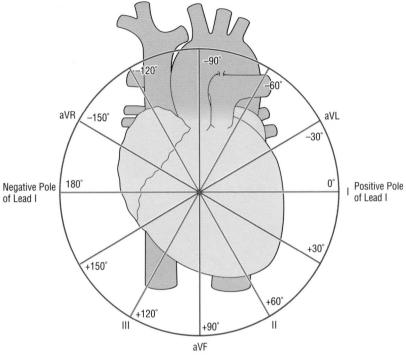

Figure 3-10: The hexaxial system.

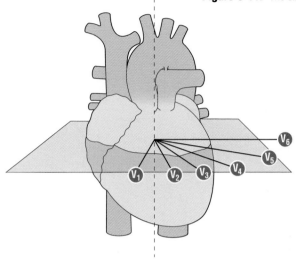

Figure 3-11: The six precordial leads.

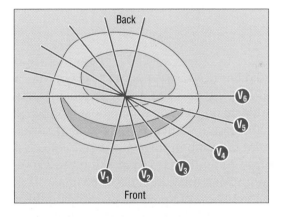

The Precordial System

Remember the precordial leads — the ones on the chest itself? Think of these leads as sitting on a plane that is perpendicular to the limb leads. Again imagine a glass sheet, this time splitting the body through the center of the heart, into top and bottom halves. This is called a sagittal plane. The result is a cross section, with six leads produced by the six chest electrodes (Figure 3-11).

The Heart in Three Dimensions

If you have followed us so far, what would be the logical next step? Right . . . we combine it all! Cutting the heart into both coronal and sagittal planes give a three-dimensional picture of the heart. What can you use this bit of knowledge for? Well, let's give you a little test.

Suppose a patient had an inferior myocardial infarction (heart attack). Where would you see the changes on an ECG? Looking at Figure 3-12, what are the leads that face the bottom of the heart? They are leads II, III, and aVF! So, if you saw ECG changes consistent with an acute myocardial infarction (AMI) in leads II, III, and aVF, you would know that the patient was having an inferior wall MI (IWMI). See? You're getting good already. Now, suppose the ECG shows changes in leads V_1 and V_2. They run along the septum — hence, a septal wall MI. V_3 and V_4 are the most anterior (anterior wall MI), and the lateral leads are I, aVL, V_5, and V_6. Get the picture? Let's look at these areas individually.

Localizing an Area: Inferior Wall

Suppose you look at an ECG and see changes in leads II, III, and aVF. Unless you have memorized the pattern, you would not know what area of the heart those changes represented. Because memorization is not the optimal way to remember (we forget 90% of what we learn that way), we need to come up with a logical way to remember this pattern. If you know the hexaxial and precordial systems, you will be able to recognize that the leads in question represent the inferior wall of the heart (Figure 3-13). Changes of ischemia or infarction on that area of the ECG would tell you that the patient was having either inferior wall ischemia or an inferior wall MI. If you know the system, there will be very few things about electrocardiography that you will not be able to work out.

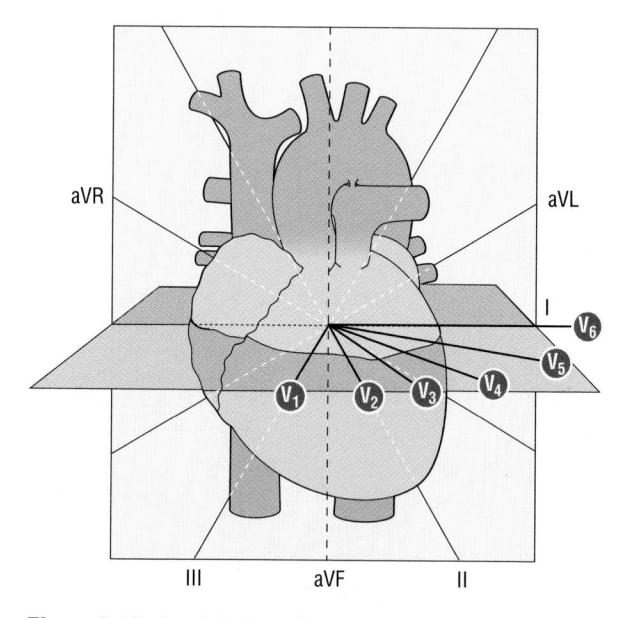

Figure 3-12: Leads in three dimensions.

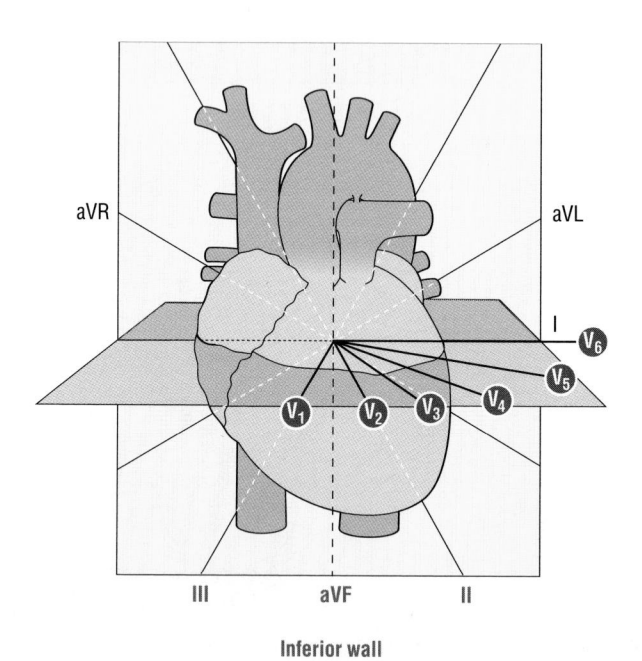

Inferior wall

Figure 3-13: Localizing the inferior wall.

Localizing Other Areas

You can also use this approach to localize the anterior, septal, and lateral walls (Figure 3-14) and events that involve more than one region — the inferolateral wall, for instance. This involves both the inferior and lateral areas. Can you figure out which leads are involved? (See Figure 3-15 for the answer.)

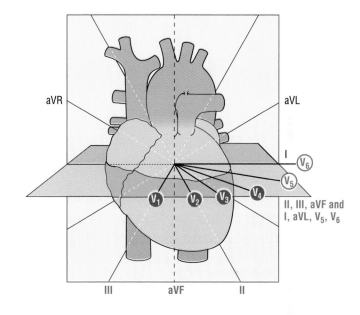

Figure 3-14: Localizing other regions.

Figure 3-15: Localizing across more than one region.

CHAPTER IN **REVIEW**

1. Which of the following is **correct:**
   A. A vector is a diagrammatic way to show the *strength* of an electrical impulse.
   B. A vector is a diagrammatic way to show the *direction* of an electrical impulse.
   C. Both A and B are correct.
   D. Both A and B are incorrect.

2. The electrical axis of the heart is a vector representing the summation of all of the individual vectors that make ventricular depolarization. True or False.

3. Which of the following statements is **incorrect:**
   A. Electrodes are sensing devices that pick up electrical activity taking place beneath them.
   B. A positive electrical wave moving toward an electrode is represented on the ECG as a positive wave.
   C. A positive electrical wave moving away from an electrode is represented on the ECG as a negative wave.
   D. A positive electrical wave moving toward an electrode is represented on the ECG as an isoelectric segment.

4. An electrical lead is like a camera taking a picture of the electrical axis from its particular vantage point. A 12-lead ECG is like a picture album representing the "shots" taken by the 12 individual leads in a systematic format. True or False.

5. V_3 and V_4 are on opposite sides of the sternum. True or False.

6. The *Angle of Louis* is the most inferior angle of Einthoven's triangle. True or False.

7. The limb leads include leads I, II, III, aVR, aVL, and aVF. True or False.

8. The limb leads are found in the hexaxial system, which electrically cuts the heart coronally. True or False.

9. The precordial leads electrically cut the heart sagitally into a top half and a bottom half. True or False.

10. We cannot use the limb leads and the precordial leads to create a three-dimensional picture of the electrical axis of the heart. True or False.

1. C 2. True 3. D 4. True 5. False 6. False 7. True 8. True 9. True 10. False

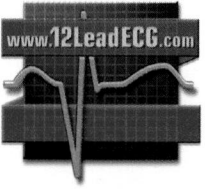 To enhance the knowledge you gain in this book, access this text's website at www.12leadECG.com! This valuable resource provides an online glossary and related web links. To learn more about the chapter topics, simply click on the chapter and view the link.

Boxes and Sizes

The pen will record the ECG waves and segments (discussed in Chapter 2) on the paper. To keep things simple, we have drawn straight horizontal lines to represent the complexes in Figure 4-1.

The ECG paper passes under the pen at a rate of 25 mm/sec. Each little box is, therefore, 1/25th of a second, or 0.04 seconds. Because a big box is made up of five little boxes, it represents 5 x 0.04 sec = 0.20 sec, so five big boxes make 1 second. Each lead is represented for 3 seconds, and the full ECG is 12 seconds long.

The paper is also broken down into either three or four strips. The top three strips are broken down, as mentioned above, into the twelve leads. Each lead is appropriately labeled for easy identification. The fourth strip, found at the bottom, is a rhythm strip. On many

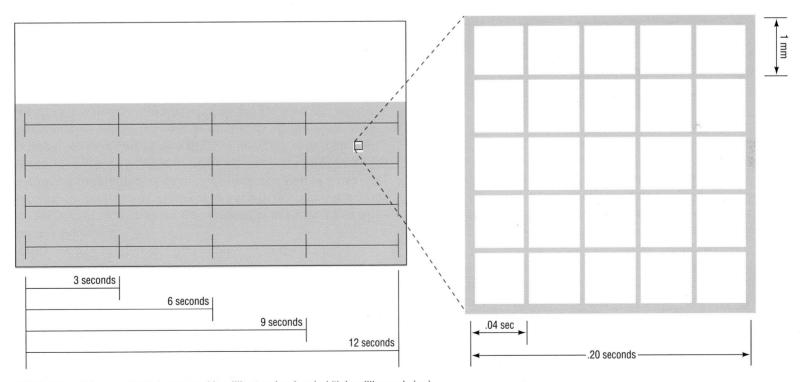

Figure 4-1: ECG paper. Height is measured in millimeters (mm) and width in milliseconds (ms).

machines, the rhythm strip is synchronized with the leads directly on top of it. On other machines, the rhythm strip will not be synchronized. We'll discuss this further later on in this chapter.

When we talk about the vertical height of a wave or segment, we use millimeters; for instance, a wave that is five little boxes high would, in reality, be five millimeters high. Likewise, a darker big box is five millimeters high.

It will be very useful to keep these measurements in mind, especially when we discuss rates and widths of waves and segments. Everything on the ECG is measured in millimeters or milliseconds, and you will use these measurements to describe your findings when examining the ECG.

As an example, a wave can be described as being 15 mm high and 0.06 seconds wide. This would tell us that the height of the wave is 15 little boxes or three big boxes, and the width is 1.5 little boxes. With a bit of practice, you'll have this mastered.

Calibration

At the end of each ECG strip, you will usually find a steplike structure called a calibration box. The standard box is 10 mm high and 0.20 seconds wide (Figure 4-2, A). The calibration box is there to confirm that the ECG conforms to the standard format.

Occasionally, you will find that an ECG has been formatted in half-standard calibration (Figure 4-2, B). This is usually done when the complexes are so tall that they run into each other. You will know that it is half-standard because there will be an additional step halfway up the box that lasts for half the width of the standard box. When you see this stairlike configuration, you are at half-standard.

The only other calibration you will run across is one in which the paper speed is set to 50 mm/sec, instead of the traditional 25 mm/sec. In this case, the calibration box will be 0.40 seconds wide (Figure 4-2,C).

Where Is Each Lead Represented?

Figure 4-3 shows the placement of the various leads in the standard format for most ECGs. There is, however, great variation in this system

among the many manufacturers of ECG equipment. You should get used to the format that is used at your institution.

Some formats do not include a rhythm strip at the bottom. We believe this puts one at a great disadvantage in interpreting ECGs. Another disadvantage of some formats is that they provide a rhythm strip, but don't show it in temporal relationship to the complexes above the strip. (We'll explain temporal relationship next.) Because the appearance of the complex varies depending on the lead, it will be difficult to distinguish normal from aberrant beats on this type of ECG. In the following chapters, we'll show you plenty of examples in which the temporally matched rhythm strip is critical to the interpretation of the ECG.

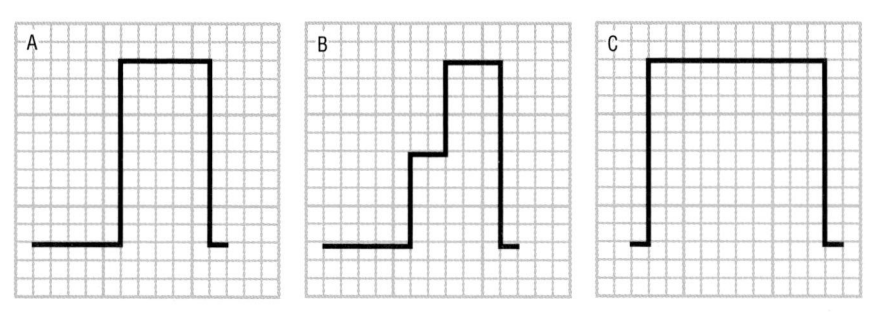

Figure 4-2: Three types of calibration.

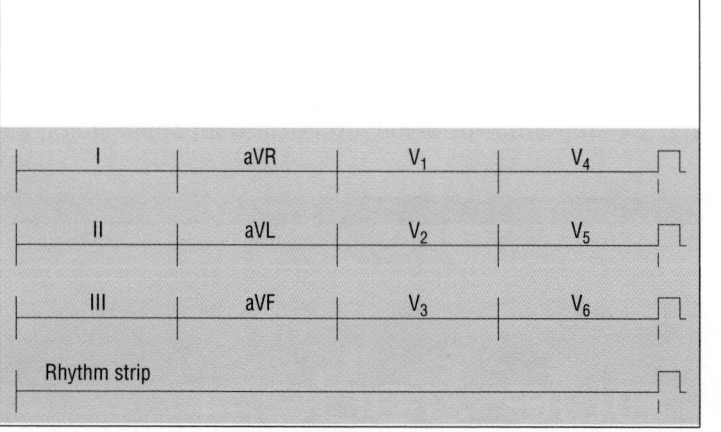

Figure 4-3: Locations of leads on the ECG paper.

Temporal Relationship of the ECG

Imagine that we have a transparent ruler with a red line running through it, placed on top of the ECG (Figure 4-4). As we move the ruler across the paper, we would encounter temporally variant spots because events at the beginning of the ECG occurred before those at the end. However, each event that is touching that perpendicular red line occurred at the same moment. The ECG machine's computer is capable of measuring three or more leads at once and representing them on the ECG simultaneously. Please note that only those events touching the red line occurred simultaneously. Always check that the tips of the complexes are found along the same vertical line on the ECG paper. This protects you against making a mistake in interpreting the complexes.

Why Is Temporal Spacing Important?

Why are we making such a big deal about this temporal spacing thing? Consider a situation such as the one shown in Figure 4-5. To simplify matters, we have represented the complexes as stars, both five- and six-pointed. Note that each lead has its own respective color, and that

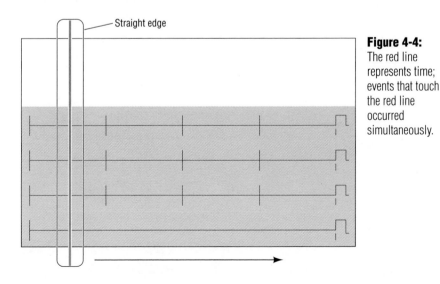

Figure 4-4:
The red line represents time; events that touch the red line occurred simultaneously.

REMINDER:
Always check the format of the ECG you are interpreting!

the rhythm strip is in the color of lead 2. As you are interpreting the ECG, you notice on the rhythm strip that the fifth and sixth complexes are different — they are six-pointed stars instead of the baseline five-pointed ones. You can use this information to alter your interpretation appropriately. If you did not have the rhythm strip to show you that these two aberrant complexes were different, you could easily misinterpret the ECG. Thanks to the rhythm strip, when you interpret the complexes appearing in leads V_1 through V_3, you will take into account that the morphology of these QRS complexes are different from the others, and you can make the right interpretation and diagnosis.

Let's make the point crystal clear: this knowledge could dramatically alter your final diagnosis. It can — and we are trying not to be too dramatic here — save the patient's life. For a great example, have a look at ECG 10-12 in Chapter 10. Among other things, temporal spacing is very important in determining rhythms, intervals, ST segment changes, premature complexes, and aberrantly conducted beats.

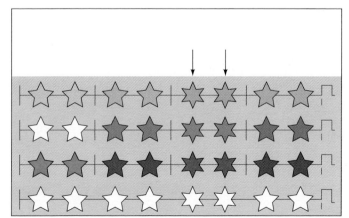

Figure 4-5:
Different types of stars represent different morphologies.

1 CHAPTER IN **REVIEW**

1. The paper on an ECG normally moves at:
   A. 50 mm/sec
   B. 75 mm/sec
   C. 25 cm/sec
   D. 25 mm/sec
   E. None of the above

2. The width of each small box represents:
   A. 0.04 seconds
   B. 0.02 seconds
   C. 0.40 seconds
   D. 0.20 seconds
   E. None of the above

3. What is the time frame occupied by one lead on a regular 12-lead ECG?
   A. 0.3 seconds
   B. 3 seconds
   C. 13 seconds
   D. 30 seconds
   E. None of the above

4. The entire ECG is:
   A. 3 seconds long
   B. 6 seconds long
   C. 9 seconds long
   D. 12 seconds long
   E. None of the above

5. The small boxes on ECG paper measure:
   A. 1 cm by 0.20 seconds
   B. 1 mm by 0.20 seconds
   C. 1 cm by 0.04 seconds
   D. 1 mm by 0.04 seconds
   E. None of the above

6. The big boxes on the ECG paper measure:
   A. 5 mm by 0.20 seconds
   B. 1 mm by 0.20 seconds
   C. 5 mm by 0.04 seconds
   D. 1 mm by 0.04 seconds
   E. None of the above

7. A wave that is 10 small boxes high and three small boxes wide is described as being:
   A. 1.0 mm by 0.3 seconds
   B. 10 mm by 0.12 seconds
   C. 12 mm by 0.3 seconds
   D. 12 mm by 0.10 seconds
   E. None of the above

8. A distance of 2 big boxes and 2 little boxes wide is described as being:
   A. 22 mm wide
   B. 0.22 seconds wide
   C. 0.48 seconds wide
   D. 4.8 seconds wide
   E. None of the above

9. If an ECG were obtained at half standard, a wave that is 20 mm high would be described as being:
   A. 10 mm high
   B. 20 mm high
   C. 30 mm high
   D. 40 mm high
   E. None of the above

10. All ECGs are formatted the same way on the paper. True or False.

1. D 2. A 3. B 4. D 5. D 6. A 7. B 8. C 9. D
10. False

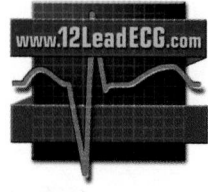 To enhance the knowledge you gain in this book, access this text's website at www.12leadECG.com! This valuable resource provides an online glossary and related web links. To learn more about the chapter topics, simply click on the chapter and view the link.

There are various tools that make reading and interpreting the ECG much easier (Figure 5-1). These include:

1. Calipers
2. Axis-wheel ruler
3. ECG ruler
4. Straight edge

We'll talk about each of these in detail in this chapter. One quick comment about tools: although tools make your job easier, it is important not to completely depend upon them. If you do, you will feel helpless when they are not available.

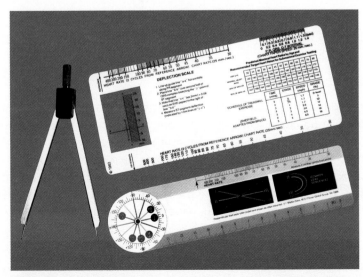

Figure 5-1: Calipers and an ECG ruler with an axis wheel and straight edge.

Calipers: The ECG Interpreter's Best Friend

In our opinion, it is almost impossible to read ECGs with any degree of accuracy if you do not use calipers (Figure 5-2). This is a strong statement, but it is true. It is possible to measure intervals and waves without calipers. It is even possible to evaluate consistency when you are evaluating the rhythm. We have seen people do all kinds of creative markings on pieces of paper to transfer the heights and widths of complexes. However, for accuracy and dependability, nothing beats the ECG calipers. If you don't own a set, go to your nearest medical bookstore or drafting supply house to get one. Always have them with you when you work clinically. It will simplify your life.

How do you use the calipers? Place one of the pins at the beginning of the object you are measuring, and move the other pin to the end. Then you can transfer that distance to an uncluttered part of the ECG to evaluate the height or the time of the measured object. Following are some simple ways to use calipers.

Figure 5-2: Measuring distances on the ECG with calipers.

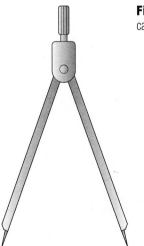

How to Use Your Calipers

Once you have measured the distance, it is easier to calculate the actual time frame on a cleaner, less cluttered area of the ECG (Figure 5-3). Remember, the big boxes are 0.20 seconds; there are two of these in Figure 5-3, for a total of 0.40 seconds. The small boxes are 0.04 seconds, and there are two and a half of these for a total of 0.10 seconds.

Now, suppose you want to see if the distance between three complexes is the same. First, measure the distance between complex A and complex B. Then, without lifting the right pin, swing the left pin to see if the distance from B to C is equal (Figure 5-4). By not moving the right pin, you are ensuring that the distances are the same. Swinging one pin over the other like this is called "walking."

You can walk the calipers back and forth across an ECG to check the regularity of the complexes. You can also take that distance and move it anywhere on the paper you want. This technique is useful in determining third-degree heart blocks and many other ECG abnormalities. Take your calipers and practice on some of the ECGs in Part 2. Make sure you do some measurements as well.

Comparing Wave Heights

You can use your calipers to measure the heights of waves and see if there is net positivity or negativity. In Figure 5-5, we see that the depth of the

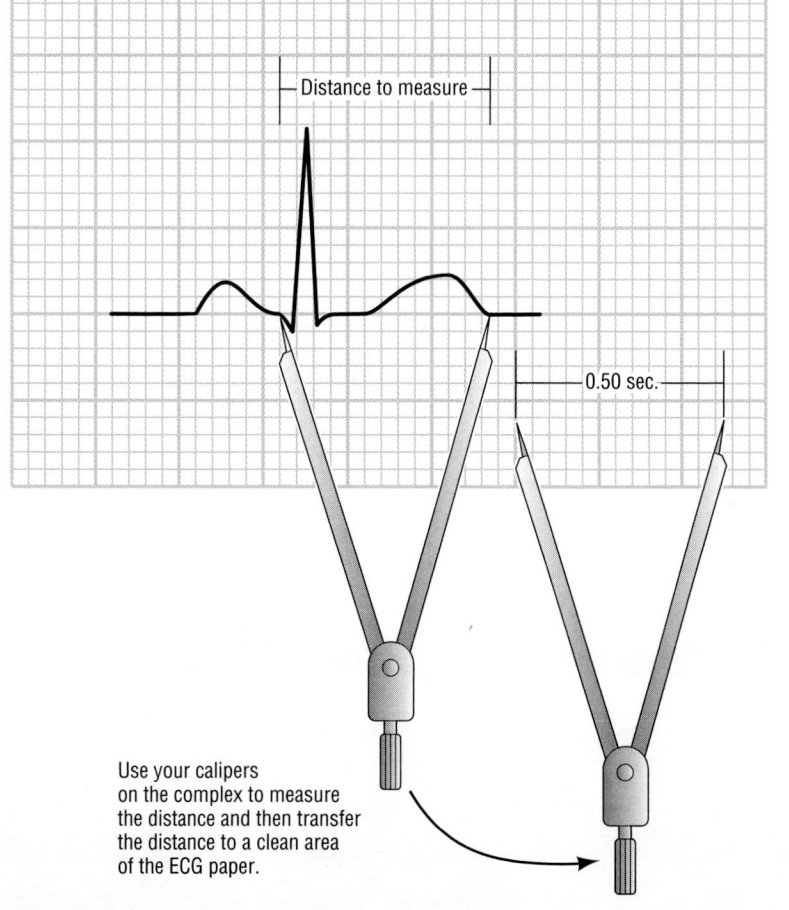

Use your calipers on the complex to measure the distance and then transfer the distance to a clean area of the ECG paper.

Figure 5-3: Total width of the complex is 0.50 seconds.

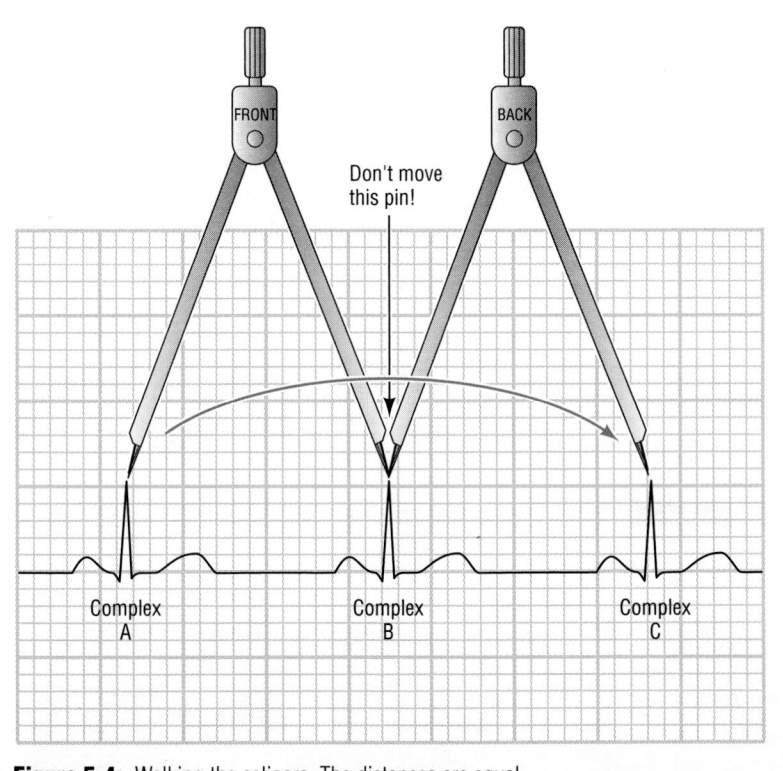

Figure 5-4: Walking the calipers. The distances are equal.

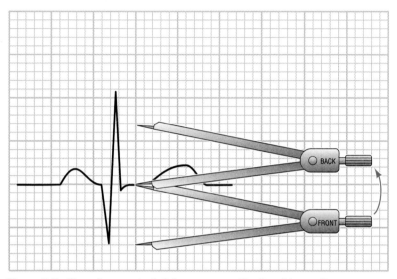

Figure 5-5: The entire complex is 3.8 mm more positive than it is negative.

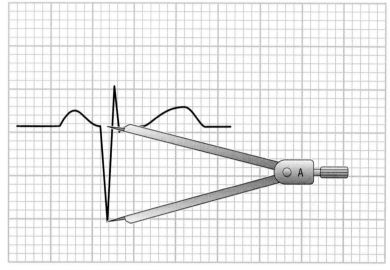

Figure 5-6: Adding the height of two waves.

negative (first) wave is 7.0 mm, and the height of the positive (second) wave is 10.8 mm. This is extremely useful when the waves are close in size. Walking the calipers up or down will tell you quickly which is the biggest. This will be useful when determining the axis of the heart.

Adding Wave Heights

Suppose you wanted to add the negative depth of one wave to the positive height of another in a different lead. You would start by measuring the negative wave of the complex in the first lead. Place your calipers as shown in Figure 5-6 and measure that distance.

Now, place your calipers — still open to that distance from A — on top of the positive complex in the second lead (Figure 5-7, B). Without moving the top pin, extend the bottom pin to the base of the wave (Figure 5-7, C). Measure this and you're done!

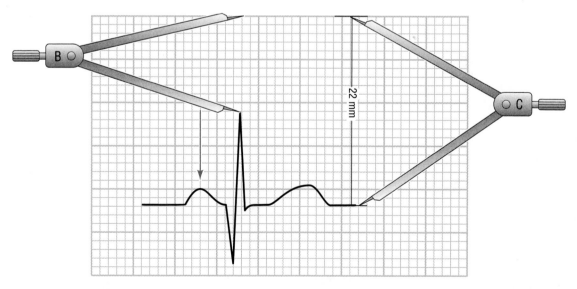

Figure 5-7: Total height is 22.0 mm.

CHAPTER **5** • ECG TOOLS

Comparing Widths

Explaining this one is a bit of overkill, but we really want you to understand the usefulness of the calipers. Suppose you wanted to see if distance A is the same as or longer than distance B (Figure 5-8). Position the calipers to measure distance A, then move them — transferring the distance accurately — to see if B is the same.

You will be using this technique for a great many comparisons in looking for atrioventricular blocks, aberrant beats, atrial premature contractions (APCs), ventricular premature contractions (VPCs), and so on. If you don't know what those things mean, don't worry about it; you will after you have reviewed the book for the first time.

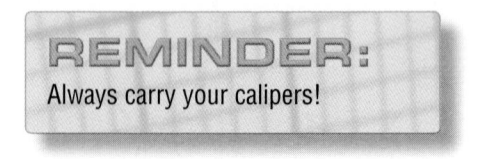

REMINDER:
Always carry your calipers!

Axis-Wheel Ruler

Axis-wheel rulers are very useful in calculating the true axis of waves and segments (Figure 5-9). They can only be obtained from drug companies, as far as we know. They show a representation of the hexaxial system on the back part of the ruler. On the front ruler are a red line and a perpendicular line with an arrow. For now, you don't need to worry about the details of how to use the wheel. A detailed description of the electrical axis, complete with figures, will be found in Chapter 12.

ECG Rulers

We believe that ECG rulers (Figure 5-10) are a waste of valuable plastic, except for the axis-wheel type ruler. They simply are not needed if you have a pair of calipers. Most rulers have one side that measures the rate, and a metric ruler on the other. If you have a set of calipers and the

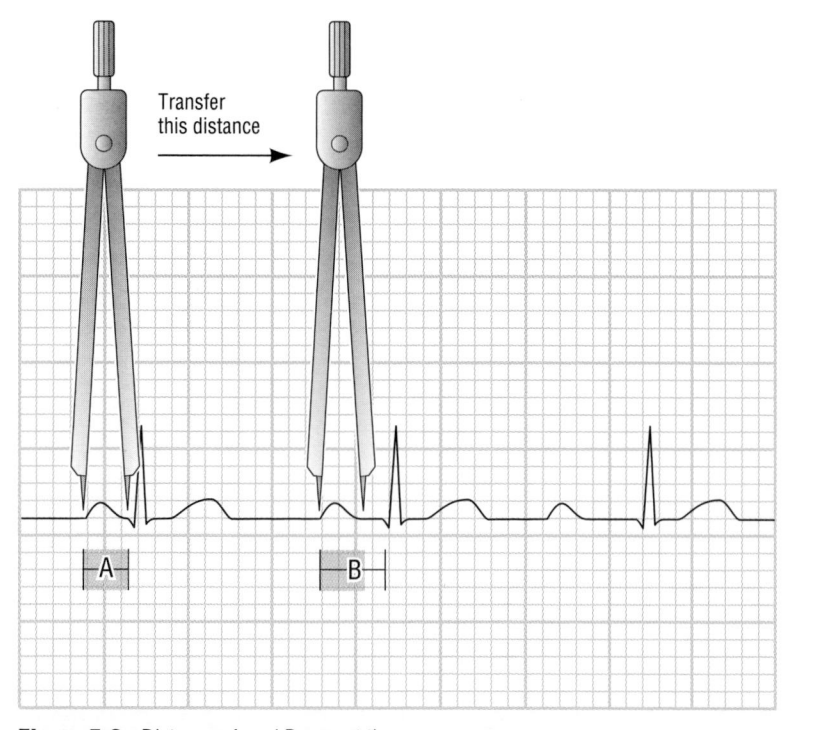

Figure 5-8: Distances A and B are not the same.

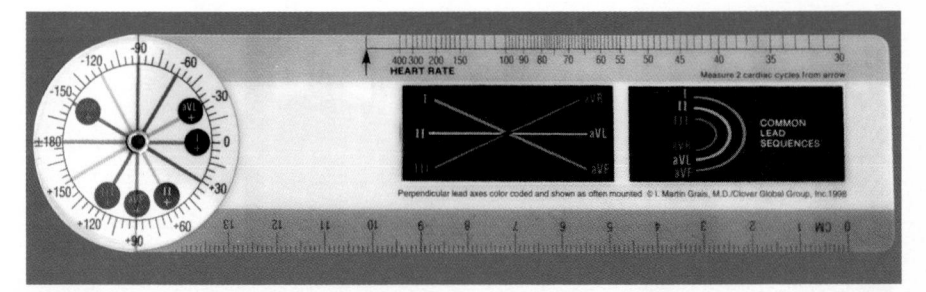

Figure 5-9: Axis-wheel ruler.

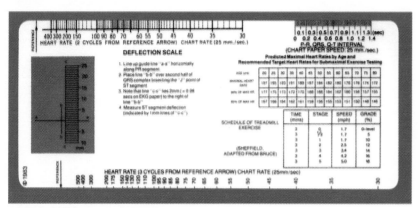

Figure 5-10: Straight edge ruler.

ECG paper, you already have the same thing. They also have some use-less bits of ECG criteria that are standard knowledge. However, if you have a lot of space and don't mind carrying the weight . . . .

Straight Edge

Straight edges are useful in evaluating the baseline and determining whether there is any elevation or depression present. You can use a piece of paper, even the ECG paper folded in on itself (without creasing the paper — messy ECGs are tough to read). The best straight edges are clear with a line in the middle so you can see the whole area in question without obstructing any of the complex. You can then use the straight line to evaluate the baseline. If you cannot find such a ruler, make a copy of the one in Figure 5-11 on overhead transparency film. Your neighborhood copy store should be able to accommodate you, preferably in color.

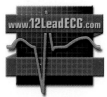

To enhance the knowledge you gain in this book, access this text's website at www.12leadECG.com! This valuable resource provides an online glossary and related web links. To learn more about the chapter topics, simply click on the chapter and view the link.

Figure 5-11: ECG straight edge.

If the QRS complex fits inside this box it is normal width. If it fits outside this box it is a bundle branch block.

0.12 seconds i.d.

First degree
Heart block

Start of QRS

0.20 sec.

CHAPTER 6

W ell, if you've gotten this far, you're ready for some true ECG interpretation! This is where we start looking at what all of those lines mean. We'll begin with the basic beat, or complex. This is one cycle of the heart represented electrocardiographically. We are going to break down the complex into its component parts. In this section of the book, we will just introduce you to the concepts involved with each of the components. In Part 2, we'll show you actual examples and their variations as they appear clinically. Let's get started . . . .

Introduction to Basic Components

Figure 6-1 shows the basic components of the ECG complex. Here are some basic definitions. A wave is a deflection from the baseline that represents some cardiac event. For instance, the P wave represents atrial depolarization. A segment is a specific portion of the complex as it is represented on the ECG. For example, the segment between the end of the P wave and the beginning of the Q wave is known as the PR segment. An interval is the distance, measured as time, occurring between two cardiac events. The time interval between the beginning of the P wave and the beginning of the QRS complex is known as the PR interval. Note that there is a PR interval, as well as a PR segment. In addition to the waves shown in Figure 6-1, there are a few others not mentioned below, such as the R' (R prime) wave and the U wave, which we will talk about individually. There are also other intervals that we are going to cover, such as the R-R interval and the P-P interval. Making sure that you understand the definitions of the basic terms will help prevent confusion. In Figure 6-1, we have labeled the waves and segments with colored letters and the intervals with black letters for easier identification.

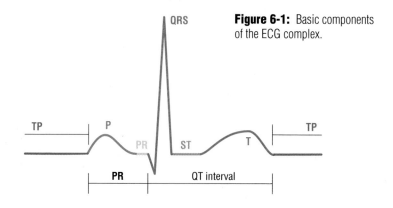

Figure 6-1: Basic components of the ECG complex.

Wave Nomenclature

A wave represents an electrical event in the heart, such as atrial depolarization, atrial repolarization, ventricular depolarization, ventricular repolarization, or transmission through the His bundles, and so on. Waves can be single, isolated, positive, or negative deflections; biphasic deflections with both positive and negative components; or combinations that have multiple positive and negative components. Waves are deflections from the baseline. What is the baseline? It is a line from one TP segment to the next.

Let's look at what that means in Figure 6-2. Note that the QRS complex is a combination of two or more waves. To be completely correct, these waves should be named according to size, location, and direction of deflection. Tall or deep waves in the QRS complex are given capital letters: Q, R, S, R'. Small waves are given small letters: q, r, s, r'. This is why the example in Figure 6-2 is called a qRs wave. This standard is unfortunately not followed as rigorously as you might expect. Many authors simply use all capital letters. In this book, we will follow the standard nomenclature with capital and small letters.

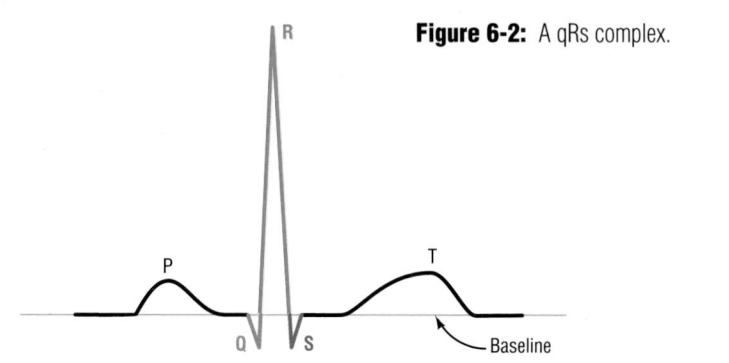

Figure 6-2: A qRs complex.

R′ and S′ Waves Just to make matters more interesting, let's look at some problems with the QRS waves. Changes occurring in the QRS complex can lead to bizarre complexes, and their waves are named

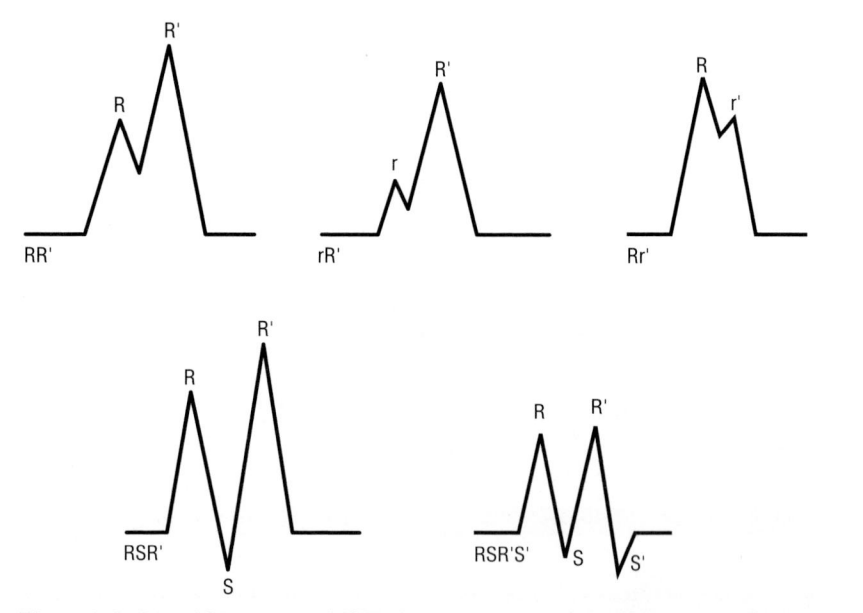

Figure 6-3: R′ and S′ complexes (NOTE: The top row does not technically contain S waves. The term S wave only applies to negative components, or components that fall below the baseline. However, it is common for people to refer to any dip in a notched R wave as an S wave, regardless of whether or not it falls below the baseline. By following this logic further, most authors and clinicians refer to the second peak as the R′ wave. Although this nomenclature is technically incorrect, it is so common that people accept this as the norm.)

differently if they change directions and cross the baseline. Such a wave is called an X′ (X prime) wave, in which X is not an actual wave, but rather a term that can stand for either an R or S wave. R′ and S′ (R prime and S prime) refer to extra waves within the QRS complex. By definition, the first negative wave that we reach after the P wave is called the Q wave. The first positive deflection after the P is the R wave. Here is where it gets tricky: an S wave is the first negative component after an R wave. If we now get another upward component, we start with R′. The next negative component is S′. A positive wave occurring after the S′ would then be an R″ wave (read as R double prime), and so on. Figure 6-3 shows some examples.

Individual Components of the ECG Complex

The P Wave

The P wave is usually the first wave we reach as we travel down the TP segment (Figure 6-4). It represents the electrical depolarization of both atria. The wave starts when the SA node fires. It also includes transmission of the impulse through the three internodal pathways, the Bachman Bundle, and the atrial myocytes themselves.

The duration of the wave itself can vary between 0.08 and 0.11 seconds in normal adults. The axis of the P wave is usually directed downward and to the left, the direction the electrical impulse travels on its journey to the atrioventricular node and the atrial appendages.

REMINDER:
Cardiac event represented by the P wave:
Atrial depolarization

Normal duration: 0.08 to 0.11 seconds

Axis: 0 to +75°, downward and to the left

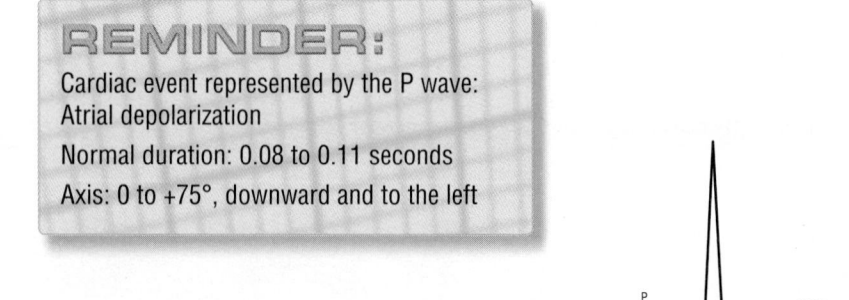

Figure 6-4: The P wave.

The Tp Wave

The Tp wave, which represents repolarization of the atria, deflects in the opposite direction of the P wave (Figure 6-5). It is usually not seen because it occurs at the same time as the QRS wave and is obscured (buried) by that more powerful complex. However, you can sometimes see it when there is no QRS after the P wave. This occurs in AV dissociation or nonconducted beats. You may also see it in PR depression, or in the ST segment depression present in very fast sinus tachycardias. It appears as ST depression because the QRS comes sooner in the cycle, and the Tp wave — if it is negative — draws the ST segment downward.

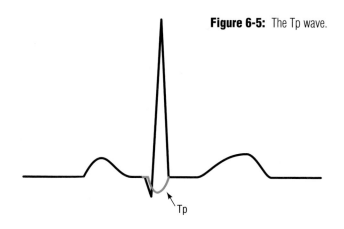

Figure 6-5: The Tp wave.

Tp

REMINDER:

Cardiac event represented by the Tp wave: Atrial repolarization

Normal duration: Usually not seen

Wave orientation: Opposite to the P wave

The PR Segment

The PR segment occupies the time frame between the end of the P wave and the beginning of the QRS complex (Figure 6-6). It is usually found along the baseline. It can, however, be depressed by less than 0.8 mm under normal circumstances; anything greater than that is pathological. It is pathologically depressed in pericarditis, and when there is an atrial infarct (a rare occurrence).

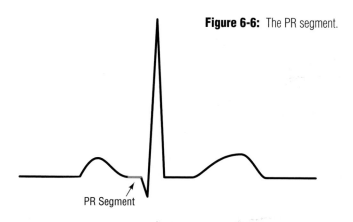

Figure 6-6: The PR segment.

PR Segment

REMINDER:

Cardiac events represented by the PR segment:

Transmission of the electrical depolarization wave through the AV node, His bundles, bundle branches, and Purkinje system

The PR Interval

The PR interval represents the time period from the beginning of the P wave to the beginning of the QRS complex (Figure 6-7). It includes the P wave and the PR segment, both discussed previously. The PR interval covers all of the events from the initiation of the electrical impulse in the sinoatrial (SA) node up to the moment of ventricular depolarization. The normal duration is from 0.12 seconds to 0.20 seconds. If the PR interval is shorter than 0.11 seconds, it is considered shortened. A PR interval longer than 0.20 seconds is a first-degree AV block, which we will talk about in a later section. The PR interval can be quite long, sometimes 0.40 seconds or greater. The term PQ interval is sometimes used interchangeably if there is a Q wave as the initial component of the QRS complex.

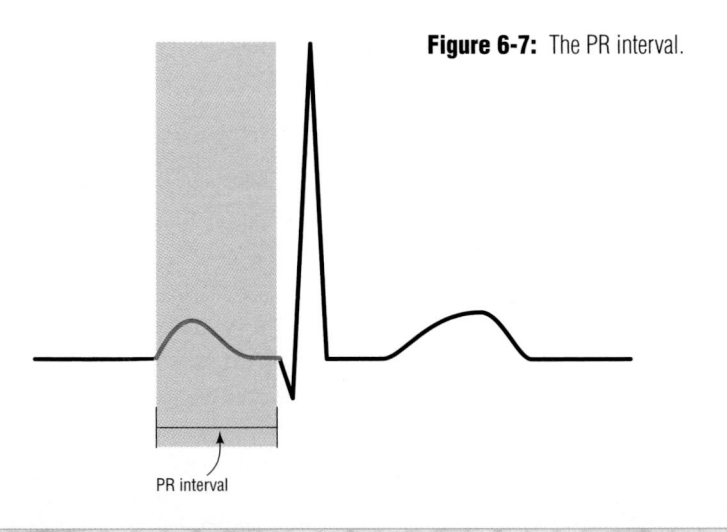

Figure 6-7: The PR interval.

PR interval

REMINDER:

Cardiac events represented by the PR interval: Impulse initiation, atrial depolarization, atrial repolarization, AV node stimulation, His bundle stimulation, bundle branch, and Purkinje system stimulation

Normal duration: 0.11 to 0.20 seconds

The QRS Complex

The QRS complex represents ventricular depolarization. It is composed of two or more waves (Figure 6-8). Each wave has its own name or label. These can become quite complex. The main components are the Q, R, and S waves. By convention, the Q wave is the first negative deflection after the P wave. The Q wave can be present or absent. The R wave is the first positive deflection after the P. This will be the initial wave of the QRS complex if there is no Q present. The first negative deflection after the R wave is the S wave. If there are additional components in the QRS complex, they will be named as prime waves (see Figure 6-3).

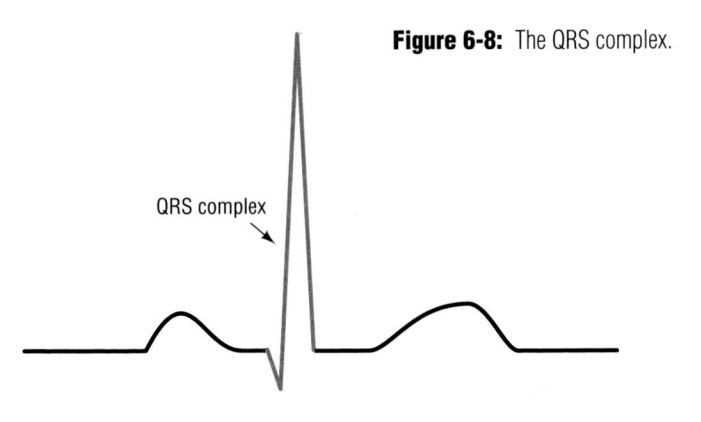

Figure 6-8: The QRS complex.

QRS complex

REMINDER:

Cardiac event represented by the QRS complex: Ventricular depolarization

Normal duration: 0.06 to 0.11 seconds

Axis: -30 to $+105°$, downward and to the left

Q Wave Significance The Q wave can be benign, or it can be a sign of dead myocardial tissue. A Q wave is considered significant if it is 0.03 seconds or wider, or its height is equal to or greater than one-third the height of the R wave. If it meets either of these criteria, it indicates a myocardial infarction (MI) over the region involved. If it doesn't, it is not a significant Q wave (Figure 6-9). Insignificant Q waves are commonly found in I, aVL, and V$_6$, where they are due to septal innervation. These are therefore called septal Qs.

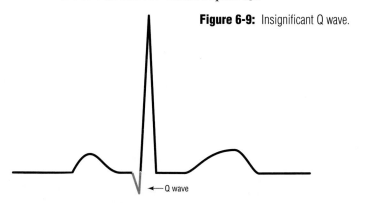

Figure 6-9: Insignificant Q wave.

← Q wave

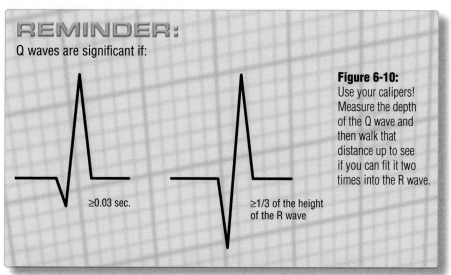

REMINDER:

Q waves are significant if:

≥0.03 sec.

≥1/3 of the height of the R wave

Figure 6-10:
Use your calipers! Measure the depth of the Q wave and then walk that distance up to see if you can fit it two times into the R wave.

The Intrinsicoid Deflection The intrinsicoid deflection is measured from the beginning of the QRS complex to the beginning of the negative down-slope of the R wave in leads that begin with an R wave and do not contain a Q wave (Figure 6-11). It represents the amount of time it takes the electrical impulse to travel from the Purkinje system in the endocardium to the surface of the epicardium immediately under an electrode. It is shorter (up to 0.035 seconds) in the right precordial leads, V$_1$ through V$_2$, because the right ventricle is thin in comparison with the left. It is longer (up to 0.045 seconds) in the left precordial leads, V$_5$ to V$_6$, because of the left ventricle's greater thickness. Now, can you imagine what would cause the intrinsicoid deflection to be prolonged? You will see a longer intrinsicoid deflection if there is a thicker myocardium, as in ventricular hypertrophy, or when it takes longer for the electrical system to conduct to that area, because of an intraventricular conduction delay such as, for instance, a left bundle branch block.

Figure 6-11: The intrinsicoid deflection.

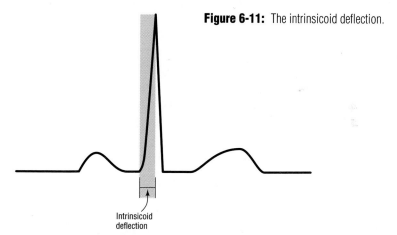

Intrinsicoid deflection

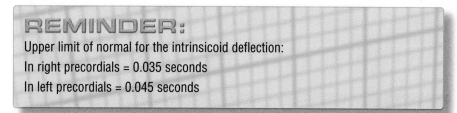

REMINDER:

Upper limit of normal for the intrinsicoid deflection:

In right precordials = 0.035 seconds

In left precordials = 0.045 seconds

The ST Segment

The ST segment is the section of the ECG cycle from the end of the QRS complex to the beginning of the T wave. The point where the QRS complex ends and the ST segment begins is called the J point (Figure 6-12). Many times, a clear J point cannot be identified because of ST segment elevation. The ST segment is usually found along the baseline. However, it can vary up to 1 mm from baseline in the limb leads of normal patients, and up to 3 mm in the right precordials of some patients. This is caused either by left ventricular hypertrophy or by what is referred to as the early repolarization pattern. This is just an introductory discussion. We will be spending much more time on this segment in Chapter 14, and we will give you the clues then that are needed to distinguish pathology from normal variants.

Now, having made the statements about ST elevation and normal variants above, we need to make a clarification that you will hear many more times. Any ST elevation in a symptomatic patient should be considered significant and representative of myocardial injury or

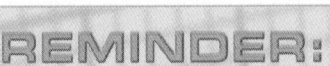

REMINDER:

Cardiac event represented by the ST segment: Electrically neutral period between ventricular depolarization and repolarization

Normal location: At the level of the baseline

Axis: Inferior and to the left

infarction until proven otherwise. Don't make the mistake of calling an acute MI a normal variant! Just because an ST segment is not elevated enough to meet the guidelines for the administration of thrombolytics (presently 1 mm in two contiguous leads) does not mean that it is benign. You must have a high index of suspicion in these cases and try to obtain an old ECG to compare.

The ST segment represents an electrically neutral time for the heart. The ventricles are between depolarization (QRS complex) and repolarization (T wave). Mechanically, this represents the time that the myocardium is maintaining contraction in order to push the blood out of the ventricles. As you can imagine, very little blood would be expelled if the ventricles only contracted for 0.12 seconds.

The T Wave

The T wave represents ventricular repolarization (Figure 6-13). It is the next deflection — either positive or negative — that occurs after the ST segment and should begin in the same direction as the QRS complex.

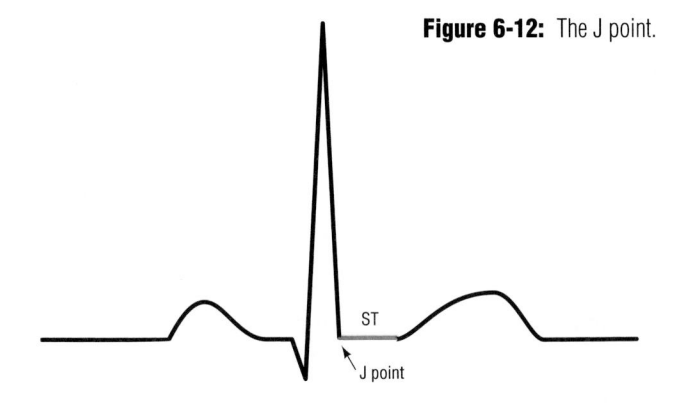

Figure 6-12: The J point.

ST

J point

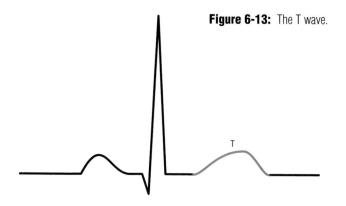

Figure 6-13: The T wave.

Why should the T wave be in the same direction as the QRS? If it represents repolarization, shouldn't it be opposite the QRS? For the answer, we need to go back to the concept of ventricular excitation. The Purkinje system is near the endocardium; therefore, electrical depolarization should begin in the endocardium and move out toward the epicardium (Figure 6-14, top arrow).

You would expect repolarization to occur in the same direction because the cell that was first depolarized should be the first to repolarize, but this is not the case. Because of increased pressure on the endocardium during contraction, the repolarization wave travels in the opposite direction, from the epicardium back to the endocardium (Figure 6-14, bottom arrow). Remember, a negative wave — and repolarization is a negative wave — traveling away from the electrode is perceived the same as a positive wave moving toward it.

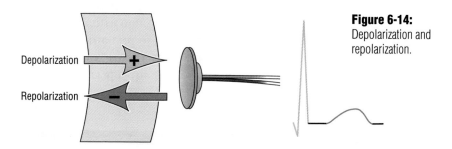

Figure 6-14: Depolarization and repolarization.

Hence, the normal T wave should be in the same direction as the QRS. There are exceptions in some pathological states.

The T wave should be asymmetrical, with the first part rising or dropping slowly and the latter part moving much faster (Figure 6-15). The way to check for symmetry of the T wave, if the ST segment is elevated, is to draw a perpendicular line from the peak of that wave to the baseline and then compare the symmetry of the two sides, ignoring the ST segment (Figure 6-16). Symmetric Ts can be normal, but are usually a sign of pathology.

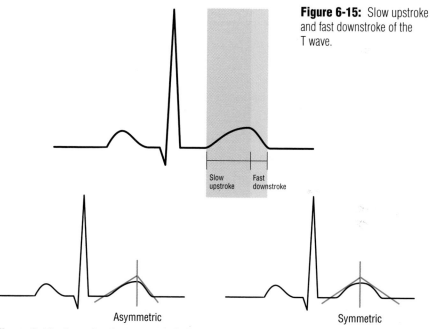

Figure 6-15: Slow upstroke and fast downstroke of the T wave.

Slow upstroke   Fast downstroke

Asymmetric   Symmetric

Figure 6-16: Assessing the symmetry of a T wave.

REMINDER:
Cardiac event represented by the T wave: Ventricular repolarization
Axis: Downward and to the left, similar to the QRS axis

The QT interval

The QT interval is the section of the ECG complex encompassing the QRS complex, the ST segment, and the T wave — from the beginning of the Q to the end of the T (Figure 6-17). It represents all of the events of ventricular systole, from the beginning of ventricular depolarization to the end of the repolarization cycle. The interval varies with heart rate, electrolyte abnormalities, age, and sex. A prolonged QT is a harbinger of possible arrhythmias, especially torsade de pointes. This is not a common occurrence, but it is life threatening. The QT interval should be shorter than one half of the preceding R-R interval (the interval between the peaks of the two preceding R waves). There are various formulas to evaluate the significance of a QT interval, but the most useful one is to evaluate the QTc (discussed next).

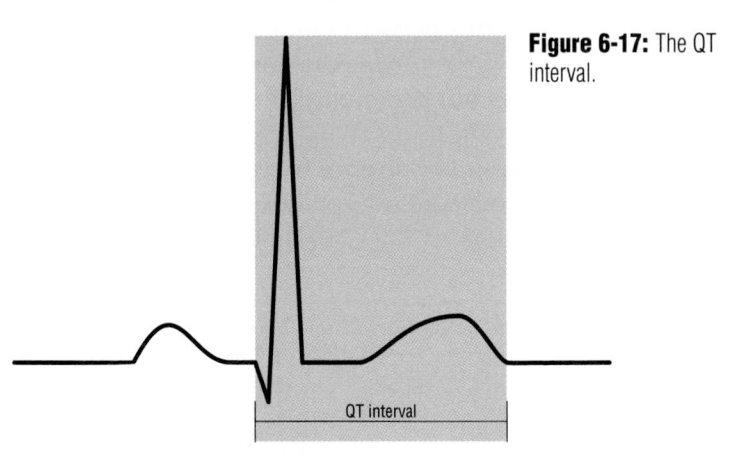

Figure 6-17: The QT interval.

QT interval

REMINDER:

Cardiac events represented by the QT interval: All the events of ventricular systole

Normal duration: Variable, especially with heart rate. Usually less than half of the R-R interval

The QTc Interval The QTc interval stands for the QT corrected interval. What is it corrected for? Heart rate. As the heart rate decreases, the QT interval lengthens; conversely, as the heart rate increases, the QT interval shortens. This makes it hard to calculate the interval at which the QT is normal. By calculating the QTc interval, we can state that normal is around 0.410 seconds or 410 milliseconds. Giving a little leeway, we will say that anything above 0.419 seconds is lengthened. The formula for calculating the QTc appears in the box that follows. Most ECG machines will automatically calculate the interval for you.

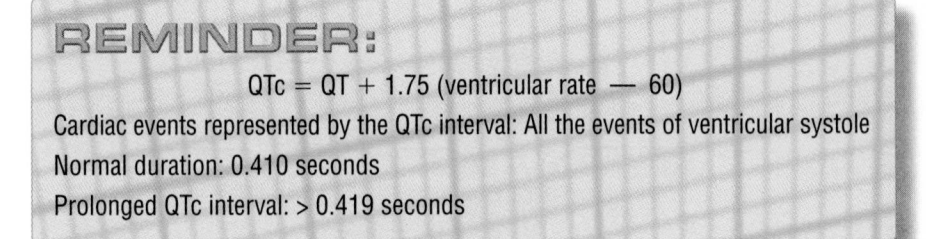

REMINDER:

$$QTc = QT + 1.75 \text{ (ventricular rate } - 60)$$

Cardiac events represented by the QTc interval: All the events of ventricular systole

Normal duration: 0.410 seconds

Prolonged QTc interval: > 0.419 seconds

The U Wave

The U wave is a small, flat wave sometimes seen after the T wave and before the next P wave (Figure 6-18). Various theories have arisen about what it represents, including ventricular depolarization and endocardial repolarization. Nobody knows for sure. It can be seen in normal patients, especially in the presence of bradycardia. It can also be seen in hypokalemia (low potassium). One valuable point is that there can be no possibility of hyperkalemia in the presence of a U wave (more about this later). The only other clinical significance of the U is that it can sometimes cause an inaccuracy in measuring the QT interval. This can lead to a longer-than-accurate value because some machines may include this interval in their measurements. ECG computers are notorious for this miscalculation.

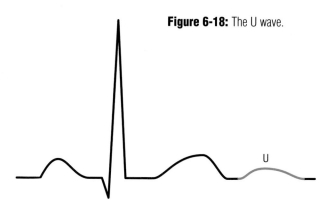

Figure 6-18: The U wave.

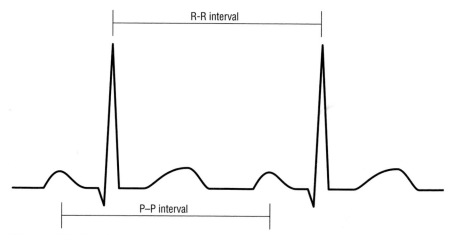

Figure 6-19: The P-P interval and the R-R interval.

REMINDER:

Cardiac event represented by the U wave: Unknown

Important points: Low voltage; deflects in the same direction as the T wave

Clinical importance: Usually benign. The most important clinical significance of a U wave is that it could potentially be a sign of hypokalemia.

CLINICAL PEARL

The true baseline of the ECG is a line drawn from the TP of one complex to the TP of another. The PR segment should fall on this line, but many times does not. Fluctuations from the baseline may signify pathology. We will discuss what these fluctuations may represent in Chapter 10.

Additional Intervals

There are a few additional intervals that we will cover as the text continues. However, let's talk about two of the most common ones now. First, there is the R-R interval, the distance between identical points (usually the peaks) of two consecutive QRS complexes (Figure 6-19). You will be measuring this often to evaluate the rhythm. Regular rhythms are those that have consistent R-R intervals.

Another is the P-P interval, the distance between two identical points on one P wave and the next (Figure 6-19). This interval will be very useful in evaluating the patient for rhythm abnormalities. Examples include Wenckebach second-degree heart block, atrial

flutter, and third-degree heart block. We will discuss these rhythm abnormalities in Chapter 8.

Looking Ahead

Each of these waves and intervals are discussed in great detail in Part 2. We hope that this has been helpful in creating some of the foundation that you will need to cover this exciting subject.

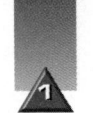

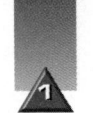
CHAPTER IN **REVIEW**

1. The baseline is a straight line drawn between the _____ of one complex to the _____ of the succeeding complex.
   A. PR segment–PR segment
   B. Beginning of one P–beginning of the next P
   C. TP segment–TP segment
   D. QT interval–QT interval
   E. None of the above

2. The P wave represents atrial repolarization and innervation of the atrial myocytes. True or False.

3. The PR segment and the PR interval both represent the same time frame. True or False.

4. The normal duration for the PR interval is _____ seconds.
   A. 0.08–0.10
   B. 0.11–0.15
   C. 0.11–0.20
   D. 0.20–0.24
   E. None of the above

5. The normal duration for the QRS interval is _____ seconds.
   A. 0.06–0.08
   B. 0.06–0.11
   C. 0.08–0.14
   D. 0.12–0.20
   E. None of the above

6. Q waves are significant if:
   A. They are ≥ 0.03 seconds (one little block) wide
   B. They are deeper than $\frac{1}{3}$ the height of the R wave
   C. Both A and B are correct
   D. Both A and B are incorrect
   E. None of the above

7. The T wave represents ventricular repolarization. True or False.

8. The T waves are usually asymmetrical. True or False.

9. The QT should always be more than $\frac{1}{2}$ the preceding R-R interval. True or False.

10. The U wave is a small, flat wave seen after the T wave and before the next P wave. True or False.

1. C 2. False 3. False 4. C 5. B 6. C 7. True 8. True 9. False 10. True

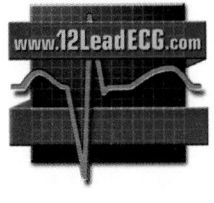 To enhance the knowledge you gain in this book, access this text's website at www.12leadECG.com! This valuable resource provides an online glossary and related web links. To learn more about the chapter topics, simply click on the chapter and view the link.

CHAPTER **7**

When evaluating the rate of the complexes, first keep in mind that the P wave rate may be different from the QRS rate. For the purposes of this discussion, we consider QRS rates only. The same principles can be applied to obtain the P wave rate, if needed.

The rate can be obtained in various ways. If you have a computerized interpretation at the top of the ECG, you can usually use the rate that is given. Keep in mind, however, that this rate may be wrong. If it appears to be the wrong rate, calculate it yourself. One way of calculating the rate is to use a ruler, such as the one mentioned in Chapter 5. There are also ways of calculating rate using the ECG and your basic knowledge of the time intervals involved. Using your calipers with these techniques will be very helpful. Let's look at some of those ways now.

Establishing the Rate

Normal and Fast Rates

The easiest way to calculate the rate is to use the method illustrated in Figure 7-1. Find a QRS complex that starts on a thick line; this will be your starting point. Next, go to the exact spot on the next QRS complex — your end point. By tradition, we try to use the tip of the tallest wave on the QRS complex. However, you can use any spot as long as it is consistent. Then just count the thick lines in between the two spots, using the numbers shown in Figure 7-1. You will have to memorize this sequence, but it is more than worth your trouble.

Another way to calculate the rate is to use your calipers to measure from the top of one complex to the top of the next. Then move the calipers — maintaining the measured distance — so that the left tip rests on a thick line, and calculate the rate as above for the distance between the two tips. The advantage here is that you don't have to hunt down a QRS that lands on a thick line to use as a starting point.

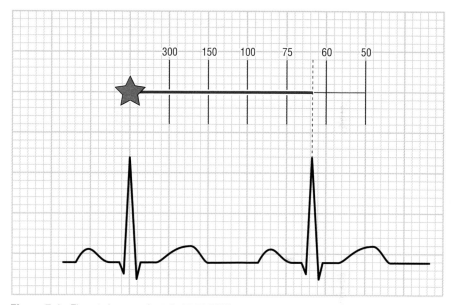

Figure 7-1: The rate is approximately 65-70 BPM.

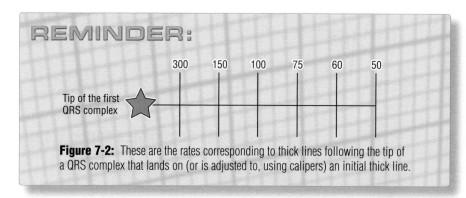

Figure 7-2: These are the rates corresponding to thick lines following the tip of a QRS complex that lands on (or is adjusted to, using calipers) an initial thick line.

Bradycardic Rates

Do you remember the concept in Figure 7-3, from Chapter 4? Knowing these time intervals will be very useful when you are calculating bradycardic rhythms. Can you think of how to use these intervals to calculate the rate generally, but especially in irregular and slow rhythms?

It's simple. Just count the number of cycles present in a 6-second strip, and multiply that number by 10. This will give you the number of beats in 60 seconds. You could also count the number of cycles in a 12-second strip and multiply by 5. Remember to use the fractional parts of cycles in your calculations, for example, 3.5 cycles in 6 seconds gives a rate of 35 beats per minute (3.5 cycles × 10 = 35 BPM).

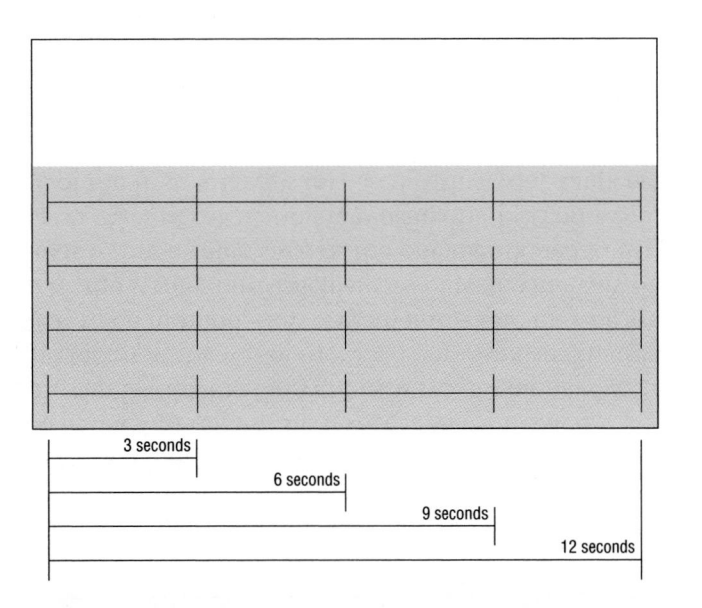

3 seconds
6 seconds
9 seconds
12 seconds

Figure 7-3: ECG paper.

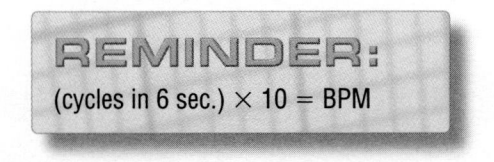

REMINDER:
(cycles in 6 sec.) × 10 = BPM

Let's practice calculating some rates. . .

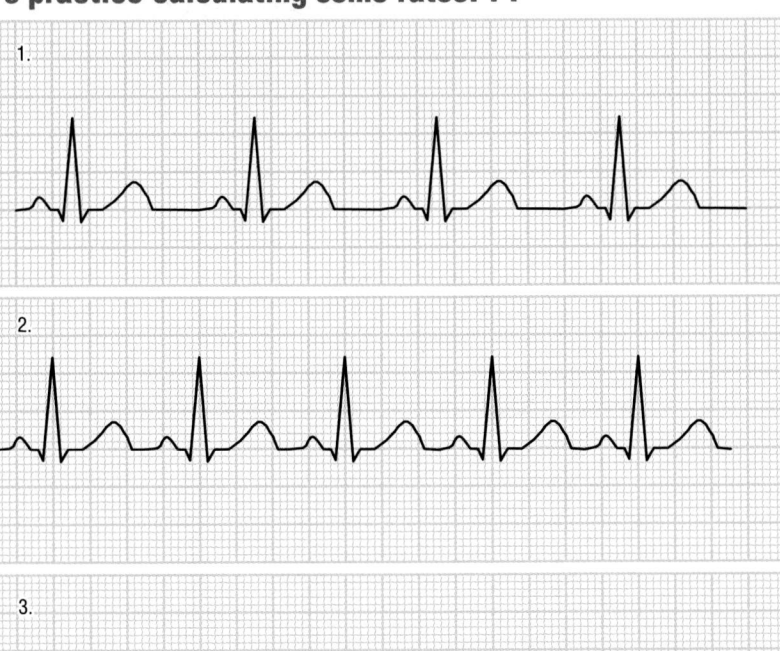

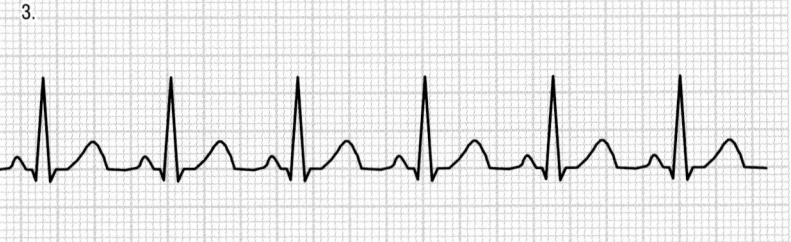

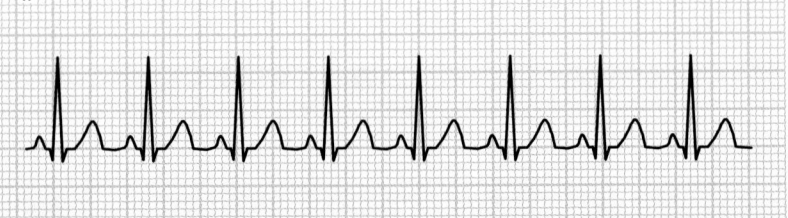

Figure 7-4

Answers: **1.** 60 BPM, **2.** 75 BPM, **3.** About 80–85 BPM, **4.** Approximately 130 BPM

Calculate the rates . . .

For simplicity, we will use a star to represent each complex.

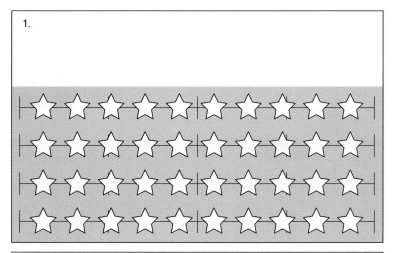

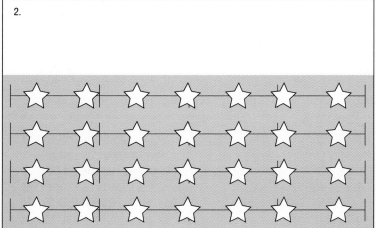

Figure 7-5

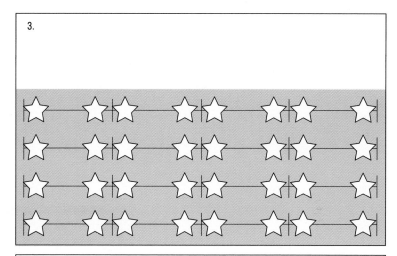

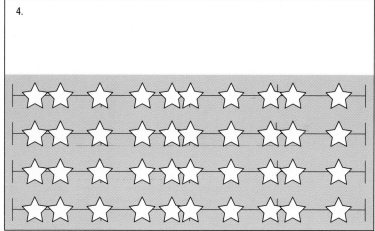

Figure 7-5: Continued

Answers: **1.** Because the rhythm is regular, we can use either the 6-second or 12-second strip to figure out that there is a rate of: 5 (the # of beats in 6 seconds) × 10 = 50 BPM. **2.** This set has approximately 3.5 beats × 10 = 35 BPM. **3.** When the beats are irregular, it is more accurate to use the 12-second strip and multiply that number by 5. This gives us a rate of: 8 beats × 5 = 40 BPM **4.** The rate is:

10 beats × 5 = 50 BPM

CHAPTER IN **REVIEW**

1. When calculating rates, the numbers to remember are:
   A. 300–160–90–75–60–50
   B. 300–150–100–75–60–50
   C. 300–150–80–70–60–50
   D. 400–160–100–75–60–50
   E. None of the above

2. When calculating bradycardic rhythms, we take the number of complexes found during a 6-second interval on the ECG and multiply that number by 10. The product is the heart rate as beats per minute. True or False.

3. What is the rate if there are 3.5 beats in a 6-second strip?
   A. 3.5 BPM
   B. 35 BPM
   C. 350 BPM
   D. 3500 BPM
   E. None of the above

4. What is the rate if there are 3.5 beats in a 12-second strip?
   A. 3.5 BPM
   B. 35 BPM
   C. 17.5 BPM
   D. 175 BPM
   E. None of the above

5. What is the rate if there are five beats in a 6-second strip?
   A. 5 BPM
   B. 15 BPM
   C. 50 BPM
   D. 150 BPM
   E. None of the above

1. B 2. True 3. B 4. C 5. C

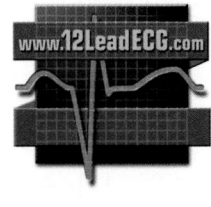

To enhance the knowledge you gain in this book, access this text's website at www.12leadECG.com! This valuable resource provides an online glossary and related web links. To learn more about the chapter topics, simply click on the chapter and view the link.

CHAPTER **8**

This chapter is dedicated to the discussion of rhythms and arrhythmias. This will be a preliminary introduction to the subject. Individual arrhythmias are discussed in greater detail as they are encountered in the text. We recommend that you read the next section (Major Concepts) once, then proceed to the discussion of the individual rhythms, and finally return to reread Major Concepts. This will help to clarify the terminology.

Major Concepts

There are 10 points you should think about in an organized manner when approaching arrhythmias:

General

1. Is the rhythm fast or slow?
2. Is the rhythm regular or irregular? If irregular, is it regularly irregular or irregularly irregular?

P waves

3. Do you see any P waves?
4. Are all of the P waves the same?
5. Does each QRS complex have a P wave?
6. Is the PR interval constant?

QRS complexes

7. Are the P waves and QRS complexes associated with one another?
8. Are the QRS complexes narrow or wide?
9. Are the QRS complexes grouped or not grouped?
10. Are there any dropped beats?

General

Is the rhythm fast or slow? Many rhythm abnormalities are associated with specific rate ranges. Therefore, it is very important to determine the rate of the rhythm in question. Decide if you are dealing with a tachycardia (> 100 BPM), a bradycardia (< 60 BPM), or a normal rate.

Is the rhythm regular or irregular? Do the P waves and QRS complexes follow a regular pattern with the same intervals separating them, or are the intervals different between some or all of the beats? This is a great tool to help you narrow down the rhythm, as you will see in the upcoming pages.

There is an additional question you must answer if the rhythm is irregular: is it regularly irregular or irregularly irregular? At first glance, this statement can be confusing. A rhythm is regularly irregular if it has some form or regularity to the pattern of the irregular complex. An example would be a rhythm in which every third complex comes sooner than the preceding two. Therefore, the intervals would be long-long-short, long-long-short, in a repeating pattern that is predictable and recurring in its irregularity.

An irregularly irregular rhythm has no pattern at all. All of the intervals are haphazard and do not repeat, with an occasional, accidental exception. Luckily, there are only three irregularly irregular rhythms: atrial fibrillation, wandering atrial pacemaker, and multifocal atrial tachycardia. This is a differential diagnosis that you should commit to memory, as it will get you out of some tight spots.

P Waves

Do you see any P waves? The presence of P waves tells you that the rhythm in question has some atrial or supraventricular component. This is another major branch of the differential diagnosis of arrhythmias. The P waves, generated by the SA node or another atrial pacemaker, will usually reset any pacemaker down the chain.

Are all of the P waves the same? The presence of P waves that are identical means that they are being generated by the same pacemaker site. Identical P waves should have identical PR intervals unless an AV nodal block is present (more later). If the P waves are not identical, consider two possibilities: there is an additional pacemaker cell firing, or there is some other component of the complex superimposed on the P wave, such as a T wave occurring at the same moment as the P wave. The presence of three or more different P wave morphologies with different PR intervals defines either wandering atrial pacemaker or multifocal atrial tachycardia, both described later in this chapter.

Does each QRS complex have a P wave? An abnormal number of P waves in comparison to QRS complexes is an important point in determining whether you are dealing with some sort of AV nodal block.

Is the PR interval constant? Once again, this is extremely useful in identifying a wandering atrial pacemaker or multifocal atrial tachycardia. It is also helpful in evaluating atrial premature contractions (APCs) with and without aberrant conduction (slow conduction from cell to cell that produces abnormally wide QRS complexes).

QRS Complexes

Are the P waves and QRS complexes associated with one another? Is the P wave before a QRS complex responsible for the firing of that QRS (associated with it)? A positive answer to this question will help determine if the entire complex is a normal beat, a premature beat, or a low-grade AV nodal block. In the discussion of ventricular tachycardia, you may note that the presence of capture and fusion beats is critical to the diagnosis. In these cases, the P wave preceding the capture or fusion beat is responsible for the complex, in contrast to the other P waves that are dissociated from their respective QRSs.

Are the QRS complexes narrow or wide? Narrow complexes represent impulses that have traveled down the normal AV node/Purkinje network. These complexes are usually found in supraventricular rhythms, including junctional rhythms. Wide complexes indicate that the impulses that did not follow the normal electrical conduction system, but instead were transmitted by direct cell-to-cell contact at some point in their travels through the heart. These wide complexes are found in ventricular premature contractions (VPCs), aberrantly conducted beats, ventricular tachycardia, and bundle branch blocks.

Are the QRS complexes grouped or not grouped? This is very useful in determining the presence of an AV nodal block or recurrent premature complexes, such as bigeminy (a repeating pattern of a normal complex followed by a premature complex) and trigeminy (a repeating pattern of two normal complexes followed by a premature complex).

Are there any dropped beats? Dropped beats occur in AV nodal blocks and sinus arrest.

Individual Rhythms

Supraventricular Rhythms

Normal Sinus Rhythm (NSR)

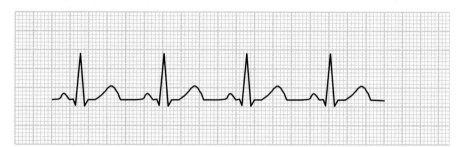

Rate:	60–100 BPM
Regularity:	Regular
P wave:	Present
P:QRS ratio:	1:1
PR interval:	Normal
QRS width:	Normal
Grouping:	None
Dropped beats:	None

Putting it all together:

This rhythm represents the normal state with the SA node as the lead pacer. The intervals should all be consistent and within the normal range. Note that this refers to the atrial rate; normal sinus rhythm (NSR) can occur with a ventricular escape rhythm or other ventricular abnormality if AV dissociation exists.

Figure 8-1: Normal sinus rhythm (NSR).

Sinus Arrhythmia

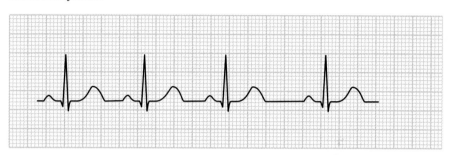

Rate:	60–100 BPM
Regularity:	Varies with respiration
P wave:	Normal
P:QRS ratio:	1:1
PR interval:	Normal
QRS width:	Normal
Grouping:	None
Dropped beats:	None

Putting it all together (see figure 8.1):

This rhythm represents the normal respiratory variation, becoming slower during exhalation and faster upon inhalation. This occurs because inhalation increases venous return by lowering intrathoracic pressure. Note that the PR intervals are the same; only the TP intervals (the interval from the end of the T wave of one complex to the beginning of the P wave of the next complex) vary with the respirations.

Figure 8-2: Sinus arrhythmia.

Sinus Bradycardia

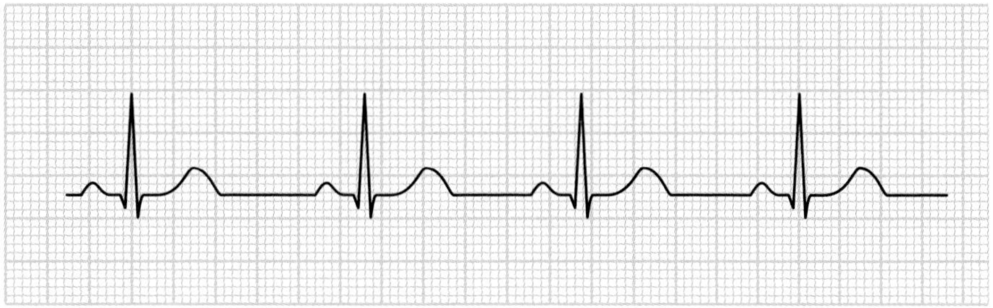

Figure 8-3: Sinus bradycardia.

Rate:	Less than 60 BPM
Regularity:	Regular
P wave:	Present
P:QRS ratio:	1:1
PR interval:	Normal to slightly prolonged
QRS width:	Normal to slightly prolonged
Grouping:	None
Dropped beats:	None

Putting it all together:

The sinus beats are slower than 60 BPM. The origin may be in the SA node or in an atrial pacemaker. This rhythm can be caused by vagal stimulation leading to nodal slowing, or by medicines such as beta blockers, and is found normally in some well conditioned athletes. The QRS complex, and the PR and QTc intervals, may slightly widen as the rhythm slows below 60 BPM. However, they will not widen past the upper threshold of the normal range for that interval. For example, the PR interval may widen, but should not widen over the upper range of 0.20 seconds.

Figure 8-3: Sinus bradycardia.

Sinus Tachycardia

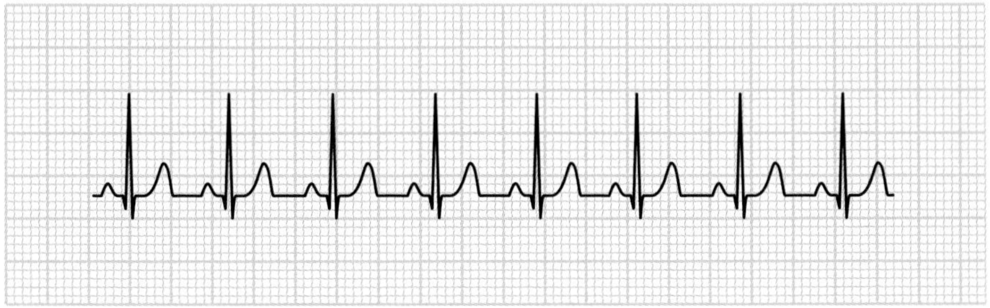

Rate:	Greater than 100 BPM
Regularity:	Regular
P wave:	Present
P:QRS ratio:	1:1
PR interval:	Normal to slightly shortened
QRS width:	Normal to slightly shortened
Grouping:	None
Dropped beats:	None

Putting it all together:

This can be caused by medications or by conditions that require increased cardiac output, such as exercise, hypoxemia, hypovolemia, hemorrhage, and acidosis.

Figure 8-4: Sinus tachycardia.

Sinus Pause/Arrest

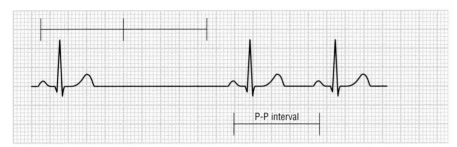

Rate:	Varies
Regularity:	Irregular
P wave:	Present except in areas of pause/arrest
P:QRS ratio:	1:1
PR interval:	Normal
QRS width:	Normal
Grouping:	None
Dropped beats:	Yes

Putting it all together:
A sinus pause is a variable time period during which there is no sinus pacemaker working. The time interval is not a multiple of the normal P-P interval. (A dropped complex that is a multiple of the P-P interval is known as an SA block, discussed next.) A sinus arrest is a longer pause, though there is no clear-cut criterion for how long a pause has to last before it is called an arrest.

Figure 8-5: Sinus pause/arrest.

Sinoatrial Block

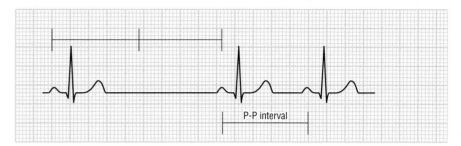

Rate:	Varies
Regularity:	Irregular
P wave:	Present except in areas of dropped beats
P:QRS ratio:	1:1
PR interval:	Normal
QRS width:	Normal
Grouping:	None
Dropped beats:	Yes

Putting it all together:
The block occurs in some multiple of the P-P interval. After the dropped beat, the cycles continue on time and as scheduled. The pathology involved is a nonconducted beat from the normal pacemaker.

Figure 8-6: Sinoatrial block.

Atrial Premature Contraction (APC)

P-P interval | P-P interval

P-P interval

Rate:	Depends on the underlying sinus rate
Regularity:	Irregular
P wave:	Present; in the APC, may be a different shape
P:QRS ratio:	1:1
PR interval:	Varies in the APC, otherwise normal
QRS width:	Normal
Grouping:	Sometimes
Dropped beats:	No

Putting it all together:

An atrial premature contraction (APC) occurs when some other pacemaker cell in the atria fires at a rate faster than that of the SA node. The result is a complex that comes sooner than expected. Notice that the premature beat "resets" the SA node, and the pause after the APC is not compensated; the underlying rhythm is disturbed and does not proceed at the same pace. This noncompensatory pause is less than twice the underlying normal P-P interval.

Figure 8-7: Atrial premature contraction (APC).

Ectopic Atrial Tachycardia

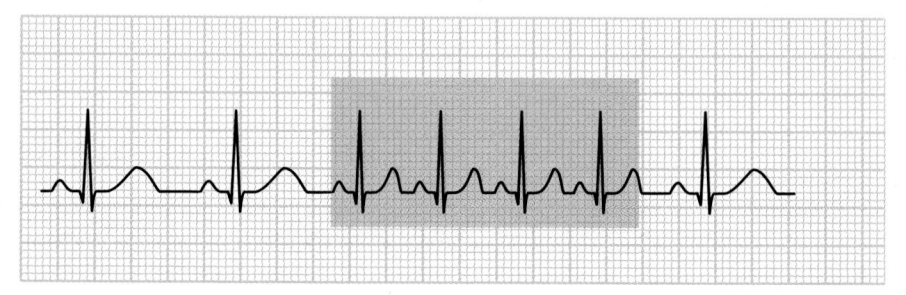

Rate:	100–180 BPM
Regularity:	Regular
P wave:	Morphology of ectopic focus is different
P:QRS ratio:	1:1
PR interval:	Ectopic focus has a different interval
QRS width:	Normal, but can be aberrant at times
Grouping:	None
Dropped beats:	None

Putting it all together:

Ectopic atrial tachycardia occurs when an ectopic atrial focus fires more quickly than the underlying sinus rate. The P waves and PR intervals are different because the rhythm is caused by an ectopic atrial pacemaker (a pacemaker outside of the normal SA node). The episodes are usually not sustained for an extended period. Because of the accelerated rate, some ST- and T- wave abnormalities may be present transiently.

Figure 8-8: Ectopic atrial tachycardia.

Wandering Atrial Pacemaker (WAP)

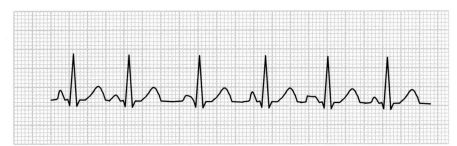

Rate:	100 BPM
Regularity:	Irregularly irregular
P wave:	At least three different morphologies
P:QRS ratio:	1:1
PR interval:	Variable depending on the focus
QRS width:	Normal
Grouping:	None
Dropped beats:	None

Putting it all together:
Wandering atrial pacemaker (WAP) is an irregularly irregular rhythm created by multiple atrial pacemakers each firing at its own pace. The result is an ECG with at least three different P wave morphologies with their own intrinsic PR intervals. Think of each pacer firing from a different distance, with a different P wave axis. The longer the distance, the longer the PR interval. The varying P wave axis cases differences in the morphology of the P waves.

Figure 8-9: Wandering atrial pacemaker (WAP).

Multifocal Atrial Tachycardia (MAT)

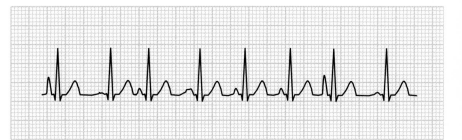

Rate:	Greater than 100 BPM
Regularity:	Irregularly irregular
P wave:	At least three different morphologies
P:QRS ratio:	1:1
PR interval:	Variable
QRS width:	Normal
Grouping:	None
Dropped beats:	None

Putting it all together:
Multifocal atrial tachycardia (MAT) is merely a tachycardic WAP. Both MAT and WAP are commonly found in patients with severe lung disease. The tachycardia can cause cardiovascular instability at times and should be treated. Treatment is difficult, and should be aimed at correcting the underlying problem.

Figure 8-10: Multifocal atrial tachycardia (MAT).

Atrial Flutter

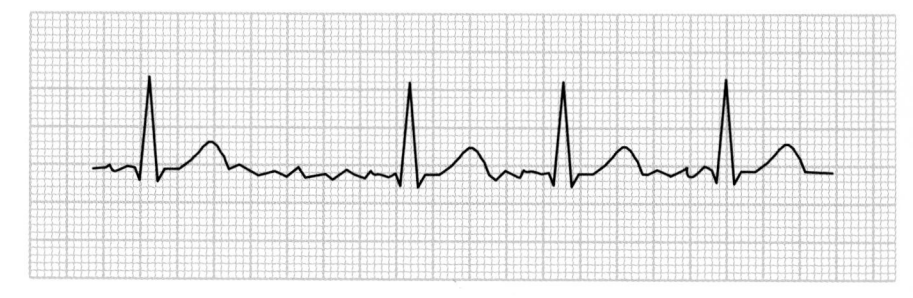

Rate:	Atrial rate commonly 250–350 BPM Ventricular rate commonly 125–175 BPM
Regularity:	Usually regular but may be variable
P wave:	Saw toothed appearance, "F waves"
P:QRS ratio:	Variable, most commonly 2:1
PR interval:	Variable
QRS width:	Normal
Grouping:	None
Dropped beats:	None

Putting it all together:

The P waves appear in a saw toothed pattern such as those in Figure 8-11. (QRSs have been removed from strip B to reveal P wave shape.) The QRS rate is usually regular and the complexes appear at some multiple of the P-P interval. The usual QRS response is 2:1 (this means that there are 2 P waves for each QRS complex). We call this an atrial flutter with 2:1 block (some of the P waves are blocked and do not cause any ventricular response), and so on. The ventricular response can also occur slower at rates 3:1, 4:1, or higher. Sometimes the ventricular response will be irregular.

Looking more closely at these cases, you will see that they also occur at some multiple of the P-P interval. The rate of the intervals, however, can vary, with some occurring at a rate of 2:1 and some occurring at a rate of 3:1, and so on. We call this atrial flutter with varying 2:1 and 3:1 block. This is an example: the ratios will vary depending on the rhythm. Rarely, you will have a truly variable ventricular response that does not fall on any multiple of the P-P interval. We call this an atrial flutter with a variable ventricular response.

In closing, keep in mind that the sawtoothed appearance may not be obvious in all 12 leads. Whenever you see a ventricular rate of 150 BPM, look for the buried P waves of an atrial flutter with 2:1 block!

Figure 8-11: Atrial flutter.

Atrial Fibrillation

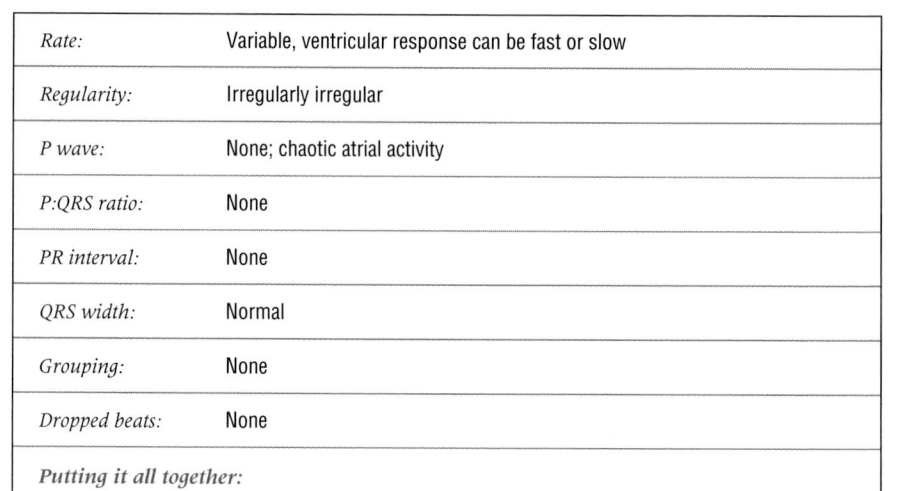

Rate:	Variable, ventricular response can be fast or slow
Regularity:	Irregularly irregular
P wave:	None; chaotic atrial activity
P:QRS ratio:	None
PR interval:	None
QRS width:	Normal
Grouping:	None
Dropped beats:	None

Putting it all together:

Atrial fibrillation is the chaotic firing of numerous pacemaker cells in the atria in a totally haphazard fashion. The result is that there are no discernible P waves, and the QRS complexes are innervated haphazardly in an irregular pattern. The ventricular rate is completely guided by occasional activation from one of the pacemaking sources. Because the ventricles are not paced by any one site, the intervals are completely random.

Figure 8-12: Atrial fibrillation.

Junctional Premature Contraction (JPC)

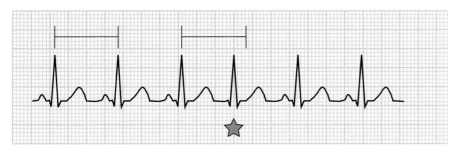

Rate:	Depends on underlying rhythm
Regularity:	Irregular
P wave:	Variable (none, antegrade, or retrograde)
P:QRS ratio:	None; or 1:1 if antegrade or retrograde
PR interval:	None, short, or retrograde; if present does not represent atrial stimulation of the ventricles.
QRS width:	Normal
Grouping:	Usually none, but can occur
Dropped beats:	None

Putting it all together:

A junctional premature contraction (JPC) is a beat that originates prematurely in the AV node. Because it travels down the normal electrical conduction system of the ventricles, the QRS complex is identical to the underlying QRSs. JPCs usually appear sporadically, but can occur in a regular, grouped pattern such as supraventricular bigeminy or trigeminy. There may be an antegrade or retrograde P wave associated with the complex. An antegrade P wave is one that appears before the QRS complex. The PR interval is very short in these cases, and P-wave axis will be abnormal (inverted in leads II, III, and aVF; more on these types of P waves in Chapter 9). A retrograde P is one that appears after the QRS complex.

Figure 8-13: Junctional premature contraction (JPC).

Junctional Escape Beat

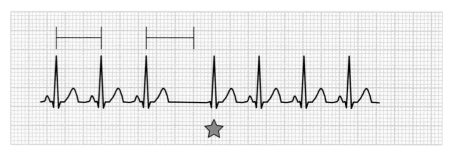

Rate:	Depends on underlying rhythm
Regularity:	Irregular
P wave:	Variable (none, antegrade, or retrograde)
P:QRS ratio:	None; or 1:1 if antegrade or retrograde.
PR interval:	None, short, or retrograde; if present, does not represent atrial stimulation of the ventricles.
QRS width:	Normal
Grouping:	None
Dropped beats:	Yes

Putting it all together:

An escape beat occurs when the normal pacemaker fails to fire and the next available pacemaker in the conduction system fires in its place. Remember that this is discussed in Chapter 1. The AV nodal pacer senses that the normal pacer did not fire. So when its turn comes up and it reaches its threshold potential, it fires. The distance of the escape beat from the preceding complex is always longer than the normal P-P interval.

Figure 8-14: Junctional escape beat.

Junctional Rhythm

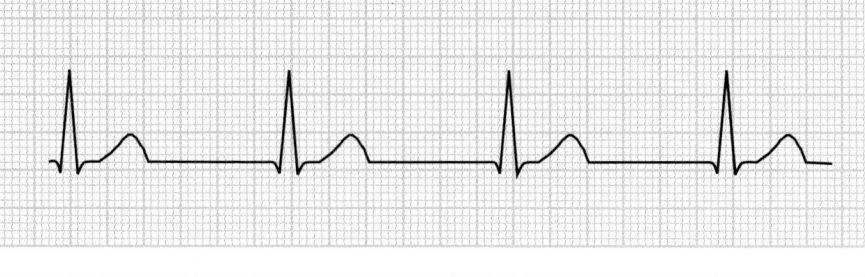

Rate:	40–60 BPM
Regularity:	Regular
P wave:	Variable (none, antegrade, or retrograde)
P:QRS ratio:	None; or 1:1 if antegrade or retrograde
PR interval:	None, short, or retrograde; if present, does not represent atrial stimulation of the ventricles.
QRS width:	Normal
Grouping:	None
Dropped beats:	None

Putting it all together:

A junctional rhythm arises as an escape rhythm when the normal pacemaking function of the atria and SA node is absent. It can also occur in the case of AV dissociation or third-degree AV block (more on this later).

Figure 8-15: Junctional rhythm.

Accelerated Junctional Rhythm

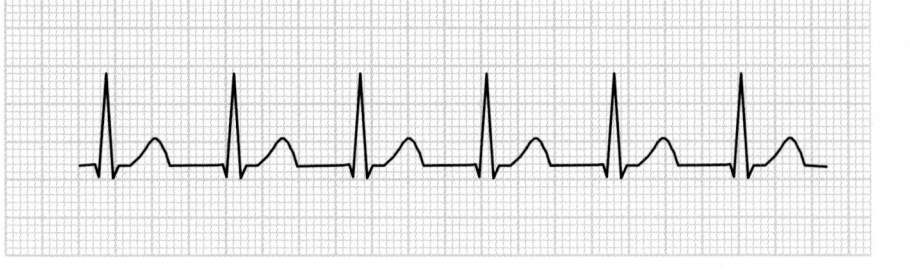

Rate:	60–100 BPM
Regularity:	Regular
P wave:	Variable (none, antegrade, or retrograde)
P:QRS ratio:	None; or 1:1 if antegrade or retrograde
PR interval:	None, short, or retrograde; if present, does not represent atrial stimulation of the ventricles.
QRS width:	Normal
Grouping:	None
Dropped beats:	None

Putting it all together:

This rhythm originates in a junctional pacemaker that, because it is firing faster than the normal pacemaker, takes over the pacing function. It is faster than expected for a normal junctional rhythm, pacing in the range of 60–100 BPM. If it exceeds 100 BPM, it is known as junctional tachycardia. As with other junctional pacers the P waves can be absent or conducted in an antegrade or retrograde fashion.

Figure 8-16: Accelerated junctional rhythm.

Ventricular Rhythms

Ventricular Premature Contraction (VPC)

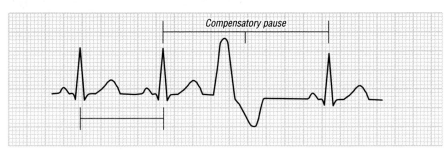

Compensatory pause

Rate:	Depends on the underlying rhythm
Regularity:	Irregular
P wave:	Not present on the VPC
P:QRS ratio:	No P waves on the VPC
PR interval:	None
QRS width:	Wide (=0.12 seconds), bizarre appearance
Grouping:	Usually not present
Dropped beats:	None

Putting it all together:
A VPC is caused by the premature firing of a ventricular cell. The ventricular pacer fires before the normal SA node or supraventricular pacer, which causes the ventricles to be in a refractory state (not yet repolarized and unavailable to fire again) when the normal pacer fires. Hence, the ventricles do not contract at their normal time. However, the underlying pacing schedule is not altered, so the beat following the VPC will arrive on time. This is called a *compensatory pause*.

Figure 8-17: Ventricular premature contraction (VPC).

Ventricular Escape Beat

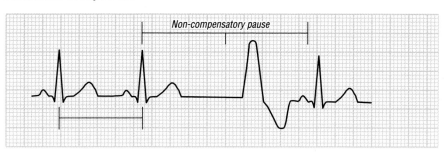

Non-compensatory pause

Rate:	Depends on the underlying rhythm
Regularity:	Irregular
P wave:	None in the VPC
P:QRS ratio:	None in the VPC
PR interval:	None
QRS width:	Wide (=0.12 seconds), bizarre appearance
Grouping:	None
Dropped beats:	None

Putting it all together:
A ventricular escape beat is similar to a junctional escape beat, but the focus is in the ventricles. The pause is *non-compensatory* in this case because the normal pacer did not fire. (This is what led to the ventricular escape beat.) The pacer then resets itself on a new timing cycle, and may even have a different rate.

Figure 8-18: Ventricular escape beat.

Idioventricular Rhythm

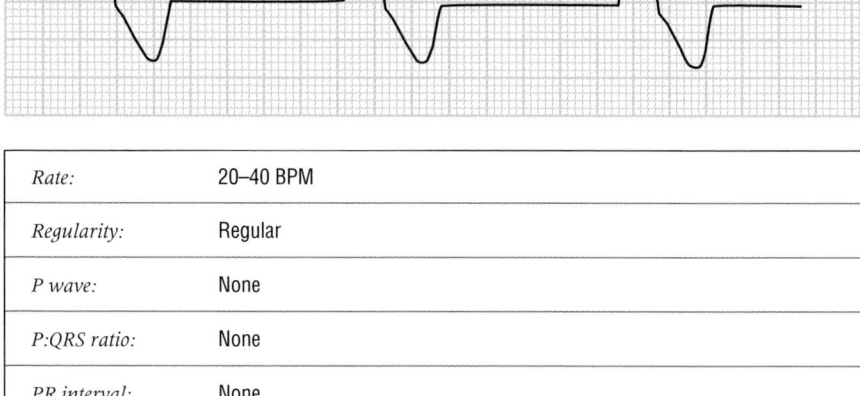

Rate:	20–40 BPM
Regularity:	Regular
P wave:	None
P:QRS ratio:	None
PR interval:	None
QRS width:	Wide (≥0.12 seconds), bizarre appearance
Grouping:	None
Dropped beats:	None

Putting it all together:

Idioventricular rhythm occurs when a ventricular focus acts as the primary pacemaker for the heart. The QRS complexes are wide and bizarre, reflecting their ventricular origin. This rhythm can be found by itself, or as a component of AV dissociation or third-degree heart block. (In these latter cases, there may be an underlying sinus rhythm with P waves present.)

Figure 8-19: Idioventricular rhythm.

Accelerated Idioventricular Rhythm

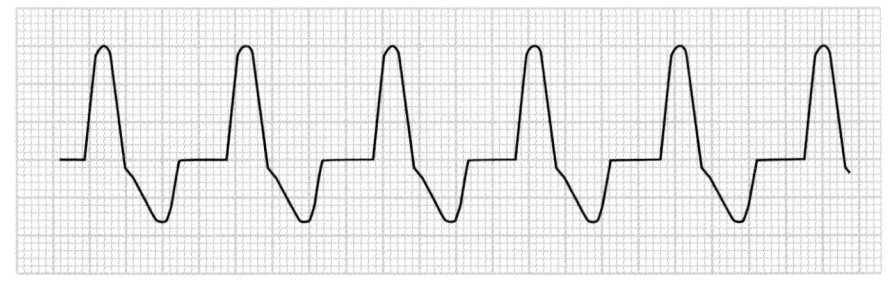

Rate:	40–100 BPM
Regularity:	Regular
P wave:	None
P:QRS ratio:	None
PR interval:	None
QRS width:	Wide (≥0.12 seconds), bizarre appearance
Grouping:	None
Dropped beats:	None

Putting it all together:

This is, basically, a faster version of an idioventricular rhythm. There are usually no P waves associated with it, in keeping with the ventricular source of the pacing. However, they can be present in AV dissociation or third-degree heart block.

Figure 8-20: Accelerated idioventricular rhythm.

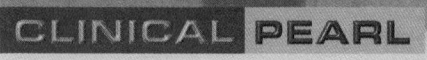
CLINICAL PEARL

We usually try to stay away from treatment, but a word of caution: Do not treat this rhythm with antiarrhythmics! If you are successful in eliminating your last pacemaker, what do you have? Asystole.

Ventricular Tachycardia (VTach)

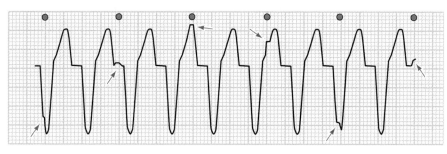

Rate:	100–200 BPM
Regularity:	Regular
P wave:	Dissociated atrial rate
P:QRS ratio:	Variable
PR interval:	None
QRS width:	Wide, bizarre
Grouping:	None
Dropped beats:	None

Putting it all together:

Ventricular tachycardia (VTach) is a very fast ventricular rate that is usually dissociated from an underlying atrial rate. In Figure 8-21, you will notice irregularities of the QRS morphologies at regular intervals. These irregularities are the underlying sinus beats. (Blue dots indicate sinus beats, and arrows pinpoint the irregularities.) There are many criteria related to VTach, which we'll take a look at now.

Figure 8-21: Ventricular tachycardia (VTach).

Capture and Fusion Beats Occasionally, a sinus beat will fall on a spot that allows some innervation of the ventricle to occur through the normal ventricular conduction system. This forms a fusion beat (Figure 8-22), which has a morphology somewhere between the

abnormal ventricular beat and the normal QRS complex. This type of complex is literally caused by two pacemakers, the SA node and the ventricular pacer. Because two areas of the ventricle are being stimulated simultaneously, the result is a hybrid — or fusion — complex with some features of both. It may help to think of this in terms of the following analogy. If you mix a blue liquid with a yellow liquid, the result is a green liquid. A fusion beat is like the green liquid; it is the fusion of the two complexes.

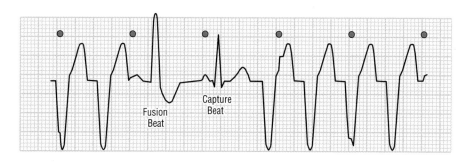

Figure 8-22: Fusion and capture beats in VTach.

A capture beat, on the other hand, is completely innervated by the sinus beat and is indistinguishable from the patient's normal complex. Why is it called a capture beat instead of a normal beat? Because it occurs in the middle of the chaos that is VTach, and is caused by chance timing of a sinus beat at just the right millisecond to "capture" or transmit through the AV node and depolarize the ventricles through the normal conduction system of the heart.

Fusion and capture beats are hallmarks of ventricular tachycardia; you will usually see them if the strip is long enough. If you see these types of complexes with a wide-complex, tachycardic rhythm, you have diagnosed VTach.

More VTach Indicators There are some additional signs we should look at. You don't need to remember the names, but you should know about Brugada's and Josephson's signs (Figure 8-23). Brugada's sign is that, in VTach, the interval from the R wave to the bottom of the S wave is ≥ 0.10 seconds. Josephson's sign, which is just a small notching near the low point of the S wave, is another indicator of VTach.

Some additional aspects in VTach include a total QRS width of ≥ 0.16 seconds, and a complete negativity of all precordial leads (V_1-V_6). Why are we spending so much time on VTach? It is a life-threatening arrhythmia that is difficult to diagnose under the best of circumstances.

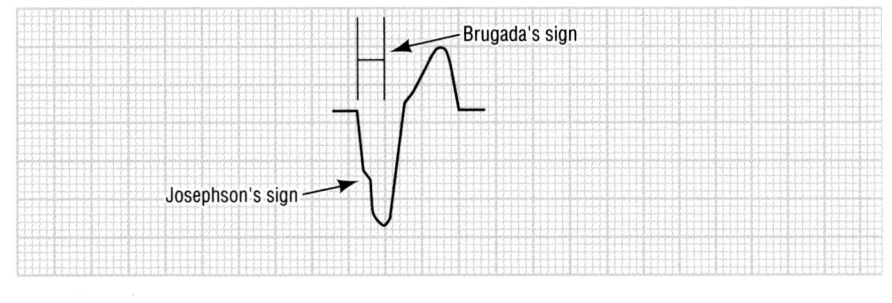

Figure 8-23: Brugada's and Josephson's signs in VTach.

CLINICAL PEARL

A word to the wise: When confronted with any wide-complex tachycardia, treat it as VTach unless you have very strong evidence to the contrary. Do not assume it is a supraventricular tachycardia with aberrancy, a common error with potentially disastrous consequences.

REMINDER:

Criteria for diagnosing ventricular tachycardia:

- Wide-complex tachycardia
- Fusion and capture beats
- Duration of the QRS complex ≥ 0.16 seconds
- AV dissociation
- Complexes in all of the precordial leads are negative
- Josephson's and Brugada's signs

Torsade de Pointes

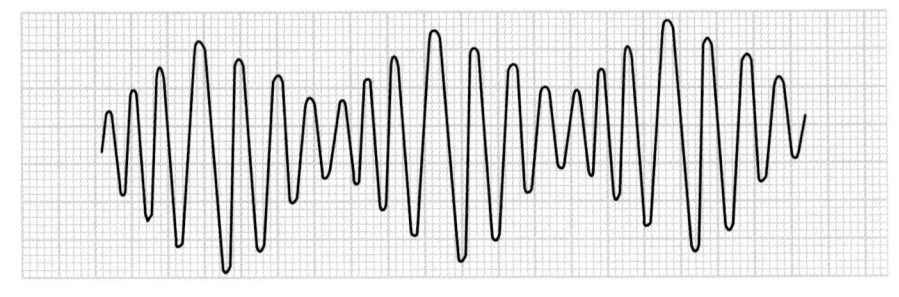

Rate:	200–250 BPM
Regularity:	Irregular
P wave:	None
P:QRS ratio:	None
PR interval:	None
QRS width:	Variable
Grouping:	Variable sinusoidal pattern
Dropped beats:	None

Putting it all together:

Torsade de pointes occurs with an underlying prolonged QT interval. It has an undulating, sinusoidal appearance in which the axis of the QRS complexes changes from positive to negative and back in a haphazard fashion. (The name, torsade de pointes, means twisting of points). It can convert into either a normal rhythm or ventricular fibrillation. Be very careful with this rhythm, as it is a harbinger of death!

Figure 8-24: Torsade de pointes.

Ventricular Flutter

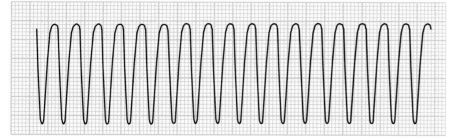

Rate:	200–300 BPM
Regularity:	Regular
P wave:	None
P:QRS ratio:	None
PR interval:	None
QRS width:	Wide, bizarre
Grouping:	None
Dropped beats:	None

Putting it all together:
Ventricular flutter is very fast VTach. When you can no longer tell if it is a QRS complex, a T wave, or an ST segment, then you have VFlutter. The beats are coming so fast that they fuse into an almost straight sinusoidal pattern with no discernible components.

Figure 8-25: Ventricular flutter.

CLINICAL PEARL

When you see VFlutter at a rate of 300 BPM, you should think about the possibility of Wolf-Parkinson-White syndrome (WPW) with 1:1 conduction of an atrial flutter. (We know this may not mean much now, but it will later on.)

Ventricular Fibrillation (VFib)

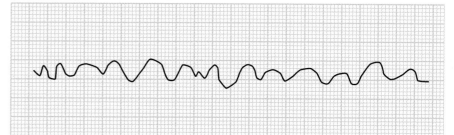

Rate:	Indeterminate
Regularity:	Chaotic rhythm
P wave:	None
P:QRS ratio:	None
PR interval:	None
QRS width:	None
Grouping:	None
Dropped beats:	No beats at all!

Putting it all together:
If you were going to draw a picture of cardiac chaos, this would be it. The ventricular pacers are all going haywire and firing at their own pace. The result is that you have many small areas of the heart firing at once with no organized activity. The heart literally looks like shaking gelatin. This is a very bad rhythm (cardiac arrest), and you should try to get your patient out of this as soon as possible.

Figure 8-26: Ventricular fibrillation (VFib).

CLINICAL PEARL

If your patient looks fine and is wide awake and looking at you, a lead has fallen off and this is artifact, not VFib.

Heart Blocks

First-Degree Heart Block

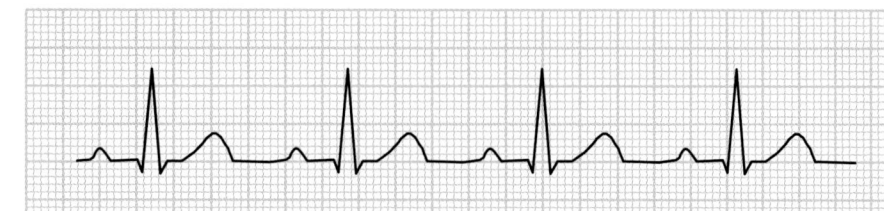

Rate:	Depends on underlying rhythm
Regularity:	Regular
P wave:	Normal
P:QRS ratio:	1:1
PR interval:	Prolonged > 0.20 seconds
QRS width:	Normal
Grouping:	None
Dropped beats:	None

Putting it all together:

First degree heart block occurs from a prolonged physiologic block in the AV node. This can occur because of medication, vagal stimulation, disease, among others. The PR interval will be greater than 0.20 seconds.

Figure 8-27: First-degree heart block.

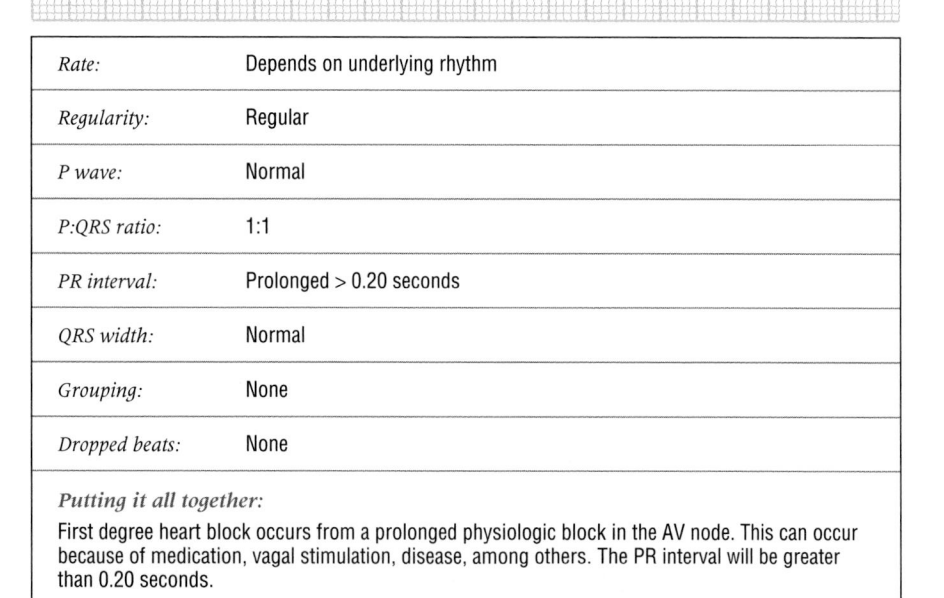

NOTE

A word of caution about the nomenclature of blocks: The rhythm disturbances we are looking at here are *AV nodal blocks.* There are also *bundle branch blocks,* a very different phenomenon. This can be confusing for beginners, but bear with us through the AV blocks and we'll get to bundle branch blocks later.

Mobitz I Second-Degree Heart Block (Wenckebach)

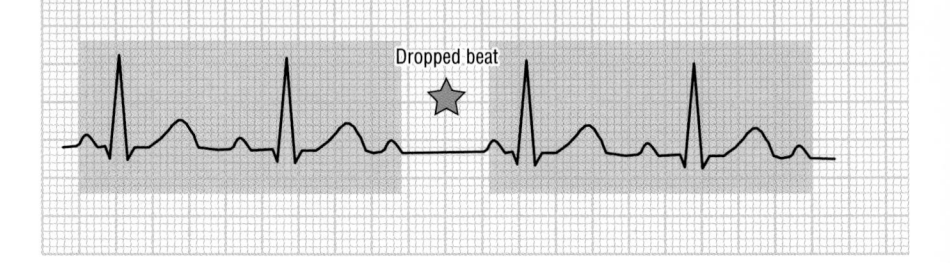

Dropped beat

Rate:	Depends on underlying rhythm
Regularity:	Regularly irregular
P wave:	Present
P:QRS ratio:	Variable: 2:1, 3:2, 4:3, 5:4, etc.
PR interval:	Variable
QRS width:	Normal
Grouping:	Present and variable (see blue shading in Figure 8-28)
Dropped beats:	Yes

Putting it all together:

Mobitz I is also known as Wenckebach (pronounced WENN-key-bock). It is caused by a diseased AV node with a long refractory period. The result is that the PR interval lengthens between successive beats until a beat is dropped. At that point the cycle starts again. The R to R interval, on the other hand, shortens with each beat. We'll discuss Mobitz I further in Chapter 10.

Figure 8-28: Mobitz I second-degree heart block (Wenckebach).

Mobitz II Second-Degree Heart Block

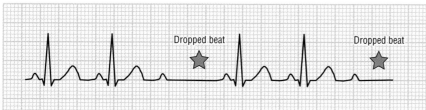

Rate:	Depends on underlying rhythm
Regularity:	Regularly irregular
P wave:	Normal
P:QRS ratio:	X:X–1; e.g. 3:2, 4:3, 5:4, etc. The ratio can also be variable on rare occasions.
PR interval:	Normal
QRS width:	Normal
Grouping:	Present and variable
Dropped beats:	Yes

Putting it all together:

In Mobitz II, there are grouped beats with one beat dropped between each group. The key point to remember is that the PR interval is the same in all of the conducted beats. This rhythm is caused by a diseased AV node, and is a harbinger of bad things to come — namely, complete heart block.

Figure 8-29: Mobitz II second-degree heart block.

CLINICAL PEARL

What if there is a 2:1 ratio of Ps to QRSs? Is this Mobitz I or Mobitz II? In reality, you can't tell. This example is named a 2:1 second-degree block (no type is specified). Because you can't tell, assume the worst — Mobitz II. You cannot go wrong by being overly cautious with a patient's life.

Third-Degree Heart Block

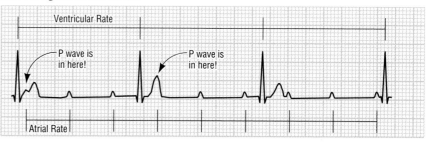

Rate:	Separate rates for the underlying (sinus) rhythm and the escape rhythm. They are dissociated from one another.
Regularity:	Regular, but P rate and QRS rate are different
P wave:	Present
P:QRS ratio:	Variable
PR interval:	Variable; no pattern
QRS width:	Normal or wide
Grouping:	None
Dropped beats:	None

Putting it all together:

This is complete block of the AV node; the atria and ventricles are firing separately each to its own drummer, so to speak. The sinus rhythm can be bradycardic, normal, or tachycardic. The escape beat can be junctional or ventricular and so their morphology will vary.

Figure 8-30: Third-degree heart block.

NOTE

Semantics alert: If there are just as many P waves as there are QRSs, but they are dissociated, it is known as AV dissociation rather than third-degree heart block.

1. Sinus arrhythmia is a normal respiratory variant. True or False.

2. A regular rhythm with a heart rate of 125 BPM with identical P waves occurring before each of the QRS complexes is:
   A. Sinus bradycardia
   B. Normal sinus rhythm
   C. Ectopic atrial tachycardia
   D. Atrial flutter
   E. Sinus tachycardia

3. If an entire complex is missing from a rhythm strip but the underlying rhythm is unchanged and maintains the same P–P or R–R interval (excluding the dropped beat), it is known as:
   A. Sinus bradycardia
   B. Atrial escape beat
   C. Sinus pause
   D. Sinoatrial block
   E. Junctional escape beat

4. An irregularly irregular rhythm of 65 BPM with at least three varying P-wave morphologies and PR intervals is known as:
   A. Atrial fibrillation
   B. Wandering atrial pacemaker
   C. Multifocal atrial tachycardia
   D. Atrial flutter
   E. Accelerated idioventricular rhythm

5. In atrial flutter, the flutter waves usually occur at a rate of 250–350 BPM. True or False.

6. Atrial fibrillation is an irregularly irregular rhythm with no discernable P waves in any lead. True or False.

7. An irregularly irregular rhythm at 195 BPM with no discernable P waves is known as:
   A. Atrial fibrillation with a rapid ventricular response
   B. Multifocal atrial tachycardia
   C. Atrial flutter
   D. Ectopic atrial tachycardia
   E. Accelerated idioventricular rhythm

8. An accelerated junctional rhythm is a junctional rhythm over 100 BPM. True or False.

9. An idioventricular rhythm is caused by a ventricular focus acting as the primary pacemaker. The usual rate is in the range of 20–40 BPM. True or False.

10. Ventricular tachycardia is associated with:
    A. Capture beats
    B. Fusion beats
    C. Both A and B
    D. None of the above

11. A wide-complex tachycardia should always be considered and treated as ventricular tachycardia until proven otherwise. True or False.

12. Ventricular fibrillation has discernable complexes on close examination of the strip. True or False.

13. A grouped rhythm with PR intervals that prolong until a beat is dropped is known as:
    A. Wandering atrial pacemaker
    B. First-degree heart block
    C. Mobitz I second-degree heart block, or Wenckebach
    D. Mobitz II second-degree heart block
    E. Third-degree heart block

14. A grouped rhythm with dropped QRS complexes occurring either regularly or variably is known as:
    A. Wandering atrial pacemaker
    B. First-degree heart block
    C. Mobitz I second-degree heart block, or Wenckebach
    D. Mobitz II second-degree heart block
    E. Third-degree heart block

15. A rhythm with dissociated atrial and ventricular pacemakers, in which the atrial beat is faster than the ventricular rate, is known as:
    A. Wandering atrial pacemaker
    B. First-degree heart block
    C. Mobitz I second-degree heart block, or Wenckebach
    D. Mobitz II second-degree heart block
    E. Third-degree heart block

1. True 2. E 3. D 4. B 5. True 6. True 7. A 8. False 9. True 10. C 11. True 12. False 13. C 14. D 15. E

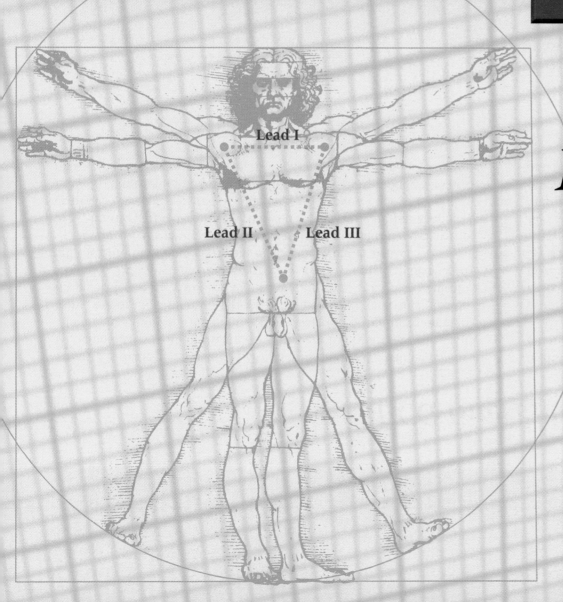

Lead I

Lead II   Lead III

ECG
Interpretation

ECG Interpretation

Part 2 is dedicated to actual ECG interpretation. We will be reviewing actual ECGs in all of their glory. They are full of artifact and small meaningless motion irregularities that occurred for reasons ranging from patient movement to serious pathologies. We have included these irregularities to get you used to interpreting "real" ECGs. In clinical scenarios, ECGs will have these irregularities. You need to be able to tell the difference between what is real and what is artifact.

If you are a beginner, read the Level 1 boxes and then review the ECGs for the particular process that you are learning in that chapter. For example, the topic covered in Chapter 9 is P waves. Look at all of the ECGs in that chapter and evaluate their P wave morphology. The ECG may contain other interesting pathology, but do not spend a lot of time trying to understand the additional issues. You will be looking at the additional information progressively as you proceed to Levels 2 and 3.

If you are at an intermediate level, review the Level 1 material and proceed to learn the Level 2 material thoroughly. Review the ECGs based on your level of information. Once again, stay away from Level 3 material until you are ready.

This is where the real fun begins! It is an exciting journey into the world of information that is available to you from such a simple test. Be patient with yourself, because it takes time to become proficient at interpretation. When you are done this section, make sure to visit our web site, www.12leadECG.com, to test your knowledge with some practice ECGs.

Overview

The P wave, shown in Figure 9-1, represents depolarization of the atria. It is the first wave in the complex, beginning when the wave leaves the baseline and ending on its return to baseline before the PR interval. The depolarization normally starts in the sinoatrial (SA) node and spreads throughout the atria until it reaches the atrioventricular (AV) node, as shown in Figure 9-2. This process lasts 0.08 to 0.11 seconds.

P waves are normally positive in leads I, II, and V_4 to V_6; negative in aVR; and either positive or negative in the other leads.

Figure 9-1: The P wave.

P wave

Internodal pathways

SA node

AV node

Figure 9-2: Transmittal of the P wave from the SA node to the AV node.

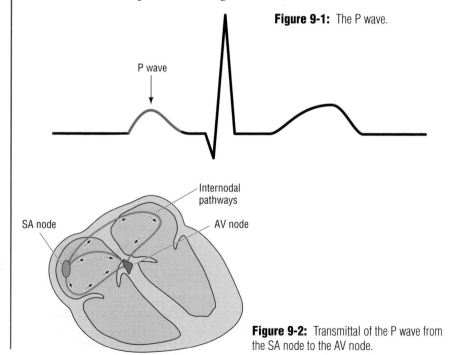

---

② QUICK REVIEW

1. The P wave is the ___1st___ wave in the complex.
2. The P wave represents depolarization of the atria. True or False.
3. The electrical impulse travels from the ___SA___ node, through the atria, to the ___AV___ node.
4. The P wave is usually upright in aVR. True or False.

1. First 2. True 3. SA-AV 4. False

---

③

Normal conduction of the impulse from the SA node to the AV node takes place through specialized conduction fibers known as the anterior, middle, and posterior internodal pathways (*red tracts* in Figure 9-2). The Bachman Bundle is an internodal pathway connecting the two atria. The pathways act similarly to the Purkinje system of the ventricles in that they rapidly transmit the impulse through the atria and cause the synchronized innervation of the atrial myocardial cells.

Inverted P waves are found when the pacing or initial impulse originates at or below the AV node; for example, junctional rhythms and idioventricular rhythms with retrograde conduction, etc. In these cases, the depolarization wave of the atria will spread in a retrograde manner causing the axis of the P wave to be directed upward. This P wave axis shift is represented by the inverted P waves in leads II, III, and aVF of the ECG because the impulse is traveling away from the positive poles of these leads.

ECG CASE STUDY: *P Wave Basics*

2

ECG 9-1 Look only at the P waves while studying this chapter. The Ps in the ECG 9-1 are clearly marked on the rhythm strip by the blue dots. The rhythm strip corresponds to the complexes in both the limb and the precordial leads above it. The blue vertical line in the first full complex demonstrates this.

Now, take your calipers and place the pins on the very tips of two P waves, then march them through to see that all the P-P intervals are equal. This confirms that the rhythm is regular. The fact that each of the QRS complexes has a P wave in front of it makes it a sinus rhythm. Therefore, this is a normal sinus rhythm at about 80 beats per minute.

Evaluate the shape, height, and width of the P waves. Are they all the same? Remember to come back and revisit this ECG after you've finished the chapter.

> **REMINDER:**
> Evaluate the shape, height, and width of the P waves.
> Are they all the same?

3

ECG 9-1 This is a good example of biatrial enlargement. The P wave in lead II is an example of P-pulmonale, a finding compatible with right atrial enlargement (RAE). The second half of the biphasic component in V_1 has a *height* x *width* product of greater than or equal to 0.3 mm sec, highly suggestive of left atrial enlargement (LAE).

In addition, this patient has an incomplete right bundle branch block (IRBBB) because the QRS width is approximately 0.11 seconds. The right axis, with an S in lead I and a q wave in lead III, suggests a left posterior fascicular block (LPFB). However, there is a P wave measuring 3 mm, a P-pulmonale, and an increased R:S ratio in V_1 consistent with RVH. The presence of the RAE and RVH excludes the possibility of a LPFB. Also note that the T wave in lead III is flipped. This completes the $S_1Q_3T_3$ pattern found in leads I and III. In this case, the $S_1Q_3T_3$ pattern represents a right ventricular strain pattern and is not due to an acute pulmonary embolus or a LPFB. The patient also has inferolateral ST segment depressions consistent with ischemia.

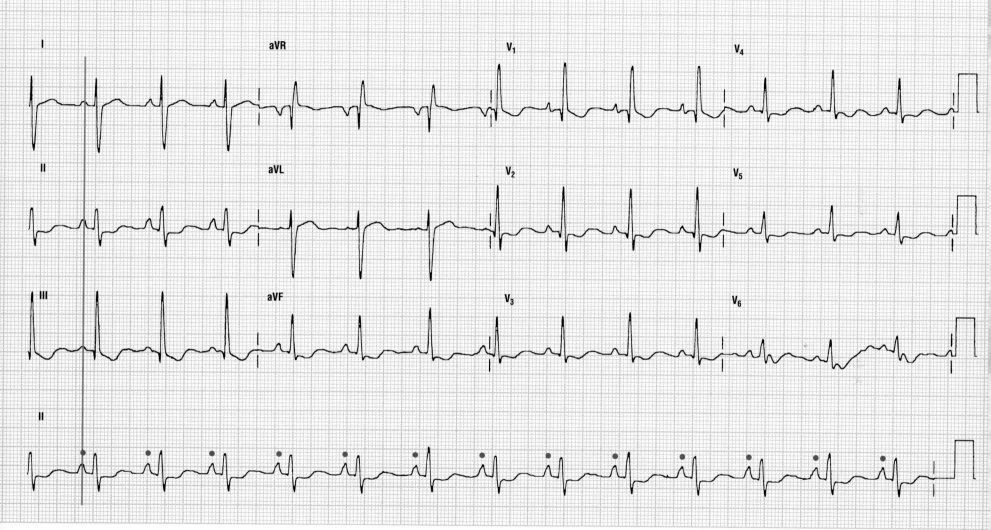

ECG 9-1

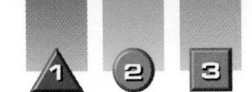

P Wave Morphology

The morphology of the P waves will vary in any one lead depending on the location of the area acting as the pacemaker. Let's look at the example in Figure 9-3. If the SA node acts as the pacemaker, the morphology of the P wave will look like that noted in the box representing pacemaker A. If the impulse originates at pacemaker B, the P wave morphology and the PR interval will both be different. Pacemaker C provides another example. Because many areas can act as secondary pacemakers, a wide variety of P wave morphologies are possible.

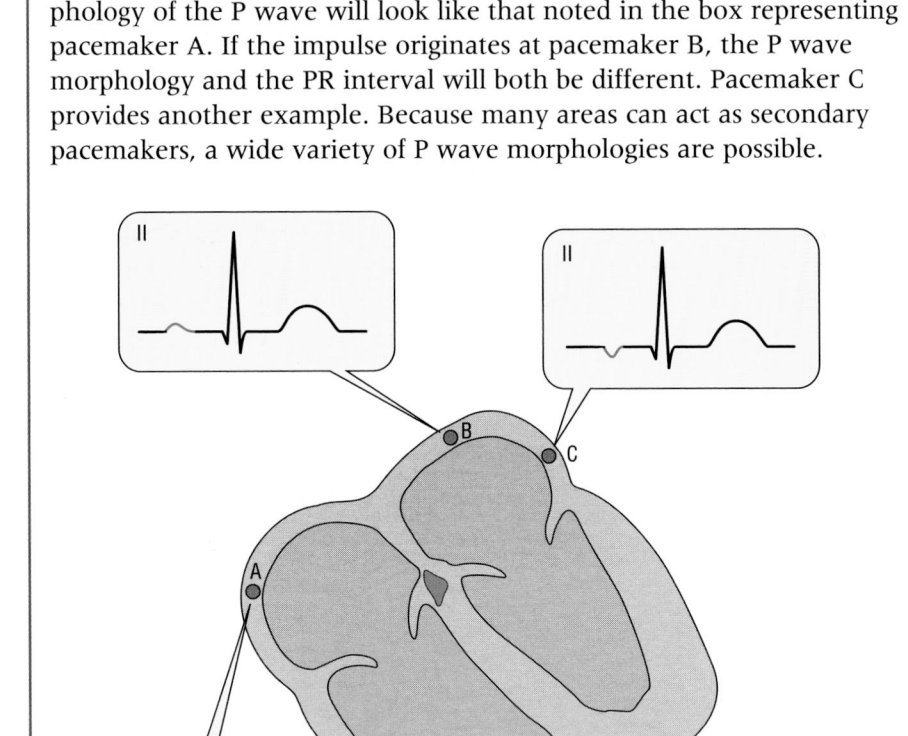

Figure 9-3: Three different P wave morphologies depending on the location of the pacemaker.

Noting the different morphologies helps to label beats that originated in another focus, such as atrial premature complexes (APCs). Because an APC originates in an area other than the original pacemaker, its P wave morphology will be different from the rest. If that focus causing the APC is irritable and continues to fire intermittently, you will see frequent APCs, all with the same P wave morphology. Can you find the APC in ECG 9-2?

Wandering atrial pacemaker and multifocal atrial tachycardia have at least three different morphologies because of the many irritable areas found in the atria. This leads to the traditional criteria for identifying these rhythm abnormalities.

> **REMINDER:**
> P wave morphology varies depending on the area of the atria acting as the pacemaker.

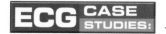 ***P Wave Morphology***

ECG 9-2 This ECG has an APC. Can you find it? Remember, an APC has a different morphology and PR interval than beats that originate in the SA node. The third beat, marked by the green line, is different than the other P waves. The morphology difference is evident in leads I, II, and III.

The beat is called premature because it originates sooner than expected. The interval between the P waves, known as the P-P interval, is normally constant. If you place your calipers over the tips of the P waves labeled P-P interval, you can transfer that interval over to the beats in question. Let's assume that this P-P interval is X seconds long. You can clearly see that the beat with the green line over it, the atrial premature contraction, occurred X − 0.20 seconds sooner than expected. Also notice that the distance from the P wave before the APC and the one after the APC is equal to 2X seconds, or two times the normal P-P interval. What happened? The SA node was not reset by the early ectopic beat and continued to fire during its normal cycle. The AV node and the ventricles were, however, refractory and the impulse was not conducted. The SA node fired at its next scheduled time at 2X seconds. This type of pause is known as a *compensatory pause*, one that brings the next beat back into sync with the preceding ones. A *non-compensatory pause* occurs when the sinus node is depolarized. The sinus node is therefore reset and the distance is less than 2X seconds. In this case, the succeeding beats do not fall back in sync. APCs are usually non-compensatory. However, as this example clearly shows, both types of pauses can occur.

ECG 9-3 This ECG can be a little overwhelming at first glance. When you come to an ECG that has a lot of complexities, break it down to make it less formidable. Now remember, you're only looking at the P waves. Forget about the rest for now. Look at the Ps in lead II, or the first four waves on the rhythm strip. Do they look alike? Are the PR intervals the same — the intervals from the beginning of the P waves to the beginning of the QRSs? Use your calipers! No, the PR intervals are different.

Now go back to the diagram in Figure 9-3. If we had four different areas acting as pacemakers, would the result look like the first four beats of this ECG? Yes. How many more P waves with different morphologies and PR intervals can you find? Do any of them resemble each other? There are about eight, possibly 10, different types of P waves on this ECG. This is an example of a rhythm known as a wandering atrial pacemaker.

Look at the area with the star on the rhythm strip. Does the T wave of the cycle before the star look different compared with the other beats? Now look at the complex to the right of the star. Can you see the P wave? What happened here is that the P wave and the T wave both occurred at the same time. This is why that T wave looks different, and you can't find the P wave. This superimposition of waves occurs frequently, and you should think about it whenever you come upon a wave that just looks different than the rest.

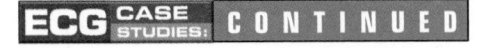

ECG CASE STUDIES: CONTINUED

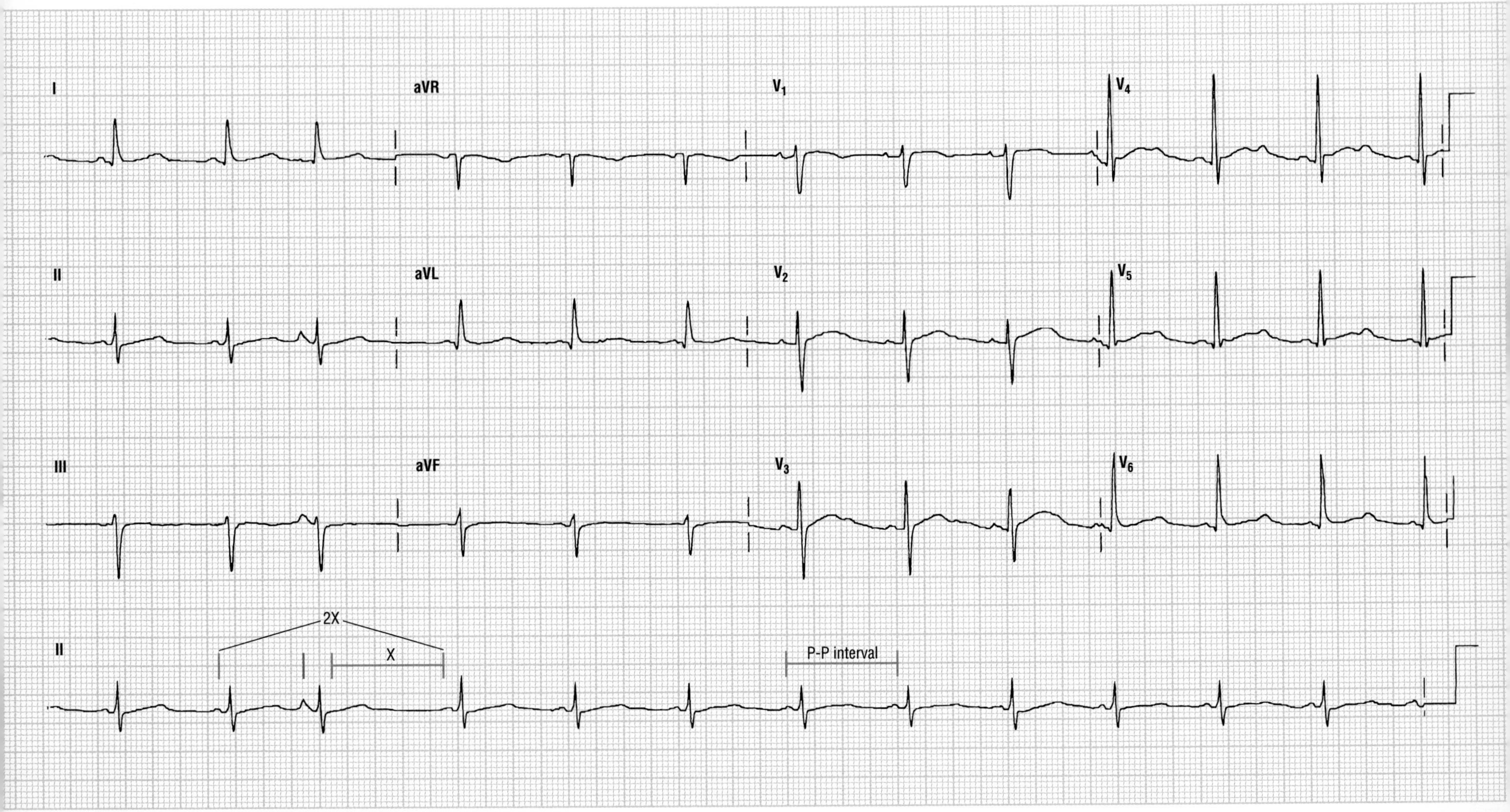
I
aVR
V_1
V_4
II
aVL
V_2
V_5
III
aVF
V_3
V_6
II
2X
X
P-P interval

ECG 9-2

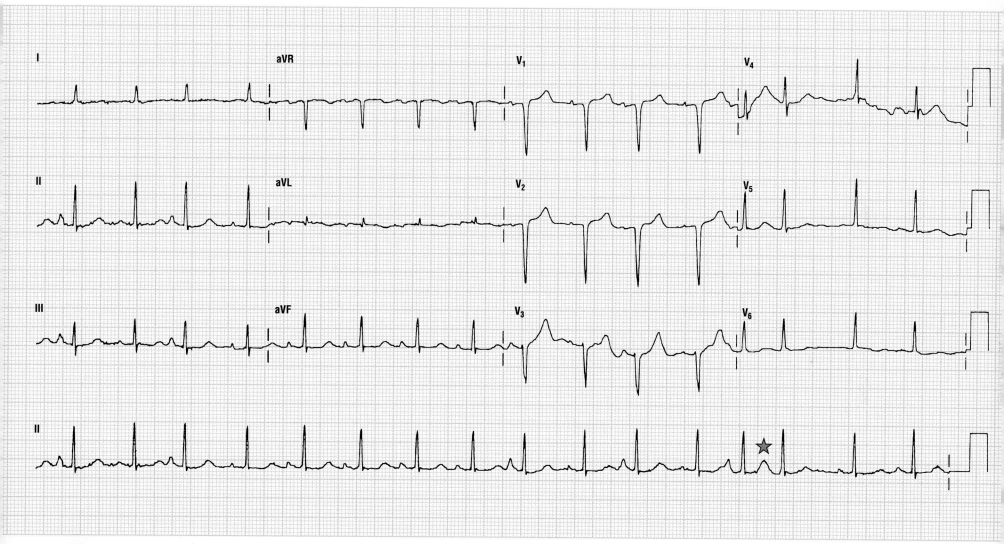

ECG 9-3

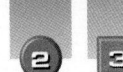
ECG CASE STUDIES: **CONTINUED**

②

ECG 9-4 Look at the P waves in all the leads in ECG 9-4. Do you notice something unusual about them or their intervals? When we look at leads II, III, and aVF, we notice that the Ps are inverted (negative, or below the baseline). We already know that normal P waves are upright in leads I and II, so something is wrong. In this case, the P waves originate at or near the AV node and the impulse spreads backwards through the atria. This reverse spread (*retrograde conduction*) of the impulse produces the inverted Ps in II, III, and aVF.

There are two rhythm possibilities in this instance. The first occurs if the pacemaker is located at the AV node. In this case, the rhythm is called a junctional rhythm with retrograde conduction of the P waves. The problem is that this usually has a short PR interval. The second possibility is that this is a low atrial ectopic pacemaker. The ectopic pacemaker in the atria would be near the AV node, before the physiologic block that occurs there, similar to pacemaker C in Figure 9-3. Because the PR interval is normal, this second possibility is more likely.

③

ECG 9-4 The criterion for left ventricular hypertrophy (LVH) is present in ECG 9-4: an R wave in aVL greater than 11 mm high. This gives the ST segments and T waves their typical LVH-with-strain pattern in the anterior precordial leads — slight ST elevation with an asymmetrical T wave.

The normal P wave axis is between 0 and 75°. In the case of junctional rhythms, the P axis will generally fall between −60 and −80°. This makes the P waves negative in II, III, and aVF, and positive in I and aVR. The Ps are variable in the precordial leads.

Could this be a junctional rhythm? Generally, the PR interval is less than or equal to 0.11 seconds in a junctional rhythm. In order for this to be a junctional rhythm, there would have to be an underlying defect in the normal or antegrade conduction through the AV node distal to the pacemaker, thereby allowing the retrograde P wave to come much earlier than the ventricular depolarization.

> **REMINDER:**
> Always look at the P waves in leads II, III, and aVF. If the Ps are inverted, then the pacemaker was either in the low (distal) atria or in the AV node. This represents retrograde conduction through the atria.

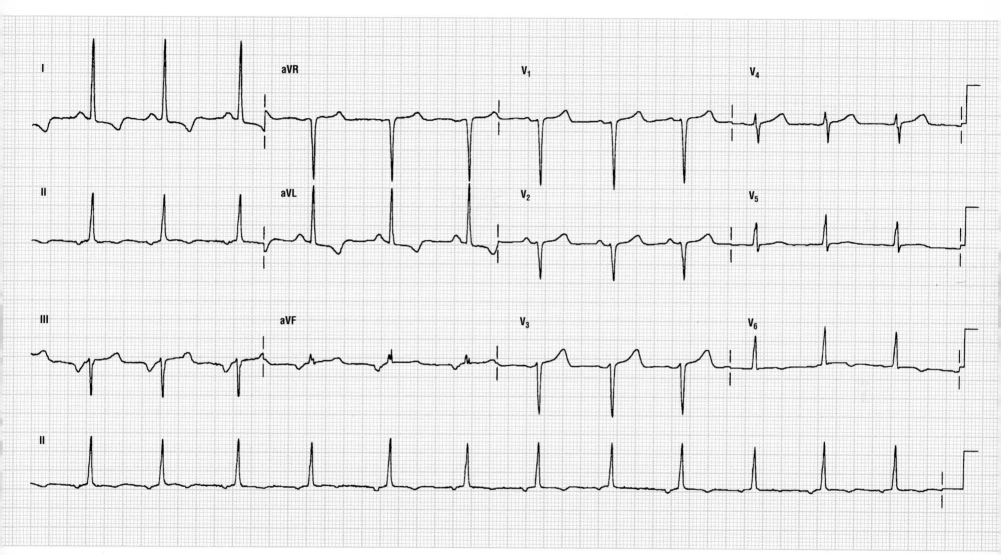

ECG 9-4

Abnormal P Waves

P-mitrale

If the P wave is greater than 0.12 seconds in the limb leads (I and II) and notched (M-shaped), it is known as a P-mitrale (Figure 9-4). This is the classic but uncommon finding in severe *left atrial enlargement (LAE)*. The space between the two humps should be greater than or equal to 0.04 seconds.

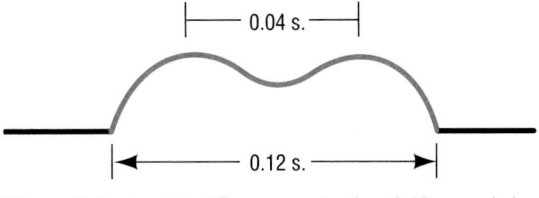

Figure 9-4: A notched P wave greater than 0.12 seconds in the limb leads indicates P-mitrale.

The notching is actually caused by the prolonged conduction times required to transmit the impulse through the enlarged left atrium. Remember that the SA node is in the right atrium. When the impulse is generated in the SA node, its faster passage through the smaller right atrium is completed before the impulse can travel through the enlarged left atrium. The final result is a double hump (Figure 9-5).

Notching can also be found in P waves less than 0.12 seconds wide. In these cases, it may not be associated with LAE.

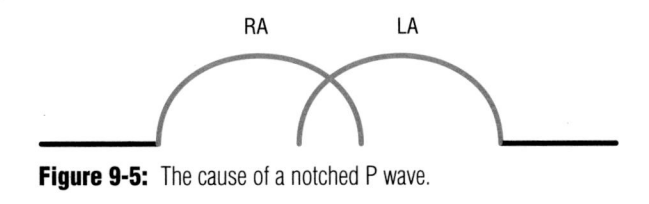

Figure 9-5: The cause of a notched P wave.

The most common cause of P-mitrale is severe mitral valve disease. This is where it gets its name (others say it is due to the M shape of a bishop's mitre). Mitral stenosis leads to left atrial enlargement by increasing the muscle mass needed to overpower the stenotic valve. Eventually, enlargement also occurs when the muscle dilates in order to compensate for the additional blood volume. Dilation is also the pathologic mechanism involved in patients with mitral regurgitation.

REMINDER:

ᴍITRALE = LAE

ECG CASE STUDIES: *P-mitrale*

②

ECG 9-5 This is a textbook example of P-mitrale. Note the biphasic component of the P wave and the characteristic width greater than or equal to 0.12 seconds with the notches greater than or equal to 0.04 seconds apart. Use your imagination and think of it as a camel's back. If you use these *mind links*, remembering the information will be easier and more fun.

③

ECG 9-5 There are flipped, asymmetrical Ts everywhere in ECG 9-5. The T-wave axis is almost directly opposite the QRS axis (T-wave axis is −120°, QRS axis is 30°). In addition, there is that large S wave with the ST elevation in lead V_1 that is about 35 mm deep. These findings are highly suggestive of LVH with strain. But why do we lose the voltage as we move to the lateral leads? The answer is unclear, but it could be caused by the loss of ventricular mass because of a previous infarct, a left pleural effusion, or obesity among other things. The Z axis is pointing about 60° posteriorly. There is an intraventricular conduction defect (IACD) noted in leads II, III, aVF, and V_2 to V_5.

You should interpret this ECG, as always, with an eye on the patient's clinical presentation. Putting it all together, this is an ECG commonly found in patients with dilated cardiomyopathy, multivalvular disease, or cardiac disease secondary to an infiltrative process. By the way, the patient was an 18-year-old woman.

②

ECG 9-6 Here is another example of a P-mitrale. Note that there can be variation in the appearance of the P-mitrale waves among different patients, just as there are different humps on different camels (Figure 9-6). We will show you additional examples so that you learn to recognize the pattern.

③

ECG 9-6 There is evidence of biatrial enlargement in ECG 9-6. We will cover this topic later in the chapter. In addition, the patient has a left axis deviation with a left anterior hemiblock (LAD with LAH). Another interesting aspect is the presence of LVH because of the height of the R wave in aVL, which is greater than or equal to 11 mm.

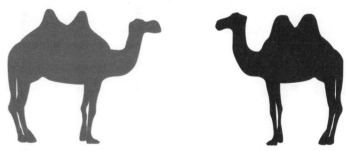

Figure 9-6: The shape of P-mitrale waves in different patients can vary.

ECG CASE STUDIES: CONTINUED

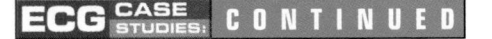

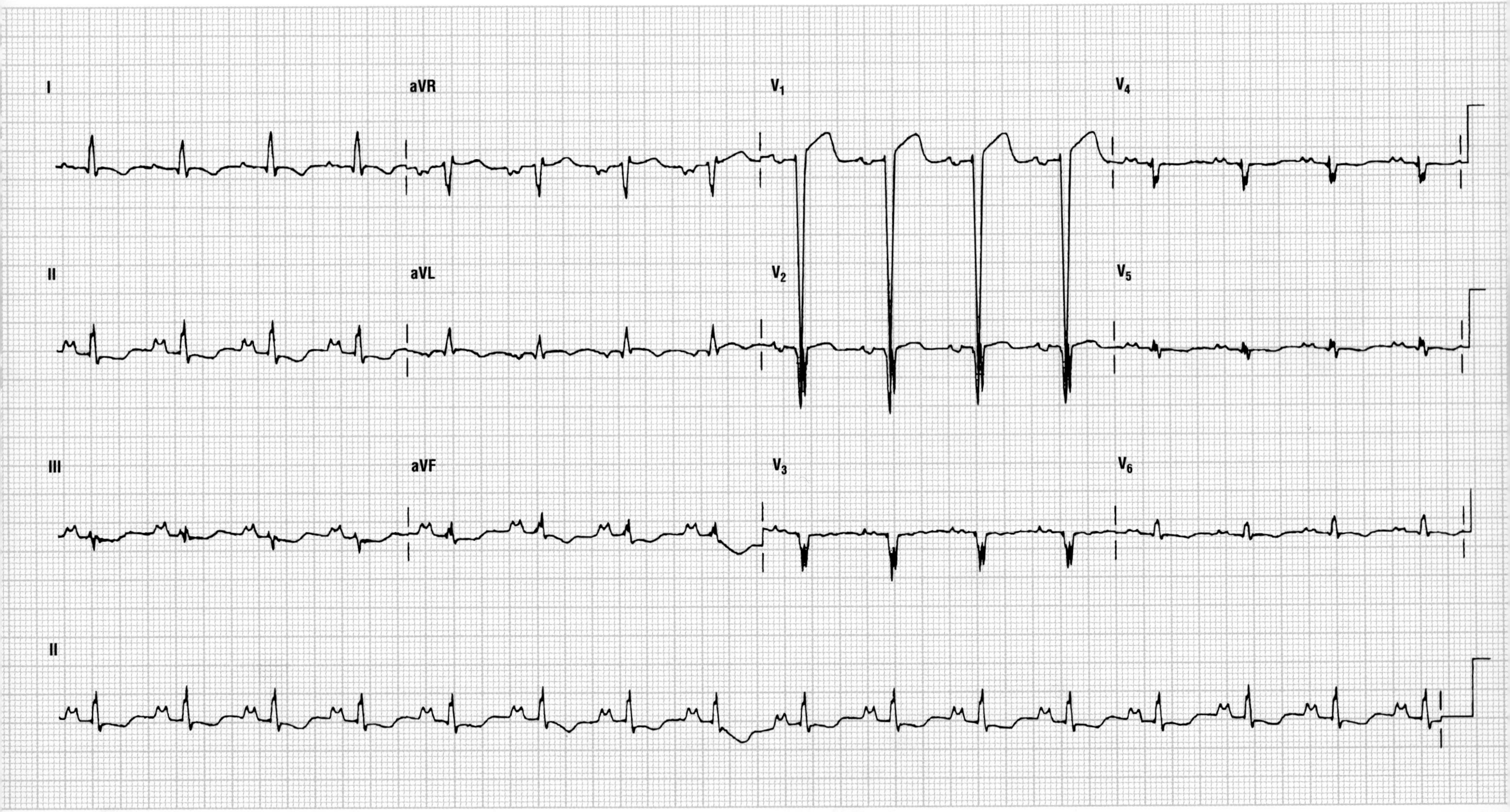
I
aVR
V_1
V_4
II
aVL
V_2
V_5
III
aVF
V_3
V_6
II

ECG 9-5

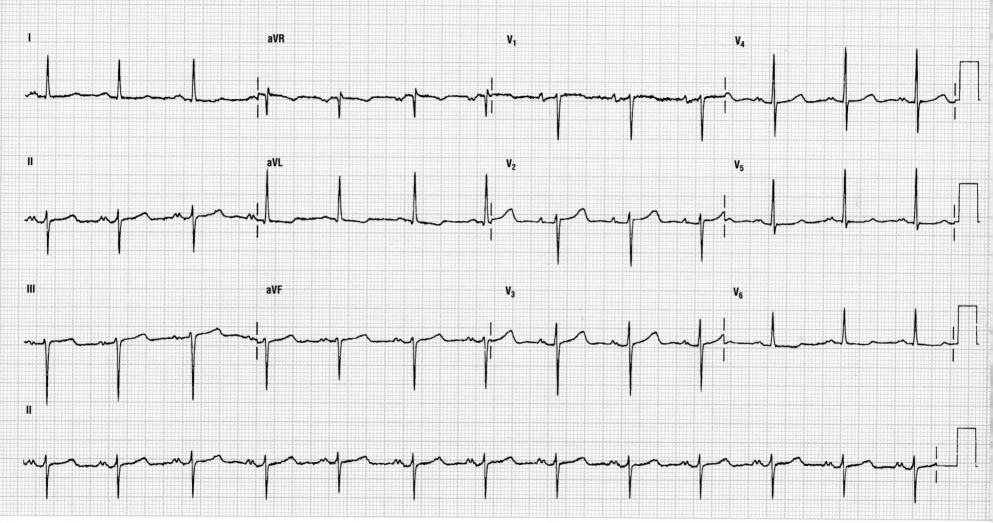

ECG 9-6

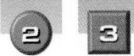

ECG CASE STUDIES: **CONTINUED**

②

ECG 9-7 The P waves in ECG 9-7 are not quite as humped as the previous ones, but they still have all of the characteristics needed to call them a P-mitrale pattern. There is a little movement during the first complex, which makes the baseline waver slightly and gives it a bizarre appearance. Don't be fooled; it is just artifact. You may have some difficulty isolating each P wave from the previous T because there is a long QT interval. The T travels both above and below the baseline, and it is very prolonged. When you have problems like this, find the lead where the P wave is clearest. In this case, it is in V_1. Measure the PR interval (from the beginning of the P wave to the beginning of the QRS) and transfer that distance to the other leads. Remember, intervals are the same throughout the entire ECG. You will quickly see which waves are the Ps.

That bizarre beat at the beginning of V_4 to V_6 is a ventricular premature complex (VPC). Apply the principles that you learned about premature beats to this complex and you will see that it fits the criteria. It is wide and bizarre because the complex originated in the ventricles instead of the atria. Because it didn't travel down the conduction system, it spread slowly, cell to cell. By itself, it is harmless. We covered this in Chapter 8 and will discuss it further a little later.

③

ECG 9-7 The QT is prolonged and biphasic in ECG 9-7. There is an early transition with a Z axis of 5 to 10° posterior. The VPC seen here may actually be a junctional premature contraction (JPC) with aberrancy, because this complex and the normal QRS both appear to start the same way and in the same direction. This is usually seen in aberrancy. For the sake of simplicity, we have elected to call it a VPC in this case.

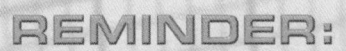

REMINDER:

Intervals are always the same throughout an ECG.

Measure the longest interval and transfer the distance using your calipers to simplify your interpretation.

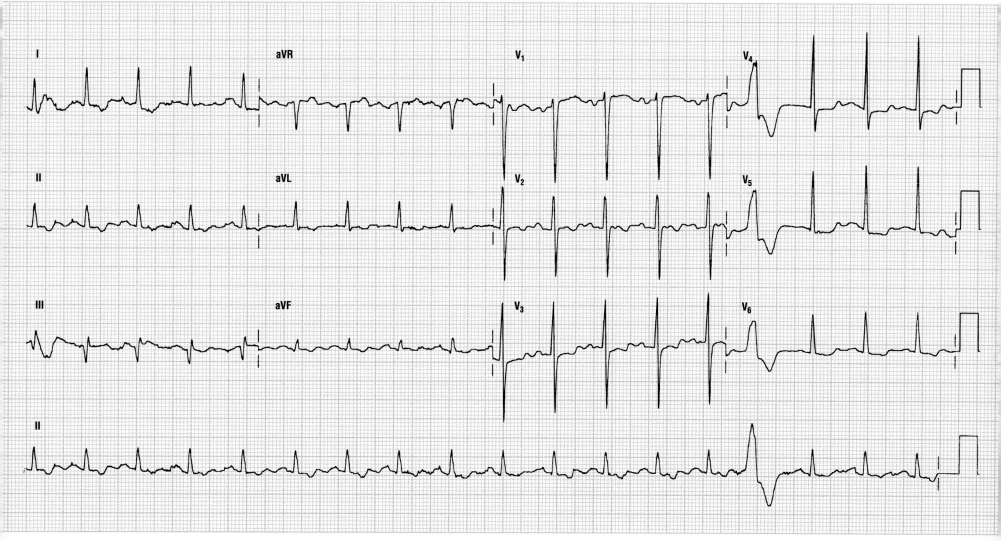

ECG 9-7

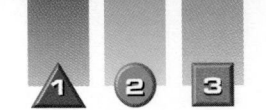

P-pulmonale

If the P wave is peaked (teepee shaped) and more than 2.5 mm high in the limb leads, it is known as a P-pulmonale (Figure 9-7). This is the classic finding in severe *right atrial enlargement (RAE)*. These Ps are most prominent, and most commonly found, in leads II and III.

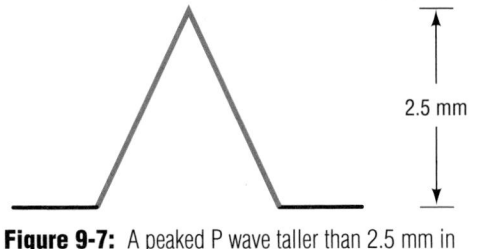

Figure 9-7: A peaked P wave taller than 2.5 mm in the limb leads indicates P-pulmonale.

A peaked P wave is one that is teepee shaped. These can also be less than 2.5 mm in height, so the P-pulmonale is a special kind of peaked P. When they are less than 2.5 mm high, peaked P waves are not associated with atrial enlargement.

REMINDER:

These waves are teepee shaped. A good way to remember the name is to remember that the last syllable of teepee stands for P-pulmonale!

QUICK REVIEW

1. P-pulmonale is a sign of _____ atrial enlargement.
2. The P wave in P-pulmonale must be at least _____ mm high.
3. A peaked P wave less than 2.5 mm high is associated with right atrial enlargement. True or False.
4. P-pulmonale is found in the precordial leads. True or False.

1. Right 2. 2.5 mm 3. False 4. False

If you find a P-pulmonale on an ECG with a right axis deviation, you cannot diagnose LPH. This is because right-sided disease can alter the axis of the heart to the right quadrant and give rise to findings that are indistinguishable from LPH. Remember, LPH is a diagnosis of exclusion. Any findings consistent with right atrial or ventricular disease exclude the diagnosis electrocardiographically.

ECG 9-8 The P waves in ECG 9-8 are more than 2.5 mm high in II and III, and they have the P-pulmonale pattern. The Ps in this case are up to 7 mm high. It is rare for Ps to be this big; if anything is going to remind you of P-pulmonale, this is it. Do you notice anything strange about the P waves in the rhythm strip? Are they all the same morphology? Are the PR intervals consistent in all of the complexes? This is another example of many different atrial pacers causing rhythm abnormality. It could be called a wandering atrial pacemaker (WAP) except for one additional problem — the tachycardia. That makes this multifocal atrial tachycardia (MAT). Another way of saying it is that a MAT is just a tachycardic WAP. We should point out that both WAPs and MATs are irregularly irregular rhythms; they come in a completely chaotic pattern.

Do you notice anything different about the beats with the dots above them? Those complexes have their Ps and Ts superimposed on each other. The P waves are firing while the ventricles are repolarizing. Now look at the three beats with the vertical lines above them. These are P waves that are coming just at the end of the T waves of the preceding complex. They are only partially superimposed on the Ts, so you can still make out the separate waves.

> **REMINDER:**
> If one T wave looks different from the rest, it is probably because there is another P wave "buried" inside of it.

ECG 9-9 The P waves in ECG 9-9 again are more than 2.5 mm high, and compatible with the P-pulmonale pattern signifying RAE. You may hear some people use the term hypertrophy. This was an older term used to describe ECG findings. According to studies, we can state only that the electrical depolarization of the atrial myocardium is proceeding by an altered route. We cannot accurately predict whether the enlargement that causes this disruption results from hypertrophy or dilatation of the muscle, so the term has changed.

ECG 9-9 The minimal ST segment elevation noted in V_1 to V_4 is troublesome because of the QS waves in V_1 to V_3 that represent an old anteroseptal infarct of indeterminate age. An old ECG would be helpful in further delineating the problem.

Note that V_1 has a completely inverted P wave. We cannot make any mention of LAE in this case.

ECG CASE STUDIES: **CONTINUED**

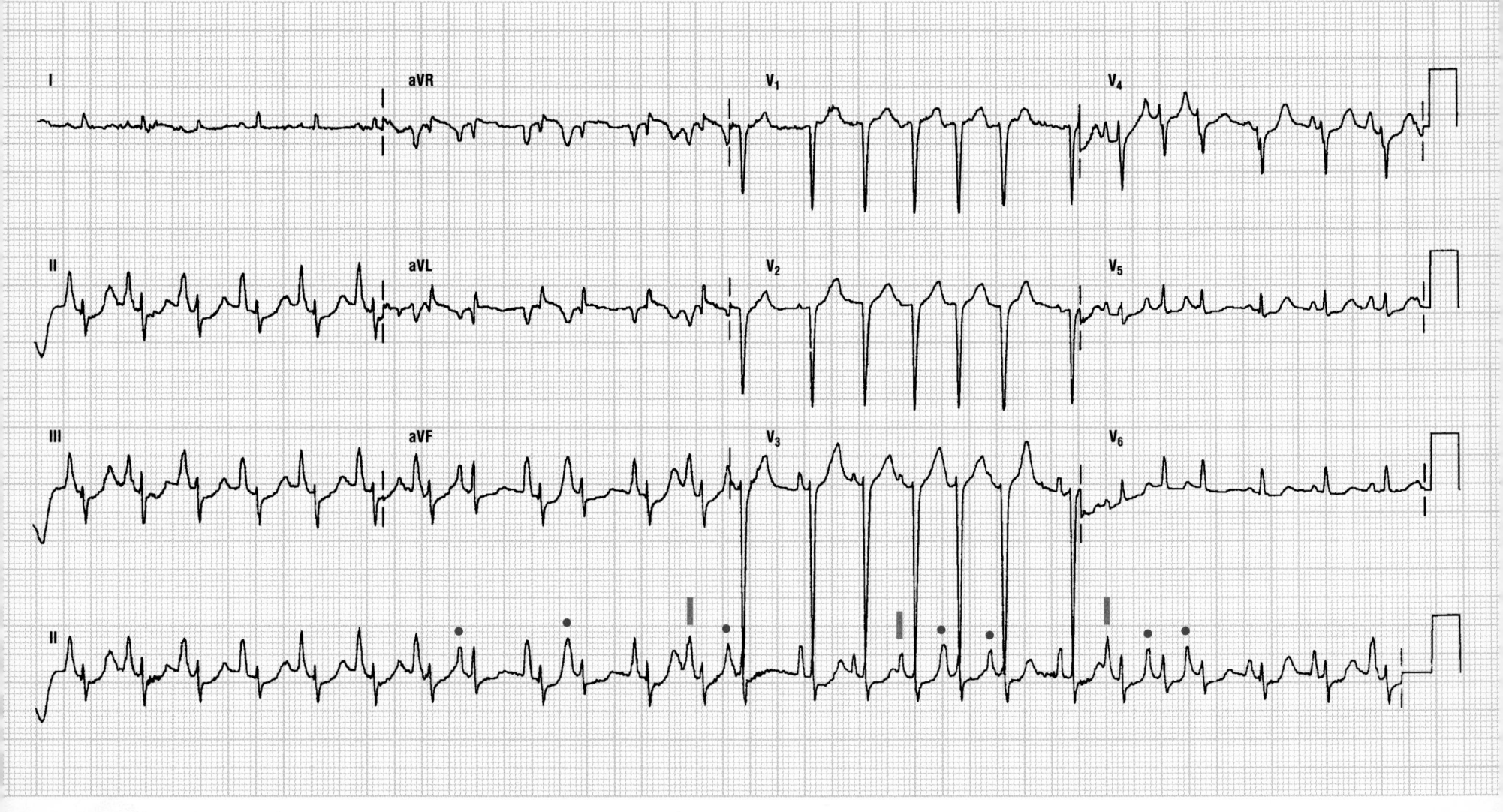

ECG 9-8

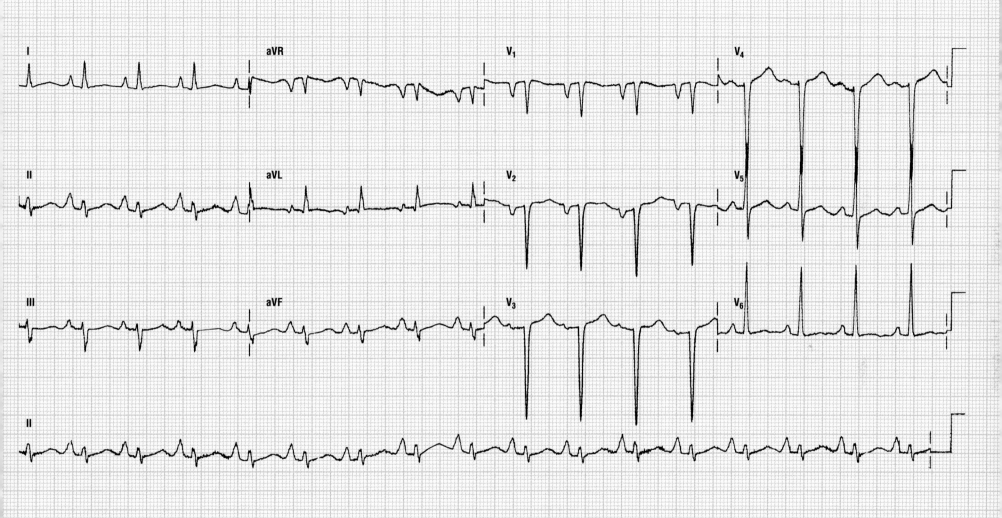

ECG 9-9

ECG CASE STUDIES: **CONTINUED**

②

ECG 9-10 These P waves also show morphology compatible with P-pulmonale. In this ECG, we do not have the luxury of a rhythm strip at the bottom. This makes interpretation a little more difficult. Look at each stacked set of three leads at one time: I, II, and III make up one set; aVR, aVL, and aVF make up another; and so forth. Do you see any abnormalities? Starting from the left, count the complexes. The third complex has an abnormal P. Check the PR and P-P intervals as we did when we were looking at APCs. Do they map through the abnormal beat? Yes. What is that beat? An APC.

Look at beat #9 and examine it the same way. Is it an APC? No. Why not? Remember that the P wave has to be upright in I, II, and V_4 to V_6, and negative in aVR. Is that P wave negative or positive in aVR? Positive — above the baseline. What else could it be? How about a JPC! Now let's look at beat #11. Is that one normal? No. What is it consistent with? An APC. By applying the principles you have learned, you can figure it out.

③

ECG 9-10 This ECG has an right bundle branch block (RBBB) configuration with a right axis. This and the P-pulmonale pattern are highly suggestive of a right ventricular strain or chronic obstructive pulmonary disease (COPD) pattern. Note that each of the PACs shows some aberrancy. The aberrancy in the third beat actually shifts the axis slightly.

REMINDER:

Compare the PR intervals and P-P intervals to spot premature beats.

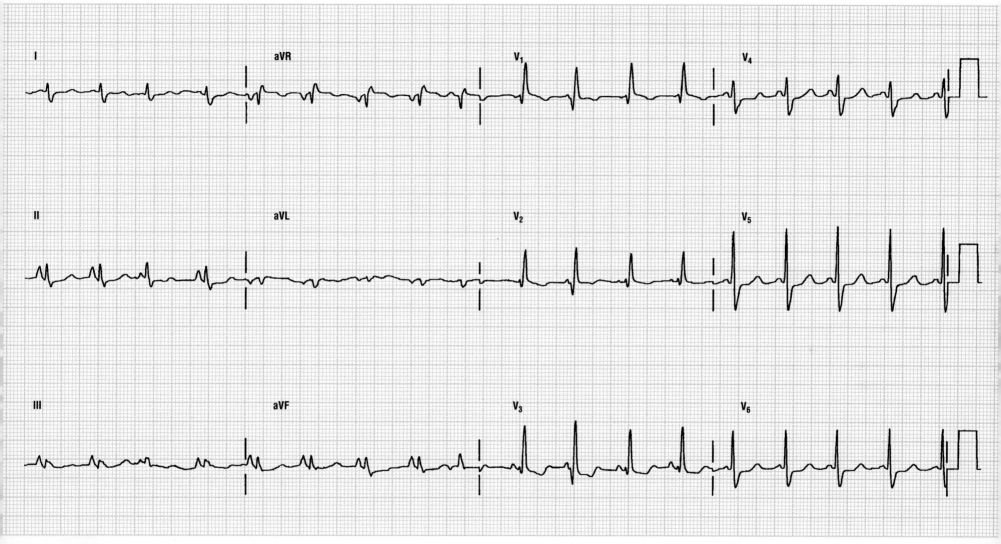

ECG 9-10

Intraatrial Conduction Delay (IACD)

You will frequently find biphasic P waves in V_1. These are evidence of intraatrial conduction delay (IACD). IACD is another way of saying that there is a non-specific conduction problem in the atria. Usually the problem is caused by atrial enlargement, although there is not enough enlargement to form the P-mitrale or P-pulmonale patterns reviewed before or to make a definitive statement about enlargement of either atria. However, there are two cases when the biphasic P can help you differentiate between left and right atrial enlargement (LAE and RAE). We will review these below.

When the first half of the biphasic P wave is taller in V_1 than the first half of the P in V_6 (Figure 9-8), RAE is likely.

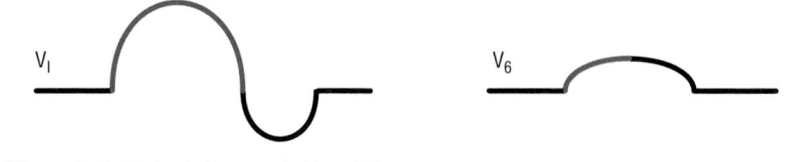

Figure 9-8: Biphasic P waves in V_1 and V_6.

When the second half of the P wave is wider and deeper than 0.04 seconds (one small block), LAE is very likely (Figure 9-9). In fact, if the product of the height times width of the last half of the P wave is greater than or equal to to 0.3 (height [mm] x width [sec] = 0.3), the probability of LAE is over 95%.

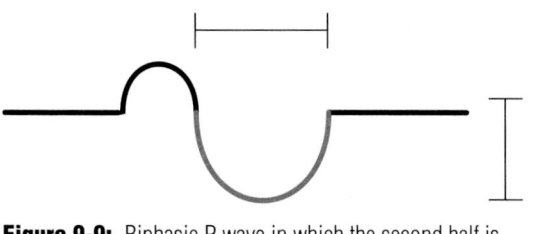

Figure 9-9: Biphasic P wave in which the second half is greater than 0.3 mm, suggesting LAE.

QUICK REVIEW

1. Biphasic P waves in V_1 are consistent with an intraatrial conduction delay (IACD). True or False.

2. When the first half of the P wave in V_1 is _____ than the first half of the P in V_6, right atrial enlargement is likely.

3. A P wave in V_1 that is 1.5 mm deep and 0.6 seconds wide is consistent with an enlarged left atrium. True or False.

4. All biphasic P waves in V_1 are examples of IACD. True or False.

1. True 2. Greater 3. True 4. True

Causes of RAE include COPD, pulmonary emboli, pulmonary hypertension, and mitral, tricuspid, or pulmonary valve disease.

Causes of LAE include severe systemic hypertension, aortic or mitral valve disease, restrictive cardiomyopathy, and left ventricle (LV) failure. In other words, anything that obstructs forward flow, such as defective valves or a stiff LV, can cause LAE.

REMINDER:

Intraatrial conduction delay is the proper term for a non-specific conduction problem in the atria.

ECG 9-11 The biphasic P waves in V_1 are consistent with RAE. Notice how the first part of the P wave is higher than the first part of the P in V_6. The limb leads have normal Ps.

ECG 9-11 The patient has LAD with an LAH. The most striking thing about the ECG is the lack of R-R progression in the precordial leads. The patient has an indeterminate Z axis because there is no transition zone anywhere in the precordials. Notice that there is a ditzel of an R wave in front of the S waves in V_1 to V_5. (We use *ditzel* to describe a miniscule, barely perceptible wave on an ECG.)

REMINDER:
Use your calipers to compare the PR and P-P intervals between differing complexes.

ECG 9-12 The P waves in the precordials are wide, at about 0.12 seconds, but there is no notching so it is not a P-mitrale pattern. The product of the width (0.7 sec) $\times$ depth (2.3 mm) of the second half of the P wave in V_1 is 1.61, far above the 0.3 value needed to classify this as LAE. There is no evidence of RAE.

Notice the fifth beat from the left. Can you figure it out? It is a JPC with aberrancy. The other possibility is that it is a VPC. In this case, it is not critical to make the distinction. Later on in the book, we will spend some time addressing the criteria used to differentiate between the two possibilities; it will sometimes be critical to differentiate between the two. If you do not remember the criteria for JPCs or VPCs, take some time to review them in Chapter 8.

ECG 9-12 Once again, for the sake of discussion, note that the fifth beat in this ECG could be an aberrantly conducted JPC. The aberrant beat begins in the same direction as the normal beats, which is suggestive of aberrancy over VPC. However, this is not a clear-cut case; arguments can be made for either option. The pause is compensatory, which means that the sinus node was not reset by the aberrant complex. This could occur in either a JPC or VPC. The uninterrupted P wave, as a matter of fact, appears during its normal cycle and is found at the beginning of the ST segment.

When considering the axis, note that the baseline is at the TP segment in lead II. Using this as the baseline, the beat is approximately 1 mm more negative (5.5 mm positive, 6.5 mm negative), which places the axis in the LAH area of -30 to $-90°$.

There is also LVH with strain and slight QT prolongation, with a QTc greater than or equal to 420.

ECG CASE STUDIES: **CONTINUED**

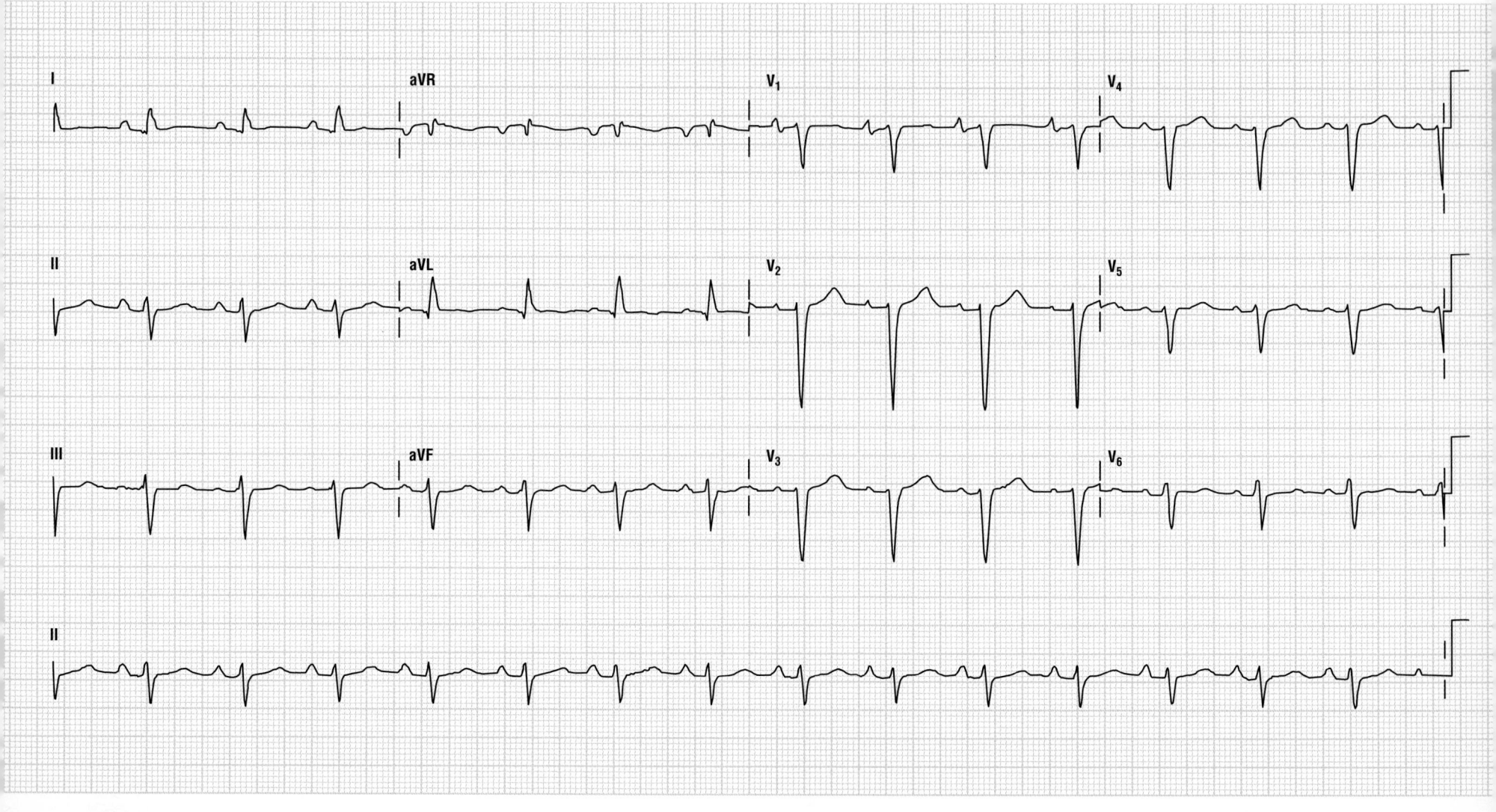

ECG 9-11

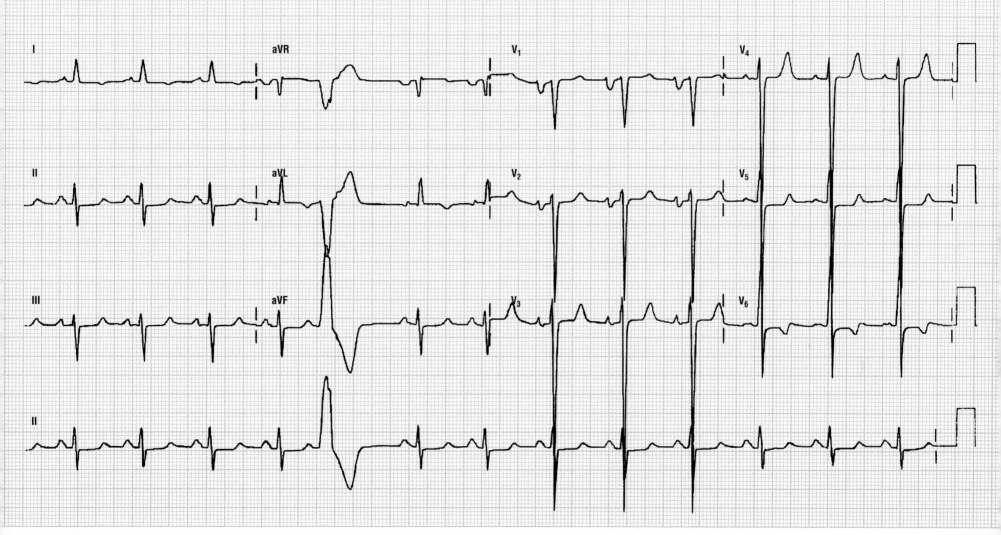

ECG 9-12

ECG CASE STUDIES: CONTINUED

ECG 9-13 The biphasic P waves in V_1 are clear evidence of LAE. The product of width (0.7 sec) × depth (1 mm) is 0.7, well above the 0.3 minimum.

What is the rhythm? Well, we know that there is a P wave before each of the QRS complexes. The P waves are normal in appearance and are upright in leads I and II. So, we can say this is a sinus rhythm. But is it normal sinus rhythm? In order for it to be normal sinus rhythm (NSR), the rate has to be between 60 and 99 beats per minute (BPM). Anything below 60 BPM is sinus bradycardia, and anything above 99 BPM is sinus tachycardia. The rate in this case is about 54 BPM, so this is a sinus bradycardia.

ECG 9-13 The T waves are symmetrical. Symmetrical T waves are commonly found in ischemic syndromes, electrolyte abnormalities, and intracranial pathology. Asymmetrical T waves are more commonly found in strain patterns and benign etiologies.

Significant Q waves are any that are wider than 0.03 seconds or deeper than one third the height of the R wave. Of these, width greater than 0.03 seconds is the more specific finding. The Q wave in II is ever so slightly greater than 0.03 seconds, making it pathological.

QUICK REVIEW

1. Biphasic P waves in lead I which do not quite meet LAE or RAE criteria can be labelled IACD. True or False.
2. In LAE, the product of width × depth must be above 0.3. True or False.
3. In RAE, the product of width × height must be greater than 2.5 mm. True or False.

1. True 2. True 3. False

ECG 9-14 The P waves in II are about 2 mm high, and at about 0.12 seconds wide. There is no notching of the Ps in the limb leads. This comes close but does not meet the criteria for P-pulmonale or P-mitrale. When you look at the biphasic P in V_1, however, the product of the width and depth values is 0.12, consistent with LAE.

ECG 9-14 The flipped T and the QRS in V_1 with an R:S ratio greater than or equal to 1 are consistent with RVH with strain pattern. Another possible criterion, ST depression in V_1 to V_2, is not present in this case.

ST and T wave abnormalities appear in the right precordials in most cases of RVH. Occasionally, they may be seen in the inferior leads. Use your judgment and an old ECG to decide if the T waves in this case are due to the RVH or ischemia. Symmetrical T-wave inversion is more consistent with ischemia.

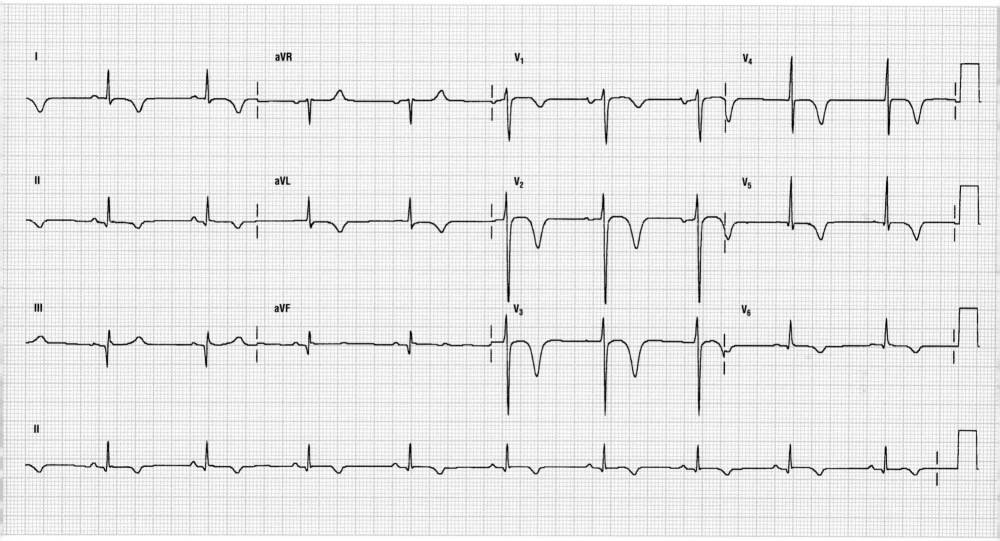

ECG 9-13

ECG CASE STUDIES: CONTINUED

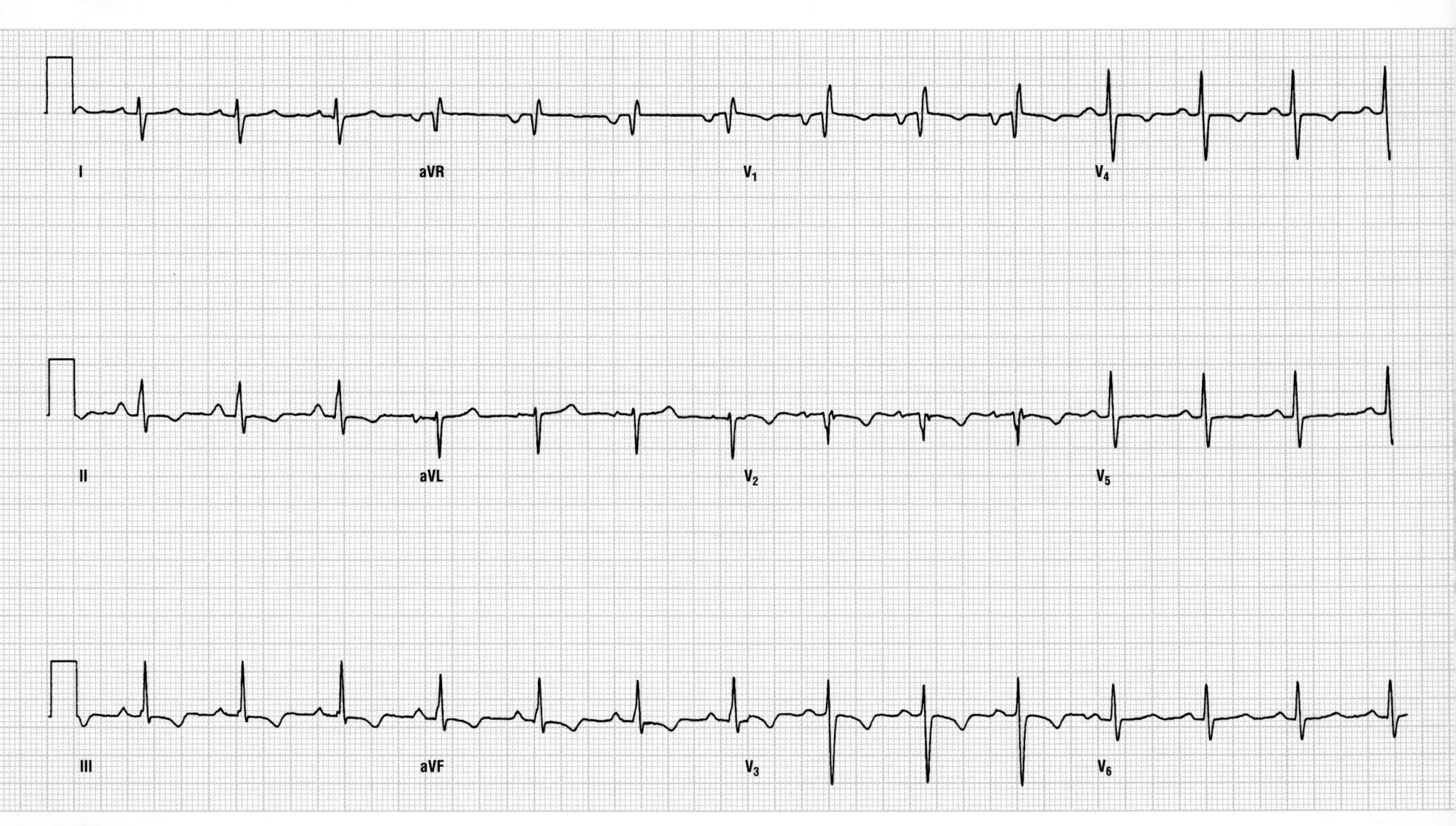

ECG 9-14

ECG 9-15 Where does the P wave start and the T wave end? Once again, we are faced with a long QT interval that brings the T wave of the previous complex right up to the P of the next. Go to a lead in which the P wave is clear, such as V_1 or V_4, then measure the PR interval with your calipers and transfer that interval to the lead in question. This way, you can be sure which wave is which.

Looking at V_1, we have a biphasic P with evidence of LAE. There is no evidence of RAE on this ECG.

ECG 9-15 The QT prolongation is impressive and obvious. Take the time to review its causes (Figure 17-3) if you cannot recall them easily. This ECG also has ST-T wave changes in the inferior and lateral leads that are consistent with ischemia.

Is there an LAH? Where is the baseline? In this case, we need to use the PR interval as the baseline. Usually the TP segment and the PR intervals are on the same line, but sometimes they are not. Using the PR interval can be dangerous; try to use the TP segment as the true baseline whenever possible. Yes, there is an LAH.

ECG 9-16 The P waves are biphasic in V_1 and meet criteria for LAE. In addition, it is obvious that the PR interval is very long (= 0.2 seconds). This is a first-degree heart block, which we will be discussing in greater detail in Chapter 10.

The rhythm is NSR. The first-degree heart block does not interfere with the criteria needed to determine the rhythm.

ECG 9-16 How many areas show evidence of infarct? Well, we have evidence of age-indeterminate infarction in the inferior, anterior, septal, and lateral leads. Qs are present in II, III, and aVF. There are QS waves in V_1 to V_5. V_6 poses a question because there appears to be a ditzel of an R wave before the S wave. The Z axis could not be determined in this ECG because no transition zone is visible.

CLINICAL PEARL

When you see structural problems on an ECG, think before you act. The presence of P-pulmonale or P-mitrale should guide you to go back and reexamine the patient. Look for evidence of pulmonary disease or heart failure. Listen to the heart for murmurs. Be careful of using certain medications in these patients that could lower preload too dramatically or alter hemodynamics negatively.

ECG CASE STUDIES: **CONTINUED**

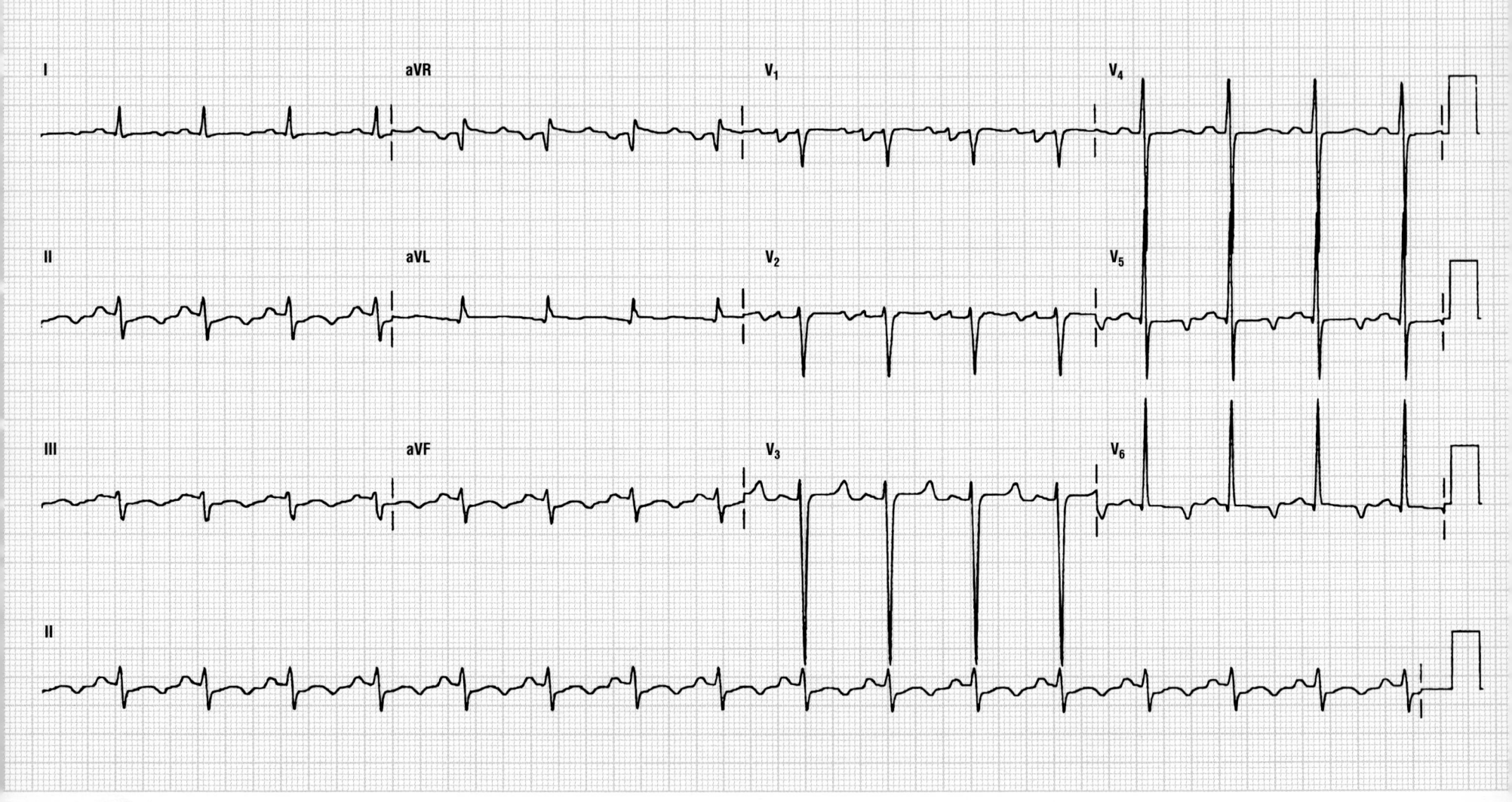

ECG 9-15

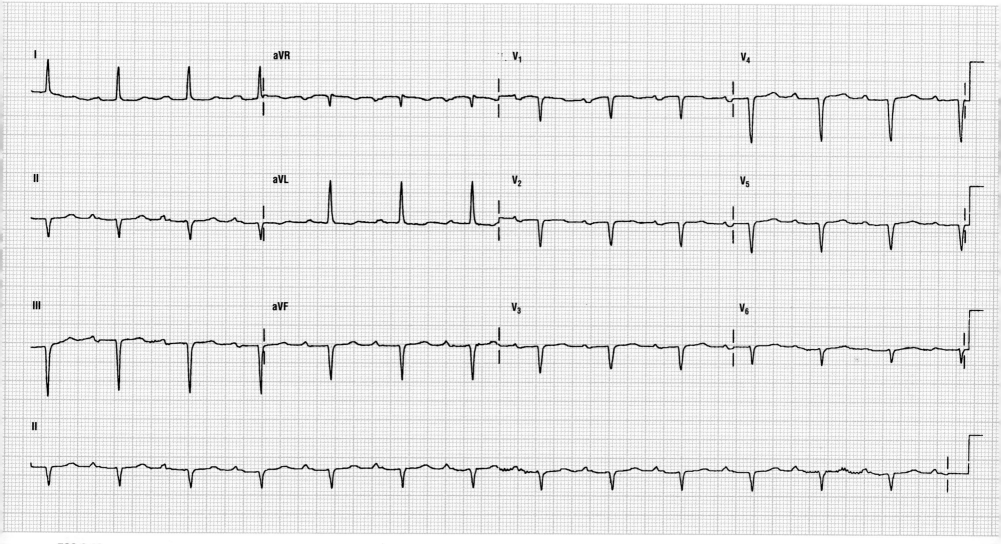

ECG 9-16

ECG CASE STUDIES: **CONTINUED**

ECG 9-17 The P waves in II are 2.4 to 2.5 mm high and therefore are borderline P-pulmonale waves. Note that at the beginning of the P waves we have the measurements above. At the end of the Ps, they are about 0.5 to 1.0 mm deeper. This is because the PR interval is slightly depressed. You always want to measure from the baseline of the ECG. That baseline is measured from the TP segment — the interval between the T of one complex and the P of the next. Always draw a line from one TP segment to the other with the item in question in between (*red line* in Figure 9-10). If you do that on lead II, you will again see minimal depression, so the measurement of the P wave height should be from baseline to the top of the wave.

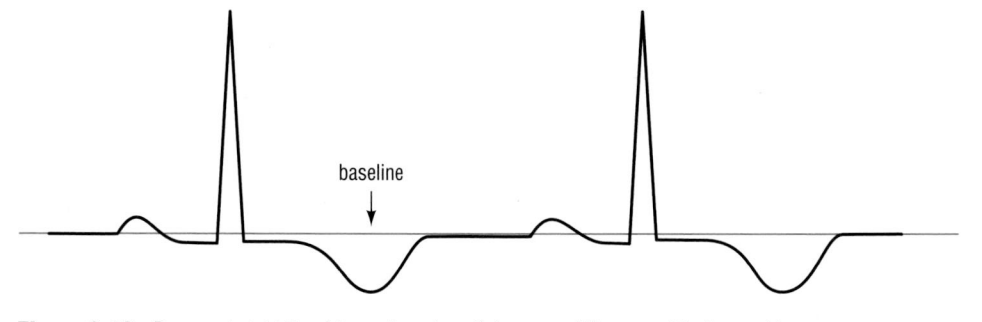

baseline

Figure 9-10: Draw a straight line (shown here in red) from one TP segment to the next to determine wave depression or elevation.

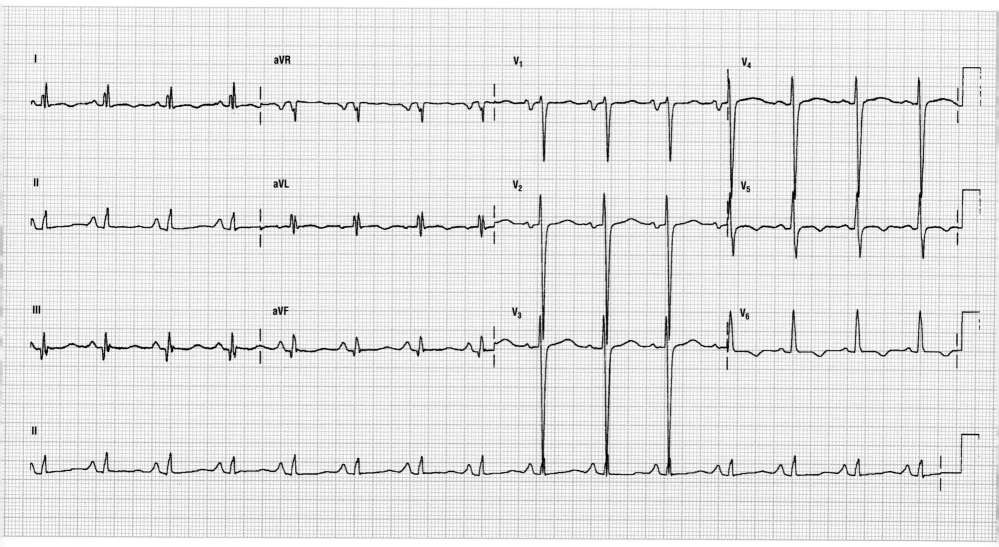

I aVR V1 V4

II aVL V2 V5

III aVF V3 V6

II

ECG 9-17

CHAPTER **9** • THE P WAVE

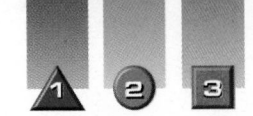

Biatrial Enlargement

Biatrial enlargement, as its name implies, occurs when there is evidence of both left and right atrial enlargement. The findings may include any of the previously reviewed criteria in any combination, such as P-pulmonale and a biphasic P with a product of width times depth greater than or equal to 0.3 seconds (see example 1 in Figure 9-11).

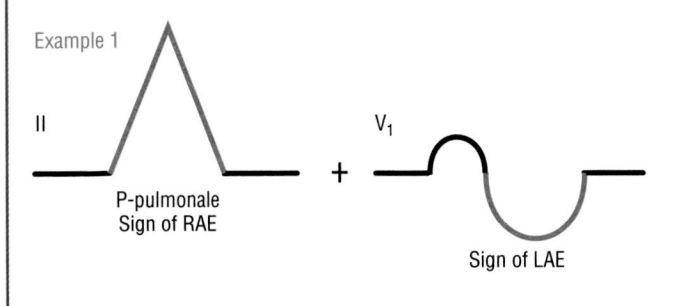

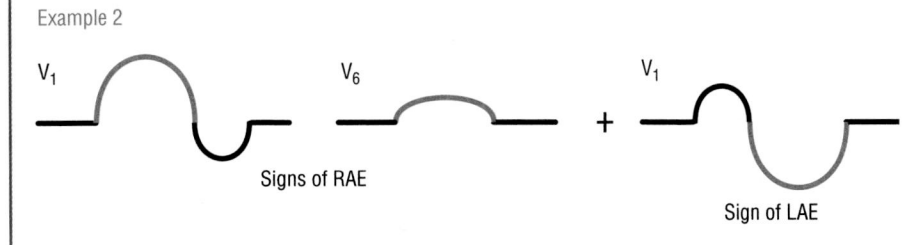

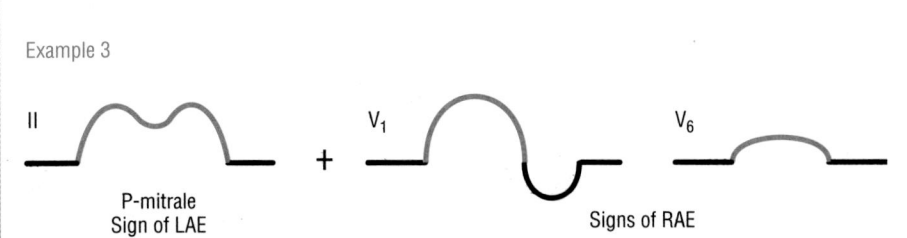

Figure 9-11: Examples showing both left and right biatrial enlargement.

③

You can use ECG signs of atrial and ventricular enlargement to help guide your diagnosis of possible valvular or structural disorders. For example, mitral stenosis (narrowing) should produce enlargement of the right and left atria and the right ventricle, and possibly signs of pulmonary hypertension. Aortic stenosis, if severe, may cause enlargement of both atria and both ventricles. Try to envision the anatomy of the heart when you are evaluating the ECG. You may get some startling results.

ECG CASE STUDIES: *Biatrial Enlargement*

2

ECG 9-18 The limb leads show a P wave that is consistent with P-pulmonale. In addition, the biphasic P waves in V₁ indicate LAE. This is an example of biatrial enlargement.

3

ECG 9-18 The patient has LVH. This accounts for the slight ST elevation in V₂ and V₃, and depression in V₅ and V₆, which are consistent with an early repolarization pattern. The patient has a troubling paucity of T waves in the limb leads, a problem that is unexplained.

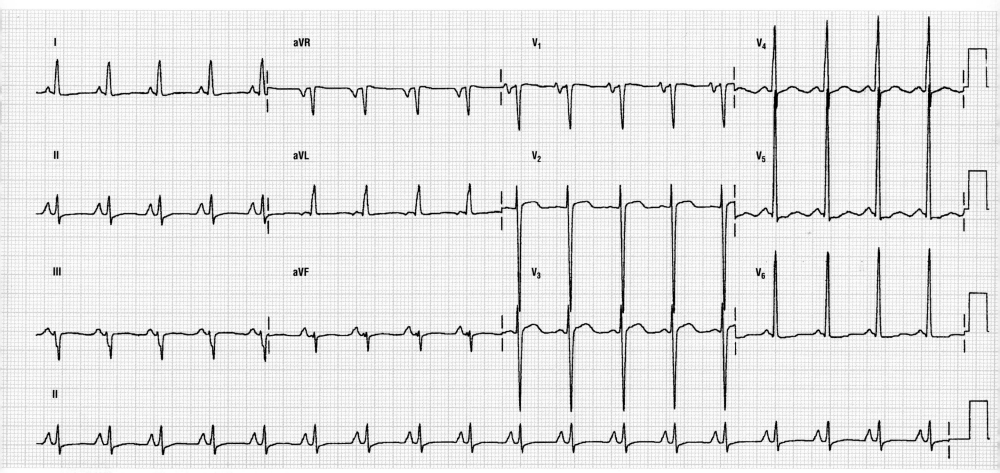

ECG 9-18

ECG CASE STUDIES: **CONTINUED**

②

ECG 9-19 This ECG shows biatrial enlargement caused by a P-mitrale and a biphasic P wave consistent with RAE. Did you notice the first-degree heart block? This is one of those ECGs that you have to study closely. Remember to focus on one thing at a time when you get to the confusing ECGs. If you break it down, it will all make sense. First, identify the P waves. Second, evaluate their morphology and pathology. Third, identify the long distance between the P and the QRS as a first-degree heart block. Why do the QRS complexes look so bizarre? This is an interventricular conduction block (IVCD), which you will learn about in later sections.

③

ECG 9-19 This is a wide, bizarre IVCD. The slurred S wave in V_6 and rabbit ears, or RSR, pattern are indicative of a right bundle branch block (RBBB). Lead I, however, should have more of a slurred S. It is unclear why the morphology is so abnormal. In addition, the patient has an LAH. (You may hear the term "trifascicular block" used to refer to a situation like this, in which there is a bifascicular block combined with a first-degree heart block. This is not a correct use of the term *trifascicular*, because the first-degree block is a *conduction block* rather than a *fascicular block*.)

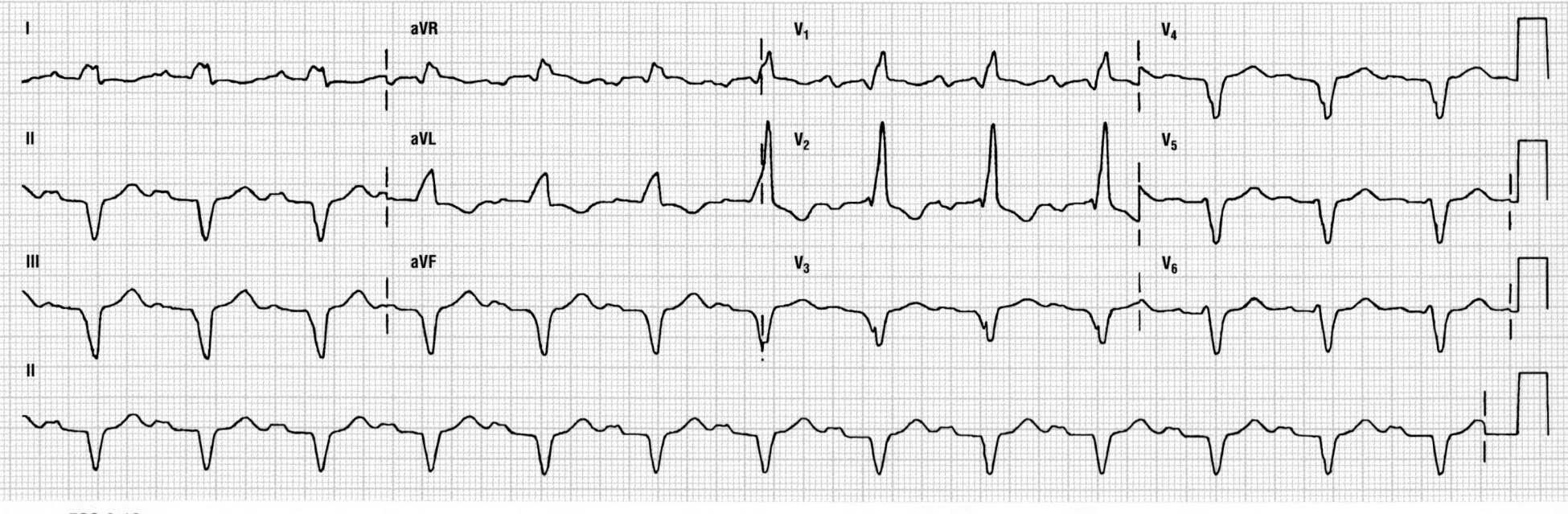

ECG 9-19

ECG 9-20 This is another case of biatrial enlargement. Can you identify why? To start with, you can readily see a P-pulmonale in lead II. There is also a biphasic P wave in V_1 with a morphology compatible with a large left atrium. The PR interval is normal. As we will discuss in greater detail in Chapter 10, the PR interval starts at the beginning of the P and ends at the beginning of the first wave of the QRS.

There is a slight variation in the Ps in V_1, a difference not seen in V_2, V_3, or II. This may reflect a slight ventilatory variation in that lead, or another benign cause.

ECG 9-20 There appears to be global ST segment depression here. The cause may be a Tp wave, or endocardial ischemia secondary to the tachycardia. This Tp wave is the atrial repolarization wave that is usually buried in the QRS complex. These are best seen in tachycardias and conduction blocks. In tachycardias, the rate is so fast that the Tp wave is noticeable as an ST depression. This is where looking at the patient is very helpful. If the patient is in extremis–hypotensive or tachypneic, for instance, ischemia is likely and you must correct the underlying problem quickly. If the patient is sitting up and looking very comfortable, this is probably a Tp wave.

ECG 9-21 The P wave in V_1 is biphasic with a very high first-half component. When you compare the height of the waves between V_1 and V_6, you clearly see the first part of V_1 as the winner. This is evidence of RAE. The second half of the P wave in V_1 is wide and deep; it meets criteria for LAE. If you don't want to multiply, here's a general rule: if the second half of the P is bigger than one total small box (1 mm high and 0.04 seconds wide), it indicates LAE. Notice that we say *one total box*. This is because of the possible scenario in which the P could be two boxes wide and half a box deep, or some other combination.

The irregularity noted in the baseline between beats 9 and 10 is caused by artifact. Use your calipers; all the intervals are the same.

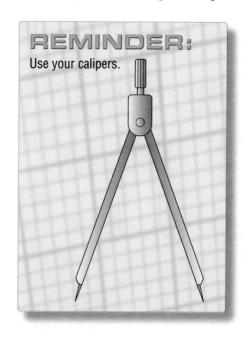

REMINDER:
Use your calipers.

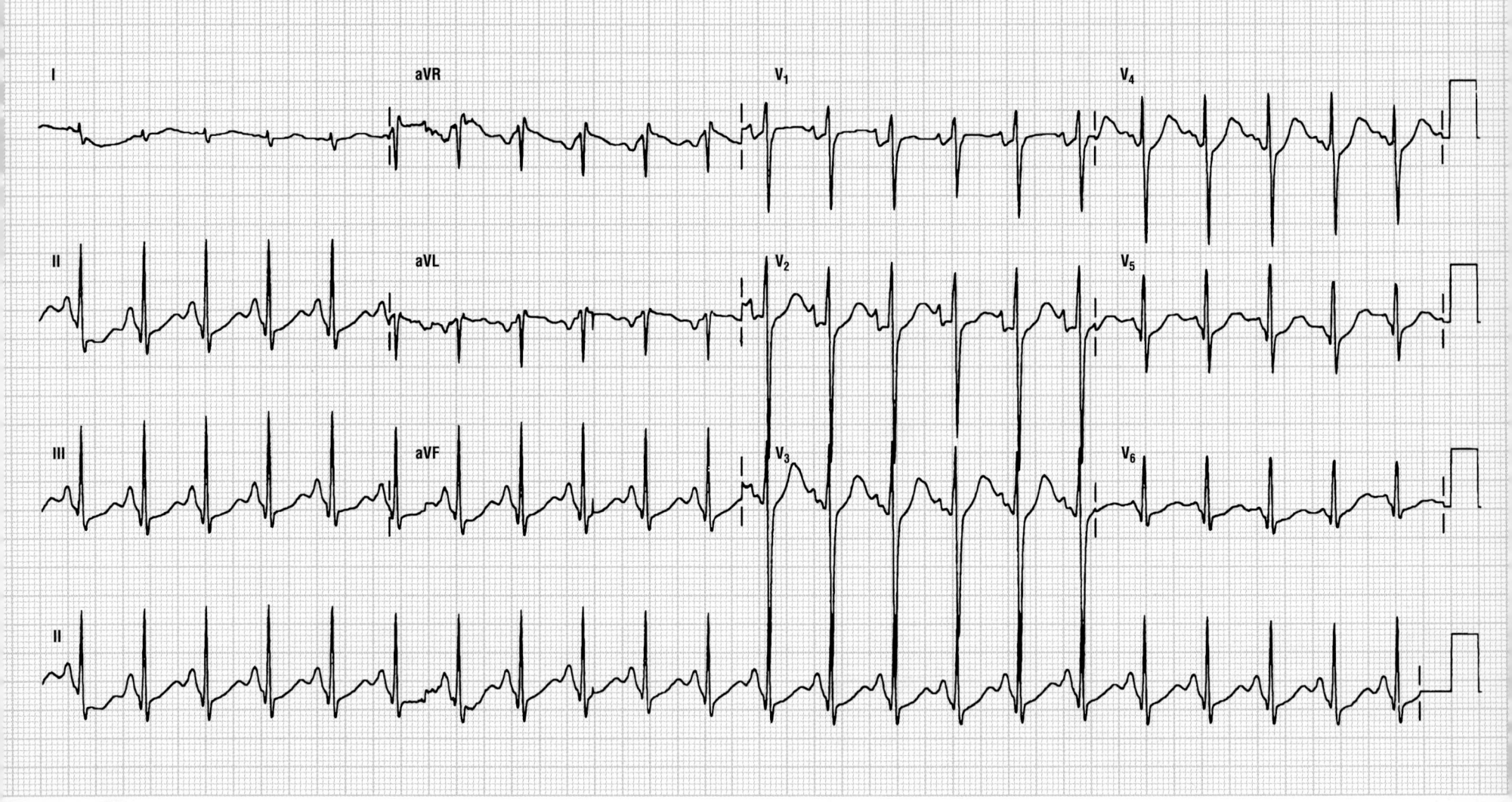

ECG 9-20

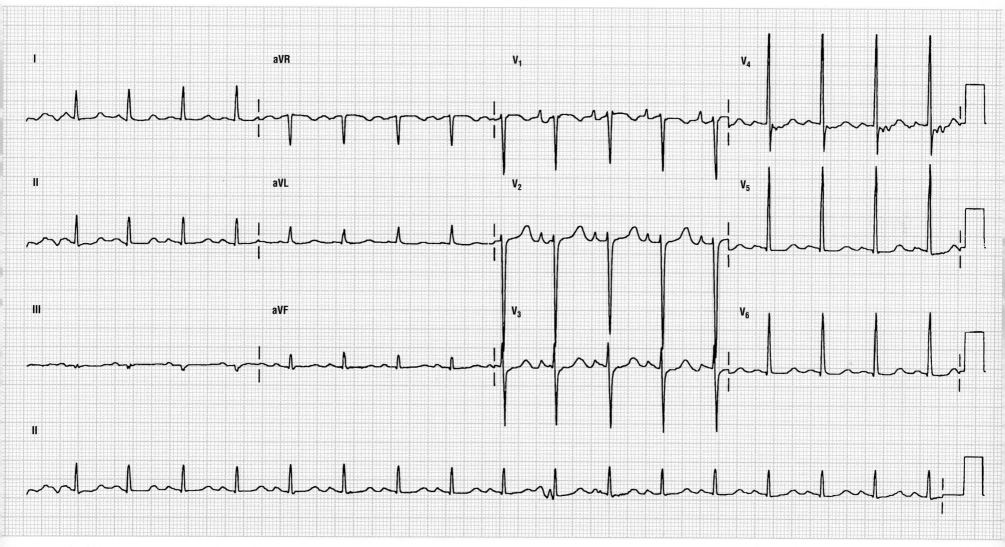

I   aVR   V₁   V₄

II   aVL   V₂   V₅

III   aVF   V₃   V₆

II

ECG 9-21

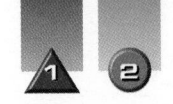
1 CHAPTER IN **REVIEW**

1. The P wave represents:
   A. Atrial repolarization
   B. Atrial depolarization
   C. Ventricular repolarization
   D. Ventricular depolarization
   E. None of the above

2. In any one lead, the morphology of the P waves will vary depending on the location of the area acting as the pacemaker. True or False.

3. Which of the following is consistent with left atrial enlargement:
   A. P-pulmonale
   B. The second half of a biphasic P wave in V_1 is wider and deeper than one small block.
   C. Both A and B are correct
   D. None of the above

4. Which of the following is consistent with right atrial enlargement:
   A. P-pulmonale
   B. The first half of a biphasic P wave in V_1 is wider and deeper than one small block.
   C. Both A and B are correct
   D. None of the above

5. Biatrial enlargement cannot be diagnosed from an ECG. True or False.

1. B 2. True 3. B 4. A 5. False

2 CHAPTER IN **REVIEW**

6. An APC has a different morphology *and* PR interval than the beats that originated in the SA node. True or False.

7. P waves are normally positive in leads:
   A. I
   B. II
   C. V_4 to V_6
   D. All of the above
   E. None of the above

8. Criteria for P-mitrale include:
   A. P wave ≥ 0.12 seconds
   B. Notching is present
   C. The space between the two humps of the notch must be ≥ 0.04 seconds
   D. All of the above
   E. None of the above

9. Criteria for P-pulmonale include:
   A. P wave ≥ 0.12 seconds
   B. Notching is present
   C. The space between the two humps of the notch must be ≥ 0.04 seconds
   D. All of the above
   E. None of the above

10. Sometimes the P waves of one complex are superimposed on the T waves of the preceding complex. True or False.

6. True 7. D 8. D 9. E 10. True

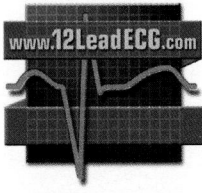

CHAPTER **10**

Conduction Overview

As mentioned in the "Basic Wave" chapter, the PR interval is the interval from the beginning of the P wave to the beginning of the QRS complex. It represents the time frame from the beginning of atrial depolarization to the beginning of ventricular depolarization.

Let's break down the events that occur during the PR interval. Figure 10-1 shows how the electrical impulse relates to the ECG. First, the atria begin to depolarize by the transmission of the electrical impulse through the specialized conduction pathway of the atria, the Bachman bundles, to the atrial myocytes. The impulse reaches the AV node before all of the atrial myocytes have depolarized because of the faster transmission down the Bachman bundles. The depolarization of all of the atrial myocytes represents a larger electrical force than depolarization of the AV node, so the force seen on the ECG tracing is the P wave.

In the AV node, the conduction slows momentarily. (See dashed rectangle; note that the rectangle is superimposed under the P wave, representing this electrocardiographically silent event.) This physiologic slowing is needed to allow the mechanical emptying of atrial blood into the ventricles. Without this block, the atria and the ventricles would beat simultaneously and the ventricles would fill only by the passive inflow of blood during diastole. This would result in a decreased volume entering the ventricles and, hence, a smaller amount ejected from the ventricles. This lack of an "atrial kick" may lead to shock in many patients.

The His bundles, the next to be activated, transmit the impulse down the left and right bundle branches. Finally, the impulse reaches the individual Purkinje fibers, which will then innervate the ventricular myocytes. This is represented by the QRS complex on the ECG tracing.

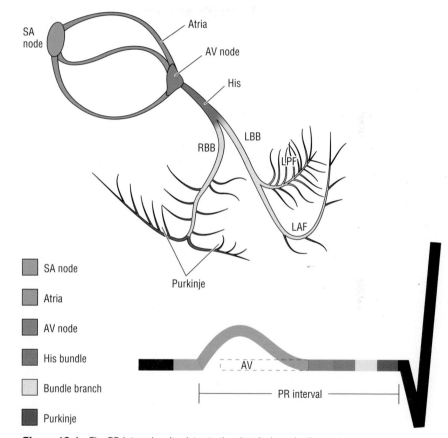

Figure 10-1: The PR interval as it relates to the electrical conduction system.

The PR segment should be on the baseline. That is, on a line drawn from one TP segment to the other.

Baseline:
TP segment to
TP segment

If the PR segment falls below the baseline, then it is said to be depressed.

If the PR segment falls above the baseline, then it is said to be elevated. This is a rare occurrence and is usually due to a poor baseline.

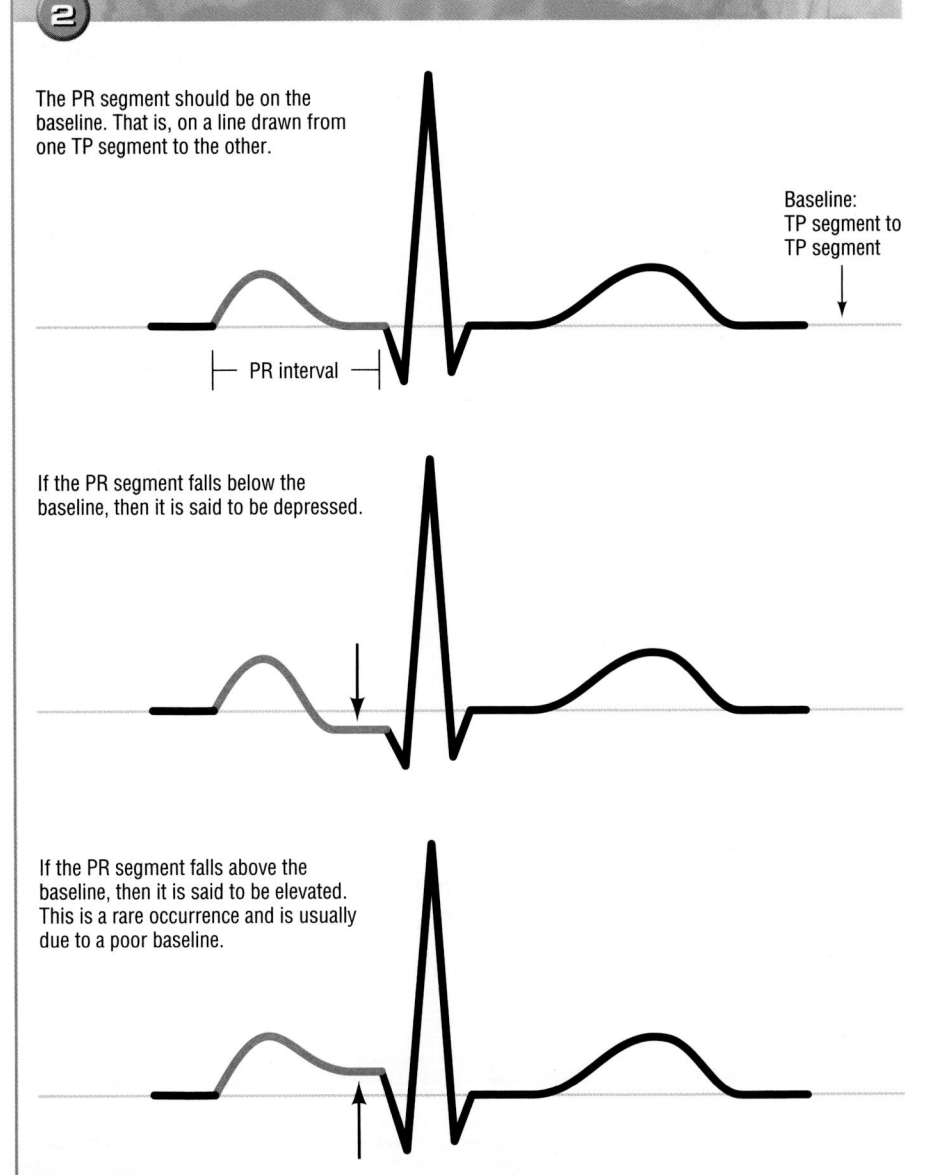

Figure 10-2: PR segment positions in relation to the baseline.

QUICK **REVIEW**

1. The baseline of the ECG is measured from TP segment to _____.

2. Should the PR segment fall on the baseline?

3. Should the ST segment fall on the baseline?

4. The baseline cannot always be measured because of rapid tachycardias that do not show a clear TP segment. True or False.

5. PR segment elevation is a common occurrence seen on most ECGs. True or False.

1. TP segment 2. Yes 3. Yes 4. True 5. False

APCs may have a shorter or longer PR interval. Why does this occur? To answer that question, look at the previous page and analyze the components of the PR interval. There are several locations where we can gain or lose a few milliseconds. We gain a few milliseconds, making the PR interval shorter, if the origin of the P wave is near the AV node, or it bypasses the AV node with its physiologic block altogether. We can lose a few milliseconds, making the PR interval longer, by having an ectopic atrial impulse transmitted from cell to cell directly rather than through the internodal pathways. Some other factors that can alter the PR interval involve prolongation of the physiologic block by vagal stimulation, drugs, or electrolyte abnormalities. The PR interval will also lengthen with prolongation of the conduction in the His bundles, the bundle branches, or in the Purkinje system caused by the same factors — or by the presence of anatomic blocks to the impulse path.

PR Depression

An example of PR depression is shown in Figure 10-3. The differential diagnosis of PR depression includes:

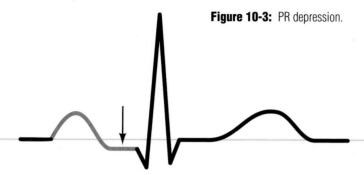

Figure 10-3: PR depression.

1. **Normal variant**

   The PR segment is usually on the baseline. However, it is sometimes found to be slightly depressed. In order for it to be considered normal, it cannot be depressed more than 0.8 mm below the baseline. This normal variant is due to atrial repolarization, which pulls the PR segment downward. The atrial repolarization wave is called the Tp wave. It is usually not seen because it is buried in the QRS wave.

2. **Pericarditis**

   Pericarditis is an inflammation of the pericardium, the fibrous sac that encircles and protects the heart. At this point, we only want you to concentrate on the PR segment when you look at the next few examples. Just remember that pericarditis is a pathological process that may or may not have PR depression that is greater than or equal to 0.8 mm. When you revisit this area as a graduate to Level 2, you will learn the other criteria.

3. **Atrial Infarction**

   This is very rare. You see it when there is significant PR depression in an ECG with signs of infarction and without any of the criteria for pericarditis.

When pericarditis is present, it presents electrocardiographically with one or more of these signs:

1. Tachycardia

2. PR depression

3. Diffuse ST segment elevation. Note that the ST elevations are usually concave up with a scooped-out appearance.

4. Notching of the terminal portion of the QRS complex, especially in the lateral precordial leads

   Look at the example ECGs that follow in the next few pages. Can you find one or more of the pericarditis criteria in any of them? The history will be very helpful in these cases, as the patient usually presents with sharp chest pain that hurts more on inspiration, coughing, or lying back. The pain will be relieved when sitting forward.

The Tp wave is usually buried inside the QRS complex and, therefore, is not seen. You can sometimes see it as the ST depression that occurs in very rapid supraventricular tachycardias, especially rapid sinus tachycardias. In general, these cases have poor baselines with TP segments that are not clearly identifiable.

Atrial infarctions are rare because of the relatively small pressures encountered in the atria and the thinness of the atrial walls. In addition, the circulation to the atria includes thebesian veins that carry blood directly to the tissues. These small veins originate in the atrial or ventricular cavities and bypass the coronary system.

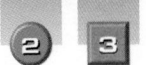

ECG CASE STUDY: *PR Interval Depression*

② ECG 10-1 Because this is the chapter on PR intervals, we want you to concentrate on them in these examples. In the following example, where is the baseline? Take a piece of paper and place the edge on the TP segments surrounding the complex you want to examine. If you placed the paper below the complex, you should not be able to see the PR interval because it is depressed. Now put the paper's edge so that the paper is on the top. (This should hide most of the QRS complex.) You should now be able to see the PR segment and calculate the amount of depression. In this case, it is about a whole block, or 1.0 mm. When you see PR depression, think of pericarditis or atrial infarct. We will discuss pericarditis further in the ST segment chapter (Chapter 14). How long is the PR interval in this ECG? Is it prolonged?

③ ECG 10-1 Notice that all of the criteria for acute pericarditis are present on this ECG, except tachycardia:

1. Diffuse ST segment elevations, which are scooped and upwardly concave
2. PR depression
3. Notching of the S wave

When you see ST elevation in the inferior and the precordials from V_3 to V_6, you should think of an inferolateral acute myocardial infarction (AMI). If the ST elevation includes V_2, it is indicative of a special kind of AMI known as an apical AMI. This is usually due to a very large right coronary dominant system.

REMINDER:
Use a straight edge or ECG ruler to calculate the baseline. Remember — it extends from TP segment to TP segment.

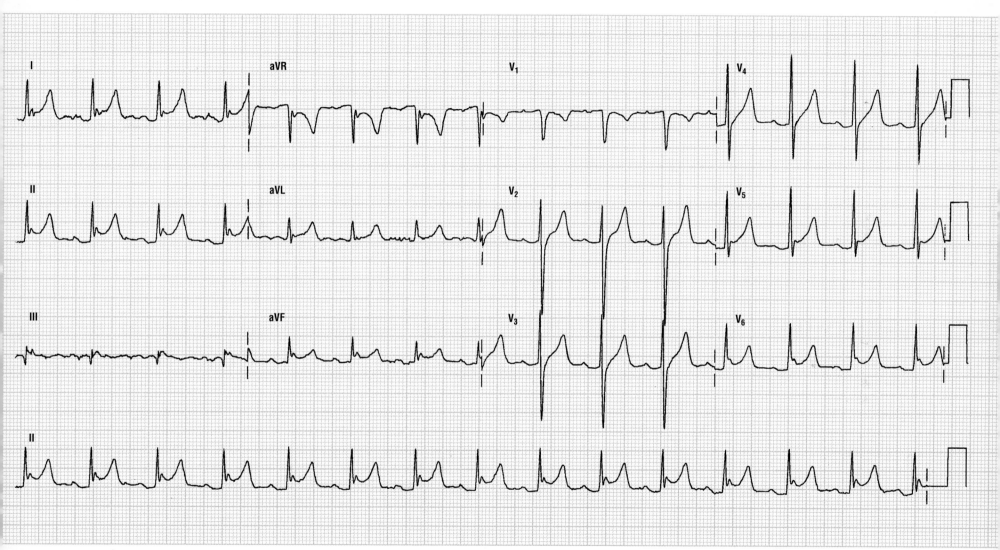

ECG 10-1

Measuring the Interval

The normal PR interval, shown in Figure 10-4, is from 0.12 seconds to 0.20* seconds in length. The PR interval is considered short when it is less than or equal to 0.11 seconds (Figure 10-5), and prolonged when it is more than 0.20 seconds (Figure 10-6). The interval should be measured in the lead with the widest P wave and the widest QRS complex in order to avoid the inadvertent omission of an isoelectric portion of a P wave. If your calculation does not take into account this isoelectric portion, it will give you a falsely shortened PR interval. You avoid the problems with isoelectric portions by using the lead with the longest PR interval to take your measurement. Remember that intervals should be the same throughout all of the leads. This will become more evident in future sections.

The PR interval is shortened in sinus tachycardia and in kids. It is usually longer in the elderly.

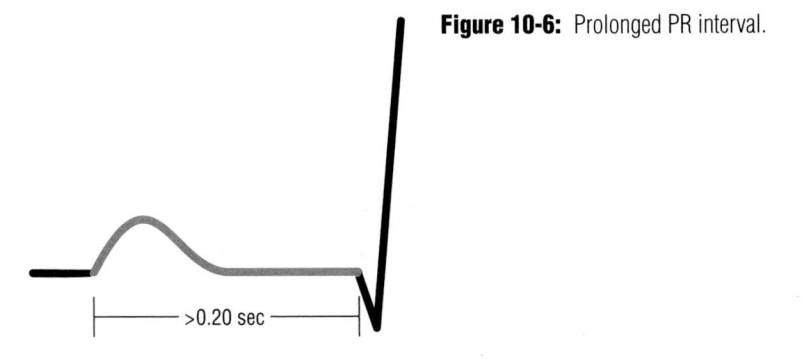

Figure 10-5: Short PR interval.

≤0.11 sec

Figure 10-6: Prolonged PR interval.

>0.20 sec

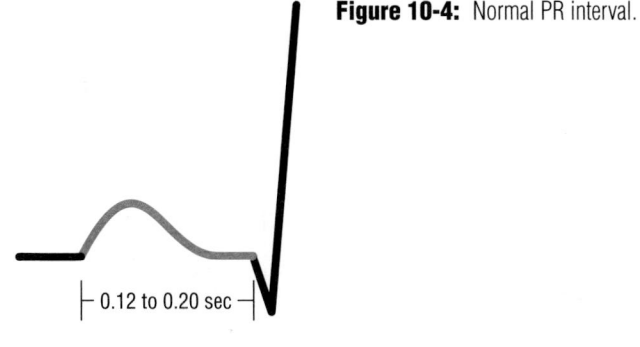

Figure 10-4: Normal PR interval.

0.12 to 0.20 sec

* Most books refer to a normal PR interval being from 0.12 to 0.20 seconds and first-degree heart block as more than 0.20 seconds. However, in their examples, they include 0.20 seconds as prolonged. In this book, we will consider 0.20 seconds as borderline PR prolongation.

1. The PR interval can be normal, short, or _____.

2. The normal PR interval is from _____ to _____.

3. The PR interval is considered short if it is less than or equal to _____seconds long.

4. Tachycardias will lengthen the PR interval. True or False.

5. The PR interval can be measured in any lead. True or False.

6. Intervals can vary from one lead to another. True or False.

1. Prolonged 2. 0.12 to 0.19 sec 3. 0.11 4. False 5. False 6. False. They can appear shorter or longer, but the intervals will always be the same in all leads!

1. Can you think of the differential diagnosis for a shortened PR interval?

2. Can you think of the differential diagnosis for a prolonged PR interval?

3. Why do we have isoelectric sections in the different leads?

1. & 2. See following sections. 3. Remember that all of the waves and segments have their own individual axes. Just as we have isoelectric segments in the QRS axis, we can have isoelectric segments of the P, ST segment, QRS, etc. Always measure the widest interval.

CLINICAL PEARL

When you have a prolonged PR interval, take a quick look at the rest of the intervals. If they are all prolonged, there may be a metabolic problem causing it; commonly it is a high potassium level.

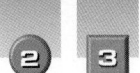

Short PR Interval

The PR interval is considered short if it is less than or equal to 0.11 seconds. There are three major mechanisms that cause a short PR interval:

1. Retrograde junctional P waves
2. Lown-Ganong-Levine syndrome (LGL)
3. Wolff-Parkinson-White pattern and syndrome (WPW)

We discussed retrograde P waves in the previous chapter. Go back and review it if you need to. It is an important point that you will run into again and again.

Lown-Ganong-Levine (LGL) syndrome is a benign condition associated with a short PR interval, a normal P wave, and a normal QRS. Some authors believe that it must be associated with tachycardias, but others disagree. Just keep in mind that the possibility of paroxysmal tachycardia or other tachycardias exists. The explanation for the short PR interval is that the impulse is transmitted through a bypass tract called James fibers, shown in Figure 10-7. These fibers bypass the upper and central portions of the AV node where the normal physiologic block

occurs. The impulse thus bypasses the normal physiologic block, shortening the PR interval. The QRS complex is normal because conduction through the His bundles and bundle branches proceeds normally.

We will discuss WPW syndrome shortly.

 Q U I C K **REVIEW**

1. What are the major causes of a short PR interval?
2. Retrograde P waves are easily identifiable on an ECG because the P waves are inverted in leads II, III, and aVF. True or False.
3. What is the name of the syndrome that features a short PR interval with a normal QRS complex?
4. What is the name of the bypass tract associated with LGL syndrome?
5. Would you be surprised if a patient with a short PR interval and a normal QRS complex reported episodes of very rapid heart rate?

1. See Level 2 material just above these questions. **2.** True **3.** LGL syndrome **4.** James fibers **5.** No

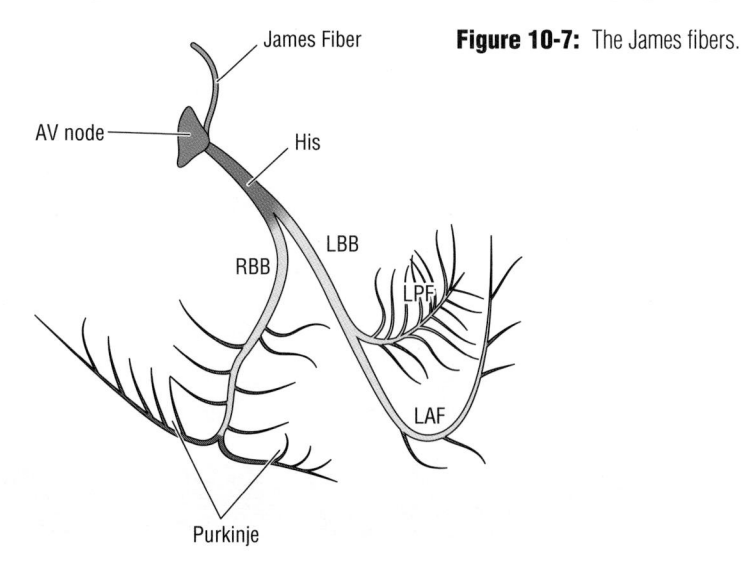

Figure 10-7: The James fibers.

There are two other types of bypass tracts besides James fibers. Can you name them? They are the Kent bundle and the Mahaim fibers. Mahaim fibers are a short bypass tract that connects the lower AV node or the His bundles with the interventricular septum. The Mahaim fibers are associated with a delta wave and can account for some of the cases of WPW. These two fiber tracts can coexist in the same patients, although it is rare.

Note that in patients with Mahaim fibers, the PR interval should be normal because the normal physiologic block has been maintained. The Kent bundle bypasses the AV node, and thus can have a shortened PR interval.

②

ECG 10-2 That's a short PR interval! It is about 0.8 seconds long. This is an example of LGL syndrome. It contains a very short PR interval and normal waves in the complex. What is the significance of this? Not much, except that it may be associated with tachycardias. Why are we spending the time to go over LGL and WPW (next section)? Simply because they are conditions that are commonly overlooked. We had one patient who presented to the emergency department 36 times with a complaint of syncope (fainting). He had about 20 ECGs done during those visits. The man was sent to a psychiatrist, who placed him on antidepressants and antipsychotics. This all led to a downward spiral in the patient's life that could have been avoided by recognizing WPW.

③

ECG 10-2 The underlying rhythm is a sinus arrhythmia. There is not a lot more to say about this ECG. So, we're going to talk about the need to know and remember the differential diagnosis of the various findings. To be a great clinician, you have to think of all of the possibilities related to the patient's condition. The only way to make the correct diagnosis is to have thought about it. Use the information you have to rule in or out the specific conditions. Make some 3x5 cards with the differentials we give you in this book and carry them with you. Review the cards for a few days and you'll never forget them.

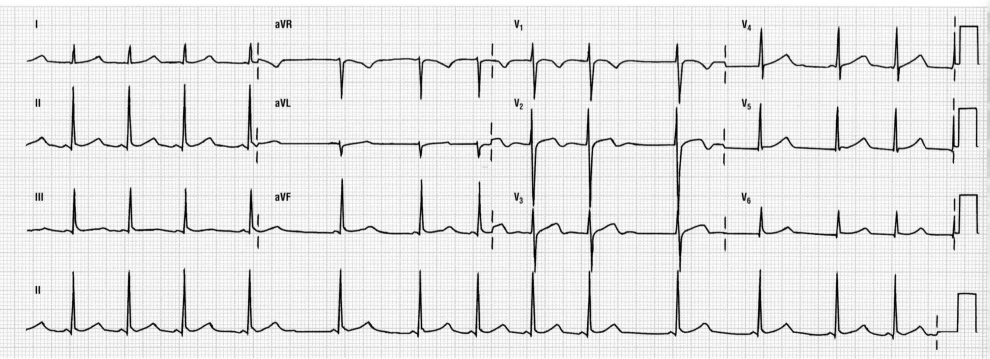

ECG 10-2

Wolff-Parkinson-White Syndrome (WPW)

The syndrome of Wolff-Parkinson-White is defined by:

1. Shortened PR interval (< 0.12 seconds) with a normal P wave
2. Wide QRS complex (≥ 0.11 seconds)
3. The presence of a delta wave
4. ST-T wave changes or abnormalities
5. Association with paroxysmal tachycardias

Patients with WPW have a tract that bypasses the AV node altogether known as the Kent bundle, shown in Figure 10-8. Now imagine the impulse traveling down through the atria. It reaches the Kent bundle and the AV node just about simultaneously. The impulse travels down the AV node and is met by the normal physiologic block. The impulse also travels down the Kent bundle, doesn't meet any block, and so begins to spread through the ventricular myocardium. This progression is slow and gives a wide pattern on the ECG tracing. This is, in reality, the same as saying that a ventricular premature contraction (VPC) (wide, bizarre complex) is starting at the terminal point of the Kent bundle. Now, remember that impulse traveling down the AV

node? It starts down the normal conduction pathway and depolarizes the myocardium that has not already been depolarized by the Kent bundle impulse. Because the AV nodal impulse is much faster than transmission of the Kent bundle impulse through the myocardium, the two waves meet and extinguish each other because of the refractoriness of the two areas. The slow Kent bundle impulse is superimposed or fused on the normal impulse and forms a fusion beat with a delta wave as shown in Figure 10-9. The actual delta wave is the initial slurring of the QRS; it represents the small amount of tissue that was stimulated by the Kent bundle impulse wave.

If the patient has all of the above findings except for tachycardia, it is known as the WPW pattern. In addition, 12% of patients have a normal PR interval. Why the big deal and the full page devoted to WPW, you ask? Well, WPW is associated with tachycardias, as mentioned above. These tachycardias can be wide (> 0.12 sec), regular or irregular, and very, very fast. The distinction between a supraventricular pattern and a ventricular tachycardia pattern is difficult, sometimes impossible. Treatment for these tachycardias is beyond the scope of this book, but we highly recommend that you spend the time to fully understand the treatment strategies and why they are important. Just remember that you should treat a wide-complex tachycardia as if it is ventricular tachycardia, until proven otherwise.

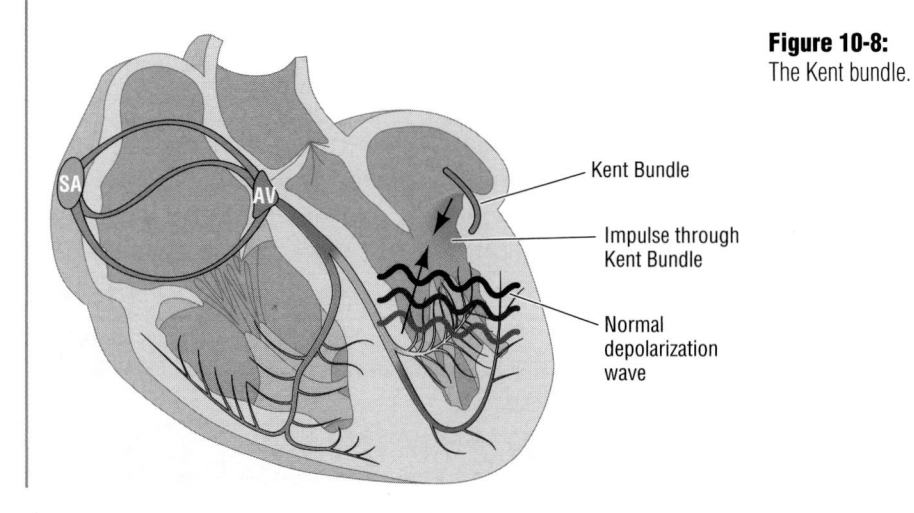

Figure 10-8: The Kent bundle.

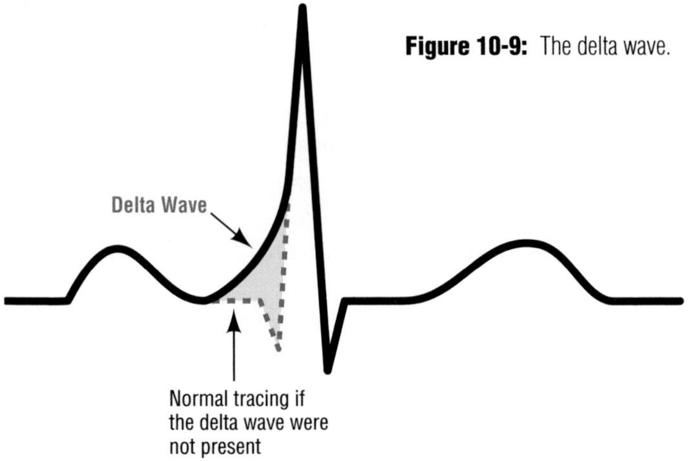

Kent Bundle

Impulse through Kent Bundle

Normal depolarization wave

Figure 10-9: The delta wave.

Delta Wave

Normal tracing if the delta wave were not present

ECG 10-3 This is a classic example of a WPW pattern on an ECG. Notice there is a short PR interval and very distinct delta waves. In this case, the delta waves are seen in all of the leads. This doesn't always occur, because some leads are isoelectric to the delta wave component. Do leads III and aVF have delta waves? Yes, but they are negative (deflected downward). If you have followed the format of the book, you should already have reviewed Q waves, and the basic infarct patterns at the end of the book. When you look at leads III and aVF, they are similar to — and sometimes confused with — Q waves. This similarity to Q waves has given rise to the term pseudoinfarct pattern. Please remember that this is not a true infarct.

Take a look at the ST and T wave changes in this ECG. Look at the ST elevation in V_1 to V_3, and the flipped Ts in I, aVL, and V_4 to V_6. Are they a sign of ischemia? Not in a patient with WPW. What happens is

that, because part of the depolarization wave travels down the accessory pathway, it causes the repolarization also to be abnormal. This abnormal repolarization gives rise to all sorts of ST and T wave abnormalities. It is therefore very hard, if not impossible, to diagnose AMI based on the standard criteria in patients with WPW. Let the history guide you in making the diagnosis, and consult a cardiologist as soon as possible if you suspect an AMI.

REMINDER:
Lown-Ganong-Levine (LGL) is usually benign. Wolff-Parkinson-White (WPW) can be life threatening!

ECG CASE STUDIES: **CONTINUED**

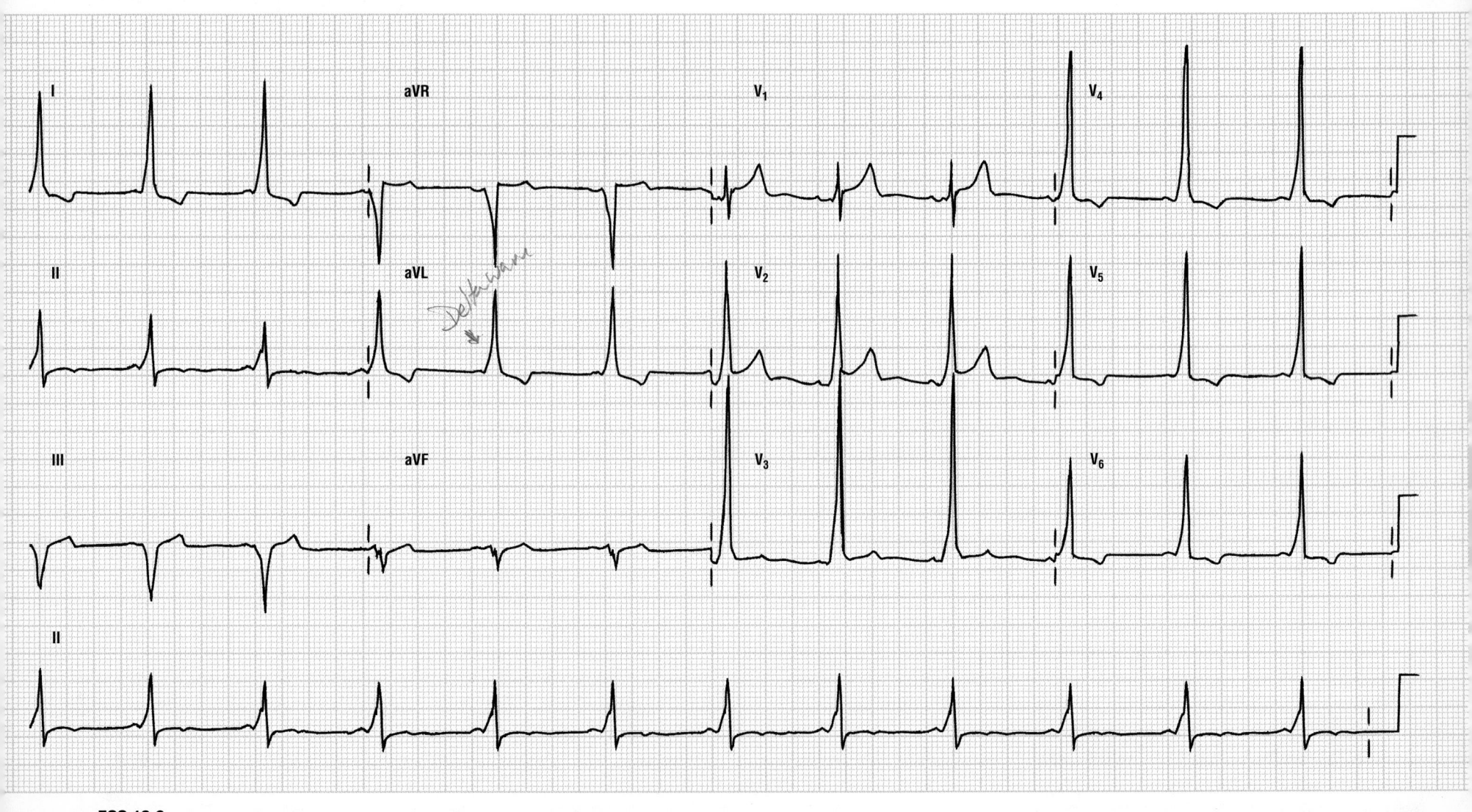

ECG 10-3

WPW Syndrome — Advanced Information

There are 3 types of WPW:

Type A: In this type of WPW, the QRS complexes are primarily upright in all of the precordial leads. A good way to remember it is to look at V_1: in type A, you can draw a small line across the QRS complex and it resembles an "A" (Figure 10-10, top). Type B, on the other hand, is negative in V_1 and V_2 and — if you use your imagination — can look like a "b" (Figure 10-10, bottom). It can sometimes resemble a right bundle branch block with an RSR' pattern, for which it is usually mistaken. The ST-T wave repolarization abnormalities are seen usually in the right precordials, and present as ST depressions and T wave inversions. Type A is usually associated with a Kent bundle on the left side of the heart.

Type B: In type B, the QRS complexes are negative in V_1 and V_2, and upright in the left-sided precordial leads. It can be mistaken for a left bundle branch block because of this pattern. The repolarization abnormalities are seen in the left precordials.

Type C: In this type of WPW, the complexes are upright in V_1 to V_4, and negative in V_5 to V_6. It starts off like WPW Type A, but does not maintain positive complexes all the way to the lateral leads. This type is very rare.

All types of WPW can be mistaken for infarcts when the delta wave is negative, because it resembles a Q wave. This is especially prominent when the deflections are negative in the inferior leads. This pattern is called pseudoinfarct because it is not associated with a myocardial infarction (see Type B diagram). Another possible relationship with AMI presents with type A, which can resemble a posterior infarction because of the tall R wave in V1.

When there is a tachycardia present, the impulse can either travel down the Kent bundle and back up the AV node, or down the AV node and back up the Kent bundle. It is called antidromic when it travels

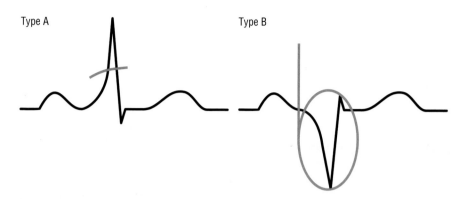

Figure 10-10: WPW Syndrome, Types A and B.

down the Kent bundle and back up the AV node. This type of circus movement gives rise to a wide-complex tachycardia that is difficult to distinguish from ventricular tachycardia. Antidromic tachycardias can be very fast, especially in cases of atrial flutter and atrial fibrillation wherein transmission can be on a one-to-one basis.

The other type of tachycardia pattern, known as orthodromic, represents transmission of the impulse down the AV node and a return to the atria through the Kent bundle. This usually presents as a narrow-complex tachycardia and is less dangerous because the AV node still exerts its influence through the physiologic block. Therefore, the tachycardia is usually slower and more controlled than it is in antidromic tachycardia.

CLINICAL PEARL

The differential diagnosis of a tall R wave in V_1 includes:

1. Right bundle branch block
2. Posterior myocardial infarction
3. Right ventricular hypertrophy
4. WPW Type A
5. Normal in adolescents and young children

ECG CASE STUDIES: **CONTINUED**

---

②

ECG 10-4 In this example, we again see the delta waves typical of WPW. But what about the PR interval? Is this a short PR interval? In this case, the PR interval is about 0.12 seconds. About 12% of WPW patients do not have a short PR interval. In some cases, there can even be first-degree heart block. Why does this happen? Remember that the delta wave just hides the underlying PR interval (see Figure 10-9). If the underlying problem is a prolonged PR interval, then the patient will have a normal or prolonged PR interval when the delta wave is superimposed.

This patient has the pseudoinfarct pattern on lead aVF, and ST-T wave abnormalities that are common to WPW.

---

③

This ECG and **ECG 10-3** are both examples of WPW Type A; the delta wave of the QRS complex in lead V_1 is positive. Type B has a negative delta wave. What do the different types mean? In general, type A is associated with accessory pathways in the left side of the heart, and type B corresponds to pathways on the right. This is not exactly true, however, because many patients have more than one pathway. The best way to find the pathway is with electrophysiologic studies.

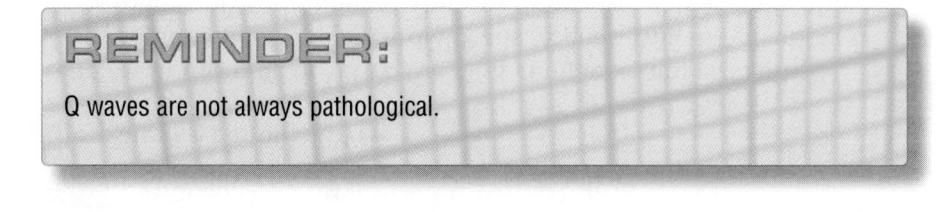

REMINDER:

Q waves are not always pathological.

---

②

ECG 10-5 This is yet another example of a WPW pattern. It has some interesting variations, however. Can you pick them out? Don't come back until you've really looked at the ECG carefully.

First of all, the sixth complex is an APC that is conducted mostly through the AV node. How do we know this? The delta wave is smaller in this complex. That means that most of the conduction occurred through the AV node.

Second, being an expert on P waves by now, you immediately see that the P waves are different in many of the complexes. In addition, the PR and RR intervals are different in many cases. Use your calipers. This is an example of wandering atrial pacemaker in a patient with WPW.

---

③

ECG 10-5 Make sure you have read the Level 2 material on this ECG and followed the directions. Were you able to pick out the rhythm and the APC? Don't get complacent. You should be using your calipers and closely scrutinizing each of these ECGs. That is the only way you are going to master reading and interpreting them.

This is an example of type B WPW. Note that the delta wave is negative in lead V_1. There is also a nice pseudoinfarct pattern in leads III, aVF, and V_1. Type B WPW is often misdiagnosed as an anterior AMI or a left bundle branch. Be careful.

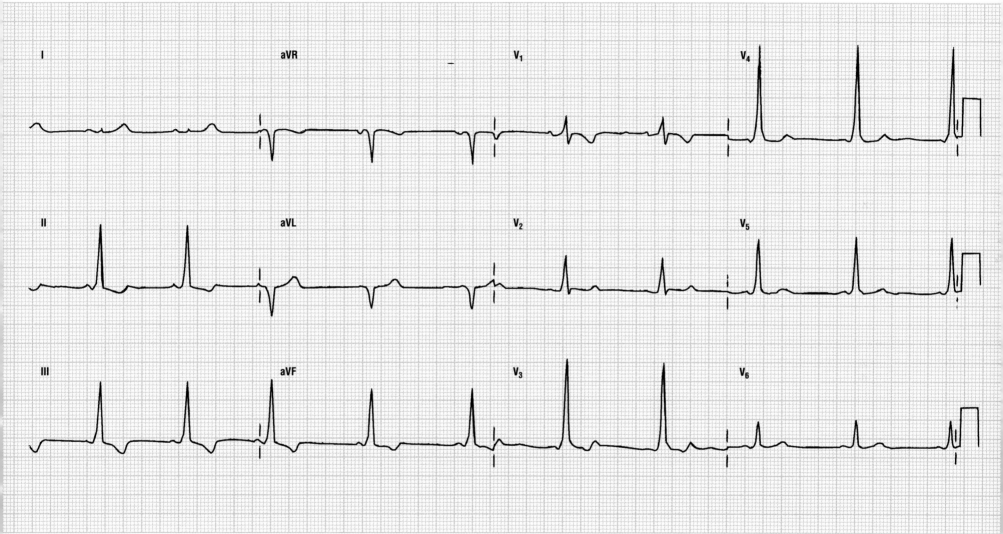

ECG 10-4

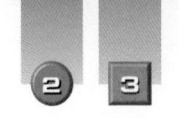

ECG CASE STUDIES: CONTINUED

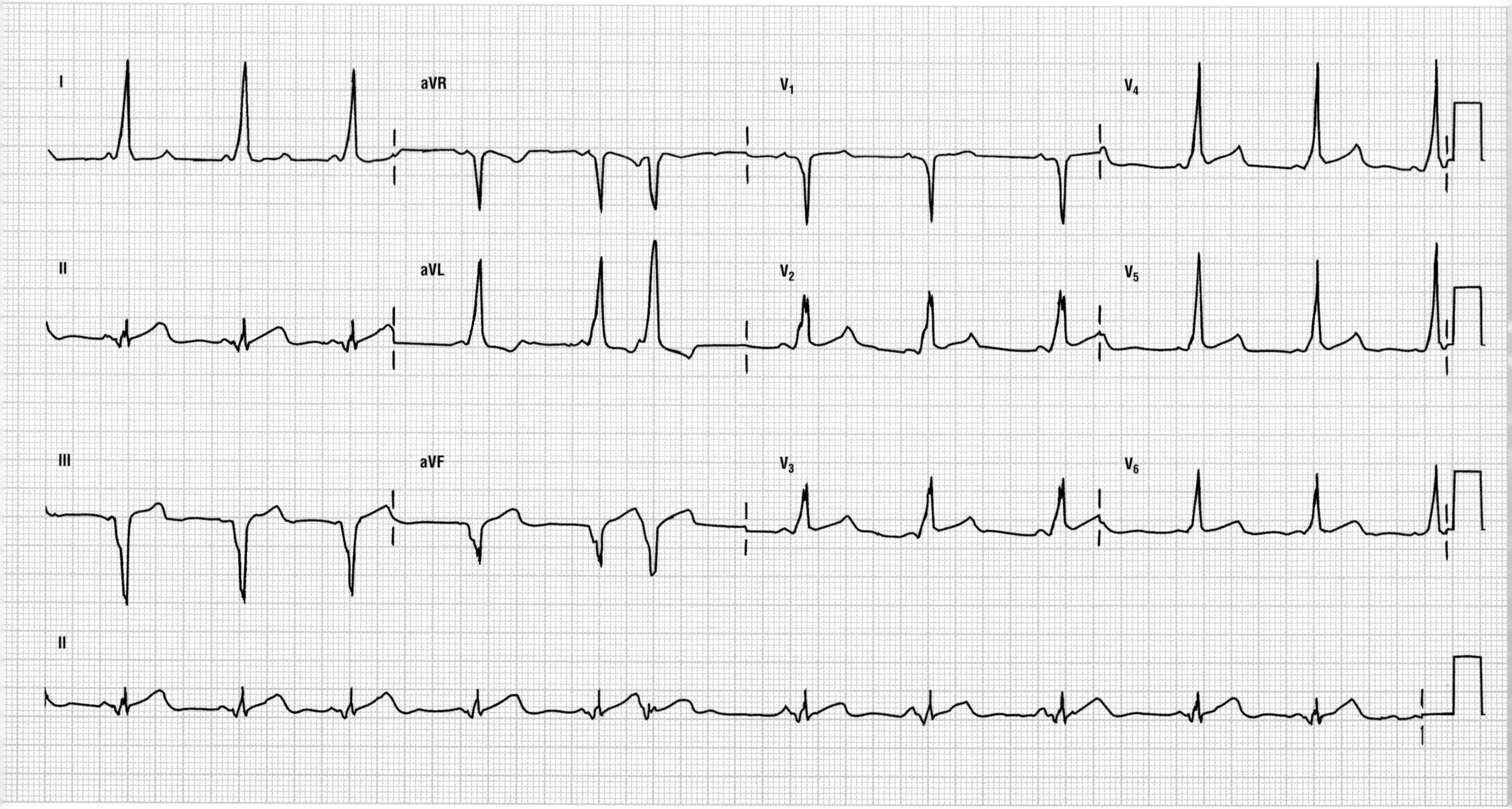

I aVR V₁ V₄

II aVL V₂ V₅

III aVF V₃ V₆

II

ECG 10-5

2

ECG 10-6 Here is another example of WPW. In this case, it is easy to see the delta wave in various leads. Once again, the PR interval is longer than expected for a WPW. Are those Q waves in leads II, III, and aVF? No. Remember that a delta wave in the inferior leads can mimic the Q waves of an inferior myocardial infarction.

3

ECG 10-6 This is once again WPW, but is it type A or type B? Well, type A has the delta wave in a positive direction in lead V_1. The problem is it should be positive in all of the precordials. Type B should have a negative delta wave in V_1, so this is obviously not the right answer. This is type C. It starts off like type A, but then has negative deltas in the left lateral precordial leads. This is a very rare form of a rare syndrome. The important thing in these cases is to diagnose the WPW and then refer the patient to a cardiologist specializing in EPS.

2

ECG 10-7 This is a different format of ECG. Note that there are calibration blocks at the start of most leads, and that there is no rhythm strip at the bottom. When you are confronted with a different format than the one that you are used to, just break it down into its components and note the leads. Although not labeled, the format for the leads is the same we are used to. If the order of the leads were different, it would have to be stated on the ECG.

This is a patient with WPW. The traditional delta wave is easy to pick out on most leads. Take a look at III and aVF. What's going on in these leads? Well, the P wave is isoelectric in these leads, or close to it, and you don't see it clearly. What you do see is a small QRS complex with a significant notch. The first part of the complex is not the P wave.

This is an example of an isolated intraventricular conduction delay. It is isolated because it does not cause any widening of the QRS complex, and you only see it in some leads. The reason the complex is so bizarre is that the conduction takes place aberrantly (through an abnormal pathway) and gives rise to a different morphology on the ECG. If the conduction disturbance occurred earlier, nearer the AV node, the length of the QRS complex could be widened and there would be more generalized changes in the QRS morphology. We will discuss this in greater detail when we get to bundle branch blocks.

CLINICAL PEARL

Remember, there is a difference between having a WPW ECG pattern and having the WPW syndrome. The syndrome is associated with paroxysmal tachycardias.

ECG CASE STUDIES: CONTINUED

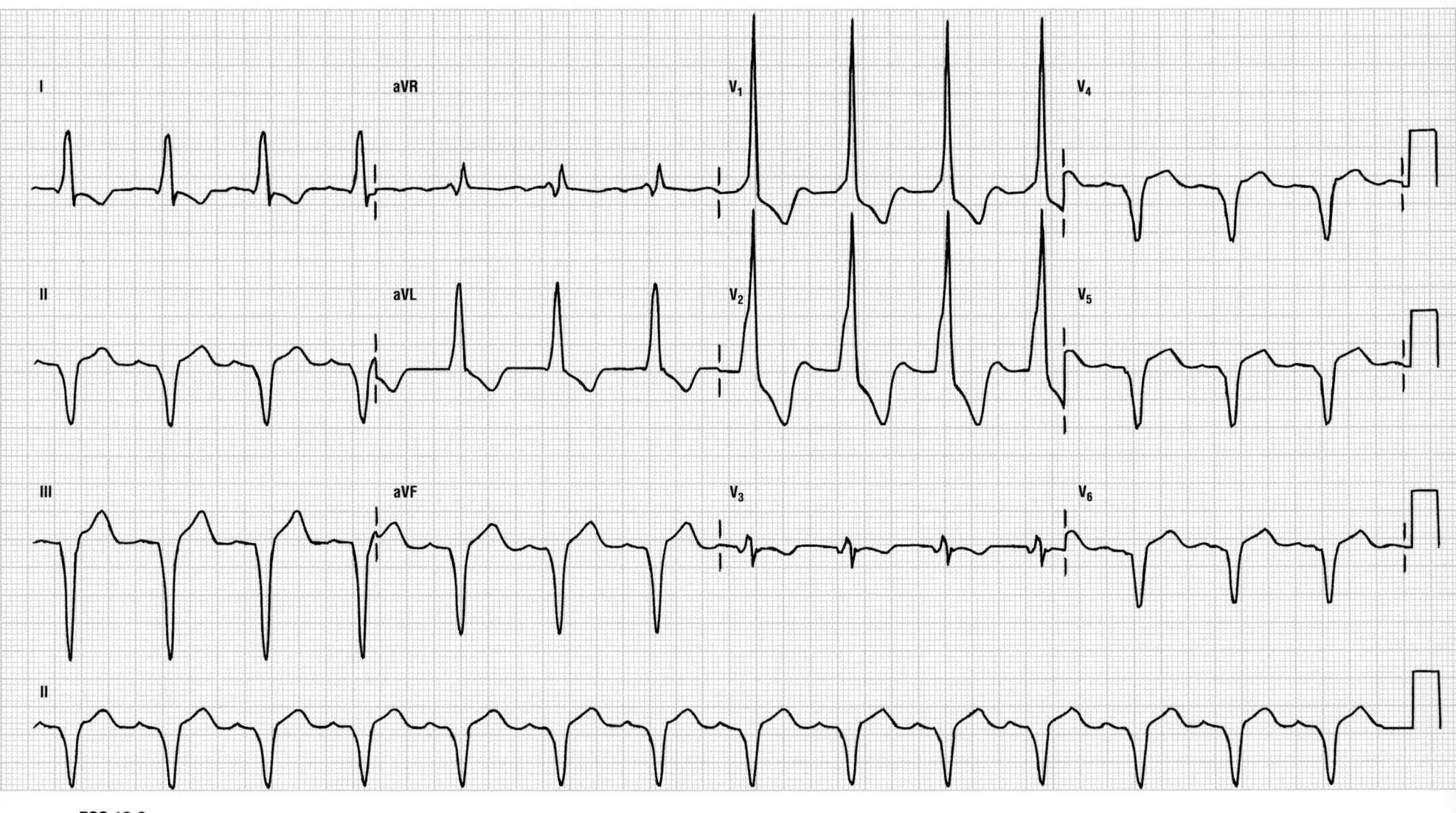

ECG 10-6

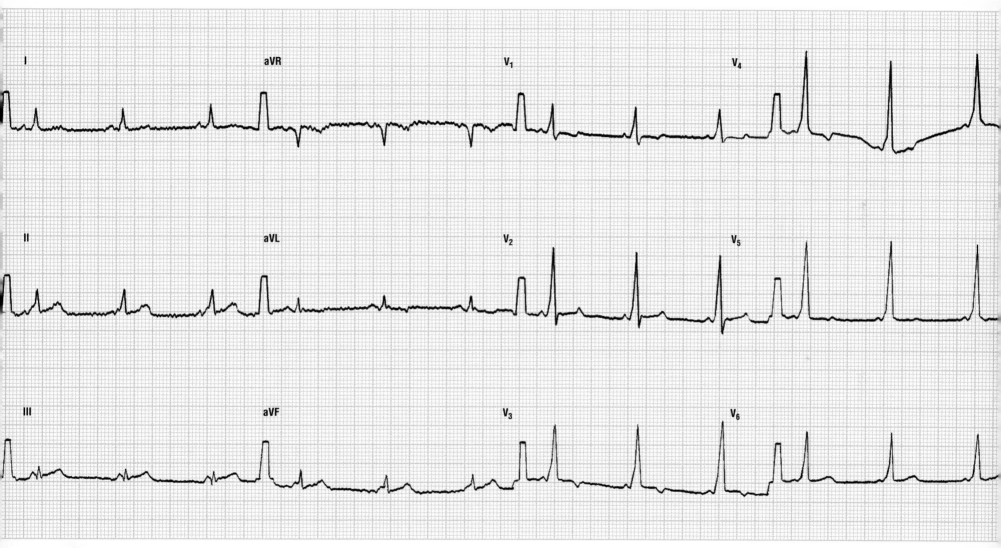

ECG 10-7

ECG CASE STUDIES: **CONTINUED**

ECG 10-8 Both this ECG and the one on the previous page are examples of type A WPW. This ECG has some interesting findings. In addition to the delta wave and ST-T wave abnormalities normally found in WPW, we have the presence of a scooping ST segment with a large upward concavity; the concave segment faces the positive part of the ECG. This concavity looks like someone just scooped it out with an ice cream scoop, as shown in Figure 10-11, doesn't it? If you don't see it, look at V_5 and V_6. This scooping is classic for digoxin drug therapy. The patient was on digoxin at the time the ECG was taken. This scooped ST segment occurs in all circumstances, not just WPW.

Notice the pseudoinfarct pattern in the inferior leads.

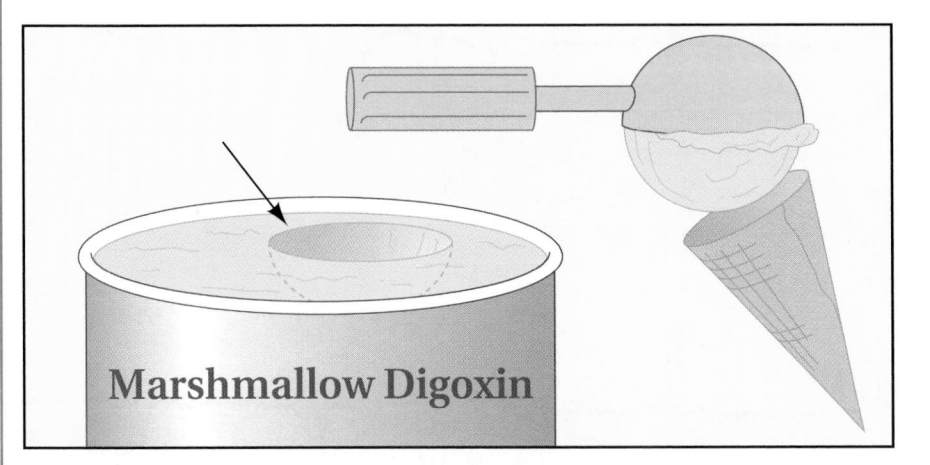

Marshmallow Digoxin

Figure 10-11: The "scoop" in the ST segment due to digoxin drug therapy.

ECG 10-9 This is an example of a wide-complex tachycardia. This patient came into the emergency department with a known history of WPW, which made his management easier. Once again, please review the management of WPW and its associated tachyarrhythmias in a medical textbook.

What is the bundle branch block pattern associated with this tachycardia? It is a right bundle branch block pattern (RBBB). The slurred S waves in leads I and V_6 are clearly evident, as are the rabbit ears — or RSR' — in V_1. Note the ECG on the next page. This is the ECG of the same patient after he was converted. The patient has a WPW type B pattern. Remember that patients with WPW type B usually have the Kent bundle on the right side. This is therefore an example of antidromic conduction leading to the RBBB pattern of the tachycardia.

A simple mnemonic is: The B of type B WPW and the R for right-sided Kent bundle are similar (Figure 10-12).

B R

Figure 10-12: The B representing type B WPW and the R representing right-sided Kent bundle create a simple mnemonic to help remember that patients with WPW type B usually have the Kent bundle on the right side.

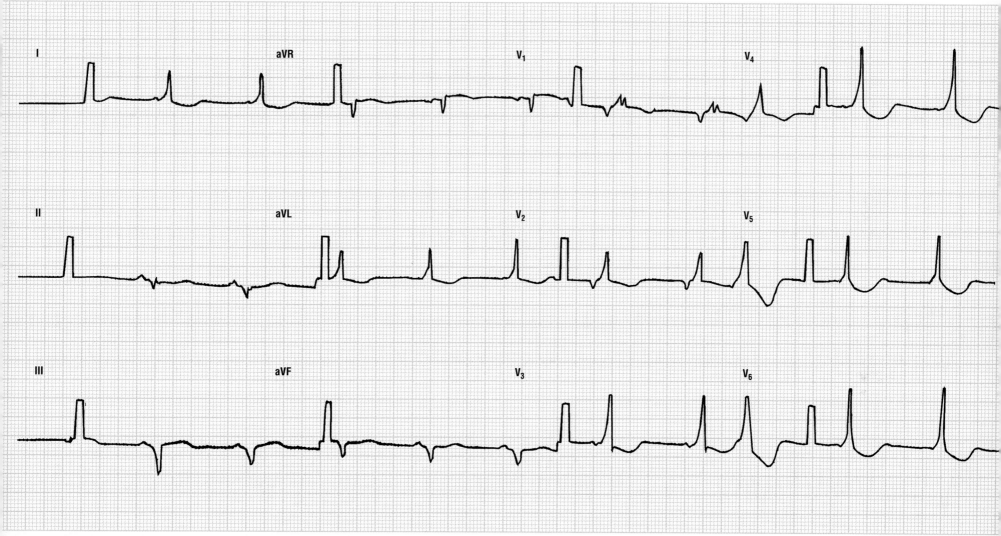

ECG 10-8

ECG CASE STUDIES: **CONTINUED**

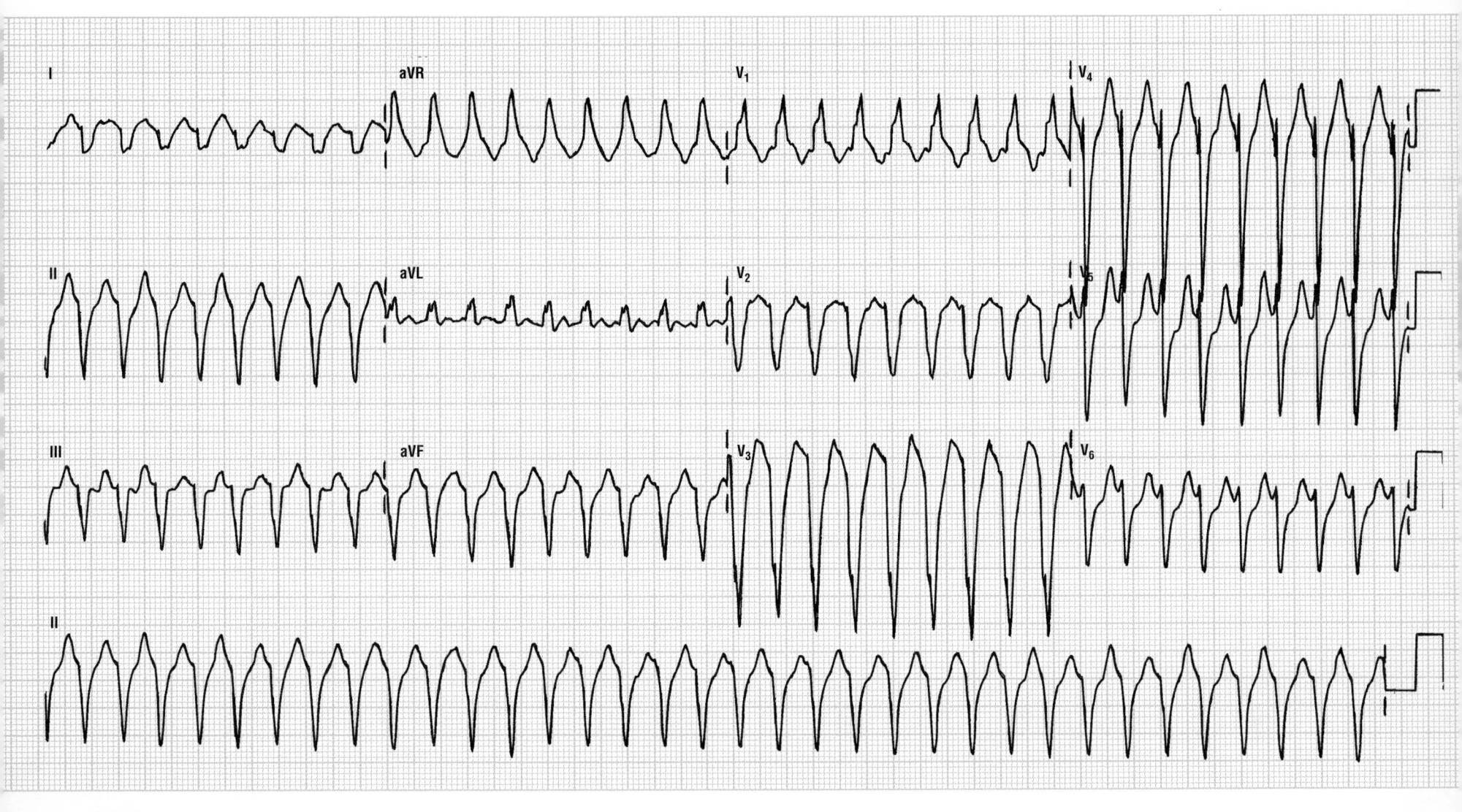

ECG 10-9

3

ECG 10-10 This ECG represents the patient's ECG after he was converted from the wide-complex tachycardia seen on the previous page. If we were to have seen this ECG by itself, it would have been easy to call it a simple left bundle branch block. This is a common problem, and we have to keep the differential diagnosis of a left bundle branch block (LBBB) pattern when we look at an ECG for the first time. The delta waves are difficult to spot because they are small, but they can be seen in many leads.

Beware of any tachycardia that is over 250 BPM, especially a wide one. If the heart rate is above 250, there is usually a bypass tract associated with it. Any tachycardia at a rate of 300 has to be associated with a bypass tract, because it is much faster than any that can be transmitted through the AV node.

When the tachycardia is above 250 BPM, it is difficult to differentiate any of the components of the complex, so diagnosis will be difficult at best. The key is to remember that there could be a bypass tract involved; you want to be careful in the drugs you use to treat this patient. A drug that further slows conduction through the AV node may worsen an already poor situation. Our advice: don't be afraid to sedate and electrically cardiovert the patient. In this situation, it is safer than the unknown problems that IV medications can induce.

REMINDER:

Be careful not to confuse a normal intrinsicoid deflection with a delta wave.

2

ECG 10-11 It's pretty obvious that this patient is very tachycardic at about 280 BPM. Remember that we mentioned that WPW is associated with fast tachycardias? Well, this is another example. Note the difference between this example and those on the two pages previous. This one is a narrow-complex tachycardia, meaning that the QRS complex is less than 0.12 seconds wide. The other one is an example of a wide-complex tachycardia with a QRS complex width more than 0.12 seconds. Take a look at the next ECG. It belongs to the same patient, except that it is much slower at this point.

3

ECG 10-11 This patient has a heart rate of about 280 BPM. As mentioned earlier, if the heart rate is above 250, think about a bypass tract. This patient spontaneously converted and was found to have intermittent WPW (see next ECG). This is an example of orthodromic conduction causing a narrow-complex tachycardia. There are no clearly discernible P waves, so the rhythm could be paroxysmal supraventricular tachycardia (PSVT) or 1:1 conduction of an atrial flutter. The atrial flutter would have to be slower than the traditional 300 BPM because the heart rate is about 280 BPM. There is ST depression everywhere on this ECG, which is probably subendocardial ischemia secondary to the tachycardia.

ECG CASE STUDIES: CONTINUED

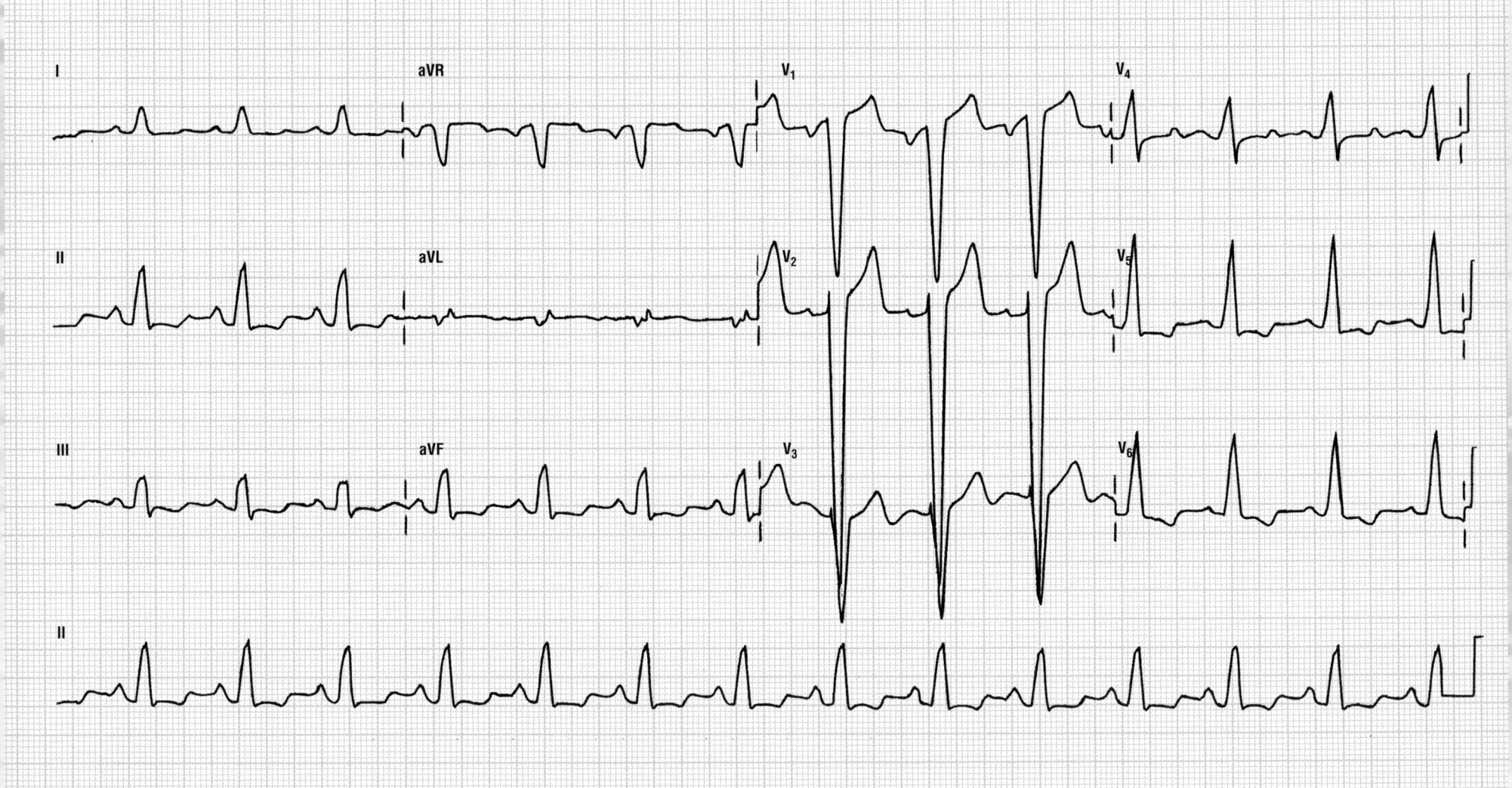

ECG 10-10

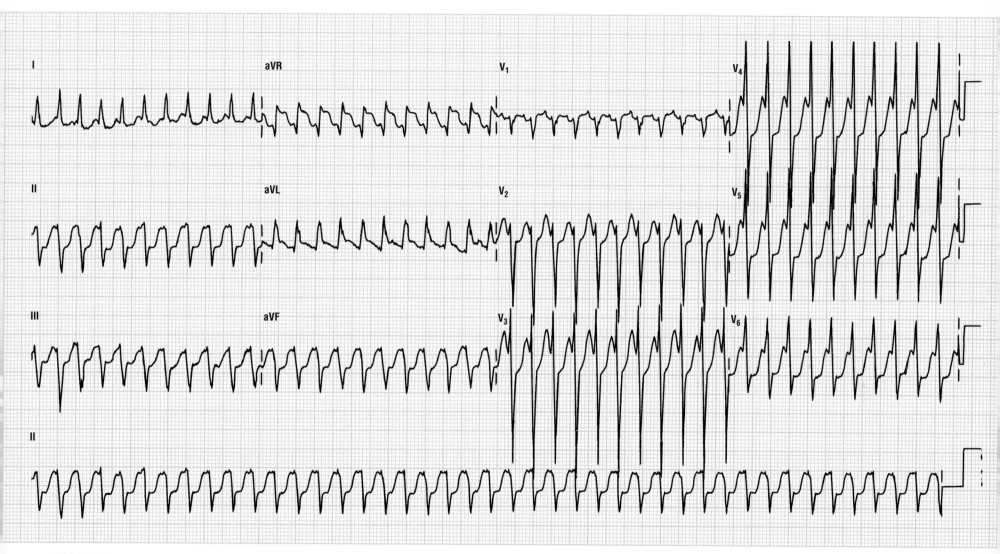

I aVR V₁ V₄

II aVL V₂ V₅

III aVF V₃ V₆

II

ECG 10-11

ECG CASE STUDIES: **CONTINUED**

② ③

ECG 10-12 This is the same patient as that of the previous ECG after his rhythm converted. So what is going on in this one? What is the rhythm? Well, this is a very tricky rhythm to figure out because it is irregularly irregular with a lot of different looking complexes throughout. The ECG complexes with the star on top show a more positive QRS complex and some slurring at the onset. If this were your only ECG, you would have a tough call, but knowing that the patient just came out of a very fast tachycardia makes it easier to diagnose intermittent WPW. So what is the rhythm? Atrial flutter with variable block. Look at the P waves in V₁, marked by the vertical black lines, and it will be clearer.

ECG 10-13 Take a really good look at the ECG below. Do you see anything unusual about the QRS complexes? This is an example of intermittent WPW. What is happening is that this patient's impulses occasionally conduct down the AV node, and at other times down the Kent bundle. The ones that conduct normally are the ones with the asterisks. It would be difficult to pick it up from the rhythm strip, but not in leads III, aVL, and V₂. In these leads, the conduction gives rise to markedly different QRS complexes.

Does it make sense that the QRS complexes of normally transmitted impulses and those transmitted through the Kent bundles are different? Sure it does! Think about the routes of transmission to the ventricles. Impulses go through two different anatomic areas to get there. They thus give rise to two different axes, because the partial transmission through the Kent bundles alters the original axis. How transmission through the Kent bundles will affect the axis depends on the anatomic location of the bundles and the size of the delta wave.

ECG 10-12 This ECG shows atrial flutter with variable block, along with intermittent WPW. The atrial rate is identical to the tachycardic rate of the previous ECG, making 1:1 conduction of an atrial flutter the answer to the rhythm in that previous ECG. V₁ is your only clue to the diagnosis. Look at the P waves and map them out with your calipers. The variability of the response to the P waves makes the morphology of the QRS complexes different. You can still see some of the delta component breaking through in some of the complexes. There is still some ST depression globally, which could be ischemia versus rate-related changes.

② QUICK **REVIEW**

1. The WPW pattern is always visible in a patient with WPW syndrome. True or False.

2. The WPW pattern is never intermittent. True or False.

3. The delta wave is caused by an early impulse transmission through the Kent bundle. True or False.

1. False. Most patients with WPW have a concealed pathway.
2. False 3. True

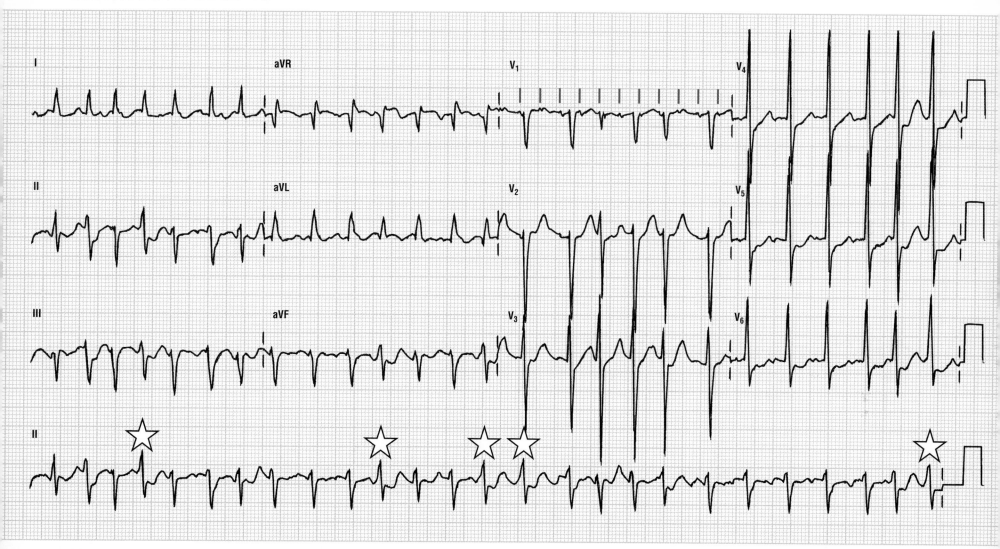

ECG 10-12

ECG CASE STUDIES: CONTINUED

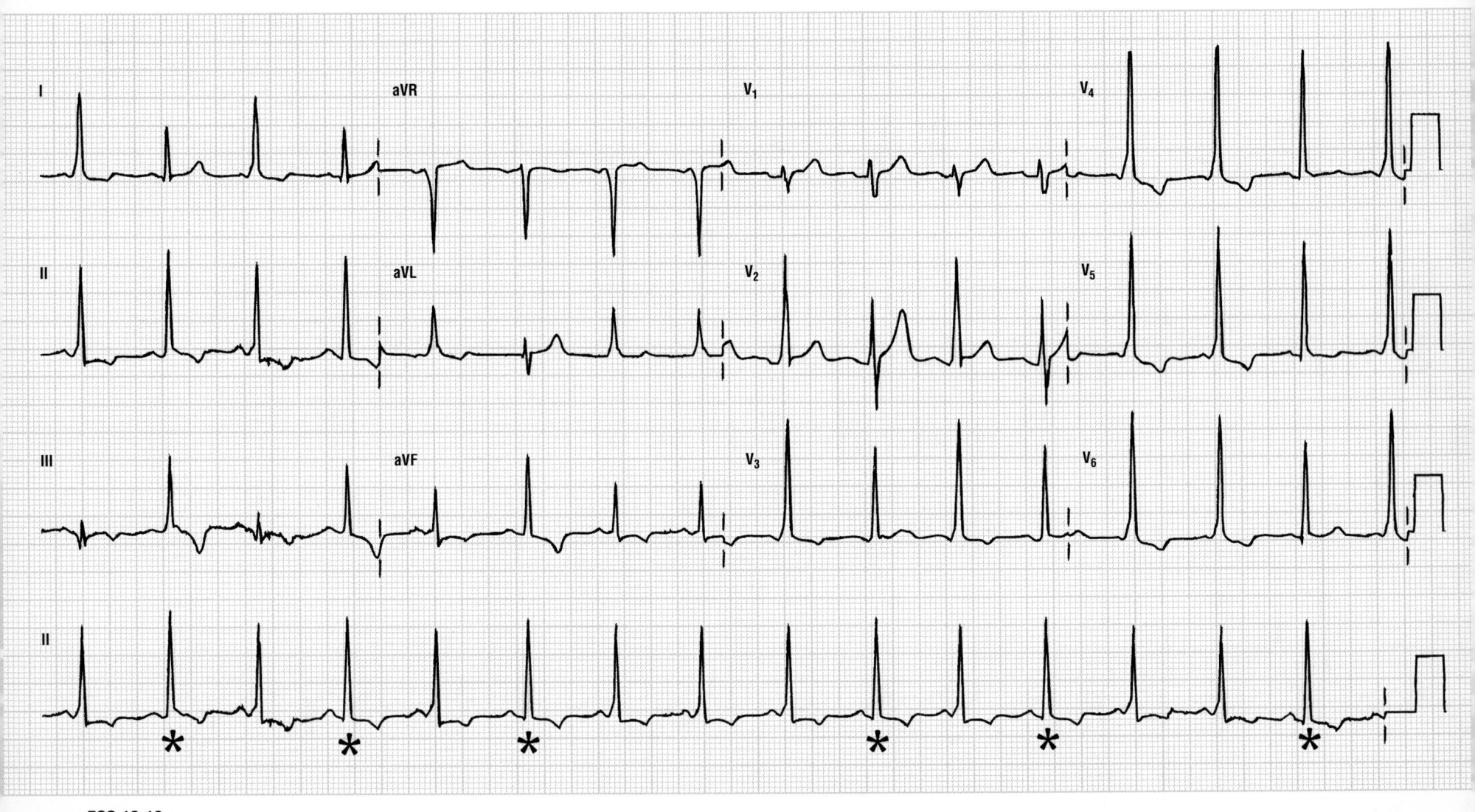

I   aVR   V₁   V₄

II   aVL   V₂   V₅

III   aVF   V₃   V₆

II

ECG 10-13

ECG 10-14 This is one of our all-time favorite ECGs. It stumps about 98% of the people who try to interpret it. Can you figure it out?

It is simpler to interpret in this book because it is in the PR interval section and, in particular, the WPW section. The key to interpreting this ECG is to look at the rhythm strip. Look especially at the last two complexes. This is another example of intermittent WPW with the transition to the normal beat occurring in those last two complexes. What makes this ECG so hard to analyze is that these two complexes are at the transition points to V_4 to V_6.

The WPW in this ECG is type B. There is a pseudoinfarct pattern in lead aVL and the usual ST-T wave changes are scattered throughout. Note that the PR interval is not shortened.

Remember, to analyze an ECG you need to be thorough and methodical. Because you are at Level 3, you should already have some method established. If you do not, we recommend that you review Chapter 17: Putting It All Together.

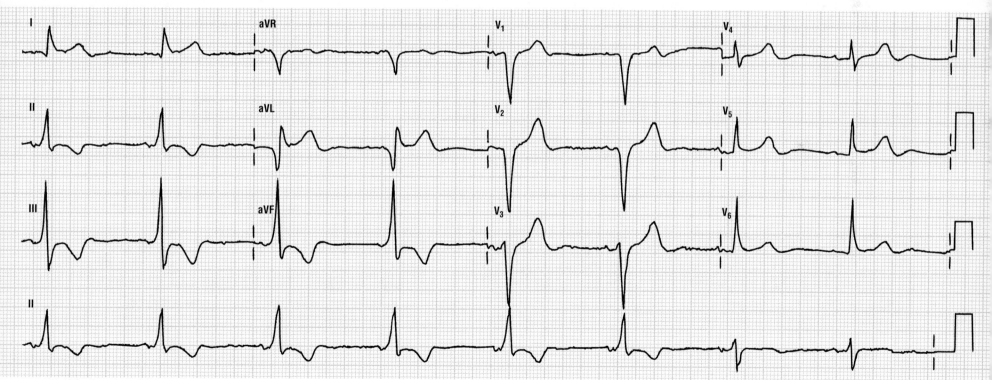

ECG 10-14

NOTE

A Few Words About Atrioventricular Blocks . . .

AV blocks are conduction disturbances in the AV node or the bundle of His. They cause abnormalities or prolongation of the PR interval, or in the extreme case, a complete disruption of impulse transmission to the ventricles. Don't get them confused with bundle branch blocks. These are blocks in either the left or right bundles or their fascicles (left anterior or left posterior), or a combination of blocks.

First-degree AV block is a prolongation of the normal physiologic block. It usually occurs at the level of the AV node itself and is caused by organic heart disease. However, it can also be caused by drug toxicity (digoxin, calcium channel blockers, tricyclic antidepressants), hypercalcemia, hypothermia, and instances of increased vagal stimulation such as inferior wall myocardial infarctions.

There are two kinds of second-degree AV blocks: Mobitz I, or Wenckebach, and Mobitz II. Mobitz I is caused by a defective AV node that has a long refractory period. When the first P waves reach the node, it gets slowed down. Because the SA node is functioning normally, it starts another beat that now reaches the AV node earlier in its refractory period. The result is that the PR interval is longer because it takes that much more time to transmit. The next P reaches it earlier and takes longer to transmit, and so on. This continues until one of the P waves reaches the node at a point when it will not conduct the impulse, so it drops a QRS. This leads you to the Wenckebach pattern, which is grouped beatings with prolongation of the PR interval until one is not transmitted. The ratio of Ps to QRSs is variable and can be 2:1, 3:1, 4:1, or more. Whenever you see grouped beating, think of Wenckebach. Some additional criteria that may help you: the R-R interval will get shorter until the dropped beat, and the distance between the QRS complexes with the dropped beats is less than twice the shortest R-R interval in the group.

Mobitz II is more dangerous and is a possible harbinger of complete block. In this type, the PR interval remains constant, but there are still intermittent dropped QRS complexes.

Note that when there is a 2:1 complex, you cannot tell if it is Mobitz I or Mobitz II. When you see such a pattern, obtain a long rhythm strip and see if there are any other groups that may help you determine the type of block. Normally, the type of block will be continuous throughout the strip.

In third-degree block, there is a complete block of the impulse at the AV node, and the P waves and the QRS complexes are dissociated from each other. Each is marching to its own drummer, so to speak. The usual atrial beat is sinus rhythm or sinus tachycardia. The ventricular beats are either junctional or ventricular in origin, and so may be either narrow or wide. There are always more P waves than QRS complexes. If there are the same number of Ps and QRS complexes, we say it is AV dissociation, not third-degree heart block. This is a fine nomenclature problem. Once again, we are not going to go into treatment, but just in case, have a temporary pacer nearby.

Prolonged PR Interval

A prolonged PR interval is one that is longer than 0.20 seconds. When you are confronted by a prolonged PR interval, ask yourself a few questions:

1. Are all of the PR intervals and P waves the same? If they are, you are probably dealing with first-degree heart block. If they are not, you have to think of premature atrial complexes, wandering pacemaker, multifocal atrial tachycardia, or another type of block.

2. Do the PR intervals vary consistently?
   (a.) Are all of the Ps the same?
   (b.) Are the PR intervals progressively lengthening?
   (c.) Do you have grouped beating (Figure 10-13)?
   (d.) Are the Ps and QRSs dissociated? If the P waves are all different, you are definitely talking about wandering pacemaker or multi-focal atrial tachycardia (MAT). If the Ps are the same, start thinking about what type of block is present. Is it Mobitz I or II? Is it third-degree AV block or AV dissociation? Should I get a rhythm strip? Finally, and most importantly, what does the patient look like? You need to put it all together to obtain the right answer.

Look at some examples on the following pages and see if you can come up with the right answer. By the way, if you disagree with us on any of the ECGs, that's OK. You're wrong, but it's OK. (Just kidding.) Remember, there are always disagreements about interpretation . . . even between your own interpretations on different days. This is a scientific fact verified in multiple studies.

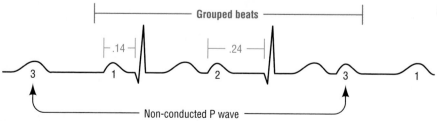

ECG 10-15 How long is the PR interval? It is a little over 0.20 seconds. This is an example of first-degree heart block. The P waves show some left atrial enlargement in V_1, but otherwise the Ps aren't remarkable. There is some slight PR depression in leads III and aVF, but these are not found in any other leads, so pericarditis is probably not present.

Remember, at this point you should only be looking at the sections of the ECG that we have reviewed in detail: the P waves and the PR intervals. When you revisit this ECG at Level 3, you will be in for some other juicy findings.

ECG 10-15 So what do you want to do with this patient? He just has some mild first-degree heart block, right? WRONG. This patient has changes consistent with an AMI in the inferior leads, and possibly involving the right ventricle. The patient has significant Q waves in II, III, and aVF, with ST segment elevation, as well. In addition, the patient has ST depression in aVL. There is some ST elevation in V_1 to V_5, with poor RR progression. The ST segment elevation in V_1 with an inferior AMI is classic for right ventricular involvement. Right-sided leads are recommended even though the ST elevation in V_1 is only about 0.5 mm.

Figure 10-13: Grouped beats.

ECG CASE STUDIES: **CONTINUED**

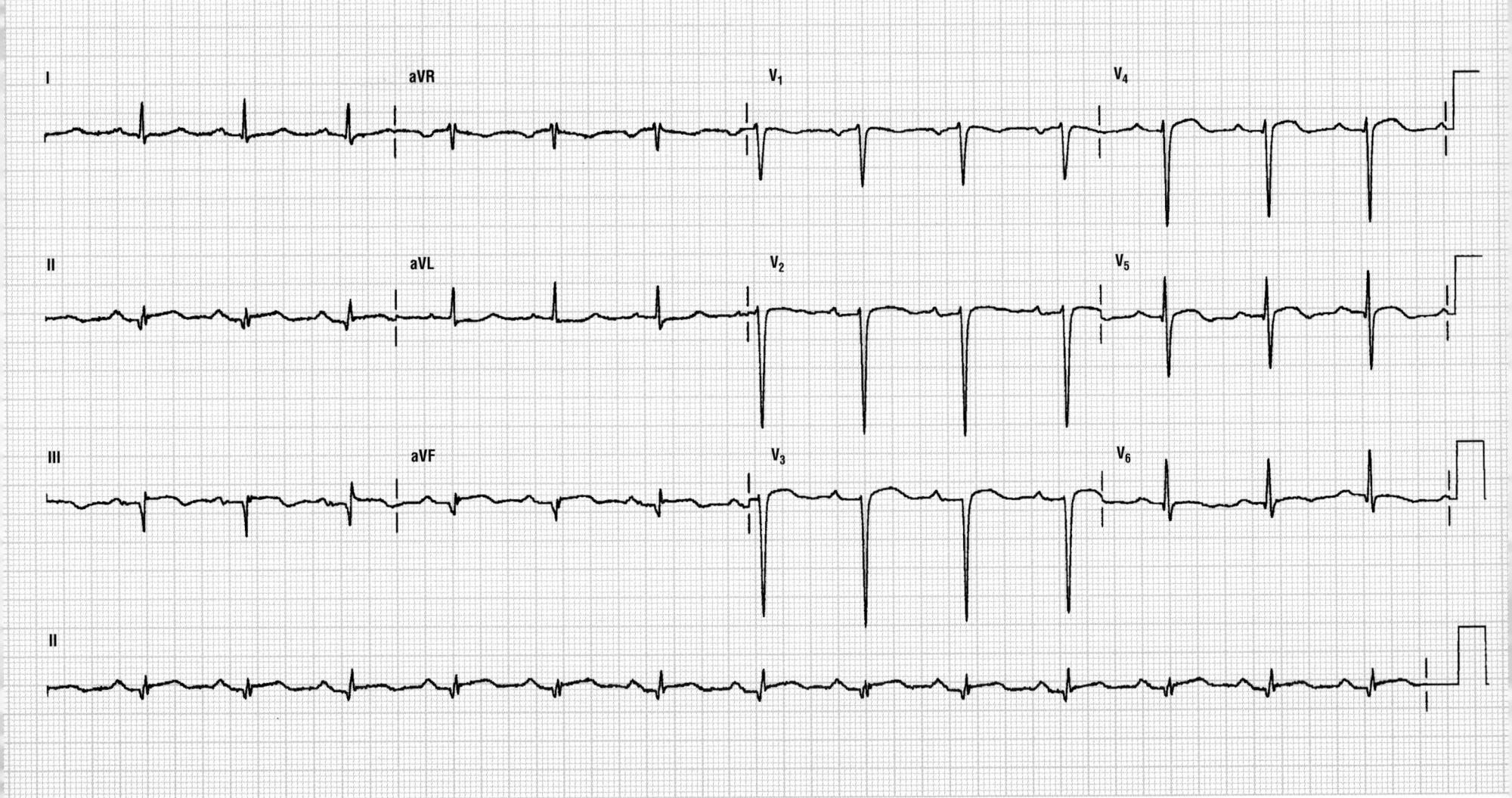

ECG 10-15

②

ECG 10-16 Here is another example of first-degree heart block. What we have tried to do in the three representative examples on first-degree block is to show you a progression of PR prolongation. Remember that this interval can vary significantly.

Did you evaluate the P waves? If you did, you saw the P-pulmonale that is present on this ECG. When you continue to go through this book, try to evaluate the ECG for all of the items covered previously. That way, when you reach the end of the book, you will be better prepared to go on to Level 3 if you wish.

③

ECG 10-16 This ECG shows an axis of about zero degrees and some lateral T wave abnormalities consistent with possible ischemia. There is also a P-pulmonale present.

> REMINDER:
>
> AV blocks and bundle branch blocks are different.

②

ECG 10-17 The right half of the ECG below shows a long first-degree heart block. How long is the PR interval in this ECG? About 0.48 seconds, which makes this a very long PR interval. Now, let's look at the first half of the ECG. The first complete complex is similar to the ones at the end of the ECG and represents a normal complex for this patient. Then there is a much longer pause between the first and second complexes. In addition, this second complex has a shorter PR interval, making you think that this was not normally conducted. It appears to be a sinus escape beat. The pause between the second and third complexes is again long, but this time the PR interval for the third complex is normal. This is not a sinus arrhythmia as it encompasses only one complex.

③

ECG 10-17 What kind of block does this patient have? It is definitely a right bundle branch block with slurred S waves in V_6 and an RSR' complex in V_1. The axis is in the extreme right quadrant. It is a wide block and has some bizarre ST-T wave abnormalities. Look at V_1 and V_2. Can you make any statements about the ST depression and the T waves? Well, you can say that the ST segments are depressed and that the T waves are concordant; they are in the same direction as the last part of the QRS complex. Could this represent a posterior AMI? Sure it could. You would need some clinical correlation and an old ECG to tell definitively.

ECG CASE STUDIES: CONTINUED

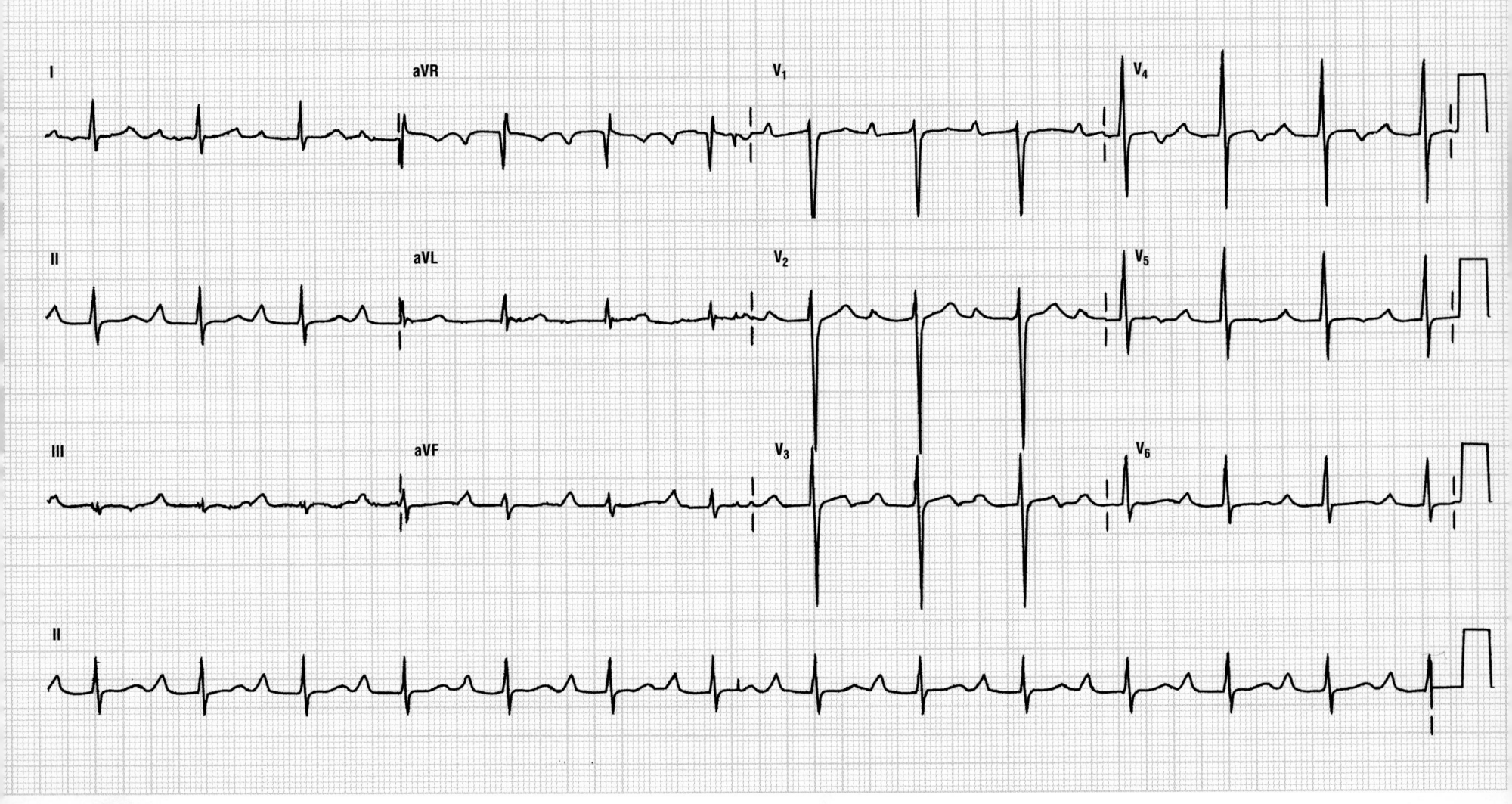

ECG 10-16

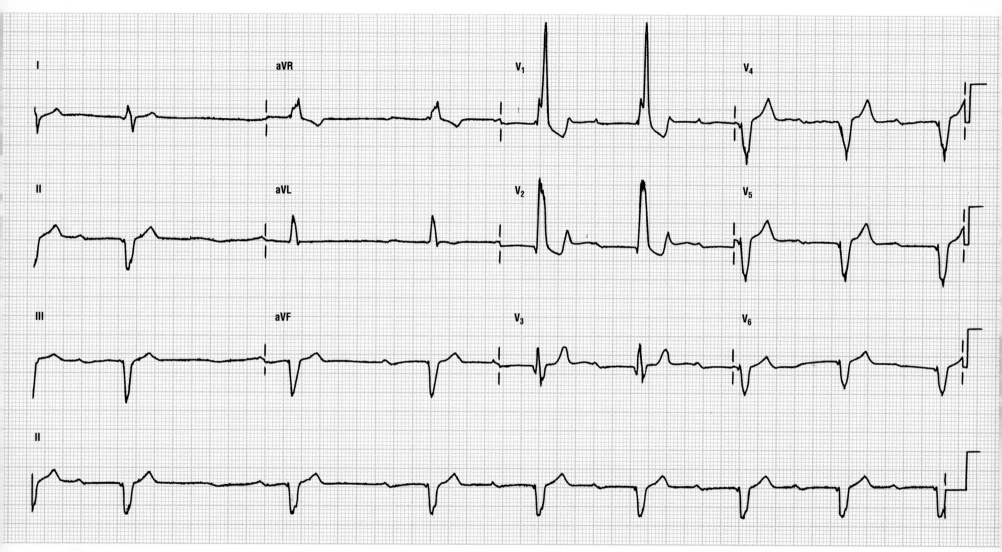

ECG 10-17

ECG CASE STUDIES: **C O N T I N U E D**

ECG 10-18 For those of you who were astute enough to pick it up, this is the same patient that was reviewed in the first-degree heart block section earlier. Now the rhythm is completely different. Do you see any grouping on this ECG? Yes, there are two full groups of three complexes each. Now, let's look at the PR intervals . . . are they the same? No, they seem to get longer in each succeeding complex. In addition, the RR intervals are shorter in each successive complex in a set. This is an example of Mobitz I or Wenckebach second-degree heart block in someone with a prolonged PR interval. Do you see the P wave of the dropped beat? No, because that P is buried inside the T wave of the third QRS complex. Whenever you see a grouped beating situation, you have to think of second-degree heart block!

ECG 10-18 What is the differential diagnosis of tall R waves in the right precordial leads?

1. Normal young children and adolescents
2. Right bundle branch block
3. Wolff-Parkinson-White syndrome
4. Right ventricular hypertrophy
5. Posterior myocardial infarction

How do you tell the difference between them? Look at the company they keep! Is the patient young? Do you have slurred S waves or delta waves? Is there any evidence of right atrial enlargement (RAE) or RAD? Does the patient look like a chronic obstructive pulmonary disease (COPD) patient or one having an AMI?

ECG 10-19 First of all, don't panic. This is yet another ECG format, and it is not much different from the ones you are used to. If you look at the top four strips and mentally erase the other two, you have the format that we usually use in this book. This format is useful in that you have three rhythm strips, and all of them are occurring simultaneously. (Note that the same beats are reflected at the same moment in time in all six strips.) This multiple-rhythm-strip capability is very helpful in studying rhythms.

Do you see groupings? Yes, they occur in sets of two complexes. Are there P waves? Yes. Are the PR intervals getting longer? Yes. Are there nonconducted P waves? Yes, the third one in each group. What is the rhythm? Mobitz I or Wenckebach second-degree heart block. Piece of cake! By the way, the patient also has first-degree heart block.

ECG 10-19 Take a look at the third P wave in each set, and look at them in all of the leads. In which lead is it easiest to see them? Leads aVL, V_1, and V_2. Can you figure out why? Because these are the leads in which the T wave is the flattest or most isoelectric. The P wave can come out in all of its glory in these leads. This concept is helpful when you order a rhythm strip. If you are looking for P waves, order a strip that includes those leads. That is what we have done in this case. When using a rhythm strip, use the leads that will yield the most useful information. You can find out which ones by getting a standard 12-lead.

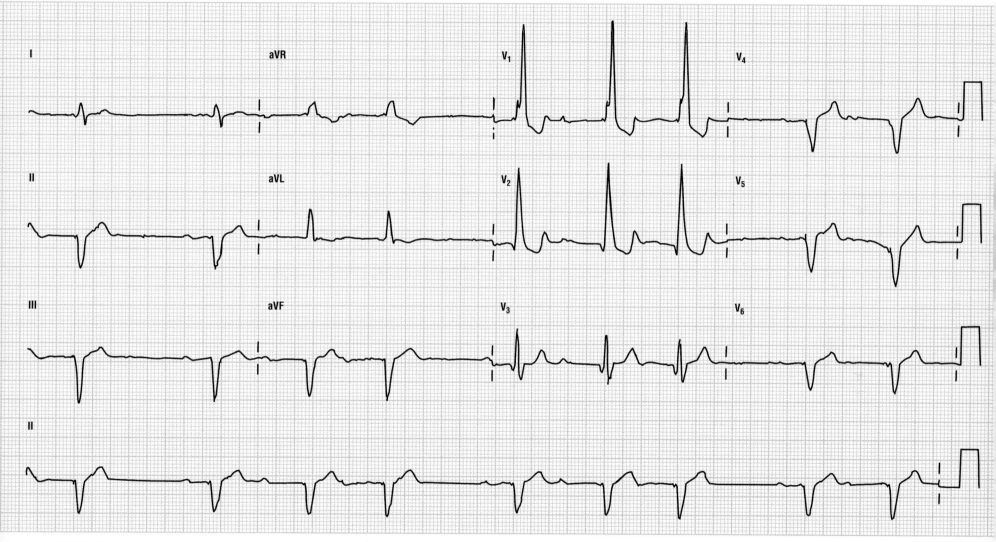

ECG 10-18

ECG CASE STUDIES: CONTINUED

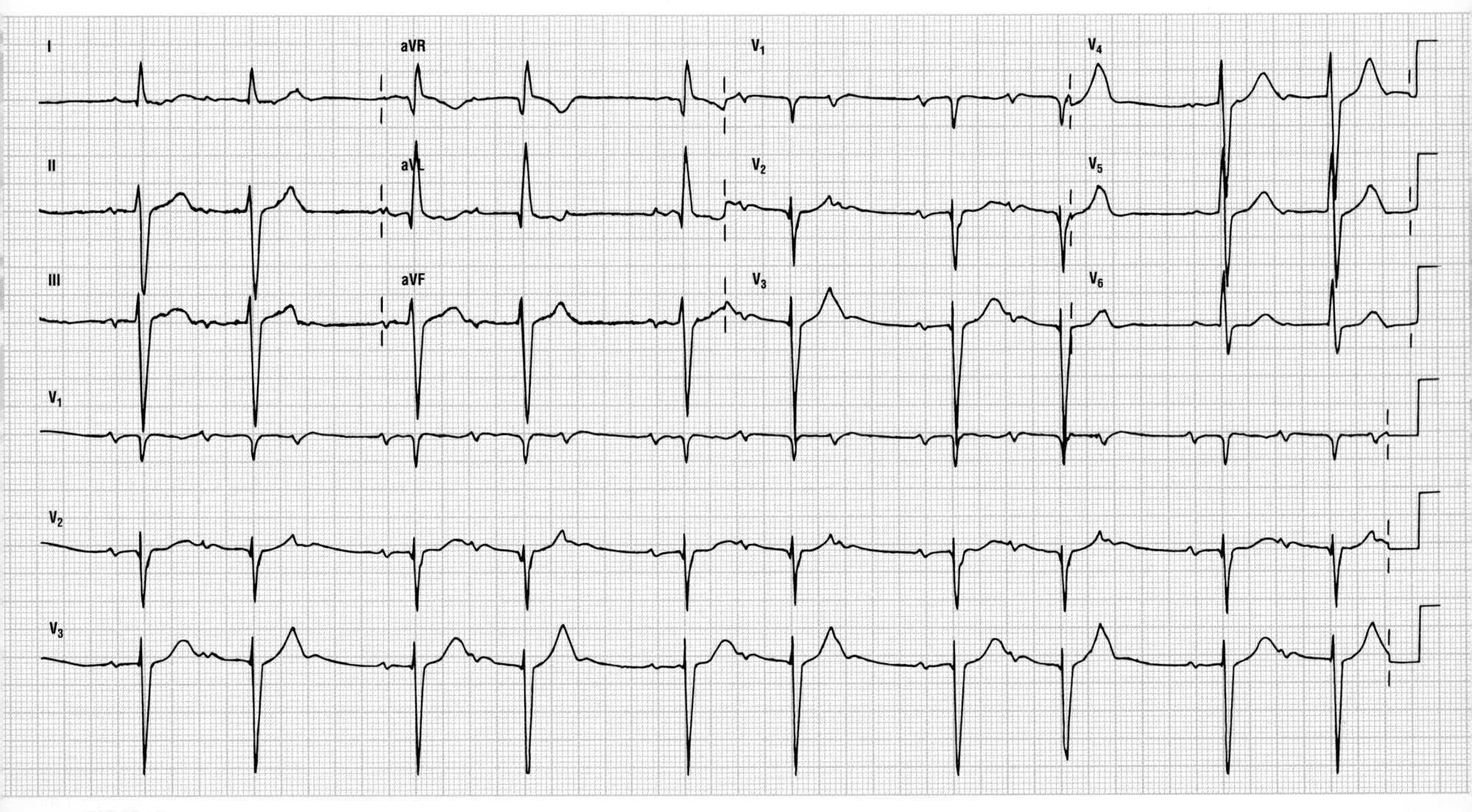

ECG 10-19

②

ECG 10-20 Let's analyze this ECG. The first thing to do is to find P waves that you can clearly identify. Now place your calipers between two of these in the first part of the ECG. Walk your calipers back and forth, identifying the rest of the P waves in the ECG. When you do that on the section covered by the blue line, you notice that the first eight beats are on time and as scheduled. The beats marked by green arrows are of a different morphology and timing than the rest. Then they go back to the same P wave morphology as the first group but at a different rate. What occurred is that two beats from an ectopic source fired and reset the underlying sinus node rate. Now look at the association between the P waves and the QRS complexes. Is there any association? NO. This is a third-degree AV block.

③

ECG 10-20 The patient has an underlying RBBB morphology with slurred S waves in I and V_6, and RSR' complex in V_1. The T waves are symmetrical and somewhat peaked in leads V_3 and V_4. Now look at the T waves in leads II, III, and aVF; these Ts are as tall or taller than the QRS complexes accompanying them. Whenever you see Ts like these, especially when there is an underlying block, you should think about hyperkalemia. We don't know clinically if this patient has hyperkalemia, but you'd better think about it and treat it if it is present. Hyperkalemic T waves are only classically tall, peaked, and narrow in 22% of cases.

②

ECG 10-21 This is an example of third-degree heart block. Notice that the sinus beat is much faster than the ventricular beats. The ventricular rhythm appears to be a junctional escape beat with a rate of about 35 BPM. Note that you cannot rule out a ventricular escape rhythm in this case, but the morphology is suggestive of a supraventricular origin.

Look at the first two complexes. Could you have diagnosed the block from these two? You could if you were looking closely at the two humps on the T waves and you noticed that the two T waves are not identical. Whenever you see two humps on a T wave you should ask yourself, "Could this be a superimposed P wave?" Use your calipers and see if it falls on the middle, or at a multiple, of the P to P interval. If the answer is yes, then it is a superimposed P wave.

③

ECG 10-21 This ECG, in addition to the beautiful example of third-degree heart block, shows a bifascicular block. The patient has a RBBB and left anterior hemiblock (LAH) pattern on his ECG. If you can just imagine that the patient has significant myocardial damage to the conduction system, enough to cause a bifascicular block, then the amount of ischemia or infarction needed to complete the block would be very little. Remember, if you have any patient with ischemia and a bifascicular block you need to keep the possibility of a complete AV block in mind. What should you do with this patient? You should have an external pacemaker available at the bedside, just in case.

ECG CASE STUDIES: CONTINUED

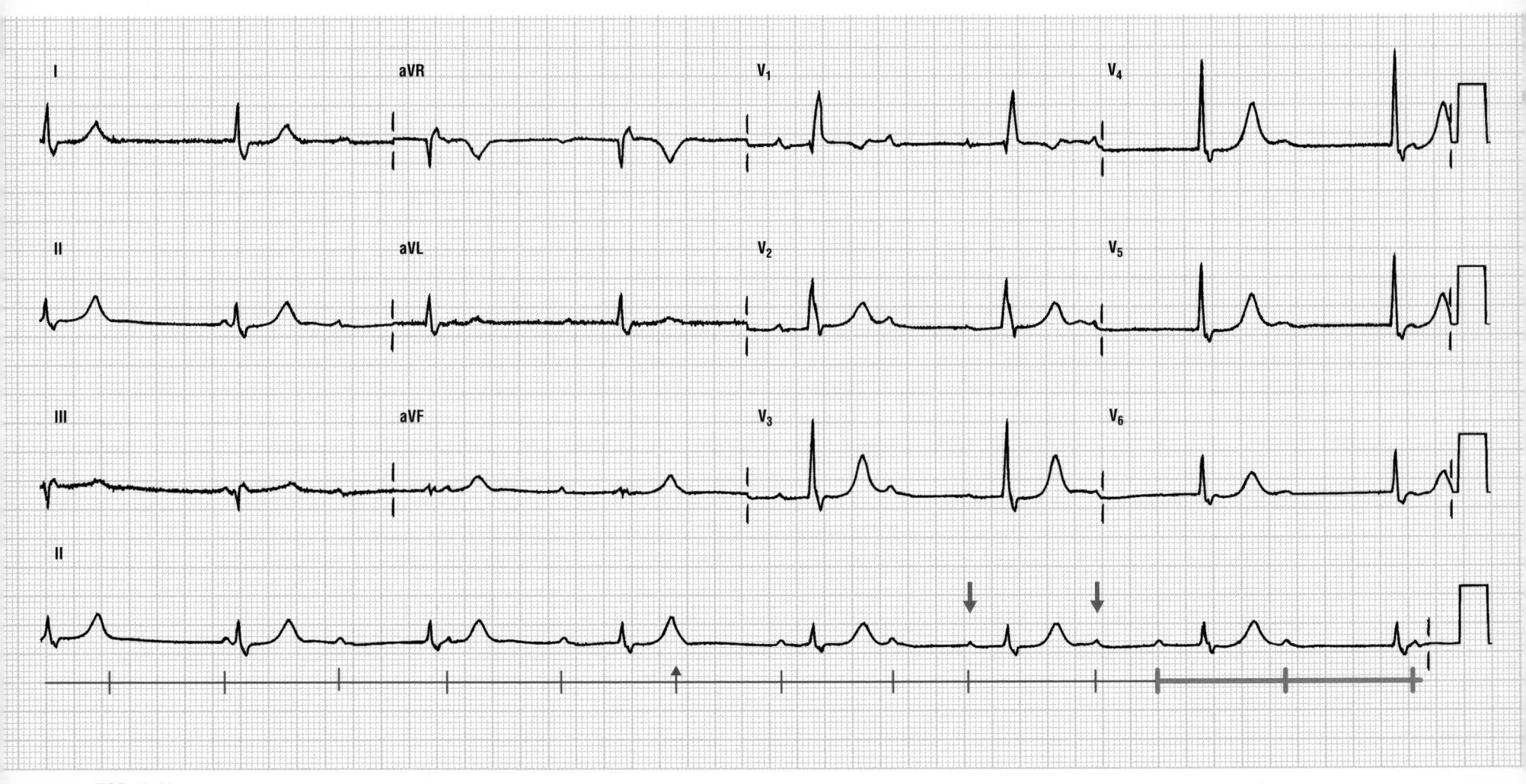

ECG 10-20

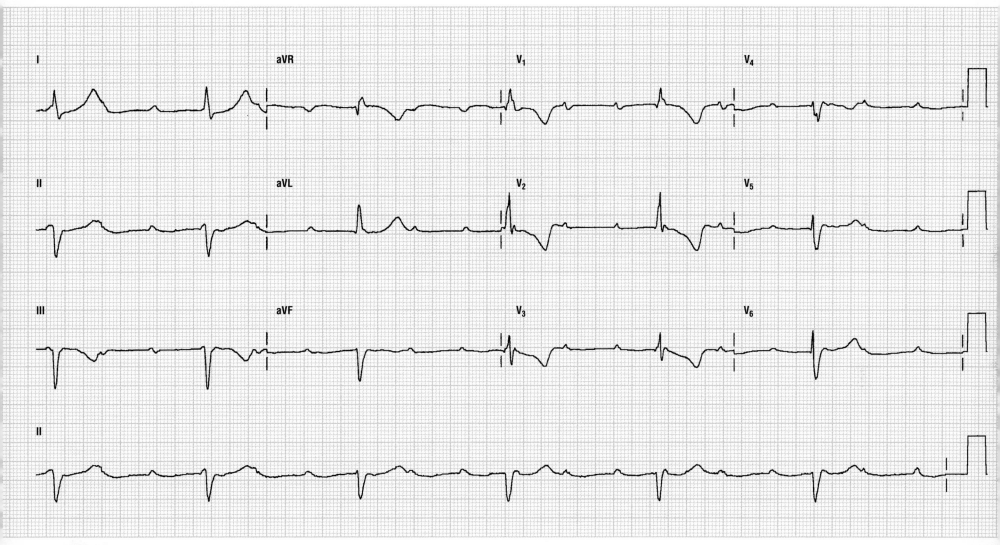

ECG 10-21

ECG CASE STUDIES: **CONTINUED**

2

ECG 10-22 What a mess! First things first: can you identify the P waves? You should be able to see them clearly on the rhythm strip. Use your calipers and map them out. Are they regular? Yes. Do they have any association with the QRS complexes? No. Are there more P waves than QRS complexes? Yes. This is an example of third-degree heart block.

Now, turn your attention to the QRS complexes. First of all, how fast is it going? The ventricular rate is about 20 BPM. Are the QRS complexes wide or narrow? Really wide. A wide-complex rhythm at a rate this slow is a ventricular escape rhythm known as an idioventricular rhythm.

3

ECG 10-22 We really try to stay away from treatment in this book, but occasionally we will make a comment for you to think about. If you had the choice of using either atropine or an external pacemaker on this patient, which would you choose? Somewhat contrary to ACLS, we suggest using the pacemaker. A pacemaker, if it captures, gives you an ability to control the ventricular rate. In contrast, what will your rate and rhythm be after you give atropine? Heaven knows! In an ischemic patient, you can cause further ischemic damage with fast tachycardic rhythms that increase oxygen demand.

REMINDER:

Remember that you can have multiple rhythm abnormalities on the same strip. For example, ECG 10-22 contains a sinus tachycardia as the underlying atrial rhythm and an idioventricular rhythm. These together form a third-degree heart block because the atrial rate is faster than the ventricular rate. All of this information can be put together into the correct and most complete label that you can give this abnormality: a paroxysmal atrial tachycardia with block. In this case, the block leads to the idioventricular rhythm.

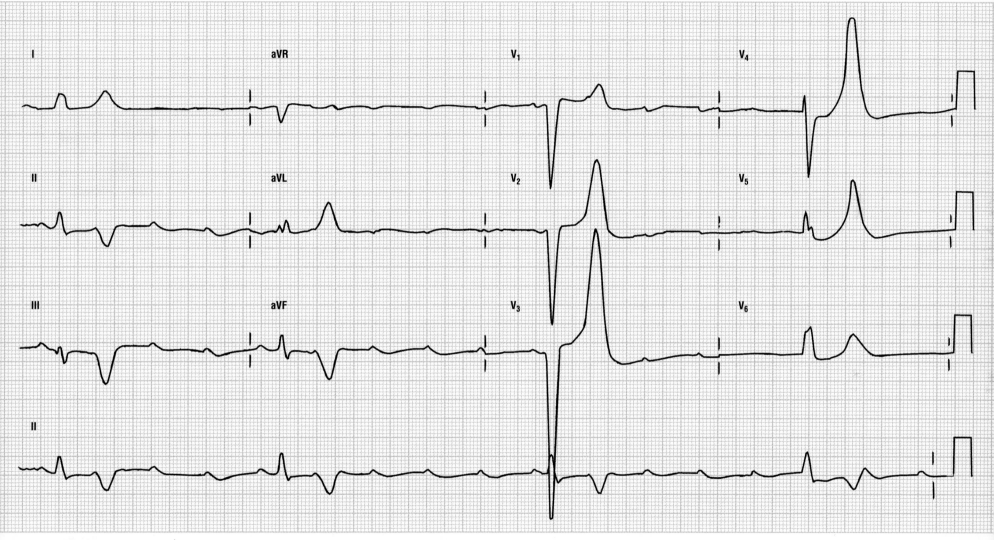

ECG 10-22

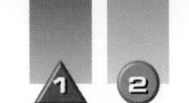

1 CHAPTER IN **REVIEW**

1. The PR interval represents the time frame from the beginning of atrial depolarization to the end of ventricular repolarization. True or False.

2. The differential diagnosis of PR depression includes:
- **A.** Normal variant
- **B.** Pericarditis
- **C.** Atrial infarction
- **D.** All of the above
- **E.** None of the above

3. If the PR interval in lead II is 0.18 seconds long and in V_1 it is 0.22 seconds long, what is the true PR interval?
- **A.** 0.18 seconds long
- **B.** 0.20 seconds long
- **C.** 0.22 seconds long
- **D.** 0.24 seconds long
- **E.** None of the above

1. False 2. D 3. C

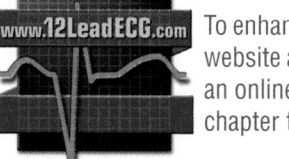

To enhance the knowledge you gain in this book, access this text's website at www.12leadECG.com! This valuable resource provides an online glossary and related web links. To learn more about the chapter topics, simply click on the chapter and view the link.

2 CHAPTER IN **REVIEW**

4. The differential diagnosis of a short PR interval includes:
- **A.** Retrograde junctional P waves
- **B.** Lown-Ganong-Levine syndrome
- **C.** Wolff-Parkinson-White syndrome
- **D.** All of the above
- **E.** None of the above

5. Which of the following is incorrect when discussing WPW syndrome:
- **A.** Shortened PR interval is always present
- **B.** Widened QRS complex ≥ 0.11 seconds
- **C.** Delta waves are present
- **D.** Associated with ST-T wave abnormalities
- **E.** Associated with paroxysmal tachycardias

6. If you see a wide-complex tachycardia, you can assume it is secondary to WPW syndrome. True or False.

7. Q waves in the inferior leads of patients with WPW are always caused by a prior myocardial infarction. True or False.

8. AV blocks and bundle branch blocks are the same. This is just a nomenclature issue. True or False.

9. Grouped beating that has progressively prolonging PR intervals until a ventricular complex is dropped is:
- **A.** First-degree heart block
- **B.** Mobitz I second-degree heart block, or Wenckebach
- **C.** Mobitz II second-degree heart block
- **D.** Third-degree heart block
- **E.** AV dissociation

10. If the sinus rate is 100 BPM, the ventricular rate is 38 BPM, and they are dissociated, we refer to this rhythm as:
- **A.** AV dissociation
- **B.** Third-degree heart block
- **C.** Both A and B are correct
- **D.** None of the above

4. D 5. A 6. False 7. False 8. False 9. B 10. B

CHAPTER **11**

How Are the Waves Made?

The QRS complex, as mentioned in Chapter 6, is composed of three different waves: the Q, R, and S waves. Normally, you do not see every wave in every complex or lead. If you remember, the complexes are just physical manifestations on graph paper of the summation of the vectors generated by the heart's electrical potentials. Depending on the angle and size of these vectors, some portions of the complex may be isoelectric; they are therefore invisible on the ECG. For an example, see the red vector component of lead II in Figure 11-1. Notice that the complexes in Figure 11-1 are displayed in a gradient of color. They slowly switch from red to yellow to blue. This is because the events in cardiac depolarization and repolarization occur sequentially, but they are not discreet events occurring separately. The events in the cycle flow from one to another in an organized pattern. The first area of the ventricles to depolarize is the septum. This area depolarizes in an anterior and rightward direction, represented by the red vector. The main ventricle then begins to depolarize, creating a large vector that is focused posteriorly and inferiorly (yellow vector). Finally, the basilar aspect of the ventricle depolarizes in a posterior-superior direction (blue vector). Note how the three vectors flow into each other to create the QRS complexes in the various limb leads.

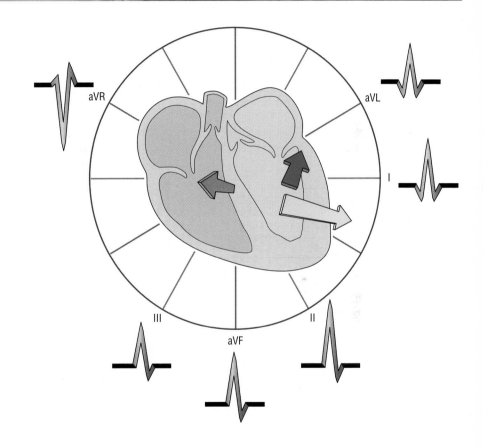

Figure 11-1: Limb leads cut the heart along a coronal plane. The color of the vector is reflected in the waves.

We also explained in Chapter 6 that the limb leads cut the heart electrically into a coronal plane (Figure 11-1), and the precordials cut the heart along a horizontal plane (Figure 11-2). Figure 11-2 demonstrates how the precordial QRSs are created. The vectors are the same as in Figure 11-1, but our view of the angles has changed because we are looking at the heart in a horizontal cross-section rather than from a frontal or coronal cross-section.

Suppose you had a really big left ventricle. What would the yellow vector look like? It would be bigger. The bigger the ventricle, the bigger the vector. Remember that the vector is represented on the ECG by its size and the direction in which it travels. Now imagine a big heart attack that infarcts the anterior wall and makes the heart incapable of producing an electrical force. What would the yellow vector look like? It would be smaller and would point more posteriorly, because there would be less force acting on the front to pull the vector around.

If there were fluid around the heart, a pericardial effusion, what would the vectors look like? The directions would be the same, but they would be represented on the ECG as small complexes because the amount of electrical force is dampened by the fluid. Think of listening to an audio speaker with a blanket on it. The sound would be the same, but lower.

If you think about how physical defects affect the vectors, you can see that the QRS complexes can appear in an infinite number of shapes and sizes.

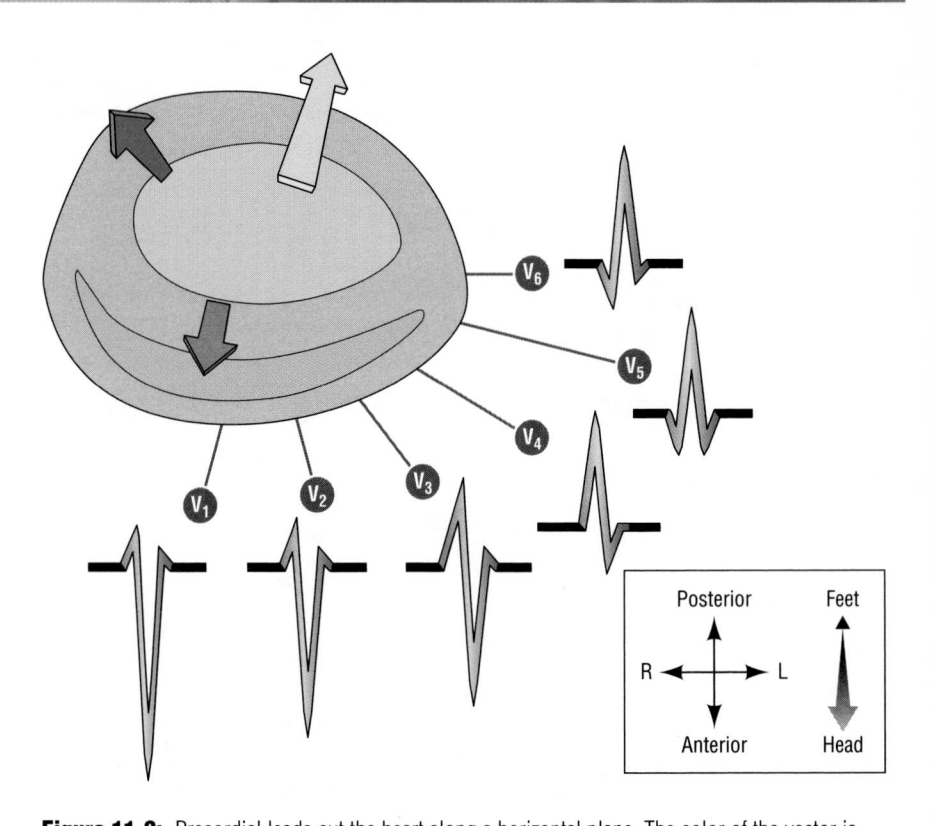

Figure 11-2: Precordial leads cut the heart along a horizontal plane. The color of the vector is reflected in the waves.

What to Look for in the QRS Complex

By now, you more or less know what the QRS complex looks like. If you are unsure, go back and review Chapter 6. This chapter discusses what you are looking at and what it all means.

There are various things to look at when interpreting the QRS complex:

1. Height, or amplitude
2. Width, or duration
3. Morphology
4. The presence of Q waves in an infarct pattern
5. The axis along the frontal plane
6. The transition zone, or Z axis

We will be looking at each one of these individually and in great detail in the next few pages. We'll also take another look at axis and transition zone in Chapter 12.

Be sure to look at the complexes in all of the leads. Don't make the mistake of looking at only one or two leads. Remember the camera analogy for the different leads? You need to have the whole picture in order to interpret the object — in this case, the heart and its vectors.

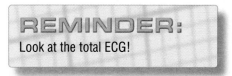

REMINDER:
Look at the total ECG!

QRS Height (Amplitude)

Many factors alter the height of the QRS complex. The main components causing a change are the size and direction of the vectors. The size of the vector reflects the number of action potentials generated by the heart in a certain direction. This, in turn, depends on the number of cells and the size of the ventricles. If the left ventricle is enlarged, or hypertrophied, we say that there is left ventricular hypertrophy (LVH). Likewise, an enlarged right ventricle is called right ventricular hypertrophy (RVH).

Another important aspect that will determine the size of the QRS complex is the direct opposition of various vectors. Remember, infarcted areas and scar tissue are electrically inert. So, when we have a vector opposite an area of infarct, it will be unopposed. Because there is nothing to dampen its size, it will appear out of proportion to the normal ECG.

We mentioned earlier that an effusion can affect the amplitude of the QRS complex. Can you think of anything else that can act like a dampener, similar to an effusion? How about body fat? Obese patients, in general, will have smaller voltages due to excess adipose tissue. Amyloid deposits work in the same way in hypothyroid patients. Can a localized pleural effusion cause decreased voltage in certain leads? Sure it can. This can sometimes be seen by decreased voltage in V_5 and V_6, the ones closest to the area where effusions usually accumulate.

In general, men have a larger amplitude than women, young people have higher amplitudes than the elderly, and the precordials have higher voltages than the limb leads because the electrodes are closer to the heart.

Abnormal Amplitude

Very tall complexes are usually caused by hypertrophy of one or both ventricles, or by an abnormal pacer or aberrantly conducted beat. In Figure 11-3, the large complex is a ventricular premature contraction (VPC).

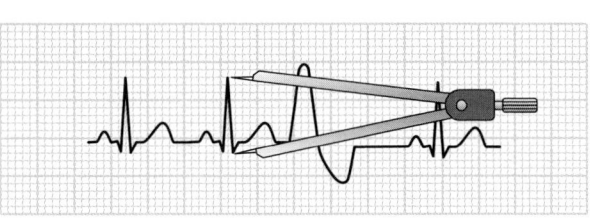

Figure 11-3: Large and small amplitudes.

Low voltage is common. What are the criteria for an abnormally small complex — caused by a pericardial effusion, for instance? A voltage in all of the limb leads of less than 5 mm is abnormal (Figure 11-4). Waves less than 10 mm high in all of the precordials are also highly abnormal (Figure 11-5). An ECG can, however, meet limb lead voltage without meeting precordial criteria. This occurs because the precordial leads are directly overlying the heart on the chest wall. A thin person with an effusion will have larger precordial leads than a more robust person with an effusion. In the heavier person, you have not only the effusion to contend with, but also the size of body wall between the heart and the electrode.

I, II, III, aVR, aVL, aVF

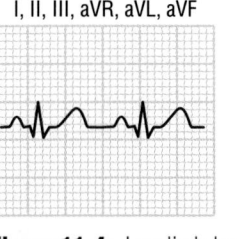

Figure 11-4: Low limb-lead voltage.

$V_1, V_2, V_3, V_4, V_5, V_6$

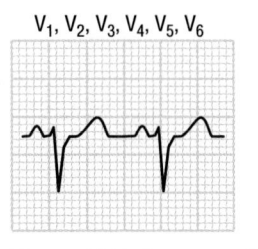

Figure 11-5: Low precordial voltage.

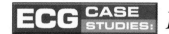

ECG 11-1 Small amounts of pericardial fluid are normal (Figure 11-6). With a larger effusion, you will see the dampening effect, shown in Figure 11-7 and ECG 11-1. ECG 11-1 is an example of this effect.

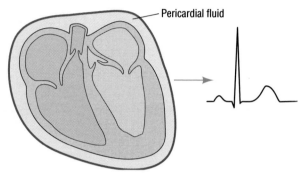

Figure 11-6: ECG wave representing a small amount of pericardial fluid.

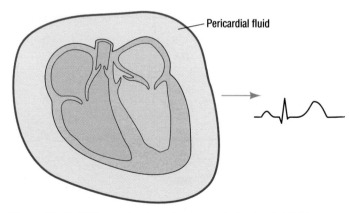

Figure 11-7: ECG wave showing a large amount of pericardial fluid.

ECG 11-2 It is difficult to apply the criteria for atrial enlargement to patients with effusions. However, remembering that all complexes and parts of the complexes are equally affected, the P waves in this patient are very big. Look at the fourth complex. What is it? If you answered a VPC, you are correct! Now, think back on most of the VPCs you've seen. Most of them were quite large because they were spread through the ventricles by direct cell-to-cell contact, and there were few, if any, opposing vectors. In this ECG, however, the VPC is normal in amplitude; the effusion causes a shrinking of the complex (see also Figure 11-8). The precordial leads are very small. Can you figure out why?*

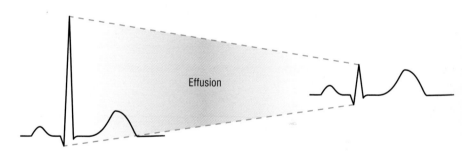

Figure 11-8: The larger the effusion, the smaller the complex!

ECG CASE STUDIES: **CONTINUED**

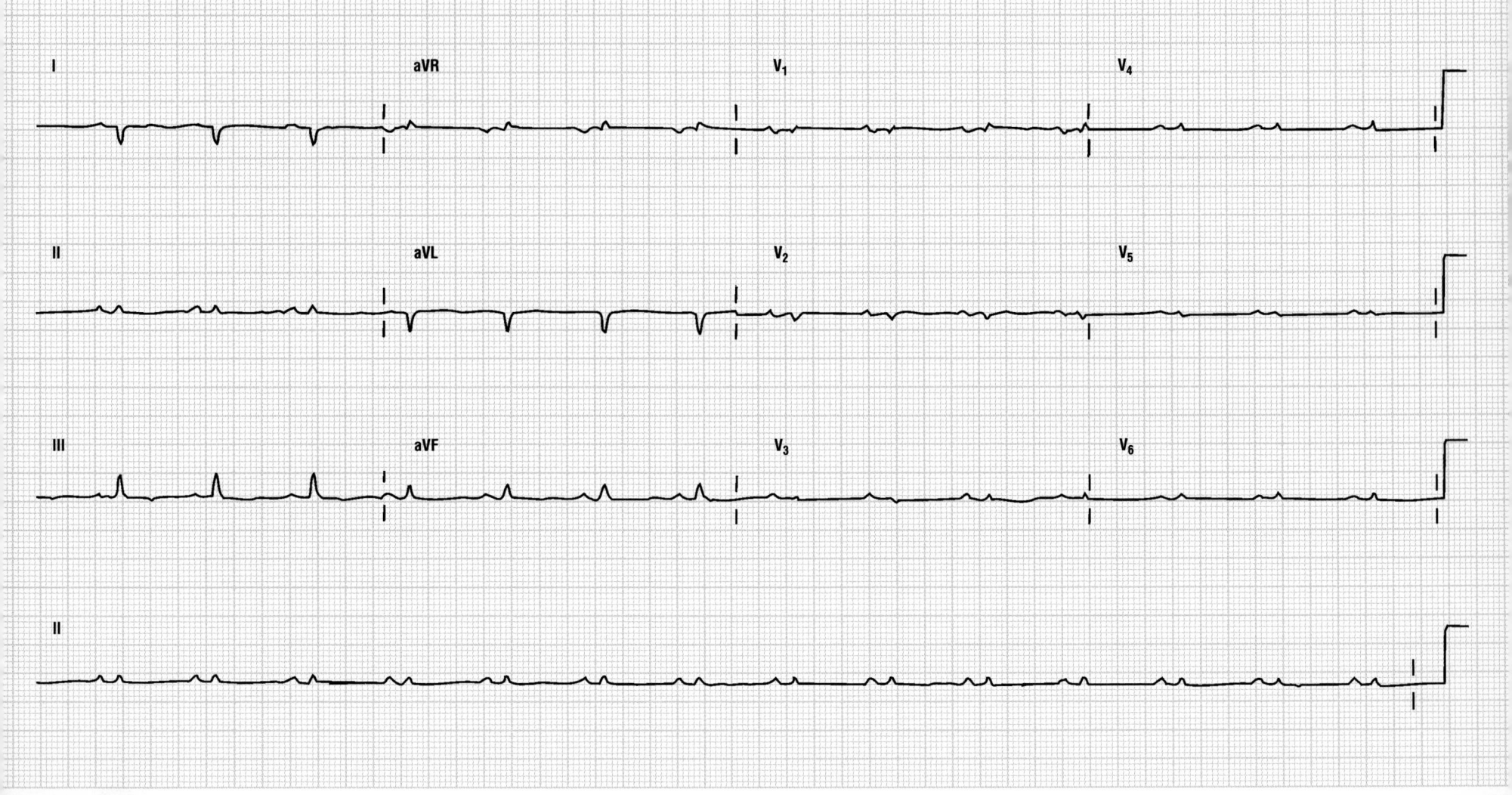

ECG 11-1

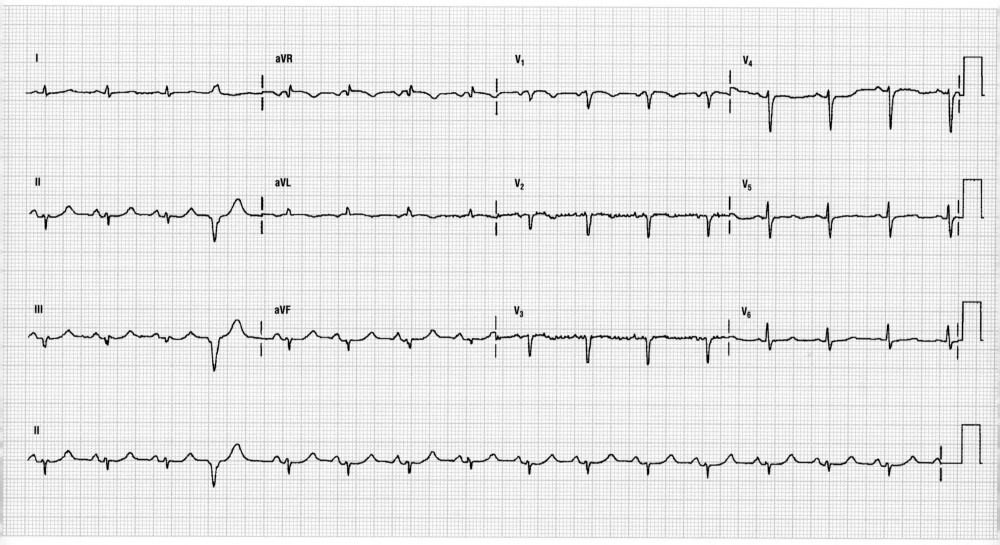

ECG 11-2

*Answer: There is some additional dampening caused by increased size of the body wall secondary to obesity or chronic obstructive pulmonary disease (COPD). This affects the precordial leads more than the limb leads. Remember, as long as the limb-lead electrodes are placed further than 10 cm from the heart, there will be very little variation in QRS size.

CHAPTER **11** • THE QRS COMPLEX

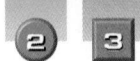

ECG CASE STUDY: *Large QRS Complexes*

2

ECG 11-3 Do you notice the small QRS complexes below? Just kidding. These are the biggest ones we've ever seen. You will probably never see anything quite this big, but it is worthwhile to examine them. The biggest lead is V_2; if you track the S wave down, you will see that it reaches the bottom of the page. The complexes are also very wide, and we will discuss this later in the chapter. There is evidence of mild biatrial enlargement in V_1. Do you notice the J point, the point of transition between the QRS complex and the ST segment? It is about 20 mm above the baseline. This is extremely high, a sign of an acute myocardial infarction (AMI) as we'll see later.

3

ECG 11-3 This is an example of left bundle branch block (LBBB). The patient's previous ECG showed LVH with a very large complex in lead V_2. The new onset of LBBB and the massive ST-segment elevation of 20 mm are consistent with an AMI in this patient. Remember, the criteria for diagnosing AMI in LBBB are:

1. ST elevation of 5 mm in the right precordials

2. ST elevation in the right precordials that is 3 mm higher than that found on the previous ECG

3. Any ST depression in V_1 to V_2

4. ST elevation in the left precordials

5. The presence of abnormal Q waves

2 QUICK **REVIEW**

1. The QRS complex is composed of multiple waves grouped together. True or False.

2. Waves are electrocardiographic representations of vectors. True or False.

3. We can only look at the heart two-dimensionally. True or False.

4. The bigger the vector, the smaller the complex. True or False.

5. Size and direction *both* matter when considering vectors. True or False.

6. In a QRS complex, we should look for:
   A. Height or amplitude
   B. Width or duration
   C. Morphology
   D. Presence of Q waves
   E. Axis in frontal plane
   F. Transition zone or Z axis
   G. All of the above.

1. True 2. True 3. False 4. False 5. True 5. G

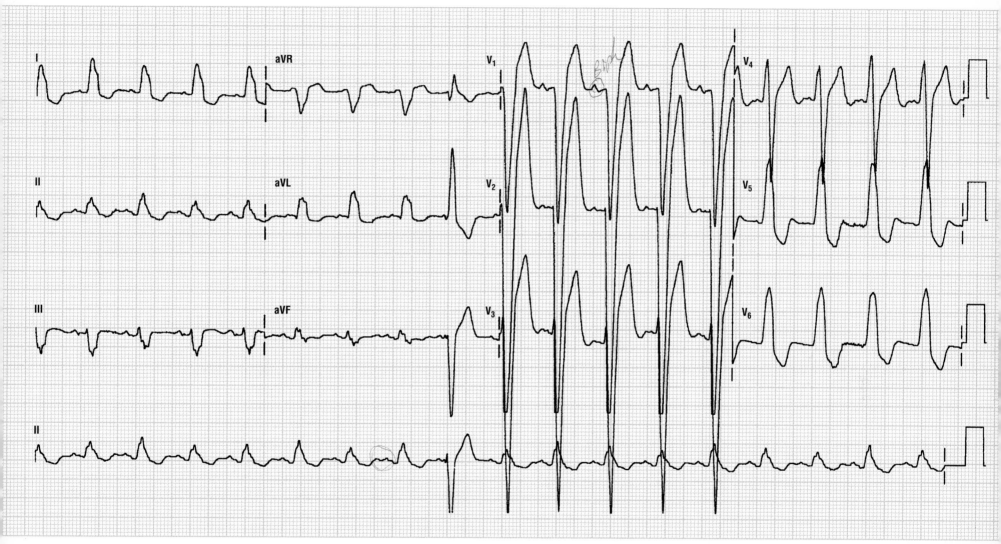

ECG 11-3

Left Ventricular Hypertrophy (LVH)

Left ventricular hypertrophy is exactly what it says: a large, or hypertrophied, left ventricle. This can be caused by either of two basic mechanisms: (1) an outflow problem, pressure overload, which develops when the ventricle has to pump harder against some resistance such as high arterial blood pressure or a stenosed aortic valve, or (2) a volume or dilation problem, volume overload, as occurs when a valve is leaking blood back into the heart after it was pumped out (aortic valve insufficiency or mitral valve regurgitation).

When confronted with the additional workload, the heart becomes larger in an effort to become stronger and pump more blood. This is similar to what happens to your muscles when you go to the gym and work out with weights. This is a simplistic view of a very complex problem, but it will suffice for our purposes.

So what happens to the ECG? As we know, the more mass or cells found in the heart, the more action potentials that are generated. This, in turn, causes a larger vector and increased amplitude on the ECG. This is especially true in the precordial leads because they are so close to the electrodes on the chest wall. Another important point is that a large left ventricle pushes the heart forward, closer to the electrodes, and thus produces a larger complex.

We are going to be using various criteria based on voltage to make the diagnosis of LVH. These criteria are not infallible, but they work pretty well. One thing to keep in mind: if electrical conduction does not occur through the normal pathways, the appearance of the QRS complex will be greatly altered and these criteria cannot be used. Some of these possible non-LVH alterations in conduction occur in LBBB, Wolff-Parkinson-White syndrome (WPW), ventricular rhythms, and certain advanced electrolyte or drug effects.

Electrocardiogram Criteria for Left Ventricular Hypertrophy

There are so many criteria for LVH that it is hard, if not impossible, to remember them all. And, authors will list various criteria depending on their preferences. That does not mean that they are right and we are wrong, or vice versa. It's just a confusing topic. Look for the criteria that have the strongest clinical correlation and are simple to remember. We recommend that you memorize only those following. (See Figures 11-9 through 11-11 for illustrations of these criteria.)

1. Add the depth of the S wave in V_1 or V_2, whichever is deepest, to the height of the R wave in V_5 or V_6, whichever is the tallest. In order to diagnose LVH, the total must be greater than or equal to 35 mm. In other words: (S in V_1 or V_2) + (R in V_5 or V_6) $\geq$ 35 mm

In addition, LVH is present if:

2. Any precordial lead is $\geq$ 45 mm.
3. The R wave in aVL is $\geq$ 11 mm.
4. The R wave in lead I is $\geq$ 12 mm.
5. The R wave in lead aVF is $\geq$ 20 mm.

In Chapter 14, we will be discussing the two differing morphologies in V_5 to V_6 for the pressure and volume overload types, as well as the effects of large QRS amplitudes in the precordials on the ST segments and the T waves — the LVH with strain presentation. This will give you some time to digest the concepts related to the QRS complexes. For now, just remember that LVH is in some cases associated with abnormal repolarization and can cause ST depression and flipped T waves. This is due to repolarization abnormalities, not ischemia.

Identifying Left Ventricular Hypertrophy, Step by Step

Here's how to measure the distances needed to determine LVH. First, measure the deepest S wave in either V_1 or V_2 (distance A in Figure 11-9). Now transfer your calipers, without changing the distance, down to the top of the tallest R wave in either V_5 or V_6 (Figure 11-10, A). Next, without moving the top pin, move the bottom pin to the baseline of the R wave that you are measuring (Figure 11-10, B). That distance is the sum of the depth of the S wave in either V_1 or V_2, and the height of the R wave in V_5 or V_6. If it is greater than or equal to 35 mm, you've identified LVH. Easy, isn't it? Figure 11-11 illustrates the other LVH criteria.

V₁ or V₂

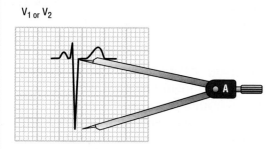

Figure 11-9: Measuring for LVH.

V₅ or V₆

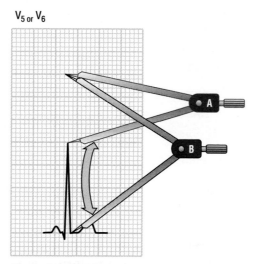

Figure 11-10: LVH criterion #1.

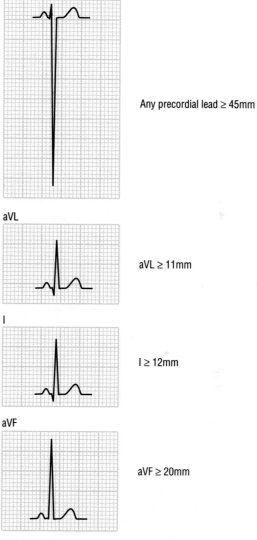

Any precordial lead ≥ 45mm

aVL

aVL ≥ 11mm

I

I ≥ 12mm

aVF

aVF ≥ 20mm

Figure 11-11: LVH criteria #2-5. Use your calipers!

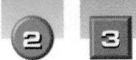

ECG CASE STUDIES: *Left Ventricular Hypertrophy*

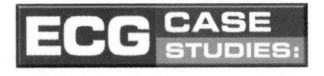

ECG 11-4 Look at the QRS complexes in leads V_1 and V_2. Which lead has the deepest S wave? Lead V_2 is the deepest, at about 25 mm. Now, look at V_5 and V_6. Which has the tallest R wave? Lead V_5 wins with a total measurement of about 13.5 mm. When we add the depth of the S wave in V_2 to the height of the R wave in V_5, we get 38.5 mm, which is consistent with LVH. That's all there is to it! Use your calipers to make it easier to calculate. You don't need to add the numbers if you add the distances using your calipers.

Look at the rest of the ECG. Do you see the P-mitrale in lead II? This is consistent with left atrial enlargement. Look at the PR intervals. Is there anything unusual? They are slightly depressed in leads II, III, aVF, and V_3 to V_6, but not significantly. This is not pericarditis.

Notice that it doesn't matter whether the R wave is big and the S is small, or vice versa, as long as the final product is greater than or equal to 35 mm, as shown in Figure 11-12. The important part is the sum, not which of the two parts is greater.

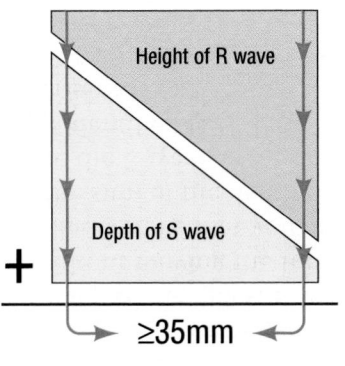

Figure 11-12: The product of R and S waves determines LVH.

ECG 11-5 Looking at ECG 11-5, we see that the two tallest leads are, once again, V_2 and V_5. Lead V_2 measures 23 mm, and V_5 measures 20 mm. By sight only, it is very hard to see whether V_5 or V_6 is tallest because there is only a 1 mm difference between the two. You need to use your calipers to measure the distances. We cannot stress the need for calipers enough. You are at a great disadvantage if you try to read an ECG without them.

The rhythm is sinus tachycardia. There is also evidence of left atrial enlargement (LAE). Are the PR segments depressed again? Slightly. Remember, less than 0.8 mm can be normal.

ECG 11-5 This is a great example of LVH with strain due to volume overload, rather than systolic or pressure overload. If you are unsure of the difference, review the criteria in Chapter 14. Briefly, LVH that is associated with a slight Q wave, and with ST segments that are upwardly concave with an asymmetrical T wave, is due to volume overload.

There are insignificant Q waves found in leads I, II, III, aVF, and V_5 to V_6. In addition, there is some ST elevation in V_2 to V_3 with upward concavity, once again suggestive of LVH with strain. The transition occurs normally between V_3 and V_4.

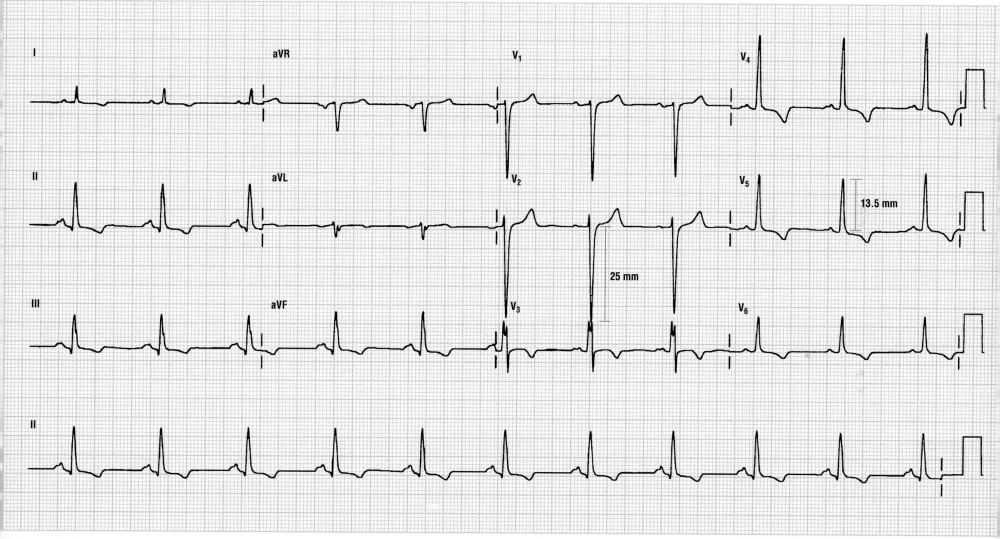

I aVR V₁ V₄

II aVL V₂ V₅ 13.5 mm

III aVF V₃ 25 mm V₆

II

ECG 11-4

CHAPTER **11** • THE QRS COMPLEX

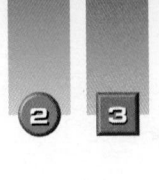

ECG CASE STUDIES: CONTINUED

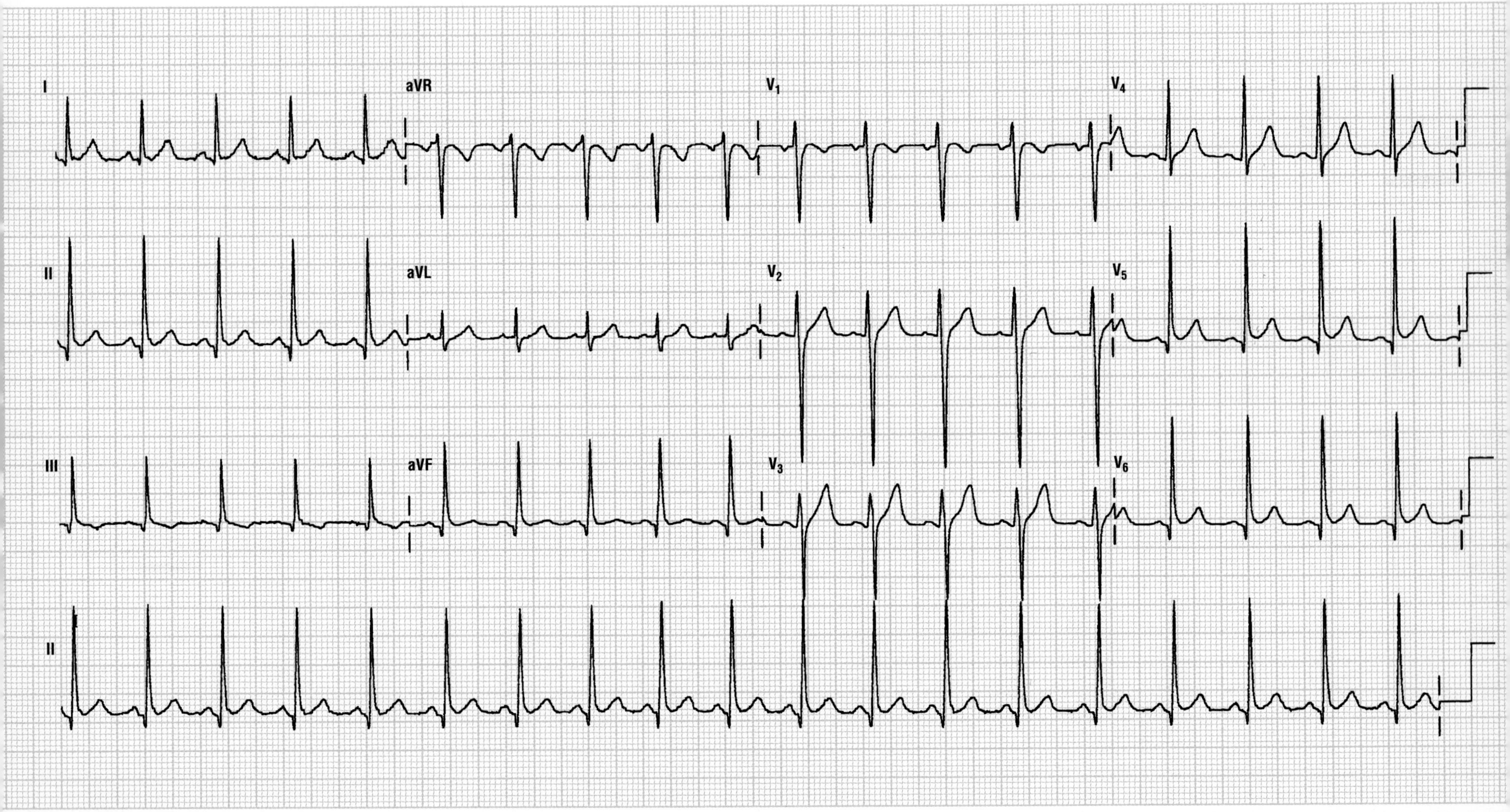

I aVR V₁ V₄

II aVL V₂ V₅

III aVF V₃ V₆

II

ECG 11-5

②

ECG 11-6 It may seem like we're beating this into the ground, but it is extremely important that you really understand LVH. It is many times mistaken for an AMI because of the ST elevation and depression associated with it. We want you to spend the time, look at these ECGs with LVH, and get to know the nuances of each one. Look at the waves and the ST segments. Notice how the tallest or deepest waves have the most ST segment variations. Observe the shapes of the waves both in the QRS and in the ST segments. Notice the rest of the ECG, as well. Did you catch the U wave in the ECG below? Be observant!

③

ECG 11-6 This example of LVH has a strain pattern in the right precordials, but the ST segments in the lateral are flat with an upright T wave. This is not the typical pattern for LVH, which has a concave downward ST segment and an asymmetrical T wave. Notice that the T waves in leads V_2 to V_6 are symmetrical. When you see the flat ST segments together with symmetrical T waves, you need to think about ischemia. Be careful of LVH with strain; it can fool you in many cases into either under- or overtreating the patient.

②

ECG 11-7 Does this patient meet criteria for LVH? The sum of the S in V_1 or V_2 plus the R in V_5 or V_6 is not greater than or equal to 35 mm. What are some of the other criteria? Are any of the precordial leads greater than or equal to 45 mm? No. Is the R wave in aVF greater than or equal to 20 mm? No. Are the R waves in aVL greater than or equal to 11 mm? Yes! Are the R waves in lead I greater than or equal to 12 mm? Yes! Those are the criteria for diagnosing LVH in this ECG. Remember to measure the waves from the baseline.

Other findings on this ECG are sinus bradycardia, U wave, and P-mitrale. The P wave is exactly 0.12 seconds in lead II and has two humps.

③

ECG 11-7 The criteria for LVH are covered in the Level 2 material here. The P waves are interesting in that there is evidence of P-mitrale in lead III, but no large terminal deflection in lead V_1. This is an unusual finding, and one for which we do not have an answer.

There are nonspecific ST-T wave changes noted with some flattening throughout. The axis is about $-20°$, and the transition is in the normal area. There is some respiratory variation to the axis; this is noted in lead III by an increasing S wave, and in aVL by an increasing R wave. This respiratory variation will be covered in more detail later in the chapter. It is a common and benign finding.

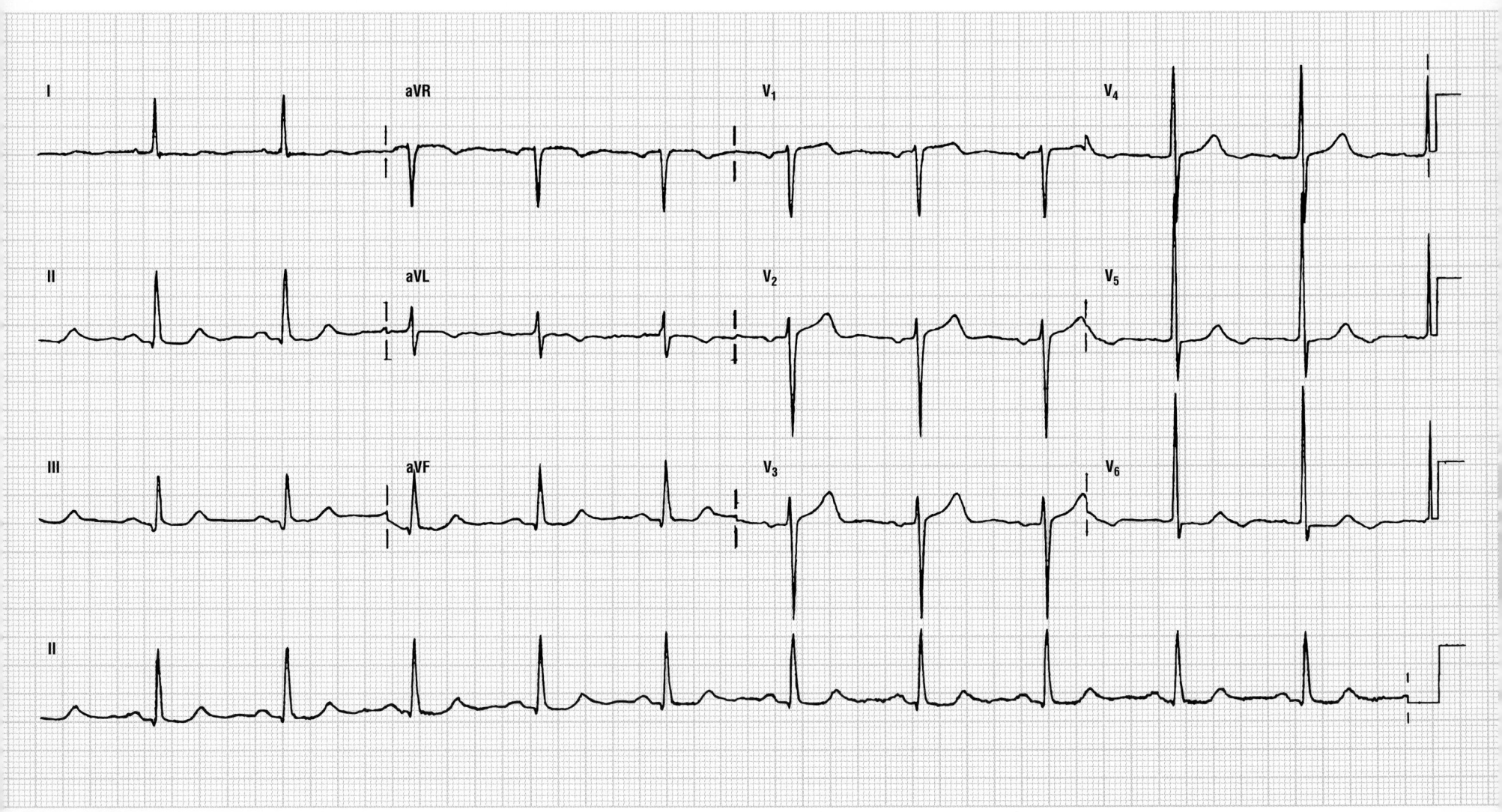

ECG 11-6

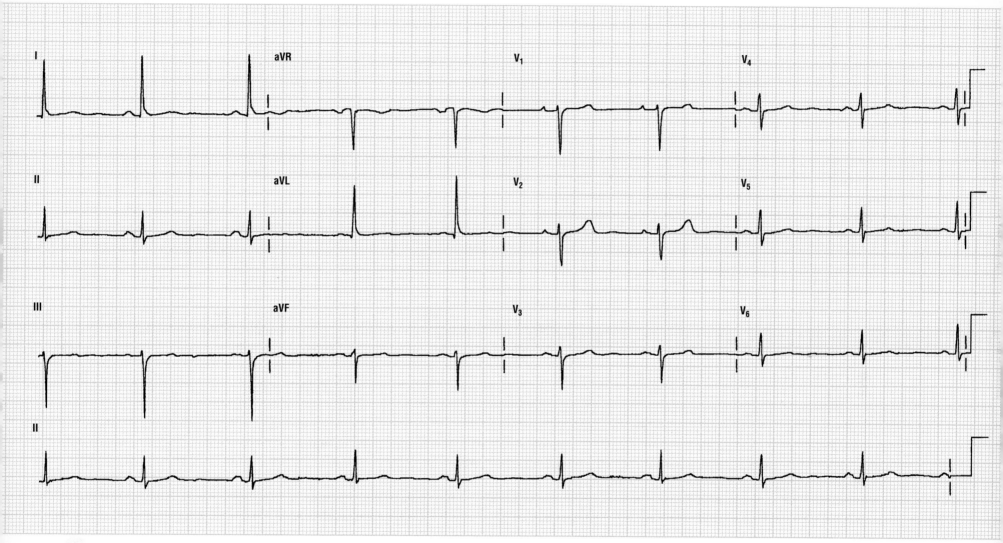

I aVR V₁ V₄

II aVL V₂ V₅

III aVF V₃ V₆

II

ECG 11-7

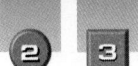

ECG CASE STUDIES: **CONTINUED**

2

ECG 11-8 Here is another fine example of LVH. This ECG meets three of the criteria. First, there is R + S = 35 mm. Second, R in aVL is > 11 mm. Third, R in lead I is > 12 mm.

Note that, in this case, most of the voltage for the > 35 mm criterion comes from V$_6$, which measures 34 mm by itself. When added to the voltage found in lead V$_1$, it surpasses the cutoff.

3

ECG 11-8 This is another example of LVH with strain pattern. The ST segments begin to take on the appearance at V$_3$ and are completely concave downward with an asymmetric T by lead V$_5$. The mild ST elevation in leads V$_1$ and V$_2$ is associated with an ST segment that is upwardly concave with an asymmetric T wave and is, therefore, consistent with LVH with strain. There are some beautiful septal Q waves in lead aVL. The flipped T waves in II, III, and aVF are probably due to the LVH. However, ischemia must be ruled out. Here is where an old ECG becomes invaluable. The main QRS axis is about −35 or −40° with a slightly late transition.

2

ECG 11-9 This patient meets LVH criteria by two mechanisms: S + R is > 35 mm, and the R wave in lead aVF is > 20 mm (24 mm, to be exact).

What is the rhythm? Sinus tachycardia. What about the PR interval? The PR interval is awfully short — generally less than 0.12 seconds. So what are the possibilities? Wolff-Parkinson-White (WPW) and Lown-Ganong-Levine (LGL) syndromes. There are no delta waves noted, so it is LGL by default. LGL can sometimes be associated with tachycardias, although it is rare. This could be one of those rare cases, or the patient may be tachycardic for some other reason.

3

ECG 11-9 The T wave abnormality noted in the inferior leads may be from one of three possible causes: (1) the LVH with very high R waves in leads II, III, and aVF, (2) the tachyarrhythmia, or (3) inferior ischemia. Numbers 1 and 2 are the most probable causes.

The LGL is noticeable, but the tachycardia cannot be blamed on the syndrome. The P waves, though peaked in the inferior wave, do not meet criteria for right atrial enlargement (RAE).

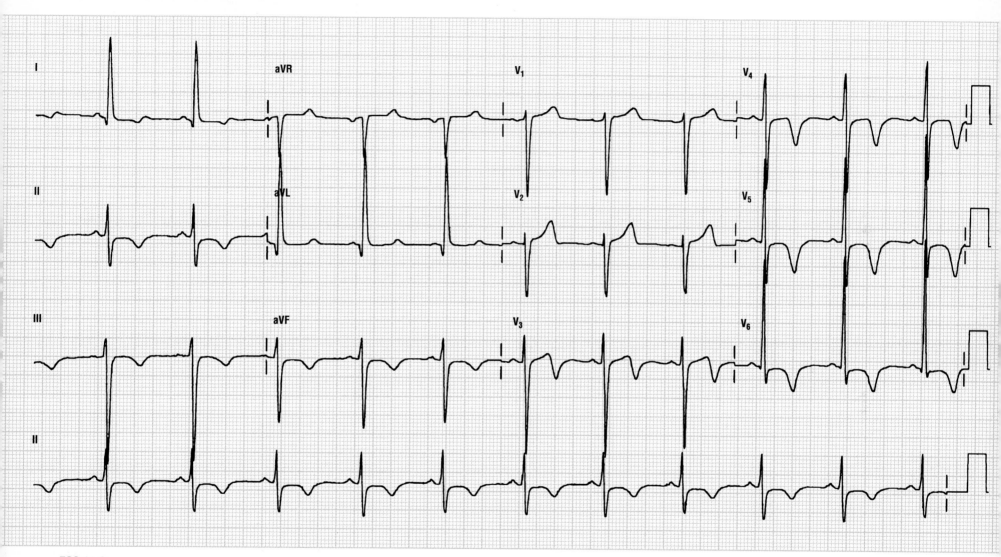

ECG 11-8

ECG CASE STUDIES: **CONTINUED**

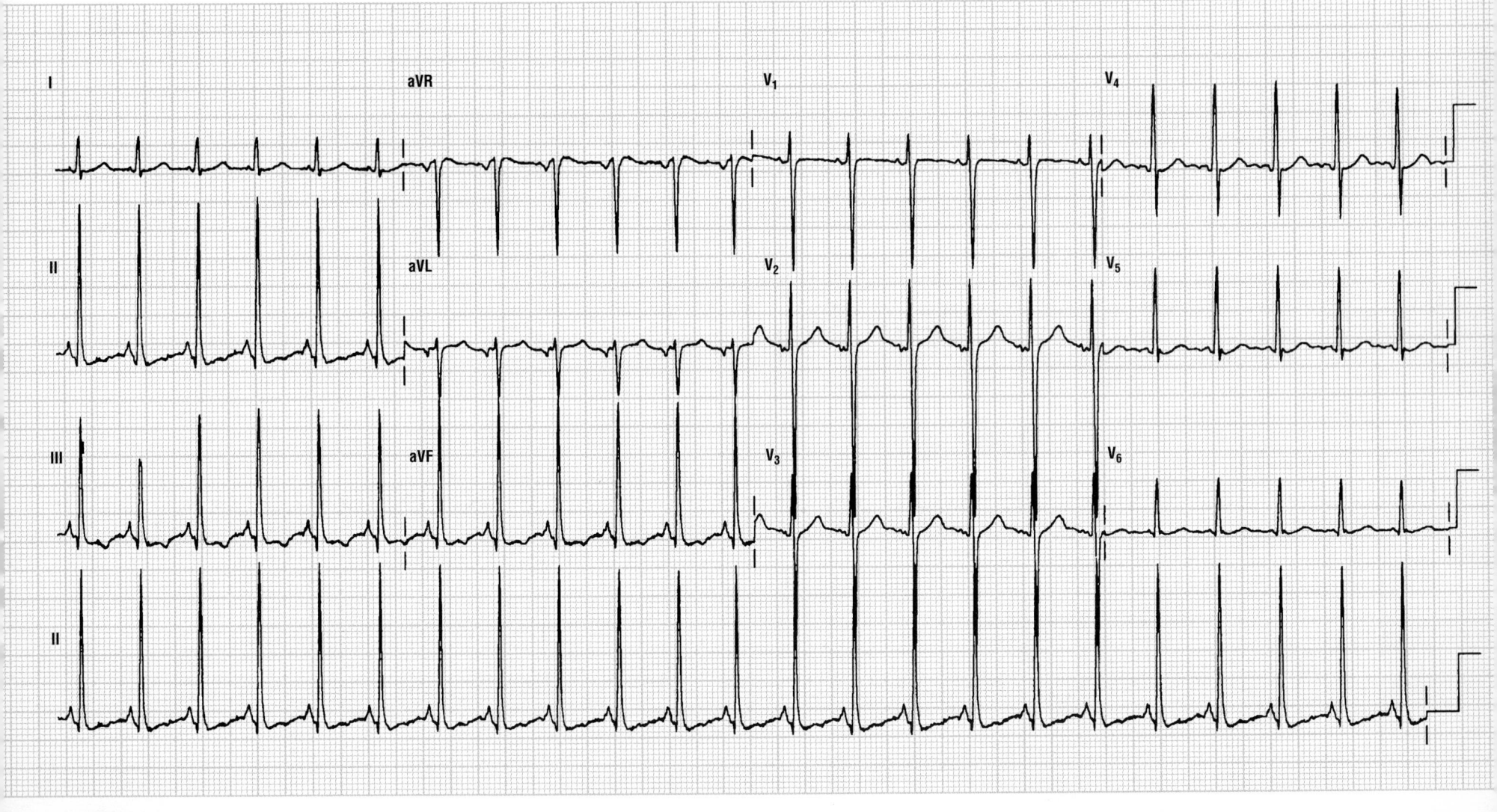

ECG 11-9

2

ECG 11-10 This patient has some huge QRS complexes in leads V_3 and V_5. The S wave in lead V_3 is 53 mm deep! The height of the R wave in V_5 is only 44 mm and so does not meet the greater than or equal to 45 mm criterion.

The patient offers a good example of P-pulmonale in lead II. There is also evidence of LAE in lead V_1, indicating biatrial enlargement. So there is evidence of enlargement in three of the four chambers. Did you notice the change in P wave morphology in the last three beats? Look at the rhythm strip to see the change clearly. This appears to be another pacemaker assuming the pacing role.

3

ECG 11-10 As noted in the Level 2 material here, there may be some speculation as to the presence of four-chamber enlargement, or cardiomyopathy. The ST segments are also interesting. There is evidence of LVH with strain in leads V_5 and V_6. In addition, there is a flattening of the T wave noted in all of the limb leads. There is a late intrinsicoid deflection found in the QRS complexes throughout the ECG.

Note the tiny r waves in lead V_2, nullifying the possibility of a QS wave extending through to V_2. There is also a small r in lead aVL.

2

ECG 11-11 This patient also has evidence of three-chamber enlargement. The patient has a P-pulmonale in lead II indicative of RAE. There is a biphasic P wave in lead V_1 with a large second component consistent with LAE. Lastly, there is LVH by three criteria. The R wave in lead V_5 alone is about 54 mm, and the top of V_4 cannot be seen. When you have LVH of this caliber, you should ask for the ECG to be done at half-standard, as seen in Figure 11-13. This will give you some measure of the true QRS complexes because you'll be able to see the whole waveform. You can then take the measurement and double that value to arrive at the true wave size.

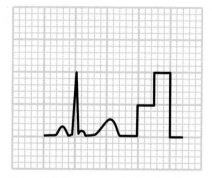

Figure 11-13: An example of half-standard. Since the QRS complex in the example on the left measures 10 mm at half-standard, the true measurement would be 20 mm if the standard were normal.

ECG CASE STUDIES: **CONTINUED**

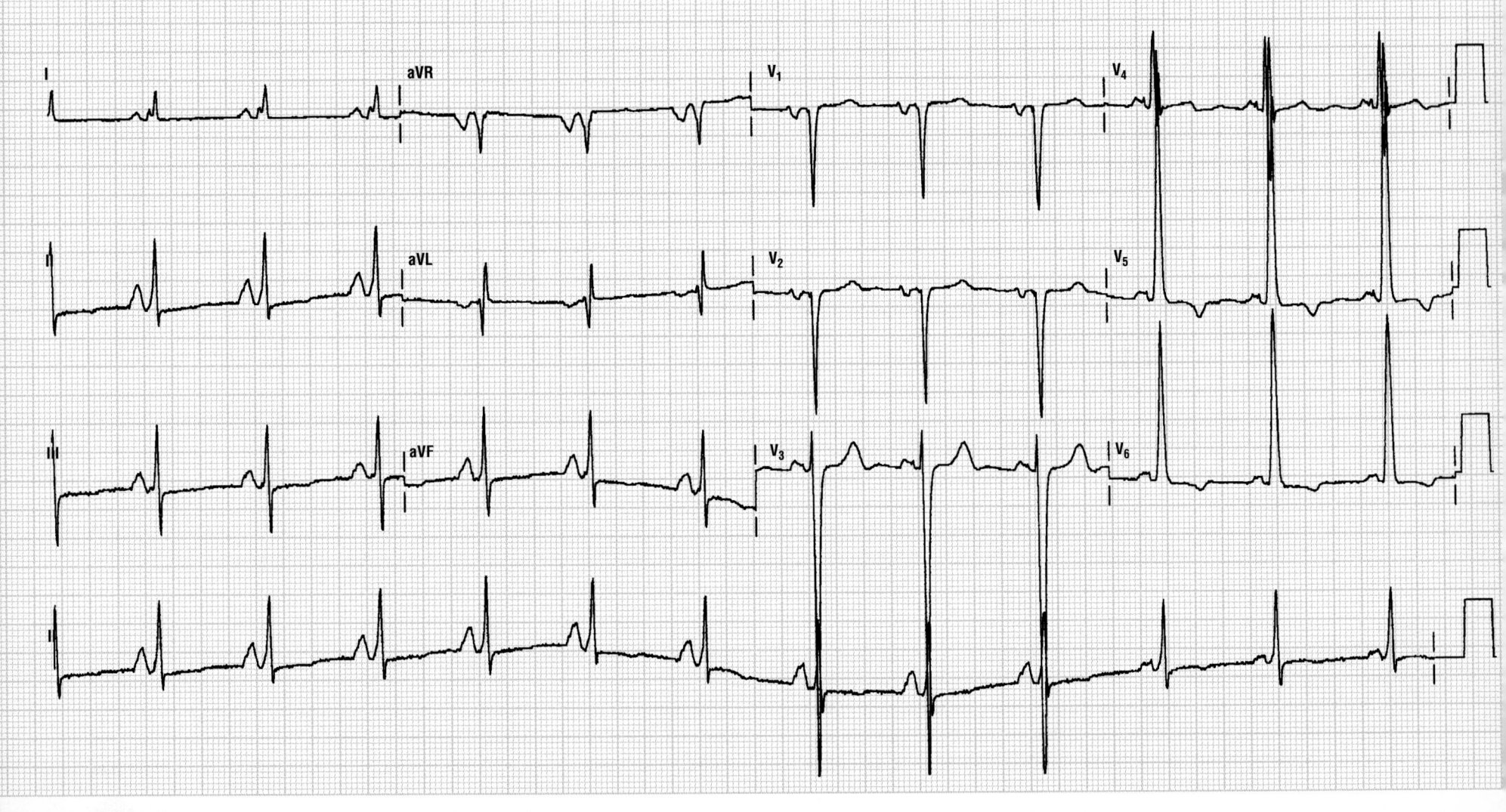

ECG 11-10

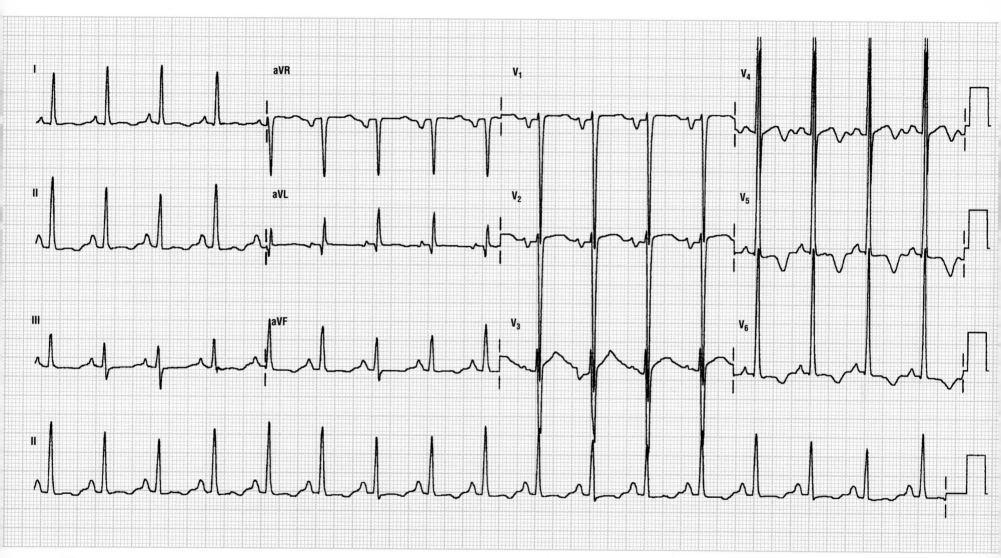

ECG 11-11

Right Ventricular Hypertrophy (RVH)

Just as the left ventricle can be hypertrophied, so too can the right ventricle be enlarged. This is usually seen in cases of right ventricular pressure overload, as occurs in pulmonary hypertension from many causes: multiple pulmonary emboli, primary pulmonary hypertension, scarring, and so on.

The electrocardiographic picture, as you would expect, is different from that of LVH because the area and the direction of the vectors created by the right ventricle are different (Figure 11-14). Those vectors are directed in the anterior and rightward directions. V_1 to V_2 are the closest leads to that direction, especially V_1. Hence, we will be looking at V_1 and V_2 to diagnose the possibility of RVH on an ECG.

Once again, we will see that the amount of change from the normal electrocardiographic pattern depends on the size of the vector produced by the right ventricle. If there is a large generation of electrical action potentials by larger myocytes, then the larger vector will produce more dramatic changes than a smaller one would.

Now, how would you expect lead V_1 to look if you had a large vector coming at it from an enlarged right ventricle? A large R wave should be the first thing you see on the QRS complex (Figure 11-15). This large R wave is a result of adding the energy generated by the initial QRS vector (due to stimulation of the interventricular septum) to the new, larger vector generated by the enlarged RV. This electrocardiographic picture is a far cry from the usual presentation of a small r in V_1 with a large S wave, seen in a normal heart. As noted, we will discuss the ST-T wave changes that occur along with the large R wave in Chapter 14.

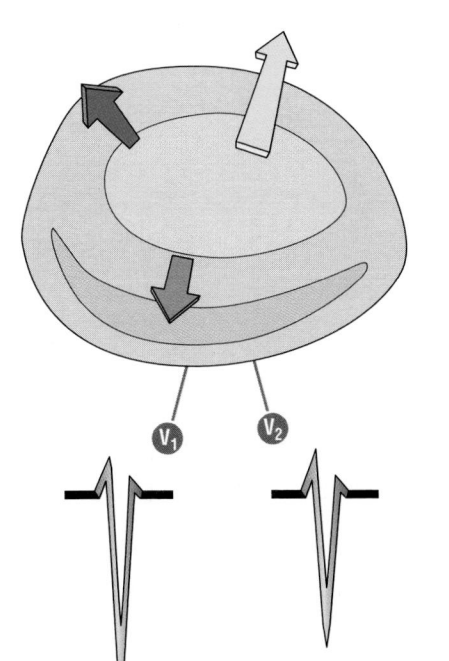

Figure 11-14: Normal state.

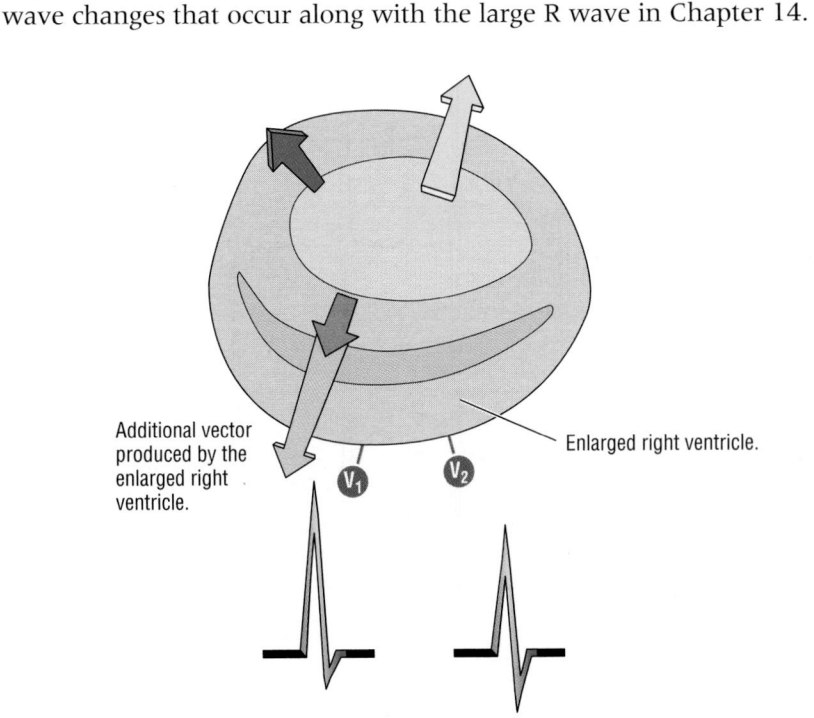

Figure 11-15: Right ventricular hypertrophy.

RVH and the ECG

In Figure 11-16, A, you will see the typical pattern for RVH in V_1. The take-home lesson is that the R:S ratio (Figure 11-17) is $\geq$ 1 in leads V_1 and/or V_2. Notice that in Figure 11-16, B, the R:S is still more than 1, but the ST and T waves look different. This is a strain pattern that we will cover in Chapter 14. For now, just concentrate on the QRS complexes. We'll be showing you various examples of how V_1 and V_2 will look in the next few pages.

There are some other electrocardiographic findings that go along with RVH. Can you think of one we have already discussed? Well, if you have a big right ventricle because of pressure overload, it should be stiff and strong, right? In order to fill that ventricle, you need to have a stronger right atrium to push more blood into it. This causes RAE. Do you remember how that looks on the ECG? If you don't, go back and review that section in Chapter 9. By the way, this logic also applies to LVH and the left atrium.

 We will later see how RVH affects the axis and the rest of the ECG. Just a teaser: it can sometimes cause right axis deviation.

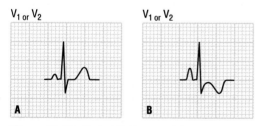

Figure 11-16: Typical RVH pattern (A) vs. RVH with strain pattern (B).

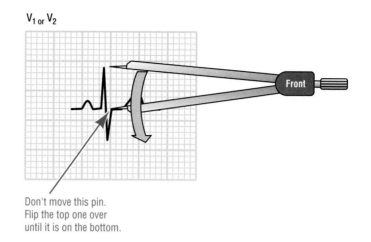

Don't move this pin. Flip the top one over until it is on the bottom.

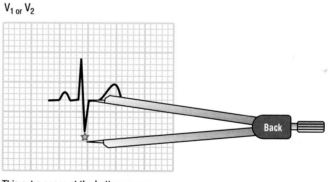

This extra space at the bottom means that the R wave had a higher amplitude than the S wave. Thus, the R:S $\geq$ 1 and meets RVH criteria!

Figure 11-17: Measuring the R:S ratio. Use your calipers!

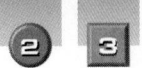

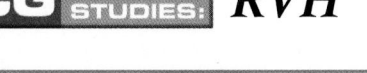 *RVH*

ECG 11-12 The ECG below has an increased R:S ratio in lead V_1 that is consistent with possible right ventricular strain. This is called a "strain pattern" because of the flipped T associated with it. (We will be reviewing this in much greater detail when we discuss ST segments in Chapter 14.) In addition, there is evidence of LAE in V_1.

ECG 11-12 Now, let's think about some of the things that can give us an increased R:S ratio in leads V_1 or V_2. We just covered RVH, so that is definitely one possibility. Can you think of any others? Here's the rest of the list:

1. Right ventricular hypertrophy
2. Right bundle branch block
3. Young children and adolescents
4. WPW type A
5. Posterior wall AMI

This list is extremely important. You should run through it every time you have an increased R:S ratio in leads V_1 or V_2. It will help you make sense of some really troublesome ECGs.

ECG 11-13 In the example below, the R:S ratio is increased in lead V_2 and is not associated with a strain pattern. As you will see, you need to keep other possibilities in mind. This ECG is not classic for RVH; there really is no other evidence of it. There are other things that can cause this pattern. The list for the differential diagnosis (DDx) of an increased R:S ratio in V_1 or V_2 appears in the Level 3 material with ECG 11-12. You don't know what some of those problems are yet, but you will soon. Upon running through the list, there is nothing else that this ECG matches, so RVH is the most probable cause. It is a process of elimination.

ECG 11-13 Let's run through the DDx of an increased R:S ratio in V_2. It is not a right bundle branch block (RBBB) pattern, as the complexes are not wider than 0.12 sec. There is no evidence of WPW on this ECG. There are no delta waves or PR shortening. What about a youth or adolescent? Well, this was a 47-year-old man. Posterior wall AMI is a possibility. However, posterior wall myocardial infarctions (PWMIs) are acutely associated with ST depression and an upright T wave. An age-indeterminate PWMI is possible, but remember that the R waves should be wider than 0.03 seconds, which they are not in leads V_1 or V_2. So what is left? RVH. The T waves are flipped and symmetrical, which could represent anteroseptal ischemia.

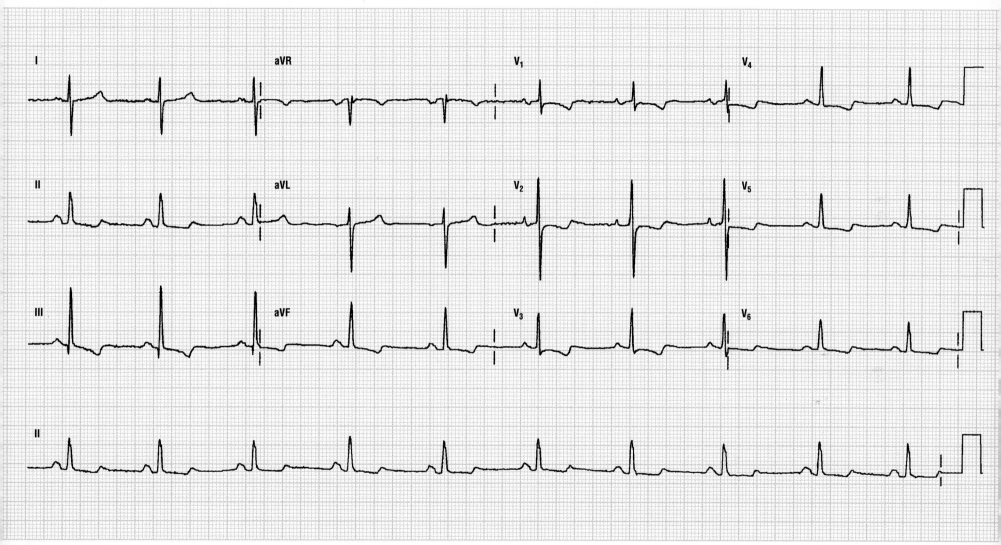

ECG 11-12

ECG CASE STUDIES: CONTINUED

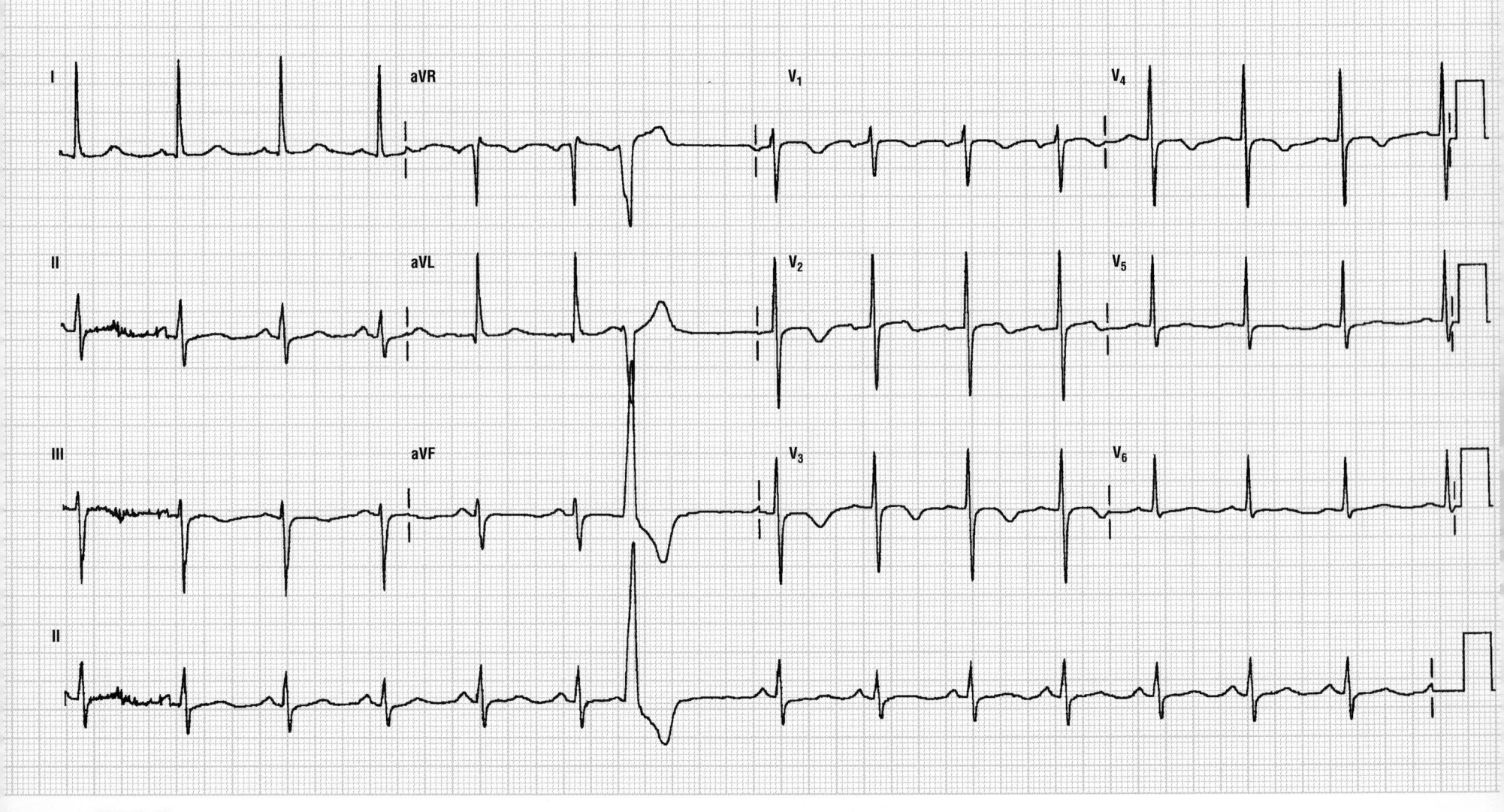

ECG 11-13

QRS Duration

You measure the duration of the QRS complex from the onset of the first deflection after the PR interval to the end of the complex. Normally, this measures between 0.06 and 0.11 seconds. If it is three small boxes or greater, it is abnormal! In the examples in Figure 11-18, you see two different types of QRS complexes. Complex A is the native, normal complex that measures 0.11 seconds. Complex B is a VPC that is 0.15 seconds wide.

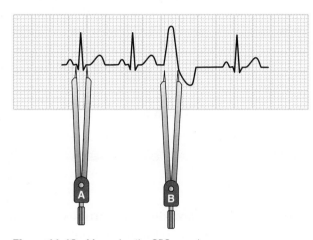

Figure 11-18: Measuring the QRS complex

   Always measure the widest QRS complex in the ECG or you will be misled as to the true duration of the complex! There are some sections of the complex that are isoelectric and graphically invisible on the ECG. If you just pick any lead, you could get a shorter duration than is really present. This can lead to serious mistakes in your interpretation. You could, for example, mistake the QRS complex for ST segment and potentially treat a patient for an AMI that is not occurring. This is especially true in cases of bundle branch blocks, as you will see later. In addition, you could mistake a U wave for a biphasic T wave. There are many instances in which the exact measurement of the interval is critical to the correct interpretation.

Not all ECGs are easy to interpret! There are a lot of cases in which there is an elevation and blurring of the start of the QRS complex or the J point. In these cases, you have to be creative. If you are lucky enough to have a multilead ECG (one with at least three leads recorded simultaneously, as in our examples), you can see if there is a sharper onset or J point on the surrounding leads. You can then follow a vertical line from that point to the lead you are trying to measure, and measure the true interval. If you still cannot get a definitive point, you may just have to take your best guess. If you do this, always assume the worst diagnosis. It is healthier for the patient if you over-analyze, rather than underanalyze, an ECG.

   Remember that any QRS complex greater than 0.12 seconds is abnormal. There are no limitations or exceptions to this rule. Thinking about your differential diagnoses in these cases is very helpful. Things that cause QRS widening include (in decreasing order of mortality):

1. Hyperkalemia
2. Ventricular tachycardia
3. Idioventricular rhythms, including heart block
4. Drug effects and overdoses (especially tricyclics)
5. Wolff-Parkinson-White
6. Bundle branch blocks and intraventricular conduction delay
7. Ventricular premature contractions
8. Aberrantly conducted complexes

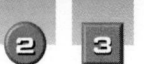

ECG CASE STUDIES: *QRS Duration*

ECG 11-14 A little wide isn't it? Is it more than 0.12 seconds? Yes! Looking at the ECG, what do you think the problem is? Well, start off with the rate, which is about 40 BPM. Are there any P waves? No. So you have a slow rate with no atrial activity. What is the most probable cause? A ventricular escape beat of some sort. Remember, when the ventricle acts as a pacemaker, the rate is usually around 35 BPM. This is an idioventricular rhythm. Do you try to suppress these ventricular complexes with lidocaine or other antiarrhythmics? Definitely not! If you suppress the ventricular complexes, you are left with _____ (a straight line).

ECG 11-14 So, you have a wide-complex rhythm. What is the cause — can you make an educated guess? Wide rhythms are caused by a few things; look at Figure 11-19 (several pages ahead) and then come back here. Is it a left bundle? Well, it's not a classic LBBB pattern because of the S wave in lead V_6 (also in lead I, if you notice). Is it an RBBB? No, because of the negative QS wave in lead V_1. By the process of elimination, it is an intraventricular conduction delay (IVCD). What is the most life-threatening cause of an IVCD? Hyperkalemia. Do you wait for the K+ level to come back before treating? No. What was his K+? Only 8.7 mEq/L!

ECG 11-15 This is an easy one — RBBB, right? Right! But what about that ST elevation in leads III and aVF consistent with inferior wall myocardial infarction (IWMI)? Would you give this patient thrombolytics? Let's take another look at the whole ECG. How wide are the QRS complexes? Well, if we take leads V_1 or aVL as the widest, we come up with about 0.14 seconds. Now, transfer that distance with your calipers to the beginning of the QRS complex in lead III and aVF. You see that the segment that looks like ST elevation is in reality part of the QRS complex! Another way to do this is to use your straight edge and bring down the lines at the beginning and end of the QRS complex in lead I. This will easily show you that they are part of the QRS complex and not ST segments.

Is there any evidence of ischemia on this ECG? Remember the rules of concordance and discordance associated with RBBB? The last portion of the QRS complex and the T wave should be opposite each other in a normal complex. This is called discordance, and discordance is the normal state in a bundle branch block. Concordance is abnormal and, if found in a regional distribution, could signify ischemia. Leads V_2 and V_3 are concordant, so they could be consistent with ischemia. You need an old ECG and clinical correlation to make a clinical decision for treatment. The last thing to point out is the PR prolongation and intraatrial conduction delay (IACD) (possible LAE).

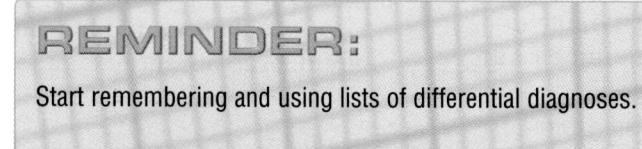

REMINDER:

Start remembering and using lists of differential diagnoses.

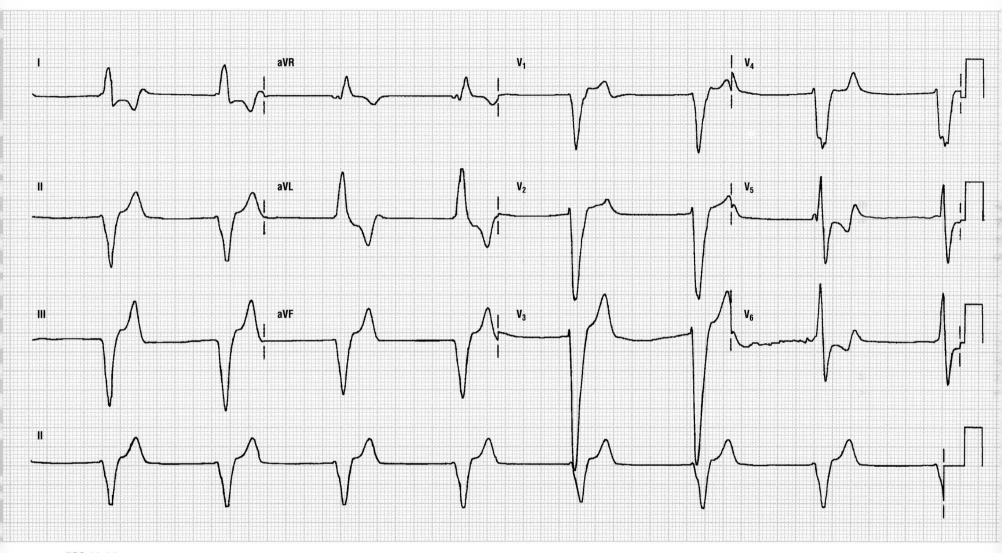

ECG 11-14

ECG CASE STUDIES: **CONTINUED**

| I | aVR | V₁ | V₄ |

| II | aVL | V₂ | V₅ |

| III | aVF | V₃ | V₆ |

| II |

ECG 11-15

2

ECG 11-16 Well, this is the kind of ECG that makes you want to run and hide, but unfortunately we can't. This ECG was obtained from a patient who was awake and talking. However, he wasn't talking one minute later as he went into cardiac arrest. What is it? A very-wide-complex tachycardia. Whenever you have a wide complex tachycardia you should treat it as you would ventricular tachycardia until proven otherwise.

2 QUICK REVIEW

1. Ventricular tachycardia always has an underlying sinus tachycardia as the atrial rhythm. True or False.

2. Fusion complexes are found in ventricular tachycardia. True or False.

3. Escape beats are found in ventricular tachycardia. True or False.

4. You should always think of hyperkalemia when you see very wide, bizarre complexes. True or False.

5. If you are unsure of the diagnosis and you have a wide complex tachycardia, you should always assume it is not ventricular tachycardia. True or False.

1. False. There is always an underlying atrioventricular dissociation, but the sinus rhythm could be sinus bradycardia, normal sinus rhythm, or atrial tachycardia. 2. True 3. True 4. True 5. False. Very false!

3

ECG 11-16 This is a tough ECG, especially when you only have a few seconds to look at it. The only thing to say is that the potassium came back at 9.4 mEq/L.

CLINICAL PEARL

Always treat a wide complex tachycardia as if it were VTach, but watch out for hyperkalemia!

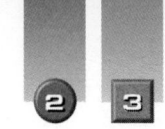

ECG CASE STUDIES: **CONTINUED**

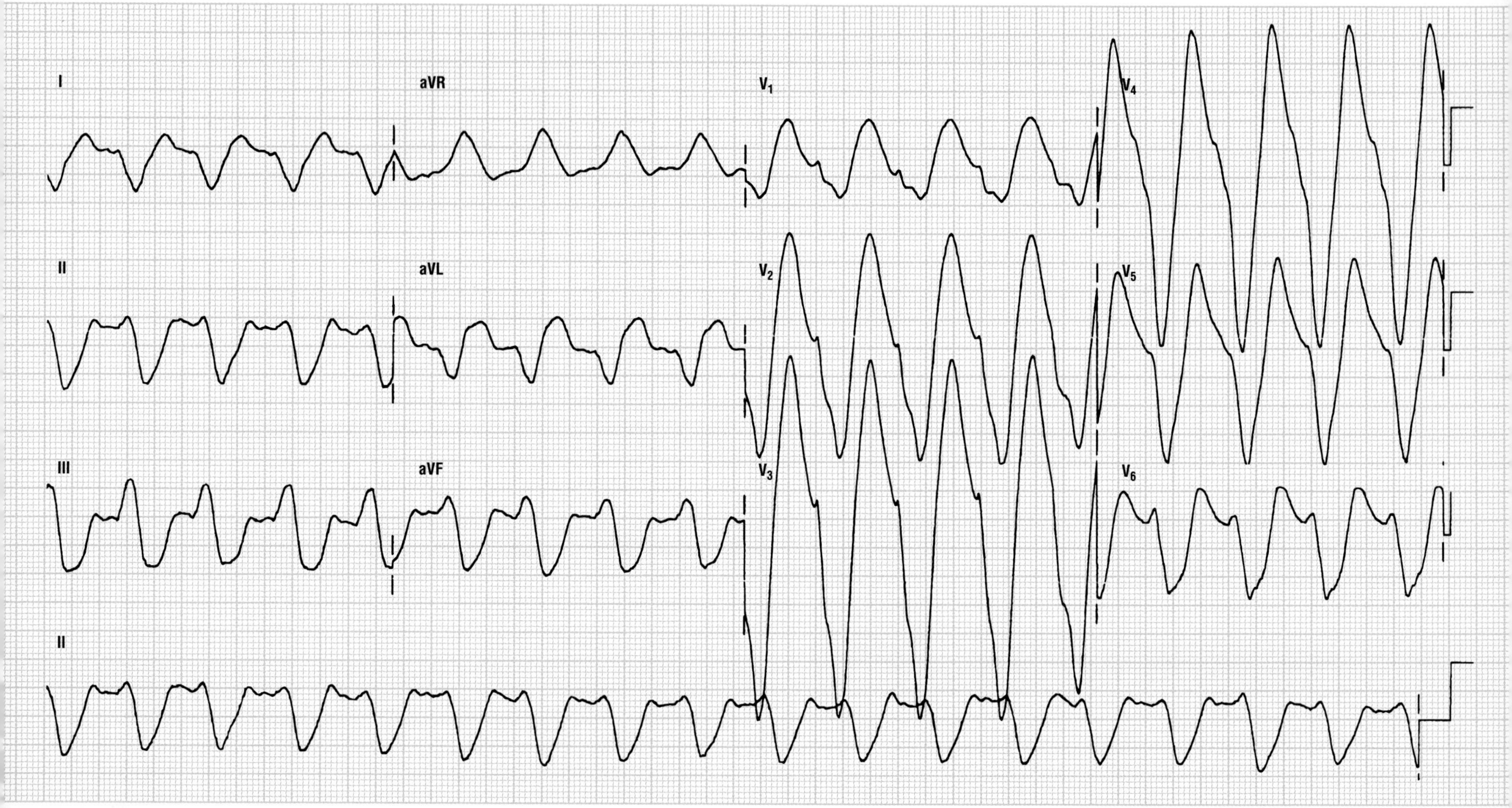

I

aVR

V₁

V₄

II

aVL

V₂

V₅

III

aVF

V₃

V₆

II

ECG 11-16

The Wide-QRS Differential, Simplified

When you see a QRS complex that is > 0.12 seconds, one of these is present (Figure 11-19):

1. Right bundle branch block
2. Left bundle branch block
3. Interventricular conduction delay

That's it, pure and simple. Look at the list on page 185 and you will see more things on the list, but they all fall in these categories (except WPW). As you will see when we cover blocks, all the beats of ventricular origin have either a left- or right-bundle configuration. In addition, hyperkalemia and drug effects are examples of IVCDs. WPW, a wide QRS caused by an abnormal conduction of the impulse through the Kent bundle, is an entity in and of itself. It is readily identified by the delta wave. So when you have a QRS complex that is greater than 0.12 seconds, think of the three possibilities above, if it is not WPW.

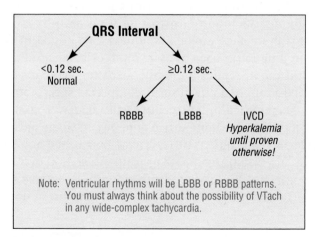

Figure 11-19: Possible causes of a QRS interval that is greater than or equal to 0.12 sec.

2

QRS Morphology

One of the main things you need to evaluate when examining the QRS complex is its morphology. Make sure the morphologies are the same in each of the complexes. If they are not, ask yourself why. In answering this simple question, you could unlock a great deal of information. For example, suppose you had an ECG with nice narrow complexes and then you saw a wide one. Is this a VPC? An aberrantly conducted beat? An intermittent WPW syndrome?

Now, suppose all of the complexes were wide and then you had a narrow one. What would that indicate? When you examine the complexes around it, you may notice that the narrow one is the only one that has a P wave clearly identified before the complexes. This would, in turn, lead you on a hunt for other P waves. You would see that there are other P waves and that they are dissociated from the QRS complexes except in the narrow beat. Your diagnosis: ventricular tachycardia. Your analysis of that one narrow complex has totally altered your management course and has saved the patient's life. Pretty cool isn't it?

CLINICAL PEARL

We the clinicians, find that all complexes are <u>not</u> created equal . . .

ECG CASE STUDIES: *QRS Morphology*

ECG 11-17 There is no such thing in this book as an easy ECG! The ECG below is an example of multiple morphologies for the QRS complexes. The first thing to note is the third-degree heart block. The first part of the ECG has one pacemaker (black arrows), and the later part has another (purple arrows). The blue arrow indicates an atrial premature contraction (APC), which causes the switch in pacemakers. The morphology of the APC is very different from the two other pacers. The two main pacemakers, however, are quite similar in morphology and therefore are probably also quite close to each other anatomically.

The first three full QRS complexes below have an LBBB morphology, and the next three show an RBBB morphology. The fifth beat (green star) is an example of a fusion beat, and the seventh (gold star) is a capture beat.

Just to make the ECG more interesting, note that the R-R intervals for the complexes with LBBB are the same, and those for the RBBB and the capture beat are the same. However, the two rates are different. The differing ventricular pacer also started at a different point than that where the atria switched rates. As mentioned above, this ECG is full of abnormalities. It is very difficult to interpret unless you spend the time to break it down.

ECG 11-18 This ECG 11-18 below is another example of a morphology shift. The blue star has a different appearance than the previous or subsequent beats. In fact, it is a fusion beat and has characteristics of both the normal and the abnormal beat (red star). This begins a short salvo of VTach for the additional five beats. There is atrioventricular (AV) dissociation in this salvo. Be careful of the lead change that occurs in the middle of the salvo.

In addition to the VTach, there are ventricular premature contractions (VPCs) and aberrantly conducted beats found throughout the rest of the ECG. The axis is in the left quadrant, with left anterior hemiblock (LAH) present. The transition occurs between leads V_1 and V_2, giving you a counter-clockwise picture. All in all, quite a confusing ECG.

REMINDER:

When you see a different morphology on the ECG, ask "Why?"

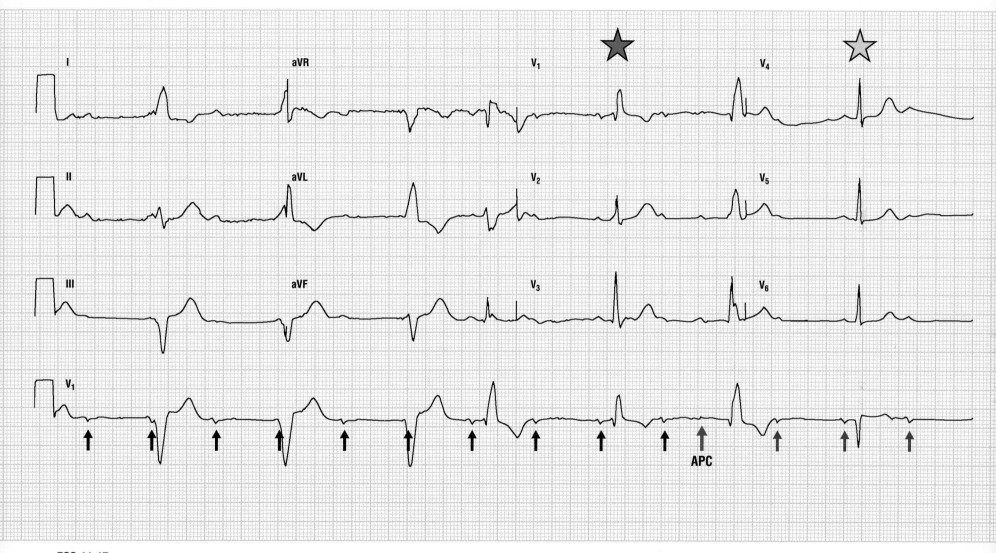

ECG 11-17

ECG CASE STUDIES: CONTINUED

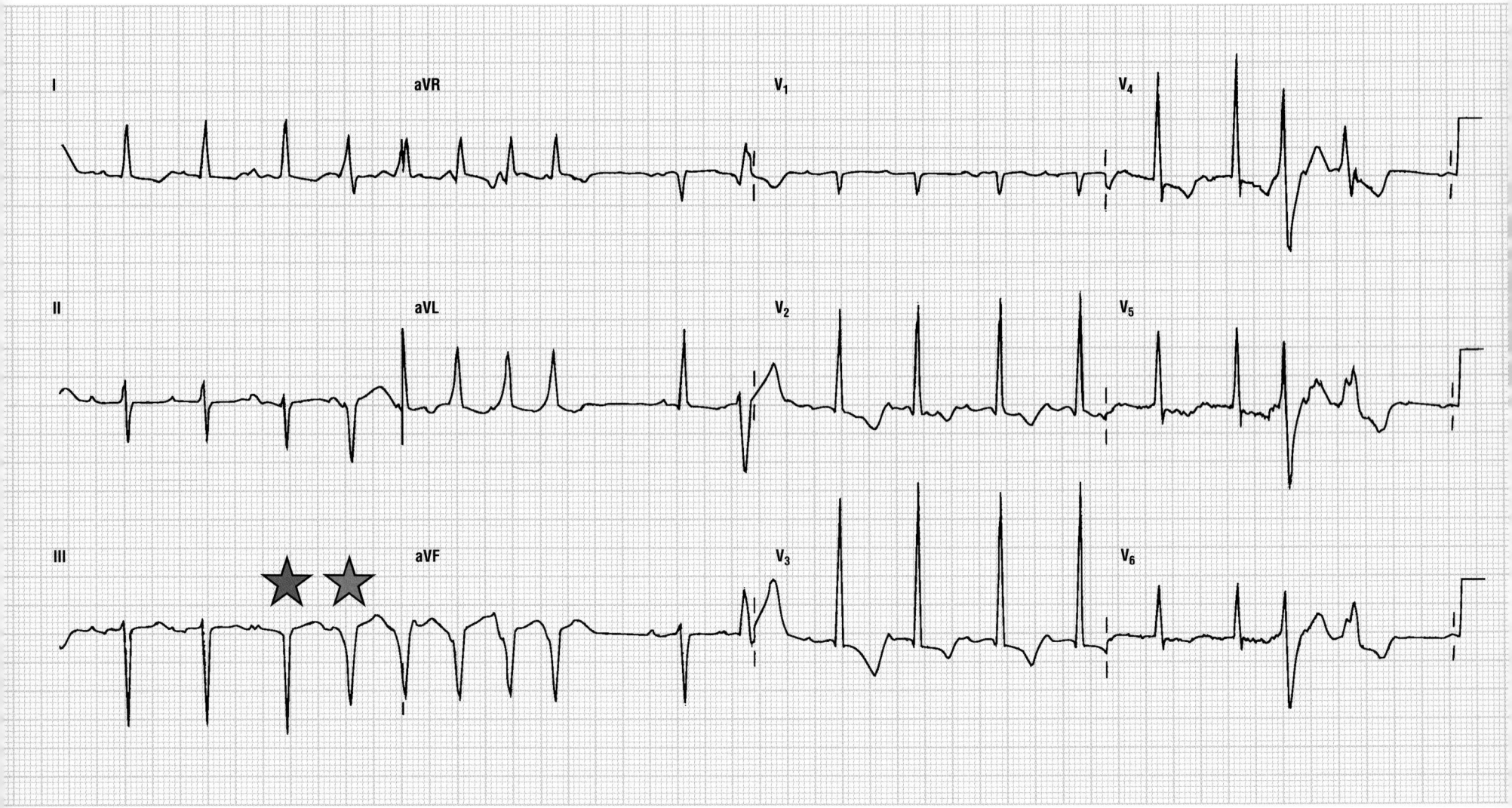

I aVR V₁ V₄

II aVL V₂ V₅

III aVF V₃ V₆

ECG 11-18

Q Wave Significance

Benign Q Waves

We touched on the Q wave in Chapter 6. We are now going to expand on the topic and discuss some of the fine points of examining Q waves.

The main interpretation of a significant Q wave is that it represents dead myocardium. Now, notice that we said a significant Q wave. Insignificant Q waves are merely a representation of the first vector of ventricular depolarization, whereas significant Q waves represent an old AMI in that regional distribution.

Insignificant Q waves are found in many places on the ECG. Septal Q waves, shown in Figure 11-20, are usually found in leads I and aVL. They are small, thin Q waves that represent the first vector of ventricular depolarization. You will see an example of one in ECG 11-19. QS waves are so named because there is no intervening R wave to break up the two, so you don't know if it is a Q wave or an S wave. QS waves, shown in Figure 11-21, are found in lead V_1 in many cases, and — if isolated to that lead — are benign. If the QS waves extend through to V_2, or especially V_3, then they are significant for an infarct of the anteroseptal areas of the heart at some time in the past, or in the present. We will show you an example of a benign QS in V_1, and an ECG with some pathological QS waves so that you can see the difference. Another example of a benign Q wave is one that is isolated to lead III only. This is usually a thin Q wave. If a significant Q wave is found in II or aVF, it is significant for an inferior wall AMI. (More on this in Chapter 15.)

I, aVL

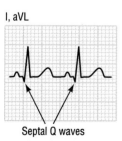

Septal Q waves

Figure 11-20: Septal Q waves

V_1 only!

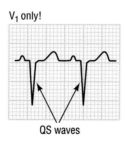

QS waves

Figure 11-21: QS waves

Respiratory Variation of Q Waves

You will sometimes see a Q wave that gets deeper and then returns to a shorter state on lead II or III of the ECG. Does this mean that the person is infarcting before your eyes in a three-second strip? No! Some people who are obese, pregnant, or full of ascites — or have another condition that makes the abdomen large — will have a horizontal heart. That is, the heart will lie along a horizontal plane. Now, what happens when they breathe? The diaphragm gets pulled down and the heart becomes more vertical (Figure 11-22). Because the vectors of the heart remain in alignment, there appears to be a deepening of the Q wave and a slight axis shift. Think of this as an electrocardiographic optical illusion! It is benign — nothing to worry about.

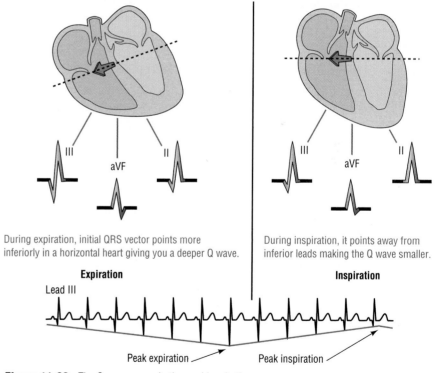

During expiration, initial QRS vector points more inferiorly in a horizontal heart giving you a deeper Q wave.

During inspiration, it points away from inferior leads making the Q wave smaller.

Figure 11-22: The Q wave on expiration and inspiration

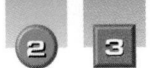

ECG CASE STUDIES: *Q Wave Significance*

ECG 11-19 We have done something different with this ECG. We took the limb leads of two patients and placed them side by side so that you can compare the Q waves present in leads I and aVL. On the example at left, you will notice that the Q waves are small and less than 0.03 seconds wide. These are examples of benign septal Q waves. In comparison, the ECG on the right has wide Q waves. These are pathologic Q waves. They do not meet the one-third height criterion, but they do satisfy the width criterion. It would be ideal if both criteria were met, but width is a bit more specific for serious pathology. It is critical that you understand the difference between pathologic and nonpathologic Q waves. Make sure you are clear on these points before leaving this chapter.

ECG 11-20 We have done something similar to ECG 11-19 with this set, to look at the differences between benign and pathologic QS waves. We are looking at the precordial leads this time. On the left, the ECG shows an example of a benign QS wave. Why is it a QS wave? Because there are no positive components to the QRS complex. Why is it benign? Because it only appears in lead V_1. If the QS complex morphology extended into lead V_2, the chance that it represented an age-indeterminate, anteroseptal AMI would be high. If it extended into lead V_3, the chances would be even higher. Notice that the ECG on the left has QS complexes extending into lead V_4. This is clear evidence of an AMI. Note the depth of the QS complex in lead V_3: Is it greater than or equal to 45 mm? Yes, it measures about 47 mm and represents a large unopposed vector aimed at the posterior wall of the heart. (We will discuss this further in Chapter 15 when we address how AMIs present electrocardiographically.)

ECG 11-19 Do you notice any additional differences between leads I and aVL on the two ECGs? The differences are subtle, but very important. Notice that the T waves are symmetrical. As discussed in Chapter 14, symmetrical T waves are more indicative of pathology — either electrolyte abnormalities, drug effect, or ischemia. The association with significant Q waves makes ischemia very likely as the cause of the underlying pathology. The ST segments are slightly elevated in lead aVL on the ECG at the right, which could also represent some injury pattern, either early or resolving.

ECG 11-20 Pathologic QS waves are indicative of AMI. The age is indeterminate unless there is evidence for an AMI with ST elevation and T wave inversion. The ST segments in the ECG on the right are more compatible with LVH-with-strain pattern, which is evident on the ECG. Note the concavity of the ST segment in most leads. The T waves, however, are symmetrical. You really need an old ECG to help you interpret this one appropriately. The other thing that would be helpful is the history of the patient at presentation. A chief complaint of chest pain would be very troublesome with this ECG because it could represent an extension of the infarct, superimposed upon the age-indeterminate infarct pattern already present on this ECG. In other words, the new infarct pattern may be overshadowed by the old infarct pattern and not be readily visible.

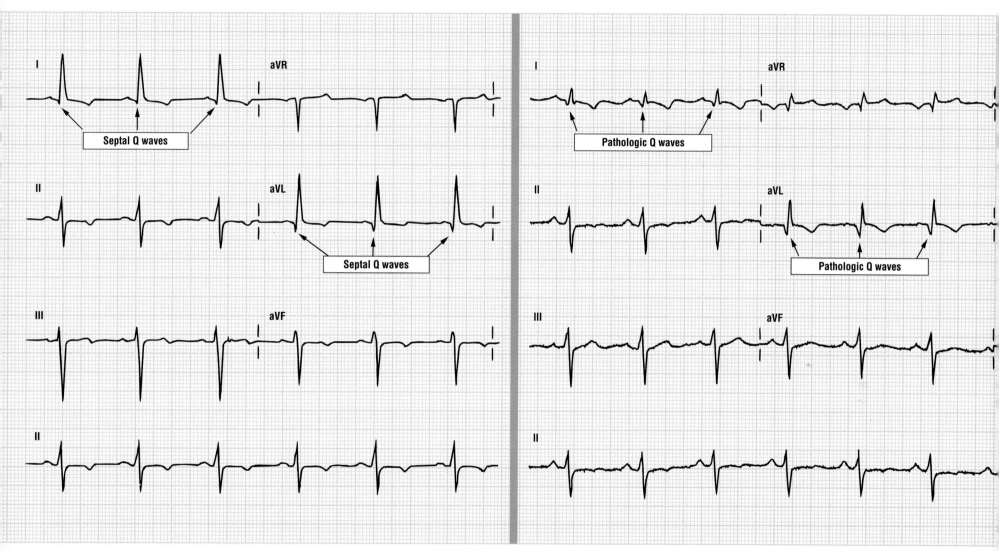

I
aVR
Septal Q waves

II
aVL
Septal Q waves

III
aVF

II

I
aVR
Pathologic Q waves

II
aVL
Pathologic Q waves

III
aVF

II

ECG 11-19

ECG CASE STUDIES: CONTINUED

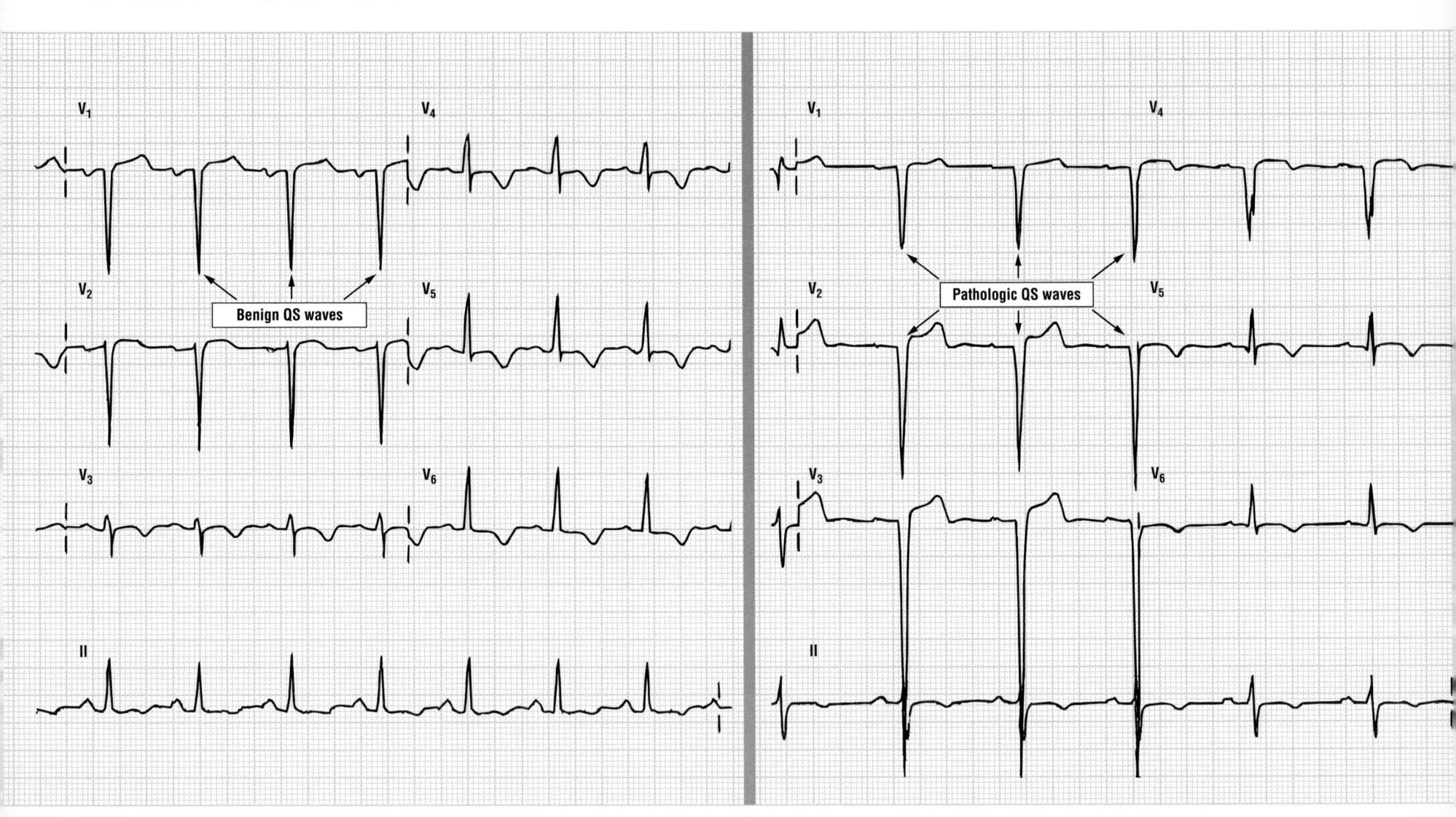

ECG 11-20

ECG 11-21 Let's look at lead III below. The Q waves are definitely changing in size from complex to complex. Looking at the rhythm strip, you'll see that the complexes with the red ovals beneath them have the shortest S waves. Why are they S waves? Because there is a tiny smidgen of an R wave preceding the negative component of each complex. Look at the undulating pattern of the length of the complex. The cycle repeats about every 3 to 4 seconds. What do we all do about every 3 to 4 seconds? We breathe. This is a respiratory variation. Changes in the respiratory pattern are reflected on the ECG. Sinus arrhythmia is also caused by the respiratory cycle.

ECG 11-21 This is not electrical alternans. Electrical alternans is associated with very different morphology and axis shifts occurring over one or a few beats. It is not just a minor and gradual shift, like the example shown below, but rather large swings in the positive and negative components of the QRS complexes. Electrical alternans is typically seen with large pericardial effusions, and with tachyarrhythmias.

There can also be electrical alternans of just the ST segments and T waves. These are typically associated with AMI, and carry a grim prognosis.

REMINDER:

There are pathological Q waves and benign Q waves. Examples of benign Q waves include:

- pseudoinfarct Q waves in WPW
- septal Q's
- benign QS complexes in V_1.

ECG CASE STUDIES: **CONTINUED**

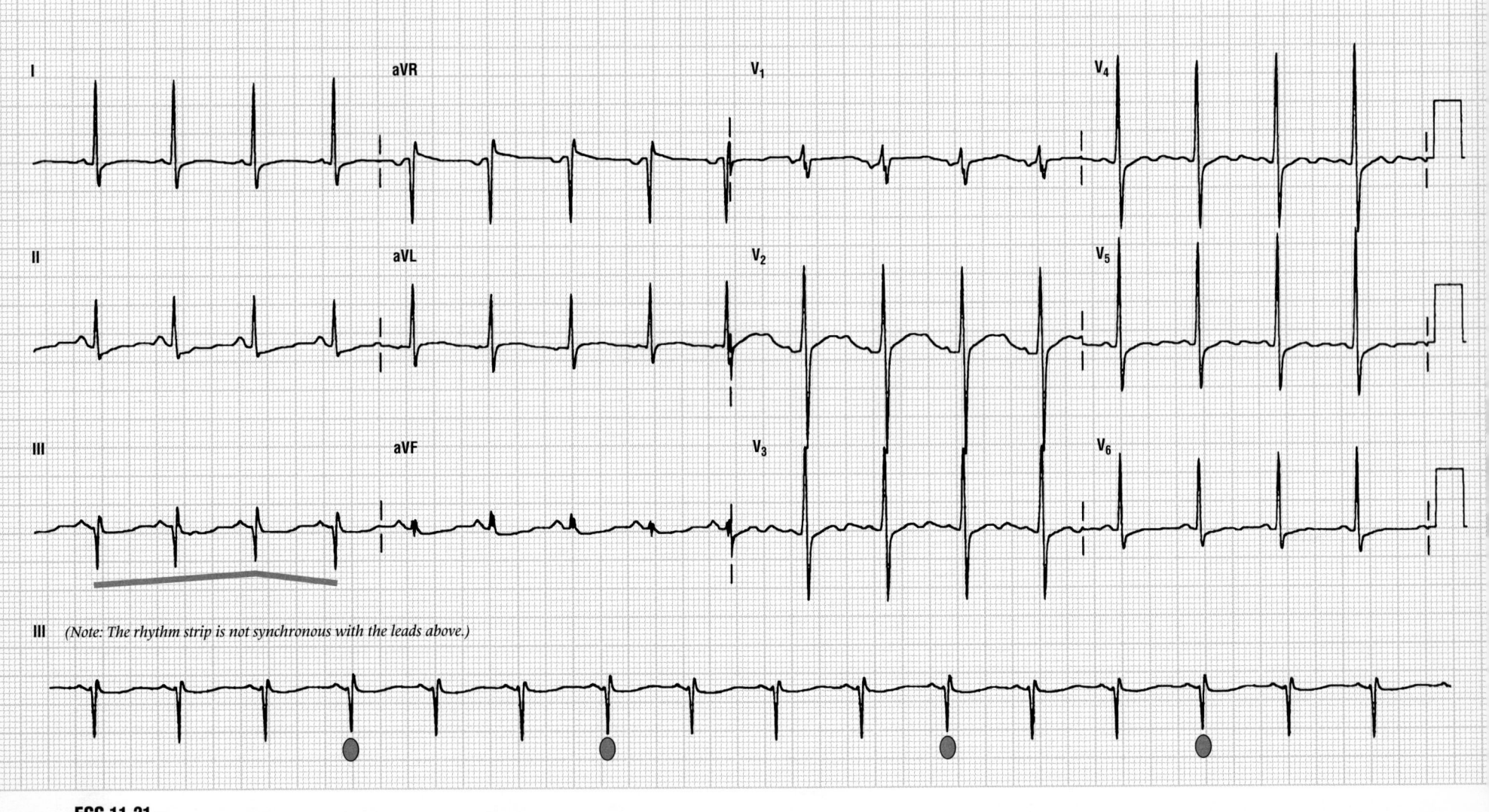

III *(Note: The rhythm strip is not synchronous with the leads above.)*

ECG 11-21

Significant (Pathological) Q Waves

So what, then, is a significant Q wave? A Q wave is significant if it is:

1. More than 1/3 the total height of the QRS (Figures 11-23 and 11-25)

2. Wider than 0.03 seconds (Figure 11-24)

It is better to have both criteria, but the second one is more significant — width more than 0.03 seconds. If it reaches one small block in duration, it is pathological.

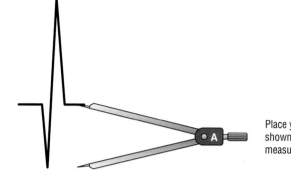

Place your calipers as shown in the diagram to measure the Q wave.

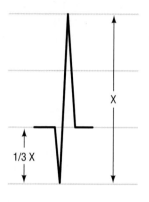

Figure 11-23: If the Q wave is more than one-third the total height of the QRS, it is a pathological Q.

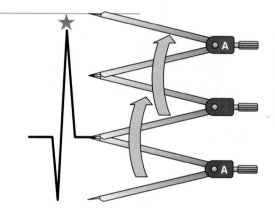

Walk your calipers up twice. If you have space between the top of the QRS complex and the top pin, then you have a pathological Q wave. This is because the Q wave is more than 1/3 the height. This is an easy way to check for the height criteria!

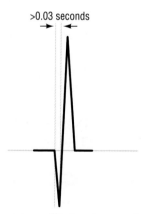

Figure 11-24: If the Q wave is more than 0.03 seconds wide, it is a pathological Q.

Figure 11-25: Measuring the Q wave.

ECG CASE STUDIES: **CONTINUED**

②

ECG 11-22 Look at this ECG and pick out the significant Q waves. Circle the leads that are affected. We start out by seeing the Qs in leads I, II, III, aVF, and V_5 to V_6. The Q waves in aVL are small but wide. The Q's in lead V_4 are essentially insignificant, but because they are part of the continuation of V_5 and V_6, they should still be considered pathological.

We're getting a little ahead of ourselves, but . . . remember when we were studying the vectors and we looked at the three-dimensional picture of the heart? We talked about some regions that could be isolated by looking at the leads. Can you see any regions in the ECG below? Leads II, III, and aVF represent the inferior leads. Leads $V_{4\,to}$ V_6, I, and aVL represent the lateral leads. Hence, this is an old infarct of the inferolateral walls.

③

ECG 11-22 The ECG shows an old infarct of the inferolateral area. There is, in addition, an anterior transition with a high R:S ratio in V_1 to V_2. The R in those leads is also wide. This is consistent with an old posterior AMI. Remember, posterior AMIs are associated with inferior AMIs because they are both under the distribution of the right coronary artery.

REMINDER:
Remember, use your differentials. If you did not go through the differential diagnosis of the increased R:S ratio in V_1 to V_2, you would have missed the PWMI.

②

ECG 11-23 Where are the pathologic Q waves in this ECG? If you answered leads III and aVF, you are correct. These are pathological because of both the width and height criteria. Now, what about leads V_1 to V_3: Are they pathological? No, a QS wave in lead V_1 is normal, and leads V_2 and V_3 have a tiny r wave at the onset of the complex. They are, therefore, not pathological.

Any other observations? Go ahead and look some more. There is evidence of LVH. Which criteria did we use to draw that conclusion? The S wave in V_2 and the R wave in lead V_6 add up to more than 35 mm.

REMINDER:
As you proceed through this book, keep in mind the things you have learned to that point. Add the new information to the old information.

Think about reading the whole ECG!

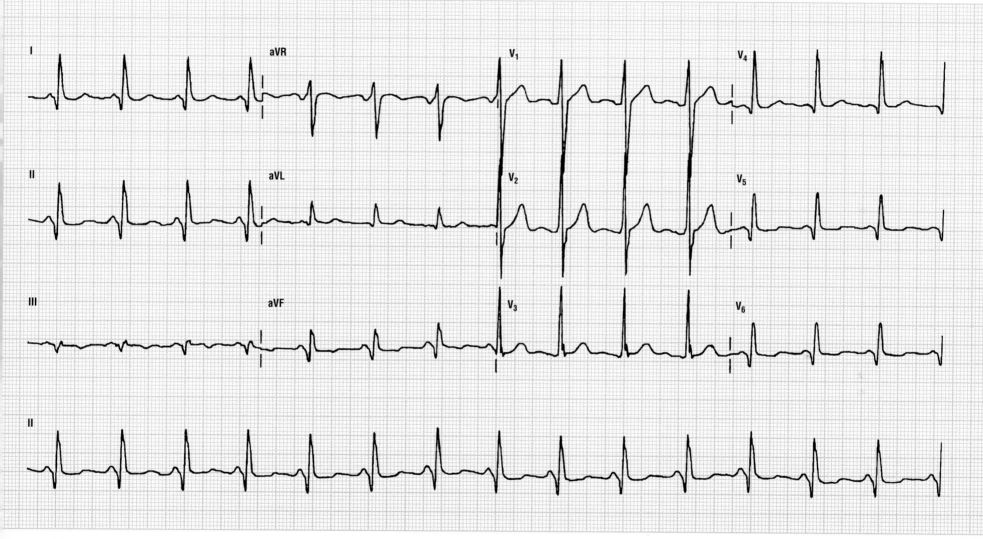

ECG 11-22

ECG CASE STUDIES: **CONTINUED**

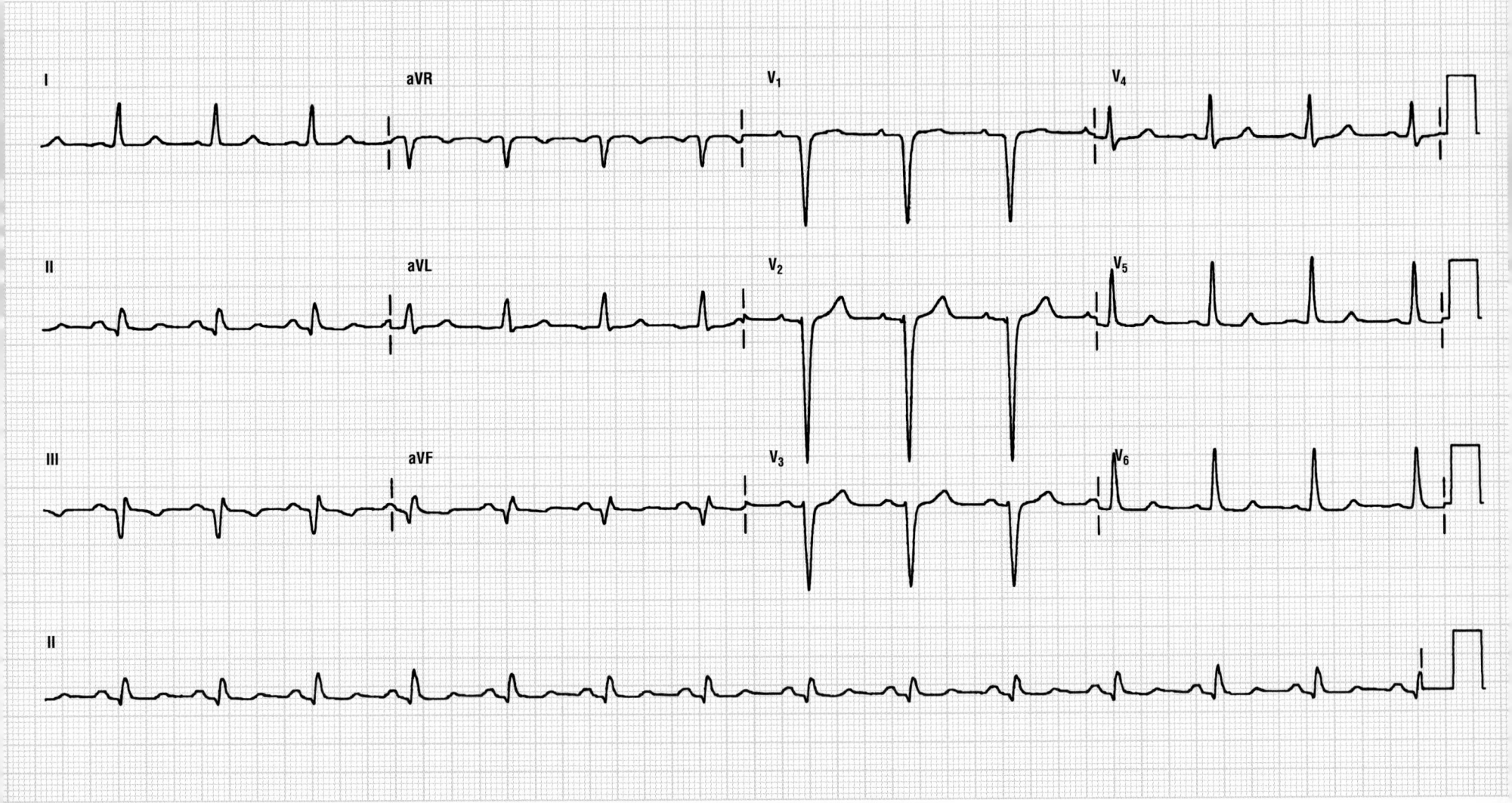

ECG 11-23

ECG 11-24 This ECG 11-24 once again has fairly easily identifiable Q waves in leads III and aVF. Lead II is also significant because it is more than one third the height of the R wave. Use the calipers the way we taught you to verify this distance.

Don't forget the rest of the ECG. There is left atrial enlargement in lead V$_1$. Did you notice the ST segments in leads II, III, and aVF? Are they normal or elevated? They are elevated. This is significant, especially in light of the pathologic Q waves in the same leads. Is there evidence for RVH? There definitely is an increased R:S ratio, but, as you will see later on, this could arise from other causes.

ECG 11-24 This is an acute AMI. It still has elevations and inverted T waves associated with the Q waves. It is not very acute, however, because the Q waves have had time to develop. Therefore, it has to be at least a few hours old.

The increased R:S ratio in lead V$_2$ could be due to RVH, or to an early PWMI. There is no way to tell which one it is unless you have an old ECG to compare. The presence of the same R wave in lead V$_2$, on both the old and the new ECG, would be consistent with RVH. A new R wave would be consistent with a PWMI.

Transition Zone

The transition zone refers to that area of the precordial leads where there is a transition from a mostly negative QRS complex to a mostly positive one. The actual transition occurs at the point where the QRS complex is isoelectric. Many times, there is one lead that is mostly negative, with the lead directly next to it mostly positive. The transition occurs somewhere between these two leads. An example is shown in Figure 11-26. (This discussion continues on page 207.)

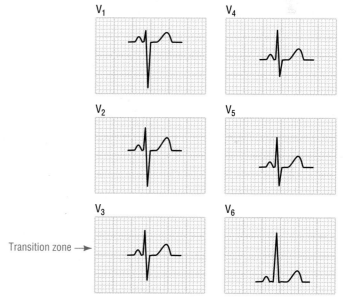

Figure 11-26: Transition zone.

ECG CASE STUDIES: CONTINUED

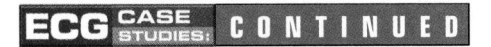

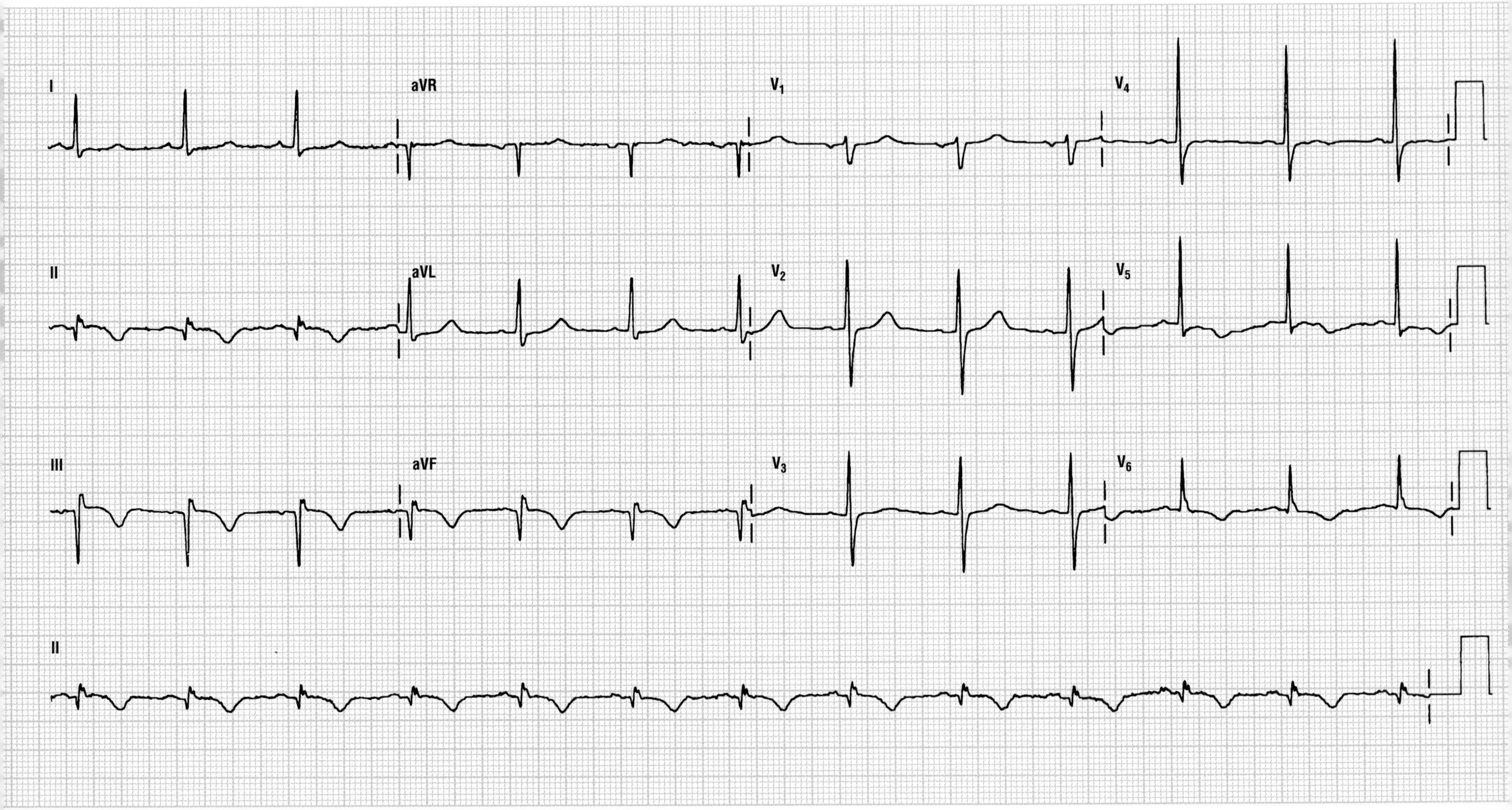
I
aVR
V_1
V_4
II
aVL
V_2
V_5
III
aVF
V_3
V_6
II

ECG 11-24

(Continued from page 205)

The normal transition occurs between V_3 and V_4 in most of the population (Figure 11-27). If the transition zone occurs before V_3, it is referred to as counter-clockwise rotation, while we call transitions after V_4 clockwise rotation, depicted in Figure 11-28. Note that clockwise and counterclockwise refer to the actual leads, as they are found on the chest wall or on the heart (if looked at from the feet), and not the ECG paper.

The transition zone will be very useful to us when we begin to discuss the Z axis and the anterior-posterior direction of the heart's main axis. We have first mentioned it in this section because of its widespread use by many authors. This will give you a superficial understanding of the concepts, and possibly avoid confusion.

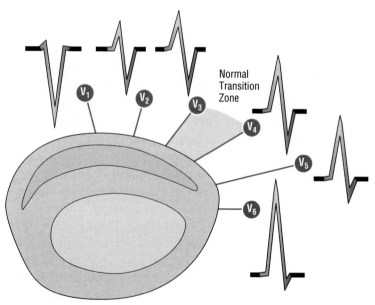

Figure 11-27: Normal transition zone

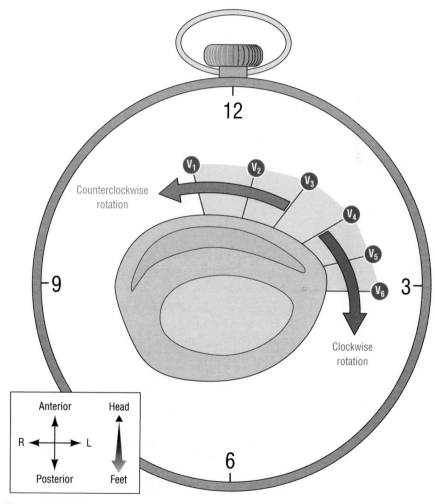

Figure 11-28: Two kinds of rotation

ECG CASE STUDIES: *Transition Zone*

ECG 11-25 Where do the precordial leads transition from negative to positive? Right after V_5. If you notice, V_5 is still slightly negative whereas V_6 is all positive. So the transition is late. This an example of a clockwise rotation.

This ECG is full of other interesting stuff. Have a closer look at it, and then come back up and we'll finish discussing some of the findings.

To begin with, there is evidence of LAE in lead V_1: a biphasic P wave with a deep second half. Is the PR interval prolonged? Remember that you have to look at the lead with the longest interval. In this case, the longest interval belongs to leads II and III. In these leads, the PR interval is just over 0.20, so it is prolonged. If you had looked at the other leads, you would have been misled.

What about the amplitude of the QRS complexes? The limb leads are just over 5 mm in leads III and aVF. So is this low voltage due to an effusion, for example? Not really, but very close! This is one of those cases in which the criteria are not met, but you still need to be awfully suspicious. Suspicion is good, especially in cardiology. There will be plenty of instances that do not meet criteria but are close. At these times, rather than making the call, state that you should correlate the history or the physical exam to evaluate the possibilities. Remember, there is always room for a small bit of error. Nothing is 100% correct or incorrect.

ECG 11-26 The transition in this ECG also occurs after lead V_5. However, this time the transition occurs about halfway between V_5 and V_6. Do you see what we mean? The S wave is about two thirds of the total amplitude in lead V_5, so it is mostly negative. In V_6, the R wave is about two thirds of the amplitude, so it is mostly positive. The exact middle is where the change occurred from negative to positive. Think of the transition as a continuum. That continuum, shown in Figure 11-29, extends from V_1 to V_6, and you are trying to find the exact spot where the transition occurred.

The PR intervals are the most interesting part of this ECG. There is diffuse ST depression and QT prolongation. There are no other criteria for pericarditis, so the cause is unclear.

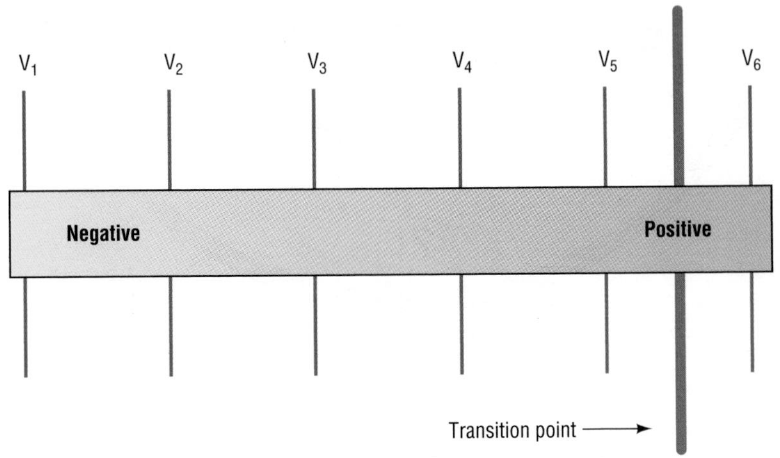

Figure 11-29: Transition point of ECG 11-26.

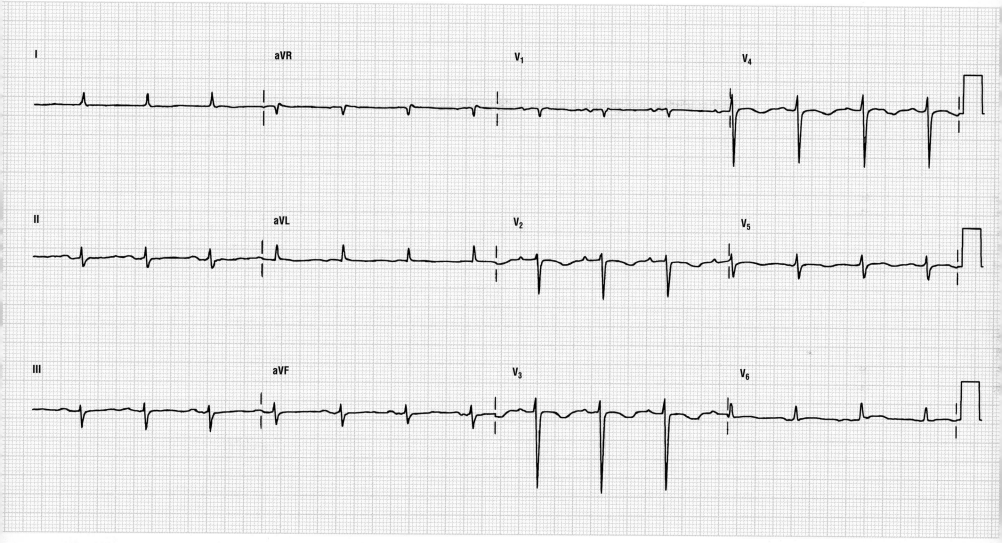

ECG 11-25

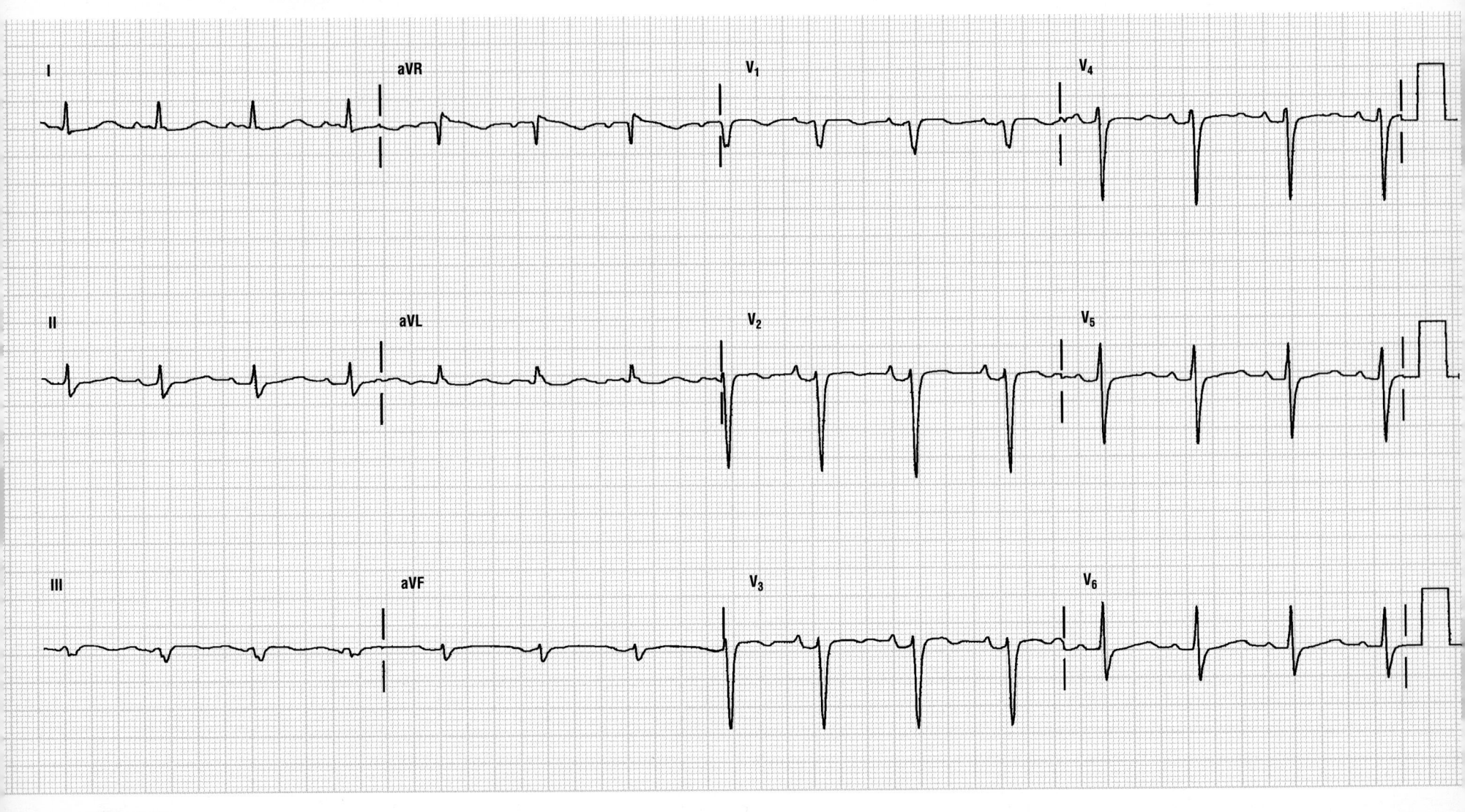

ECG 11-26

ECG 11-27 Notice on this ECG that the transition point occurs early, between V_1 and V_2. Once again, it is close to the middle of the area between the exact leads (shown in Figure 11-30).

Could this be an example of RVH? Sure it could! There is no additional evidence of right-sided hypertrophy, such as RAE, but it is definitely a big possibility. The other possibilities are that the patient is very young or an adolescent, or had a loss of posterior forces (a posterior MI).

What about LVH? Does it meet any criteria, and if so, which ones? The main ones are R in aVL that is more than 11 mm, and R in lead I that is more than 12 mm. So this patient could potentially have biventricular enlargement. Clinical correlation would be very helpful.

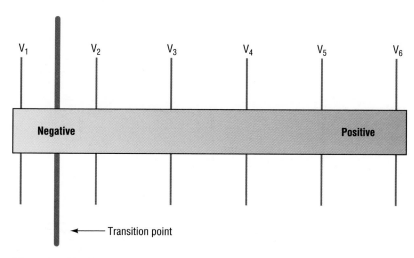

Figure 11-30: Transition point of ECG 11-27.

ECG 11-28 This ECG has a similar transition point (Figure 11-31) to the one seen in ECG 11-27, but there are some differences that make the differential diagnosis much easier here. The R wave is thinner — less than 0.03 seconds, to be exact. This knocks the possibility of a posterior wall AMI out of the picture. In addition, there are flipped T waves associated with the right precordial leads. The T waves are a bit more symmetrical than we would like for a strain pattern (see Chapter 14), but they don't have the characteristics of ischemic changes, either. In addition, there appears to be some mild RAE, because the first half of the P wave in lead V_1 is taller than that in V_6. Finally, there is some notching at the end of the QRS complex (which we'll review with ECG 11-29) that proves the ST segment changes to be non-ischemic in nature.

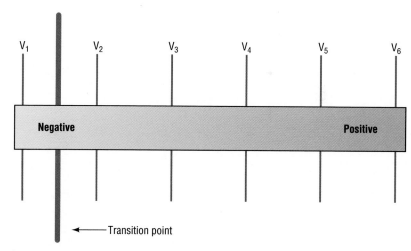

Figure 11-31: Transition point of ECG 11-28.

ECG CASE STUDIES: CONTINUED

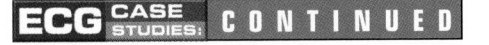

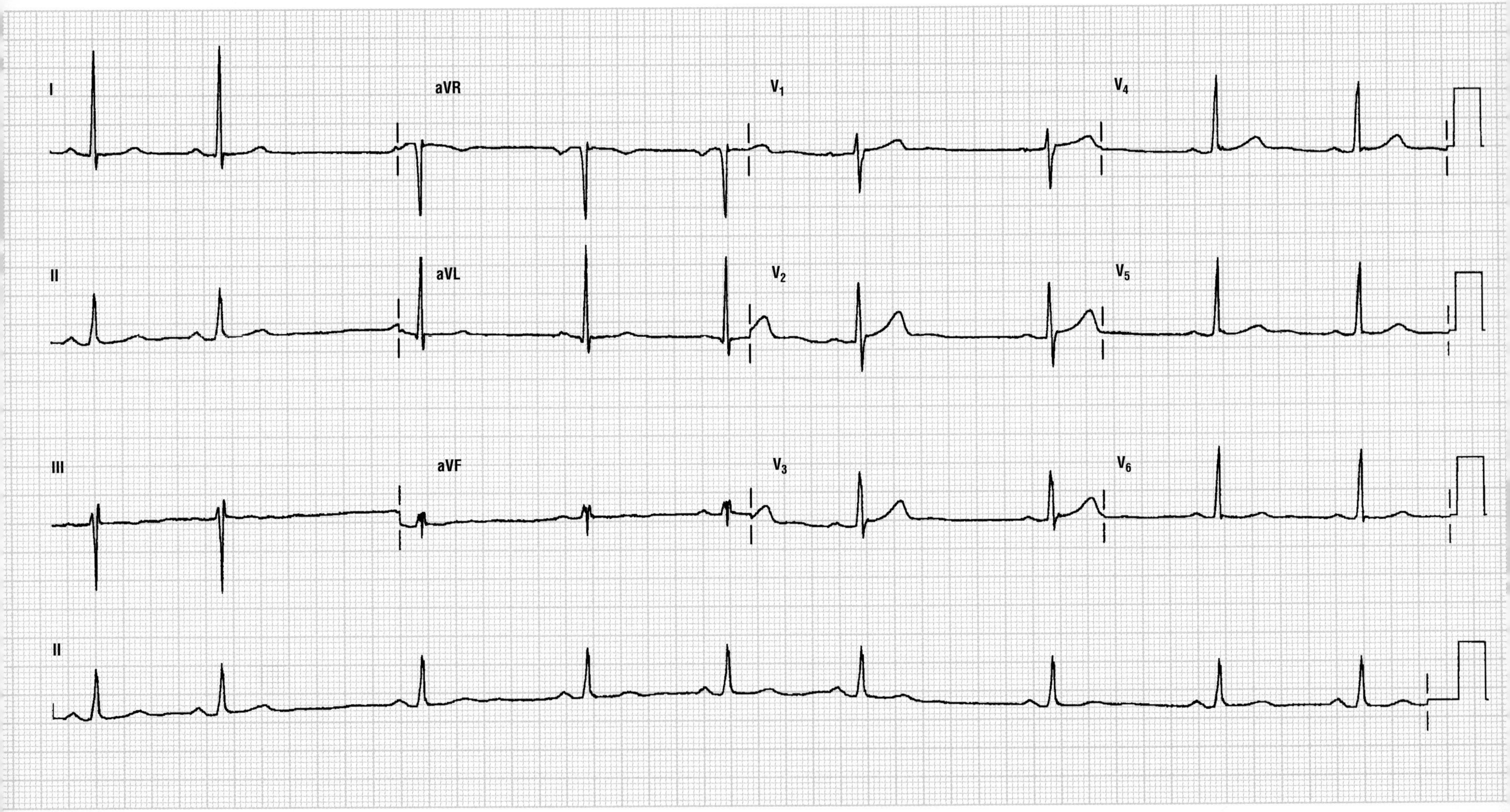

ECG 11-27

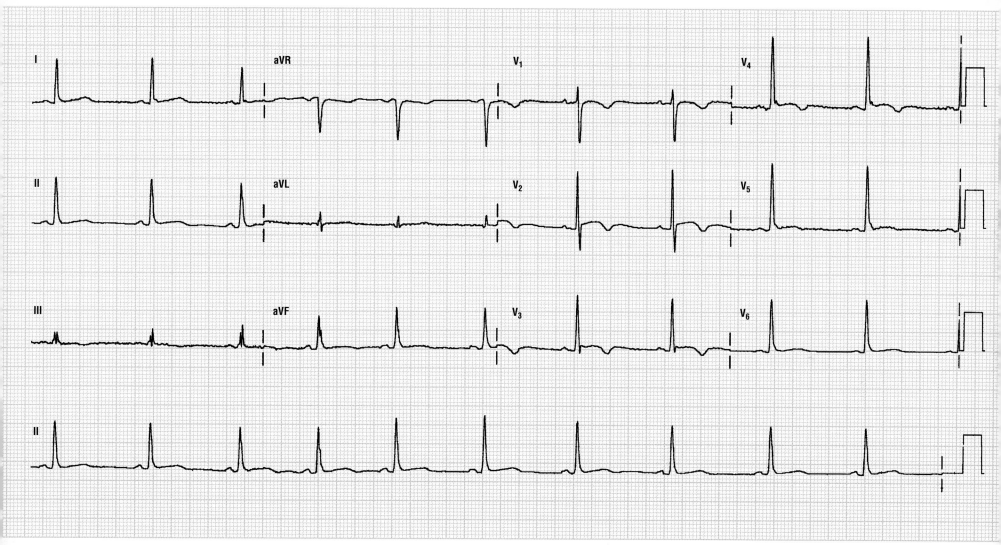

ECG 11-28

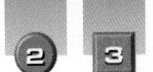

QRS Notching

Many times when you look at an ECG, you'll notice a small notch at the end of the QRS complex, as shown in Figure 11-32. The notch is almost always associated with a benign cause of ST segment elevation, such as early repolarization pattern or pericarditis (see Chapter 14). It will commonly be seen in the precordial leads, but can occur anywhere on the ECG.

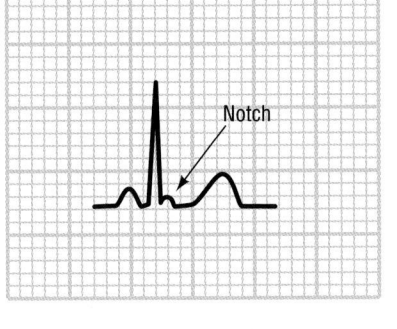

Figure 11-32: QRS notching

As with everything we do in ECG interpretation, you need to use some clinical correlation to arrive at the correct answer. You can be almost completely sure, when you see the notching, that the ST elevation afterward is benign. Some authors actually state that it is always benign. However, we have seen one case of a young man who had notching on his original ECG, then presented having a cocaine-associated AMI with additional elevation on top of his usual pattern. There are very few times when it is completely safe to say "always."

Do not confuse the notch above, which is small and looks like a bump on the QRS complex, with the Osborn — or J — wave that we'll cover next.

Osborn (J) Waves

The Osborn, or J, wave, shown in Figure 11-33, occurs in cases of severe hypothermia. It presents as a large deflection at the end of the QRS complex and could be mistaken for another wave in the QRS complex, such as RSR". The cause of the wave is not known. One thing is clear, however — the colder the patient's core temperature, the higher the Osborn wave. There can also be ST segment depression and flipped T waves seen with very tall Osborn waves. The Osborn wave is usually associated with other findings of hypothermia, such as bradycardia or atrial fibrillation.

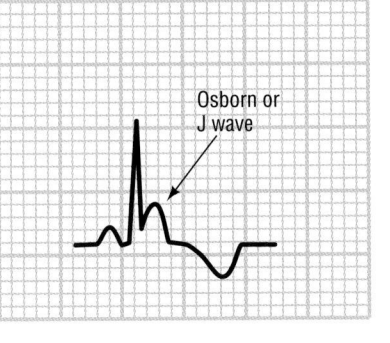

Figure 11-33: Osborn or J wave

NOTE

Hypothermia can result from many causes, including Addison's disease, sepsis, and severe hypothyroidism. The Osborn wave can occur in any circumstance associated with hypothermia, regardless of the cause! There does not have to be environmental exposure, even though this is the most common cause.

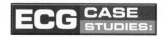

ECG 11-29 Look at the areas pointed out by the blue arrows below. These are the notches that we are talking about. Notice that they are small and not very obvious. When you see some ST elevation associated with the notch, you can be almost 100% sure that it is not due to an AMI. We say almost because there are very few things in life that are completely certain. We had said 100% up until we saw the young man with early repolarization pattern, mentioned above, who presented with a cocaine-associated AMI. The first ECG showed higher ST elevation with the notch. The second ECG, 20 minutes later, showed a more classic picture for an AMI. That first ECG, however, blew the 100% mark right out of the ballpark. We will say, though, that it is still extremely rare.

Now, what other findings do we see? There is PR depression noted in many leads. It is not major depression, but it's there. Use your ruler to verify this finding. In addition, there is diffuse ST segment elevation with a scooping, upwardly concave pattern. These findings are consistent with either early pericarditis or early repolarization. So, how can you tell which one it is? Talk to the patient. If the complaint is chest pain that increases when the patient lies back, this is pericarditis. If the patient came in with a fractured ankle, it is probably early repolarization.

REMINDER:
Clinical correlation is invaluable in interpretation!

ECG 11-30 It should have been easier to spot the notch on this ECG, now that you've seen one. You will usually notice them more often in the lateral leads, V_4 to V_6. On this ECG, the lateral leads have a fairly prominent notch.

This ECG also has some PR depression and some ST segment changes similar to those we discussed in ECG 11-29. The differential diagnosis is the same: early, mild pericarditis versus early repolarization.

 NOTE An Osborn wave is not a really big notch! One is pathological, the other is a variant found on normal ECGs.

ECG CASE STUDIES: **CONTINUED**

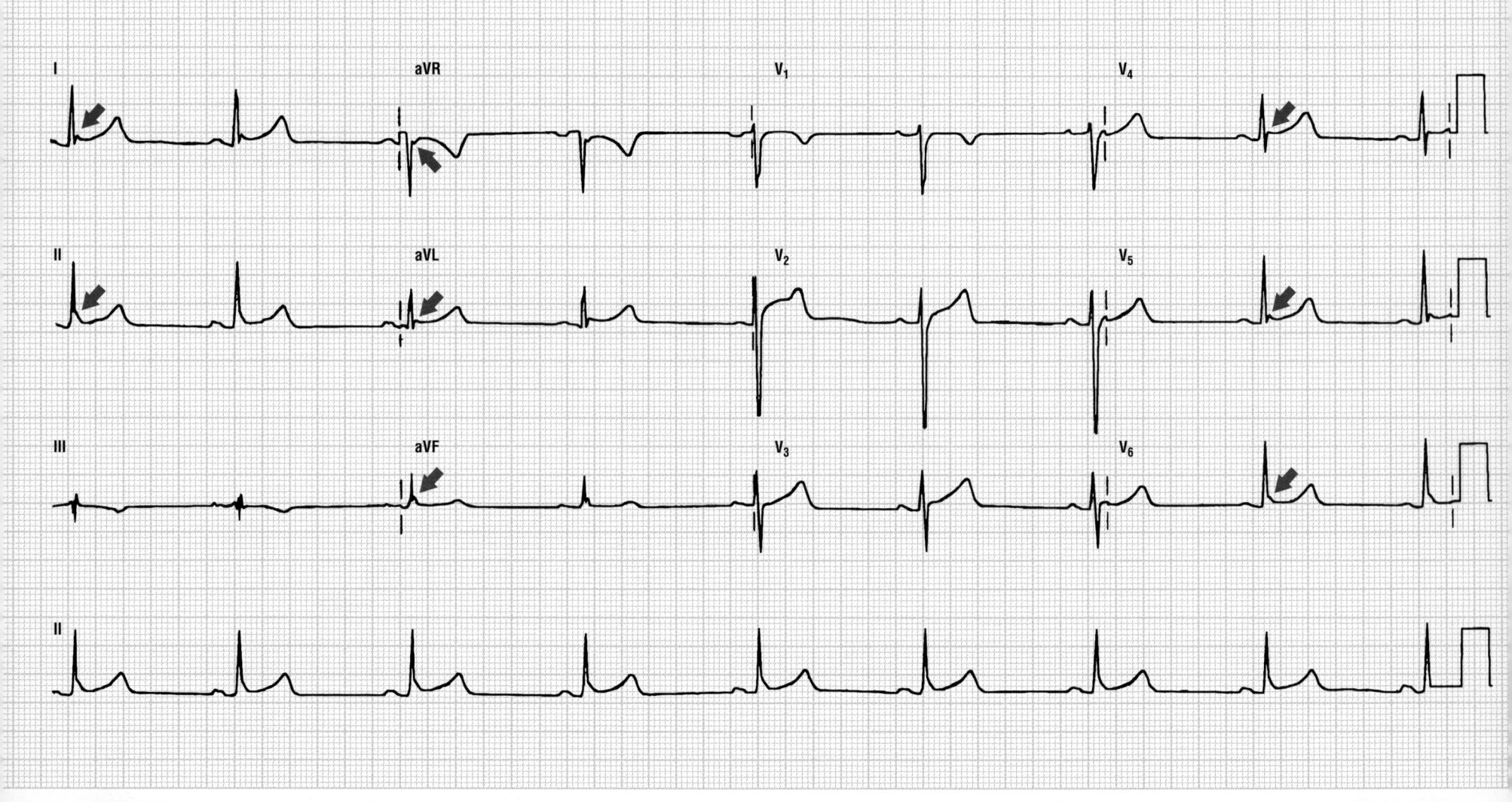

ECG 11-29

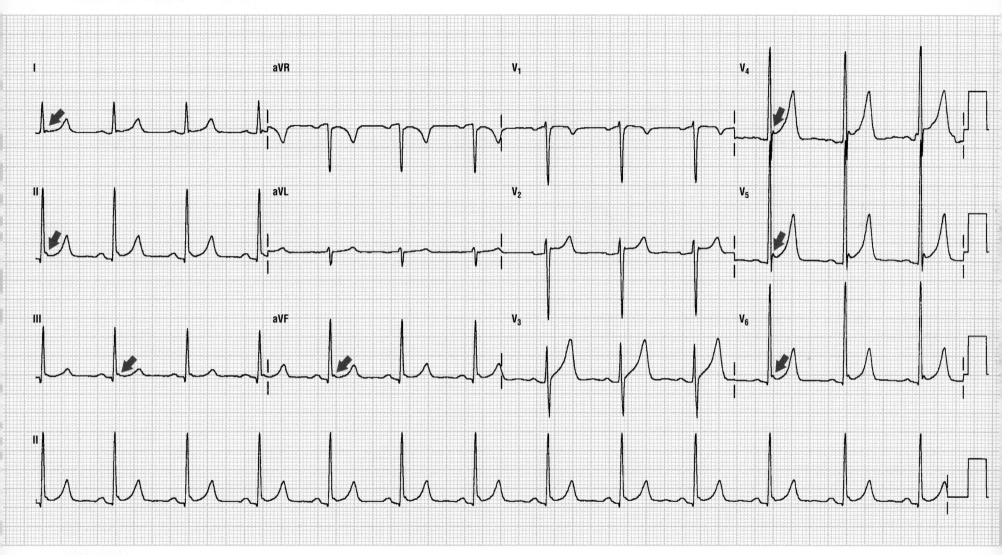

ECG 11-30

ECG CASE STUDIES: **CONTINUED**

3

ECG 11-31 We're going to show you three examples of Osborn waves in a row, so you can see some variations on a theme. Notice that they do not look alike at all. When you look at the Osborn waves below, highlighted by the blue arrows, they are much bigger than the notches we saw in ECG 11-29 and 11-30. They are not only taller, but also wider, than the benign notches.

Hypothermia has some other associated ECG findings. Bradycardia is very common because of the patient's decreased core temperature. A slight widening of the intervals occurs, but prolongation of the QT interval is usually significant, as in this case.

Did you notice the different P wave morphology on the rhythm strip? This is an APC.

ECG 11-32 The Osborn wave in ECG 11-32 is not difficult to miss. This is a great example of a diffuse Osborn wave and QT prolongation. You will notice that there is some artifact on the ECG. This is common for hypothermic patients. It is not due to shaking, because the body defenses to elevate the temperature are nonfunctional at very low temperatures. This patient was at 23.7°C on arrival in the emergency department.

The ECG is an invaluable asset in assessing these patients in the emergency department. Most of them arrive with altered mental status and intoxication, and they are cold to the touch. But most patients feel cold in winter. When you get an ECG as part of your regular evaluation, it will guide you to the appropriate therapy.

ECG 11-33 The Osborn waves in ECG 11-33 are not quite as big as the ones seen in ECG 11-32, but they are still quite obvious. Though these are narrower, many patients present with these characteristic findings.

The third complex is an APC. LVH is indicated by both the greater than or equal to 35 mm criterion (summing the S wave in V_1 to V_2 and the R wave in V_5 to V_6) and by the R wave that is greater than or equal to 20 mm in aVF.

REMINDER:
Be careful moving these patients around!

CLINICAL PEARL

Hypothermia is associated with cardiac irritability. Ventricular arrhythmias are common. Core body temperatures below 32°C make the heart irritable and vulnerable to ventricular arrhythmias, including fibrillation, when it is mechanically shaken. This occurs, for example, in moving the patient onto a stretcher or a heating blanket. When you see an Osborn wave on the ECG, be extra cautious in moving the patient!

CLINICAL PEARL

Catecholamines such as epinephrine and dopamine will not work in a hypothermic patient. You need to warm the patient to above 32°C in order for them to work. Give only one round of catecholamines in a code, until you warm the patient.

The patient is not dead until he's warm and dead!

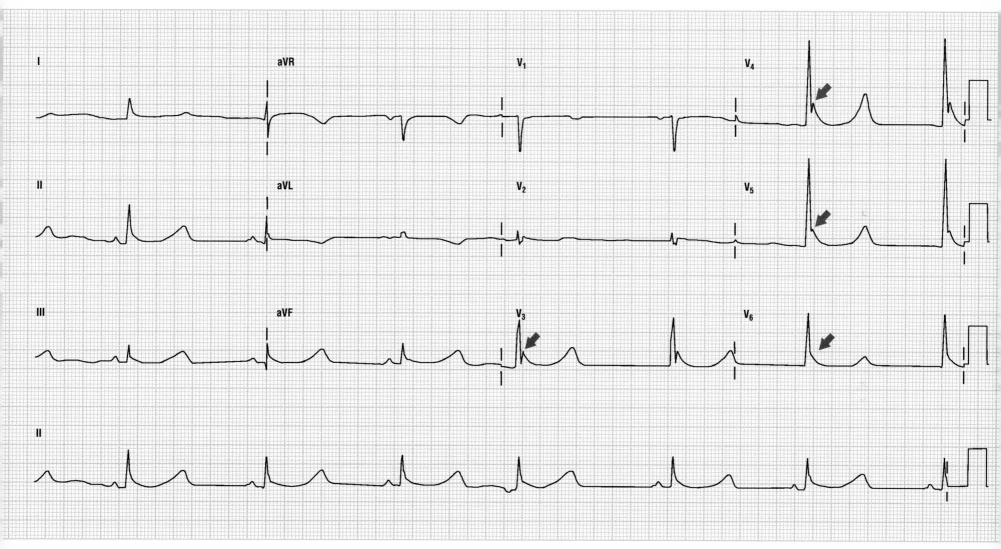

ECG 11-31

ECG CASE STUDIES: **CONTINUED**

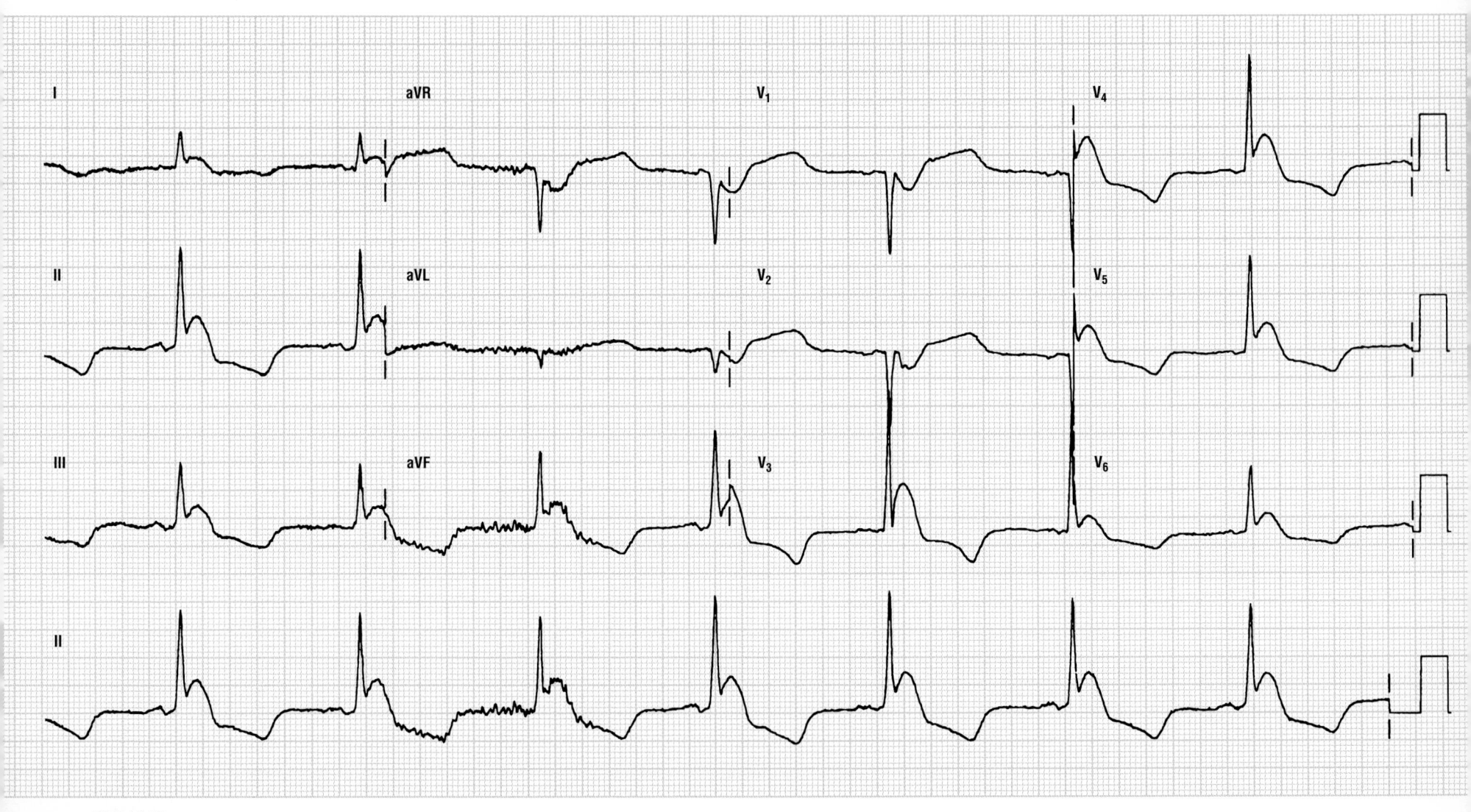

ECG 11-32

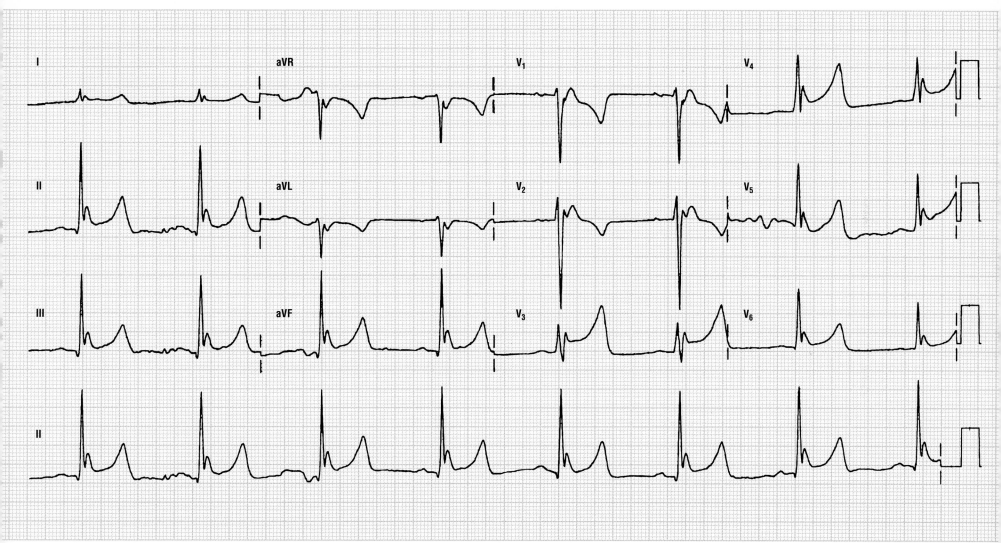

ECG 11-33

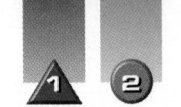

1 CHAPTER IN **REVIEW**

1. Which of the following is not important when evaluating the QRS complex:
   A. The height or amplitude
   B. The morphology of the complexes
   C. The presence of Q waves
   D. The frontal plane axis
   E. The length of the PR interval preceding it

2. Infarcted areas of myocardium add amplitude to the QRS complex. True or false.

3. The voltage in the limb leads is normally ≥ 5 mm; the voltage of the precordial leads is normally ≥ 10 mm. True or false.

4. You should always measure the widest QRS complex in the ECG, or you will be misled as to the true duration of the QRS complex. True or false.

5. Which of the following is incorrect:
   A. Septal Q waves are normally found in leads I and aVL.
   B. Septal Q waves are a normal variant.
   C. Septal Q waves are not significant.
   D. Septal Q waves represent an age-indeterminate myocardial infarction.
   E. None of the above

1. E 2. False 3. True 4. True 5. D

2 CHAPTER IN **REVIEW**

6. Which of the following is not a criteria for LVH:
   A. (S in V_1 or V_2) + (R in V_5 or V_6) ≥ 35 mm
   B. Any precordial lead ≥ 40 mm
   C. R wave in aVL ≥ 11 mm
   D. R wave in lead I ≥ 12 mm
   E. None of the above

7. In RVH, the R:S ratio is 1 in leads I and II. True or false.

8. Causes of QRS widening include all of the following except:
   A. Hyperkalemia
   B. Ventricular rhythms
   C. LGL
   D. Drug effects
   E. Bundle branch blocks

9. Make sure all of the morphologies are the same in each of the complexes on an ECG. If they are not the same, you need to ask yourself why. True or false.

10. A small notch at the end of the QRS complex is always associated with:
    A. Myocardial infarction
    B. Drug effect
    C. Temperature
    D. Infection
    E. None of the above

6. B 7. False 8. C 9. True 10. E

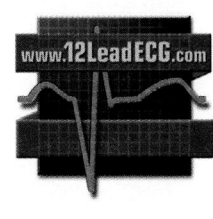

CHAPTER 12

Up until now, we have touched on the concept of the electrical axis in various chapters. This tells you that just about everything in electrocardiography is related to the electrical axis and its graphic representation in the different leads. Before you begin this chapter, you should go back and review Chapter 3 on vectors.

The electrical axis, as we discussed there, is the sum total of all the vectors generated by the action potentials of the individual ventricular myocytes. We cannot evaluate the ventricular axis directly. Instead, we have to measure the way the vector looks as it travels under each of the various electrodes. The "pictures" generated by each of the leads give us different views of this axis as it relates to the three-dimensional state, as shown in Figure 12-1. When we examine how those pictures appear, we can piece together the vector because we know the locations from which they were taken.

How do we use the axis clinically? Suppose there is hypertrophy of one of the ventricles. That ventricle would alter the ventricular axis in such a way as to assist us in diagnosing the problem. Now, imagine that an area of the heart infarcts. The ventricular axis would definitely be altered by the lack of electrical activity generated in that dead zone. Suppose a section of the electrical conduction system is diseased or blocked. Do you think that would alter the electrical axis of the ventricle? It certainly would.

For now, we are going to be reviewing the ventricular axis. Remember that there is an axis generated by each of the waves and intervals of the complex. The way they interact will reflect pathology.

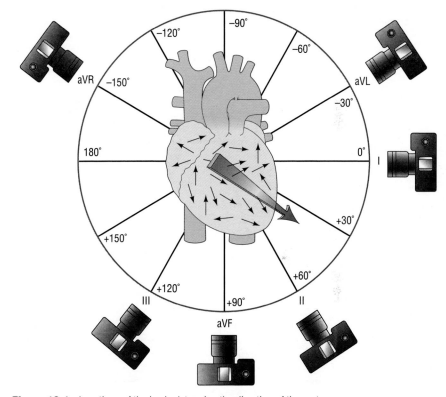

Figure 12-1: Locations of the leads determine the direction of the vector.

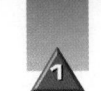

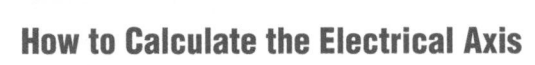

How to Calculate the Electrical Axis

There are many ways to calculate the direction and intensity of the ventricular axis. We will show you a system that we feel is easy to understand and use. In this Level 1 introduction, we will present a very simple system that breaks the hexaxial system down into four quadrants. Then we will show you how to determine the exact quadrant that holds the ventricular axis. In Level 2, we will show you how to localize that vector further in a coronal, or X-Y, plane using the limb leads. Level 3 will explain how to calculate the "Z axis" (anterior-posterior plane) using the precordial leads.

The hexaxial system is represented by a circle with all of the leads enclosed. Remember that the entire circle is composed of six leads superimposed on each other? (Review this in Chapter 3 if you don't.) Each lead has a positive half and a negative half, as shown in Figure 12-2. For simplicity, we'll make the side with color and the lead label the positive half; the white and unlabeled side will always be the negative half.

Now, notice that the dividing line between each positive and negative half of a lead happens to fall on a lead that is at an exact 90° angle from it. This lead is referred to as the isoelectric lead, meaning that it is neither positive nor negative along that line (red labels in Figure 12-2). In other words, each lead has a corresponding isoelectric lead; I is isoelectric to aVF, II is isoelectric to aVL, III is isoelectric to aVR, and vice versa. This concept of the isoelectric lead will be very useful to us later on when we want to isolate the lead to within 10°.

On the ECG, any positive vector will be represented as taller or more positive. Any negative vector will appear as a deeper or more negative complex (Figure 12-3). A lead is considered positive if it is even a smidgen more positive than negative. (Webster's defines *smidgen* as a little teeny bit.) Likewise, it is considered negative if it is even a smidgen more negative than positive.

A lead is isoelectric when it is exactly the same distance positive as it is negative. There is only one isoelectric limb lead on the ECG because there is only one ventricular axis. All the other leads are either positive or negative.

When we plot the vector on the hexaxial system, a vector that is even slightly positive will be found on the positive half of the circle. By the same token, any negative complex has to be on the negative half of the circle. If it is exactly isoelectric, then it will fall directly along

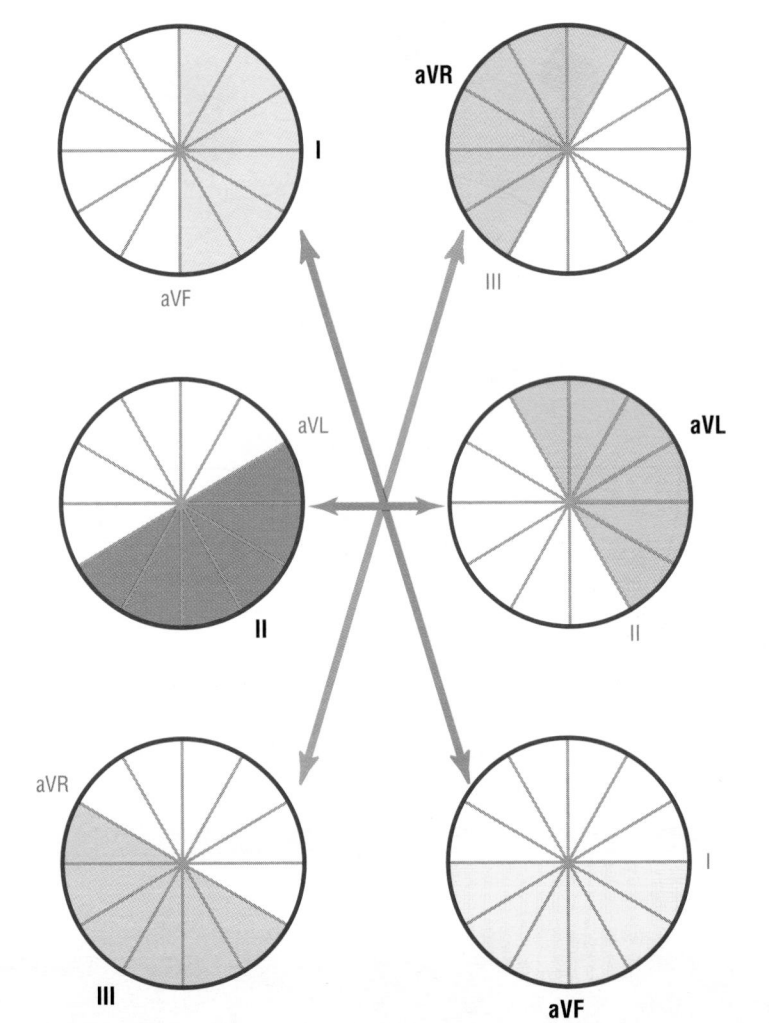

Figure 12-2: Leads and their isoelectric partners.

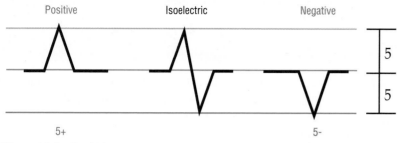

Figure 12-3: The QRS complex of positive, isoelectric, and negative leads.

the isoelectric lead. If that occurs, you have a slight problem. The vector can point in one of two directions, either toward the negative or toward the positive pole. Note that both of these directions will be exactly isoelectric to the lead in question. How can we resolve this dilemma? At this point, you need to go back to the ECG and take a look at the complexes that are found in that isoelectric lead. If those complexes are positive, then the vector will point in the direction of the positive pole of the isoelectric lead. If the complexes are negative, then the vector will point toward the negative pole. This is your first introduction into how we will always use two leads to isolate the vector. This is an important, but difficult, point to understand. In Figure 12-4, for instance, vectors A, B, and C are all positive in Lead I, and vectors D, E, and F are all negative in Lead I.

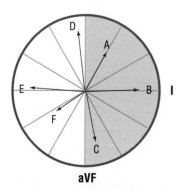

Figure 12-4: Positive and negative vectors in the hexaxial system.

Can you now see how the vector and the ECG are related? Because the vector cannot be seen, we use the complexes, and their relative positivity or negativity in each lead, to calculate the exact direction of the ventricular axis. Let's begin by seeing how to shorten the direction from 360° down to one of four 90° quadrants.

When we look at a 12-lead ECG, we do not know where the axis is pointing. To start isolating that direction, we want you to look at Leads I and aVF (notice that these leads are isoelectric to each other). First, look at Lead I and figure out whether it is positive or negative. Don't worry about how positive or negative right now; you only care about which half of the circle it falls into. If it is positive, it would have to be on the blue or positive side of the lead; if negative, it will fall in the white or negative half of the lead, as shown in Figure 12-5A. Next, look at lead aVF. Repeat the same thought process. Is it positive or negative in aVF? Place it in either the yellow or the white half, as referenced in Figure 12-5B. Because we know that yellow and blue make green, by overlapping these two circles, we create a new circle with four quadrants: one white, one blue, one yellow, and one green, as seen in Figure 12-5C.

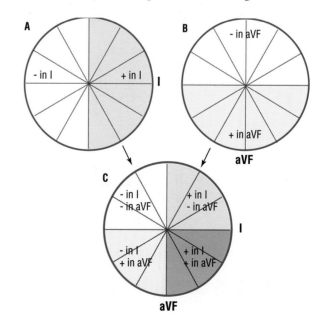

Figure 12-5: Isolating the direction of the axis

CHAPTER **12** • THE ELECTRICAL AXIS

Instead of saying positive or negative, we find it useful to say that a positive lead is taller than it is deeper, hence ↑. A negative lead is deeper than it is tall, thus ↓. Using this system, you do not have to add the heights of the complex's components algebraically.

Suppose a 12-lead has a positive Lead I and a positive Lead aVF. The only quadrant that matches this pattern is the Normal quadrant (Figure 12-6). See how easy? Next, we will isolate the axis to within 10°, but for now let's just take baby steps in determining the quadrant.

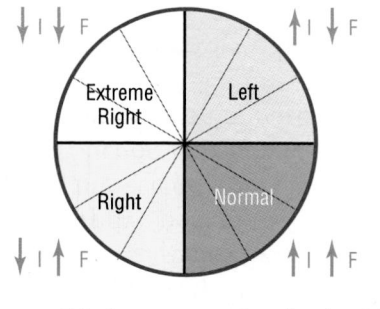

Figure 12-6: The four quadrants of the hexaxial system.

We have seen that by looking at only Leads I and aVF, we were able to break the hexaxial system down into four quadrants. We are going to name these four quadrants to make them easier to identify: Normal, Left, Right, and Extreme Right. These are shown in Figure 12-6.

These are going to be very useful to us when we get ready to calculate the true axis as closely as possible. For now, we can just state that any axis that falls outside the Normal quadrant should be considered abnormal. (In reality, the Normal quadrant extends from −20 to +100°, not 0 to +90°, but the latter is close enough for now.) If the axis falls into the Left quadrant, it is considered to have a *left axis deviation*. If it falls into either the Right or Extreme Right, it has a *right axis deviation*.

Remember, use your calipers!

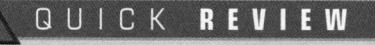

Figure 12-7: Sample ECG waves from which to calculate quadrants.

1. Normal 2. Left 3. Right 4. Extreme right 5. Normal 6. Left (−90°) 7. Extreme Right 8. Normal (90°) 9. Left 10. Right (180°)

Isolating the Axis

There are five steps to figuring out the ventricular axis:

1. Find the quadrant
2. Isolate the isoelectric lead
3. Isolate the closest lead
4. Isolate the vector
5. Double-check your findings

1. Find the Quadrant

Go back and review the Level 1 material at the beginning of this chapter. This will give you a quick and easy way to isolate the quadrant that contains the axis. Figure 12-8 once again shows the names of the four quadrants.

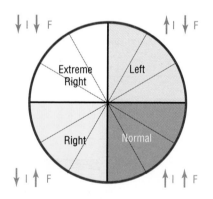

Figure 12-8: The four quadrants of the hexaxial system.

2. Isolate the Isoelectric Lead

Look at the six limb leads and decide which is the isoelectric lead. *Remember, for purposes of axis isolation, the isoelectric lead always has the smallest QRS voltage.* It doesn't necessarily have to be isoelectric. If possible, choose the smallest *and* the most isoelectric lead; if two leads are the same size, pick the one that is the most isoelectric. Figure 12-9 demonstrates vector direction in relation to wave shape.

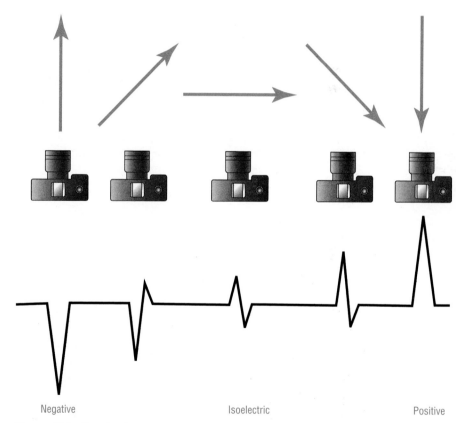

Figure 12-9: Negative, isoelectric, and positive ECG waves resulting from vectors.

CHAPTER **12** • THE ELECTRICAL AXIS

227

3. Isolate the Closest Lead

Think "T" when you go to isolate the axis to within 30°. What do we mean by that? Simply that you will be using a modified T to isolate the lead closest to the axis.

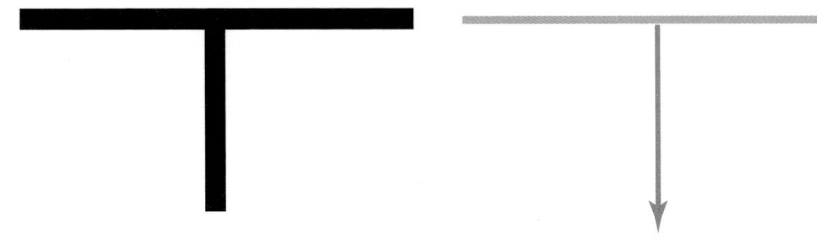

Figure 12-10: The "T" that will be used to isolate the lead closest to the axis.

Now, you notice that the T on the right in Figure 12-10 has a red arrow pointing at a 90° angle to the main line. There is only one arrow because the axis can only point in one direction on the X-Y axis. The main black line represents the isoelectric lead. You should place this black line directly over the isoelectric lead on the hexaxial system, with the red arrow pointing toward the appropriate quadrant that you isolated in step 1. This is a critical step. First, isolate the quadrant; then, when you place the arrow, it should point in that direction. If you do not follow this simple rule, you will be 180° off from the true axis.

Congratulations! If you have followed the first three steps, you should be close to the true direction of your axis — within 30° of it, to be exact. However, this is not close enough. We need to get to within 10°. We will be doing that in step 4. But first, let's go practice a little bit.

QUICK REVIEW

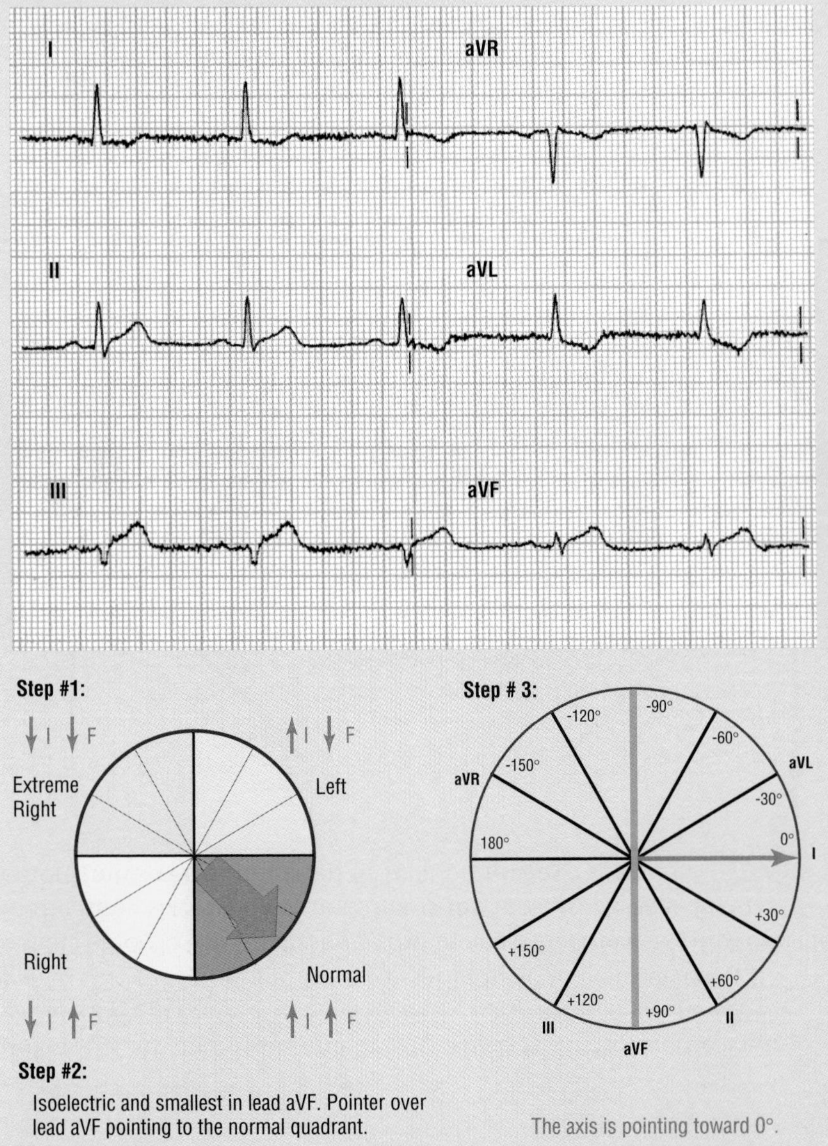

I	aVR

II	aVL

III	aVF

Step #1:

Extreme
Right

Left

Right

Normal

Step #2:

Isoelectric and smallest in lead aVF. Pointer over lead aVF pointing to the normal quadrant.

Step # 3:

-120° -90° -60°
aVR -150° aVL
-30°
180° 0° I
+150° +30°
+120° +90° +60°
III aVF II

The axis is pointing toward 0°.

Figure 12-11: Example #1

Figure 12-12: Example #2

Figure 12-13: Example #3

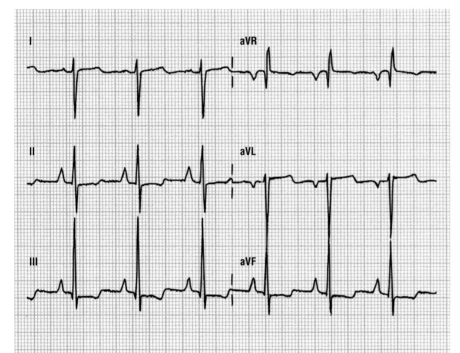

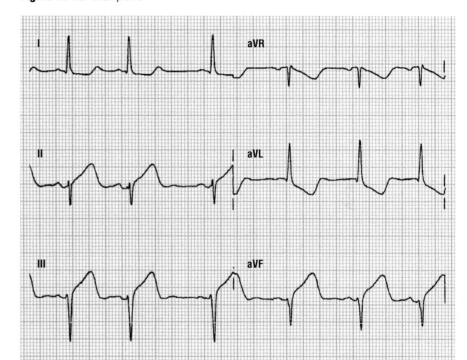

Step #1:

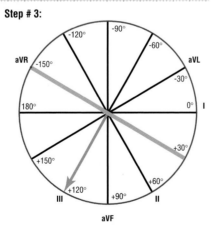

Step #2:

Isoelectric and smallest in lead aVR. Pointer over lead aVR pointing to the right quadrant.

Step # 3:

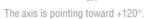

The axis is pointing toward +120°.

Step #1:

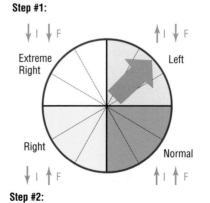

Step #2:

Smallest in lead aVR. Pointer over lead aVR pointing to the left quadrant.

Step # 3:

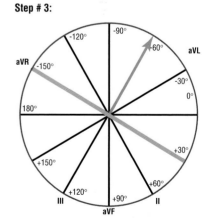

The axis is pointing toward -60°.

CHAPTER **12** • THE ELECTRICAL AXIS

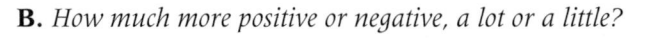

4. Isolate the Vector

Up to this point, we have narrowed down the exact location of the axis to within 30°. Why only to 30°? Well, the limb leads are 30° apart and the exact isoelectric lines may fall in between two of the leads — 45 or 50°, for example. In other words, the isoelectric limb lead and the isoelectric line are not necessarily the same. Remember we mentioned that the isoelectric limb lead had the smallest complexes, but that sometimes it didn't have isoelectric complexes? Sometimes the smallest lead is all positive or all negative. Other times it is slightly positive or negative. This occurs when the true isoelectric line falls somewhere outside the exact limb lead. Only when the limb lead is the smallest and has an isoelectric component is it the exact isoelectric lead.

We can arrive at the exact direction of the axis, or at least to within 10° of the true axis, with some simple adjustments of the isoelectric line to accommodate for the extra positivity or negativity of a lead.

The exact axis must be within 30 or 40° of the isoelectric limb lead. Otherwise, it would be isoelectric to one of the adjacent leads. For simplicity, we are going to look at 20° on either side of the isoelectric limb lead — 20° more positive or more negative. You will decide whether it is in the positive or negative direction by looking at the complexes that make up the isoelectric limb lead. If they are positive complexes, the axis will be shifted in the positive direction. If they are negative complexes, it shifts negatively. We decide whether to alter it by 10 or 20° based on the amount of the positivity or negativity of the complexes. Confused? The next few pages should help. This is the toughest part of the process, so stick with us.

Here are some simple steps to make the adjustment:

A. *Are the complexes in the isoelectric limb lead positive or negative?*

If they are isoelectric, you needn't go any further. This is your isoelectric line, and the vector is the exact measurement of the isoelectric limb lead. If the complexes are more positive or negative, then. . .

B. *How much more positive or negative, a lot or a little?*

First, measure the smaller of the two distances from the baseline. If the complex is positive, then the negative component will be the smaller. If the complex is negative, the positive component is the smaller. Next, use your calipers to transfer the measurement of the smaller component — let's name it x — to overlie the larger component. If the larger component is less than 2x in measurement, the complex is a little bit more positive or negative, about 10°. If the larger component is more than 2x in measurement, then the complex is a lot more positive or negative — 20° or so. This concept is demonstrated in Figure 12-14.

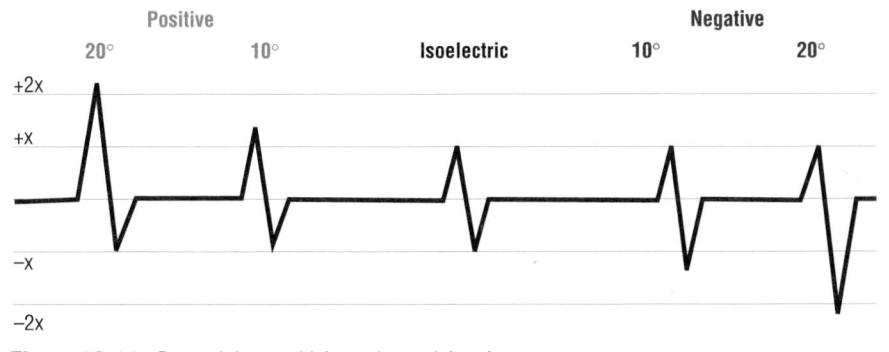

Figure 12-14: Determining positivity and negativity of vectors.

C. *Adjust the "T" bar to identify the true axial measurement!*

Now, in completing step B, we have decided that the axis is either 10 or 20° in either a positive or negative direction. But positive or negative to what? *The axial direction arrow, the red arrow of the T, needs to be moved 10 or 20° closer to the negative or the positive pole of the isoelectric limb lead!* Remember, we cannot measure the true axis; we calculate it based on the only information we know, the isoelectric line. By moving the axial direction arrow, we also move the isoelectric line. *Do not make the mistake of just algebraically adding the numbers to the degrees represented by the isoelectric limb lead!* We are using vectors and isoelectric leads, not numbers.

For example, suppose the isoelectric limb lead, aVL, is a lot more positive at 20°. Figure 12-15 illustrates the process we've just described.

The isoelectric lead is aVL. The positive pole of aVL is circled in red. Because the complex was a lot more positive (20° more), we move the axial direction arrow 20° toward the positive pole of aVL. The actual axis of the ventricle, therefore, is 40°.

With this step in hand, we can now return and finish our three examples from earlier in the chapter.

Figure 12-16: Example #1 (continued) (see Figure 12-11).

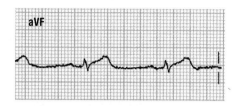

We see that aVF is the isoelectric limb lead and that it is a little bit more positive, 10°.

Figure 12-15

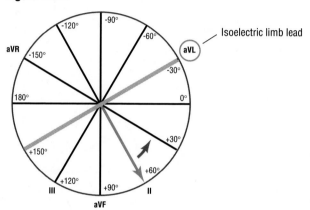

Isoelectric limb lead

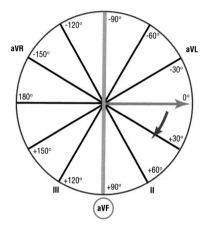

The isoelectric limb lead is aVF. So we move the axial directional arrow 10° toward the positive pole of aVF.

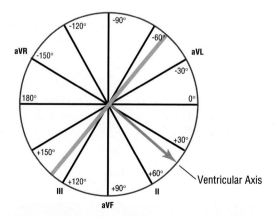

Ventricular Axis

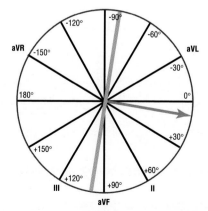

The ventricular axis is at +10°.

Figure 12-17: Example #2 (continued) (See Figure 12-12).

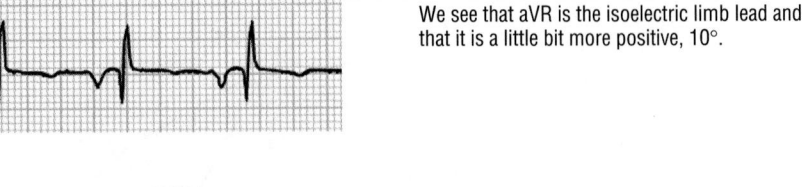

We see that aVR is the isoelectric limb lead and that it is a little bit more positive, 10°.

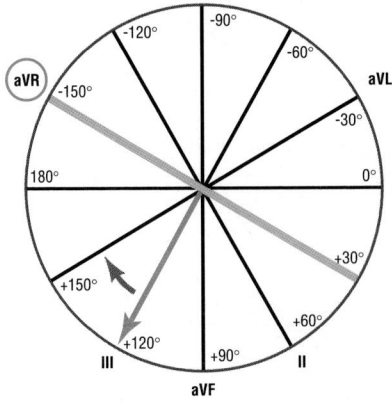

The isoelectric limb lead is aVR. So we move the axial directional arrow 10° toward the positive pole of aVR.

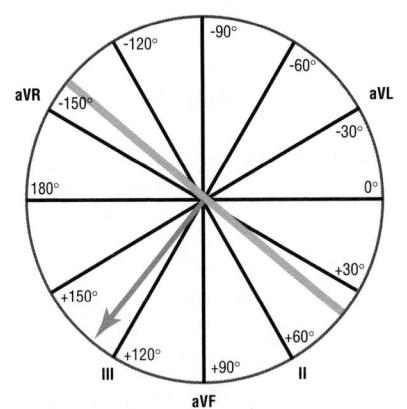

The ventricular axis is at +130°.

Figure 12-18: Example #3 (continued) (See Figure 12-13).

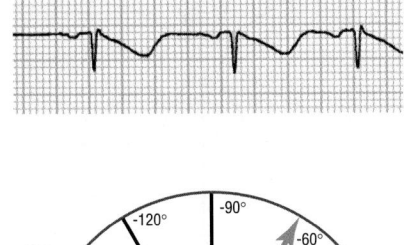

We see that aVR is the isoelectric limb lead and that it is a lot more negative, 20°.

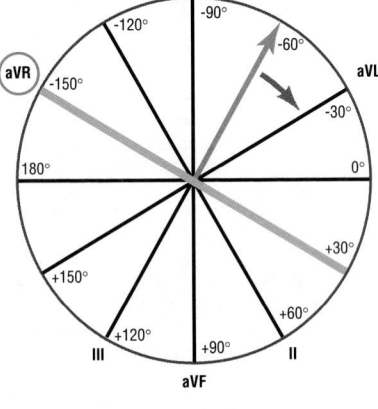

The isoelectric limb lead is aVR. So we move the axial directional arrow 20° toward the negative pole of aVR.

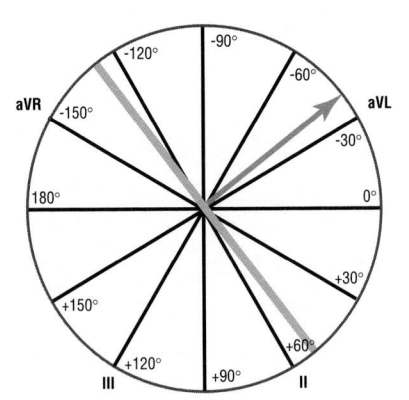

The ventricular axis is at -40°.

5. Double-check Your Findings

After you have arrived at the exact location of the ventricular axis, double-check yourself to see if you are right. This is a very easy step. Look at the lead closest to the direction that the axial direction arrow is pointing. That lead should be the tallest of all of the limb leads. Conversely, look at the lead that is directly opposite the axial direction arrow. That lead should be the deepest of all the limb leads (Figure 12-19).

This size criterion should make absolute sense. If it isn't completely clear, you can review it in Chapter 3, or see the section, *2. Isolate the Isoelectric Lead,* earlier in this chapter. This size criterion can also be used to approximate the axis in cases of indeterminate leads. These are rare cases in which the axis is difficult to pinpoint by using the system outlined in this chapter because two leads may look isoelectric.

Figure 12-19

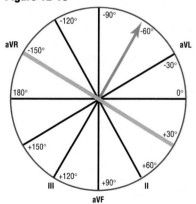

In this example, the tallest limb lead should be aVL, and the deepest should be III.

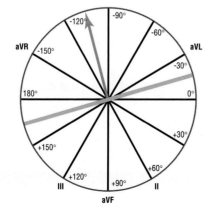

In this example, the tallest lead should be aVR, and the deepest ones should be II and aVF since the arrow is pointing away from the midpoint between them.

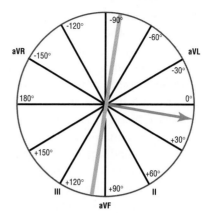

Figure 12-20: Example #1, double-check.

The tallest lead should be I, and the deepest should be aVR. Go back to figure 12-11 to see if this is right.

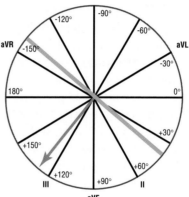

Figure 12-21: Example #2, double-check.

The tallest lead should be III, and the deepest should be aVL. Go back to figure 12-12 to see if this is right.

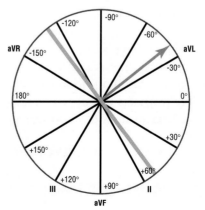

Figure 12-22: Example #3, double-check.

The tallest lead should be aVL, and the deepest should be III. Go back to Figure 12-13 to see if this is right.

Causes of Axis Deviation

Right Axis Deviation

These are the most common causes of right axis deviation (RAD):

1. Normal in adolescents and children
2. Right ventricular hypertrophy
3. Left posterior hemiblock
4. Dextrocardia
5. Ectopic ventricular beats and rhythms

Left Axis Deviation

The most common causes of left axis deviation (LAD) are:

1. Left anterior hemiblock (LAH)
2. Ectopic ventricular beats and rhythms

The most frequent cause of LAD is a LAH. We will be going into the bundle branch blocks in great depth in Chapter 13. Some people state that left bundle branch block (LBBB) also gives rise to LAD, but most patients with LBBB have a normal axis. As a matter of fact, LBBB with LAD is a poor prognostic indicator.

Since we are on this topic: Can you think of an easy way to diagnose LAH?* (Hint: Go back to the hexaxial system.)

*Answer: If you have a positive complex in lead I and a negative complex in aVF, the axis is in the left quadrant. If the complex is negative in lead II, you have isolated the axis to -30 to -90°, which is definitely abnormal. Remember your differentials. The most common cause of LAD is LAH. Therefore, if the complex is positive in I, and negative in aVF and II, you have identified LAH. More on this later.

The Z Axis

By this point in your electrocardiographic development, you should be well versed in the electrical axis and how to calculate it exactly. If you are unsure of the process, a short review trip through the beginning of this chapter should help tremendously.

What is the Z axis? Mathematicians have broken down the three dimensions into three axes. The X axis is traditionally labeled along a horizontal direction. The Y axis is labeled in a vertical direction. Together these two axes describe a plane. Now, to add a 3-D perspective, they created another axis and plane, which are perpendicular to the X-Y axis and plane, respectively: the Z axis and plane. All points in three-dimensional space, therefore, have three values that define their positions. In electrocardiography, vectors point in three dimensions and have a direction based on the X, Y, and Z axes along the frontal and cross-sectional planes. For example, suppose the frontal plane of the electrical axis points to 60°. You have no idea where along an anterior-posterior (Z) plane that the 60° vector points. It could point along a 60° angle straight down, slightly anteriorly, slightly posteriorly, and so on. The Z axis would help you isolate the true three dimensional direction of the axis.

Clinically, knowing the Z axis will be a big help to you to decide between possible differential diagnoses in certain pathological states. For example, suppose the patient had an anterior Z axis. This would indicate that the patient either had more tissue anteriorly (e.g., an enlarged right ventricle) or it could represent less tissue along the posterior wall (a posterior wall myocardial infarction). By the same token, if the patient had significant left ventricular hypertrophy or suffered a large anterior acute MI (AMI), his axis would face more posteriorly. The normal transition zone is between leads V_3 and V_4. This is numerically represented by a Z axis between 20 and 40° posteriorly. This slight posterior displacement of the Z axis occurs because most of the cardiac tissue is in the left ventricle. This causes the main axis to point in an inferoposterior direction.

We begin the process of isolating the Z axis by reviewing the origins of the A-P plane. The A-P plane, or Z plane, is calculated using the precordial leads, which split the heart in cross-section into superior and inferior portions (Figure 12-23).

The problem in deriving the three-dimensional electrical axis, once again, is that we cannot directly visualize it. Just as we used the isoelectric lead of the true axis to calculate its direction in the frontal plane, so too will we use the isoelectric component along the precordial leads to calculate the exact three-dimensional direction of the electrical axis. We start by identifying the precordial lead in which the complexes first change from negative to positive. If there is an exact isoelectric precordial lead, then that is your answer. Many times, however, you have a negative component in one lead and a positive component in the succeeding lead. In these cases, you estimate where the transition occurred. For purposes of calculation, the precordial leads are exactly 20° from each other with V_2 being the zero degree-mark. Let's look at an example. Suppose lead V_3 was completely negative and lead V_4 was completely positive, and the transition point occurred halfway between the two leads. Once you know where the transition occurs, you can look at Figure 12-24 and find the line corresponding to that precordial lead (represented by the colored circle and line). That line is actually the perpendicular of the true axis — in our example it is a line halfway between leads V_3 and V_4. Following the "T," we see that the vector will lie at either an angle that is 30° anterior or 30° posterior. That is where the frontal axis comes in. If the axis is normal or left, then the thick arrows are used. If the axis is rightward, then the thin arrows are used. The numbers at the ends of the arrows correspond to the direction of the electrical axis of the heart along the Z axis and plane. If our example were in the normal quadrant, the Z axis would face 30° posteriorly. It really isn't hard, but you do need to think three dimensionally. Let's go through it again in a little more detail . . . .

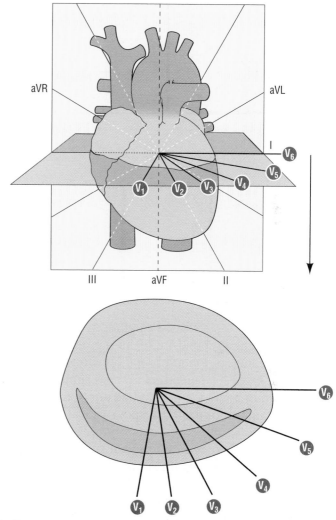

Figure 12-23: Three-dimensional view of the heart, divided by the coronal and sagittal planes.

Z-Axis Precordial Lead System

80°P

60°P

40°P

20°P

20°P

0° ———— 0°

V₆

20°A

20°A

V₅

40°A

V₄

60°A

V₁

80°A

V₂

V₃

If it falls in one
of the blue quadrants,
look at the degree markers
on the blue side above.

Extreme
Right | Left

Right | Normal

If it falls in one
of the yellow quadrants,
look at the degree markers
on the yellow side above.

Figure 12-24

The Z Axis Precordial Lead System

The complicated looking graphic in Figure 12-24 is a fast way of calculating the Z axis of any ECG. Once again, it is based on the concept of perpendiculars and a T bar similar to the one introduced in Figure 12-10. In this case, however, the perpendicular is the short bar rather than the long one, and it runs along the V leads rather than the limb leads. The arrow still points toward the true axis, though.

Let's look at lead V_2, for instance, shown in Figure 12-25. Because we cannot measure the exact axis, we need to use the perpendicular. In the case of the Z axis, the perpendiculars relate to the precordial leads. The two directions that are perpendicular to V_2 are 0° and 180°. Because these two vectors are not found at the same time (one corresponds to the Normal or Left quadrants, and the other to the Right or Extreme Right), we use 0° for both vectors.

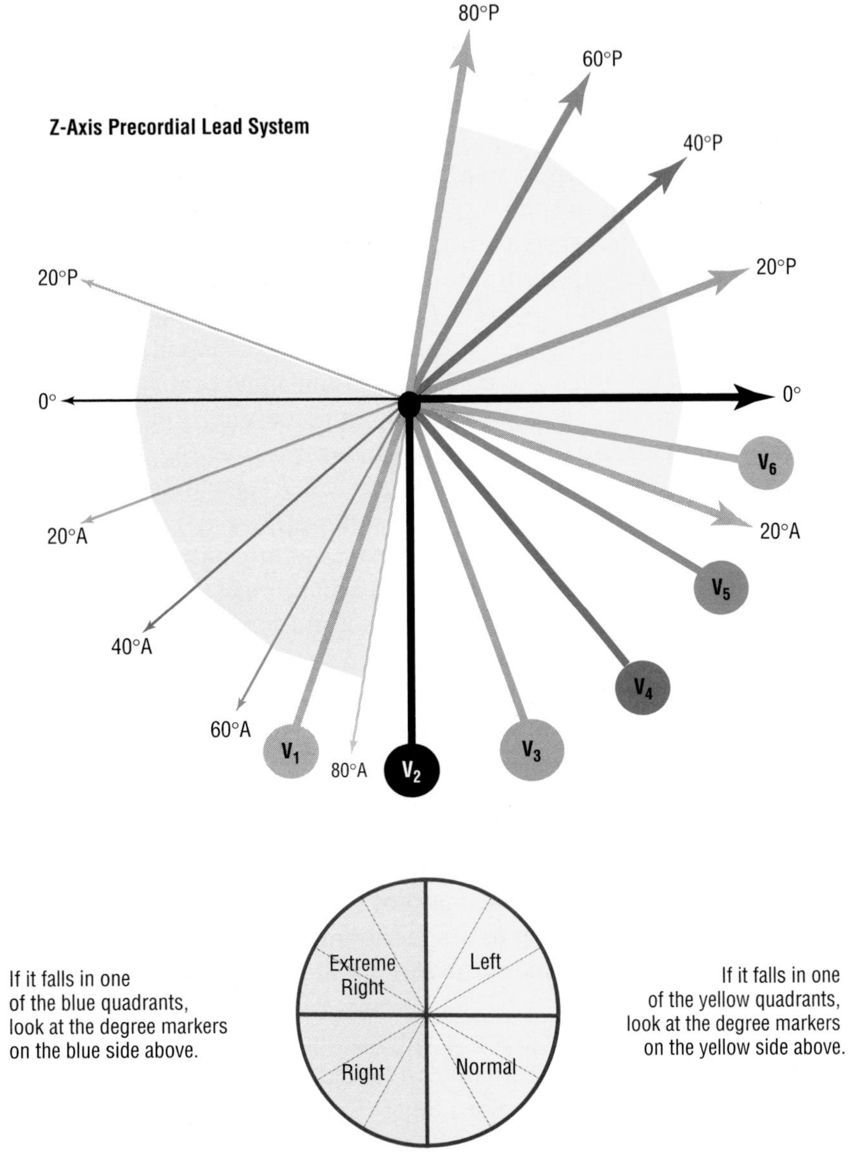

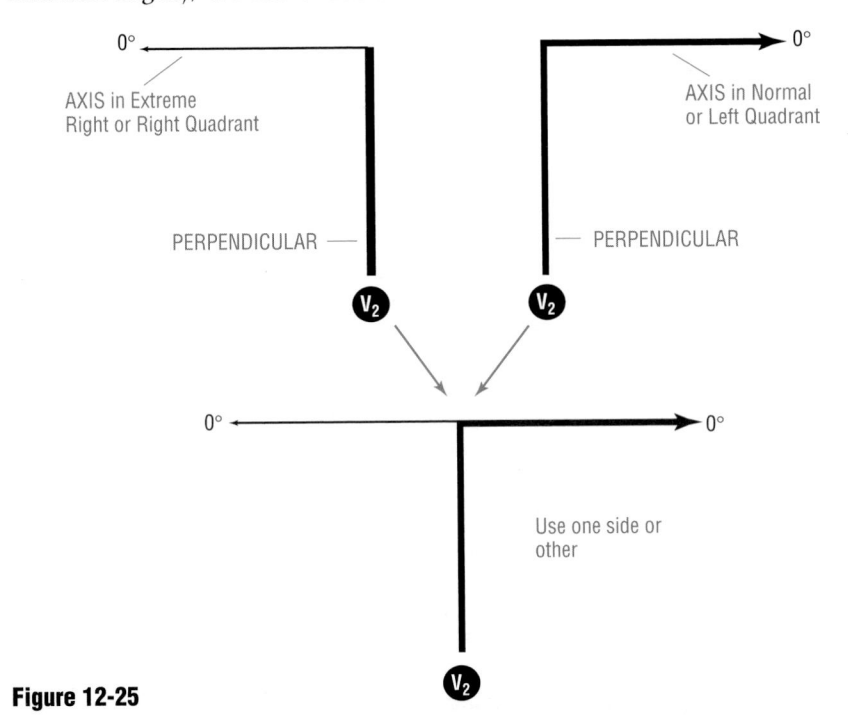

0° — AXIS in Extreme Right or Right Quadrant

AXIS in Normal or Left Quadrant — 0°

PERPENDICULAR

V₂

PERPENDICULAR

V₂

0° ———— 0°

Use one side or other

V₂

Figure 12-25

Now that we have looked at the perpendiculars, let's take a look at which side or vector we are going to use. First, decide which quadrant of the hexaxial system the axis falls into. If the axis falls into either the Left or Normal quadrant (yellow background color), you use the thick arrows on the yellow side of the system. If the axis falls into either the Right or Extreme Right quadrants (*blue background*), use the thin arrows on the blue side of the system.

If, when we look at the precordial leads, the isoelectric line falls exactly on a lead, we use the exact measurement found at the end of the corresponding vector. But suppose that the isoelectric component falls between two leads? We then need to interpolate the number of degrees from the two leads, to determine the location of the axis between the two leads. For example, if the axis falls into the Normal quadrant, and V_3 is mostly negative and V_4 mostly positive, the isoelectric line would be between the two leads. Following the system, we see that V_3 corresponds to 20° posterior and V_4 to 40° posterior. We can say that our axis will be directed 30° posteriorly. By using this interpolation, we can calculate the direction of the axis on the Z plane to within 5°.

We are going to use the first perpendicular only! This means we will use the lead where the complex first changes from negative to positive. If lead V_1 is already positive, the Z axis is indeterminate. It is also indeterminate if the leads never transition and are still negative in V_6. Other cases in which the Z axis cannot be calculated include Wolff-Parkinson-White syndrome and right bundle branch block.

We are using the hexaxial and Z systems to arrive at the three-dimensional direction of the electrical axis of the ventricles. The hexaxial system will give us the direction on a coronal cut of the heart, and the Z system will give us the direction on an A-P (cross-sectional) cut. As we go on, we will use the axis to derive the pathology that is present. It will be worth your while to master these concepts.

More Examples: Adding the Z Axis

Now that you know the whole process, let's do a few trial runs to get you some practice. Using the ECGs in Figures 12-26 through 12-28, see if you can work out both axis calculations before you look at the illustrations and answers beneath the ECGs.

Figure 12-26: Example 4, electrical axis. X-Y axis = −40°; Z axis = 5° posterior.

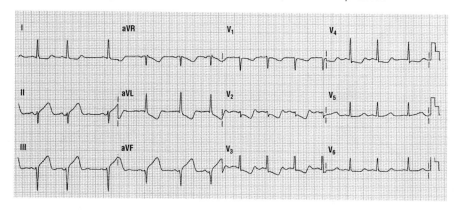

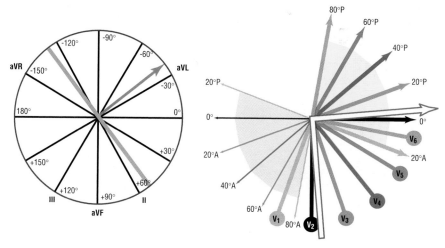

Figure 12-27: Example 5, electrical axis. X-Y axis = 10°; Z axis = 50° posterior.

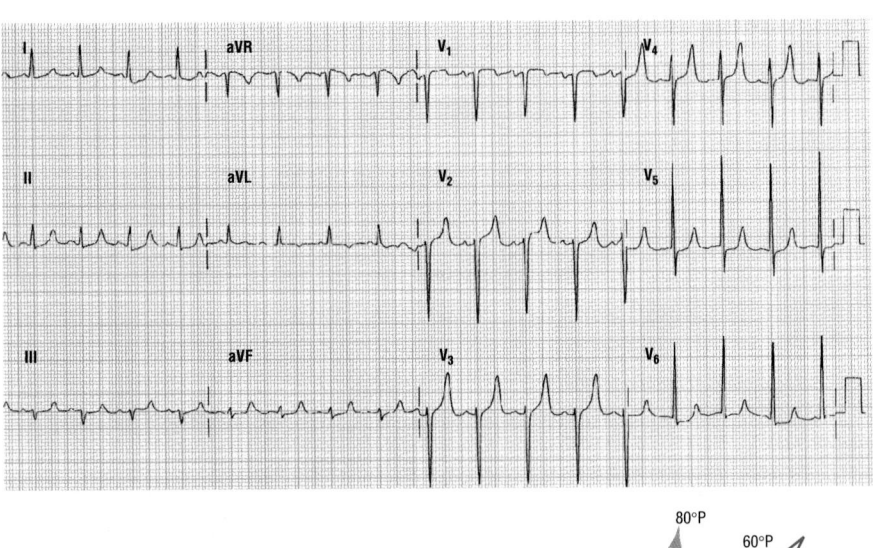

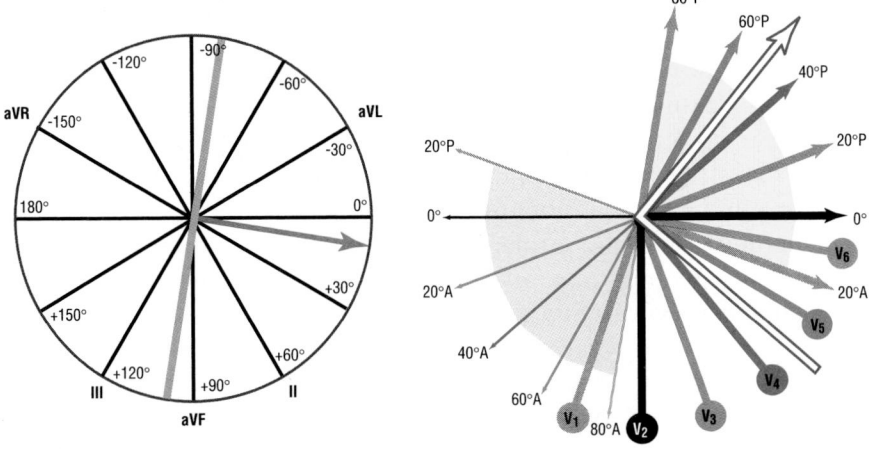

Figure 12-28: Example 6, electrical axis. X-Y axis = 0°; Z axis =70° posterior.

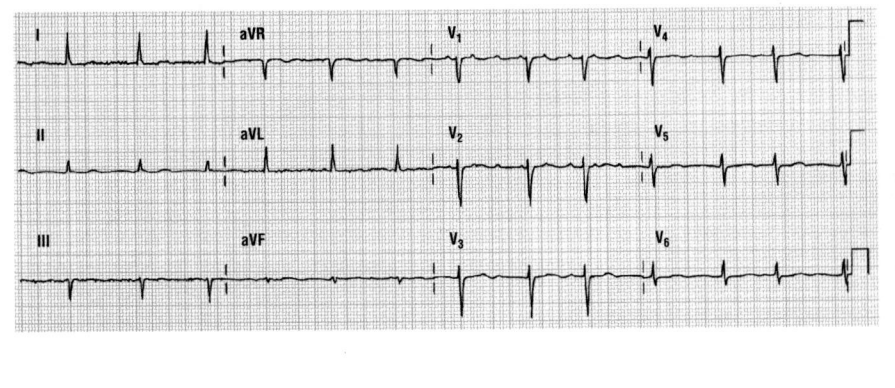

Z Axis: Other Approaches

Just in case you happen to be reading an ECG somewhere and you don't have the Z system with you, Figure 12-29 shows an easy way to figure out the Z axis. This system uses numerical values, instead of graphics, to arrive at the same answer. Just find the isoelectric lead and the corresponding number for the Z axis. When you are calculating the Z axis, use whichever system you feel comfortable with. It is important for you to understand the perpendicular concept that is the basis of the Z axis, rather than just calculating the number. That is why we showed you the Z system first. A student, JB, once told me he remembered that V_1 was anterior in the Left (and Normal) quadrants by thinking of LA. I never asked him if it stood for the city or for the left anterior.

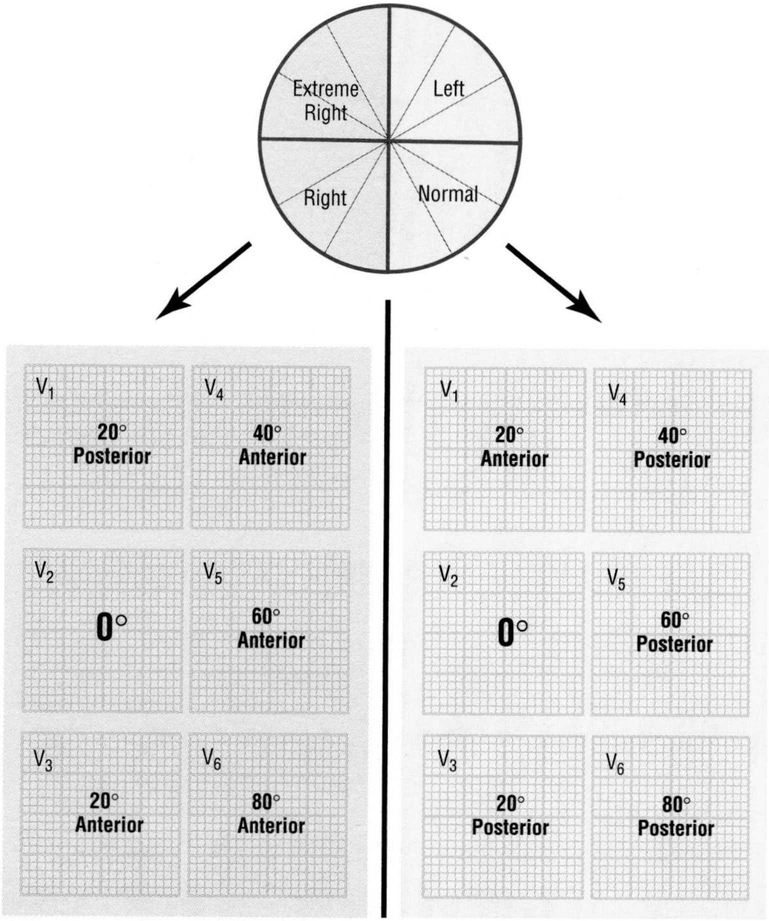

Figure 12-29: Alternative method for calculating the Z axis.

NOTE

Here's another quick memory aid . . .

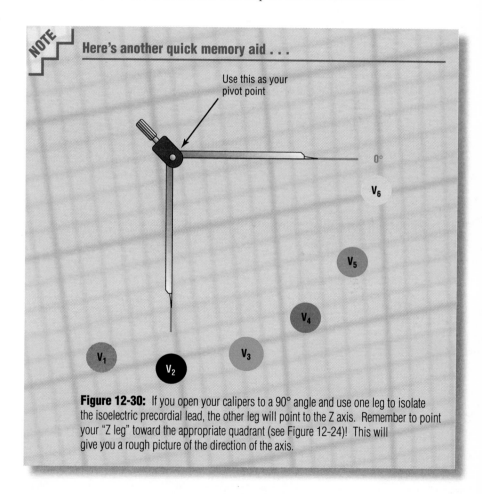

Figure 12-30: If you open your calipers to a 90° angle and use one leg to isolate the isoelectric precordial lead, the other leg will point to the Z axis. Remember to point your "Z leg" toward the appropriate quadrant (see Figure 12-24)! This will give you a rough picture of the direction of the axis.

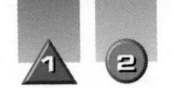

① CHAPTER IN **REVIEW**

1. The electrical axis is the sum total of all the vectors generated by the action potentials of all of the ventricular myocytes. True or False.

2. Which one is correct when we refer to the normal quadrant?
   A. Lead I is positive.
   B. Lead aVF is positive.
   C. Both A and B are correct.
   D. None of the above

3. Which one is correct when we refer to the left quadrant:
   A. Lead I is negative.
   B. Lead aVF is positive.
   C. Both A and B are correct.
   D. None of the above

4. Which one is correct when we refer to the right quadrant?
   A. Lead I is negative.
   B. Lead aVF is negative.
   C. Both A and B are correct.
   D. None of the above

5. Which one is correct when we refer to the extreme right quadrant?
   A. Lead I is negative.
   B. Lead aVF is negative.
   C. Both A and B are correct.
   D. None of the above

② CHAPTER IN **REVIEW**

6. Which of the five steps below is **incorrect** in calculating the electrical axis of the heart?
   A. Find the quadrant
   B. Isolate the isoelectric lead
   C. Isolate the closest lead
   D. Isolate the vector to 10°
   E. Double-check your findings
   F. All of the above

7. The isoelectric lead is the lead with the smallest QRS voltage. True or False.

8. When calculating the true axis, we algebraically add the numbers to the degrees represented by the isoelectric limb lead. True or False.

9. Which of the following is **not** a cause of right axis deviation?
   A. Right ventricular hypertrophy
   B. Left anterior hemiblock
   C. Dextrocardia
   D. Ectopic ventricular beats and rhythms
   E. Normal in adolescents and children

10. The most common causes of left axis deviation include:
    A. Left posterior hemiblock
    B. Ectopic ventricular beats and rhythms
    C. Both A and B
    D. None of the above

1. True 2. C 3. C 4. A 5. C

6. F 7. True 8. False 9. B 10. B

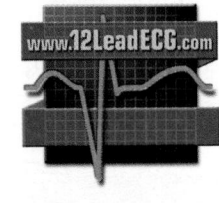

Now that you understand the electrical axis, we are ready to move into the pathological realm of bundle branch blocks (BBBs). If you remember, there are two bundle branches, left and right. The left bundle branch further subdivides into the left anterior and left posterior fascicles, shown in Figure 13-1.

Impulses generated by the pacemakers in the atria or the atrioventricular (AV) node are normally conducted down the bundle branches to innervate the myocardium in an organized fashion. Do you think that a blocked bundle would affect conduction through the heart, and, therefore, the axis? Well, picture a situation in which the electrical impulse suddenly hits an obstacle. The impulse would not be able to proceed to the cells downstream from that block through the normal conduction system; it would instead have to travel by direct cell-to-cell transmission. This is a slow and chaotic way of innervating the myocardium, the type of transmission that accounts for the wide and bizarre complex in a ventricular premature contraction (VPC) or other aberrantly conducted beat. The BBBs are similarly characterized by wide and bizarre complexes. However, there is one big distinction between a VPC and a BBB. Can you figure out what it is? The VPC is aberrantly conducted from its inception, whereas the BBB is normally conducted until it hits the block. This initial component gives the BBBs two main appearances, with minor variations: the right bundle branch block (RBBB) and left bundle branch block (LBBB) patterns.

Right Bundle Branch Block

When there is a block in the right bundle, the impulse gets transmitted normally by the left bundle to most of the left ventricle. The impulse to part of the interventricular septum and the right ventricle, however, is delayed because of the cell-to-cell depolarization imposed by the block

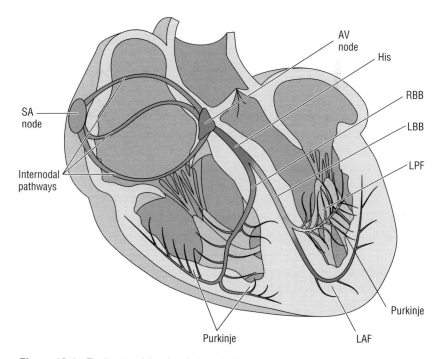

Figure 13-1: The heart and the electrical conduction system.

(*concentric circles* in Figure 13-2). This slow impulse causes a slower depolarization time, which is manifested on the ECG by a prolongation of the QRS interval to 0.12 seconds or more. (This prolongation is a trademark for any *complete* BBB.) It also manifests itself as an additional wave, or an aberration of an existing wave. In the right precordial leads of V_1 and V_2, it develops as an RSR' complex. The R' is the graphical manifestation of the additional vector, caused by the slow conduction through the interventricular septum and the right ventricle.

The main criteria for RBBB are:

1. QRS prolongation of ≥ 0.12 seconds

2. Slurred S wave in leads I and V_6

3. RSR' pattern in lead V_1, with R' taller than R

We have already seen why the QRS is prolonged, so let's look at #2 and #3 in this list. Under normal circumstances, the left ventricle gives rise to the vector that accounts for the QRS complex. The late innervation of the septum and the right ventricle in RBBB creates a new, slower vector (vector 4 in Figure 13-3) that is unopposed by the vectors from the left ventricle (*vectors 1, 2, and 3*). This new vector produces a variation in the normal ECG pattern. A new R wave appears in the right precordial leads of V_1 and V_2, because there is a new vector headed toward those leads. A deeper S wave is also seen in the leads that face the left side of the heart (V_5, V_6, and I). The S wave is slurred because of the slow transmission of the vector. *This slurring of the S wave in I and V_6 is, in our opinion, the most important criterion for diagnosing RBBB.* You will hear many people say that RSR' complex in V_1 is the key, but because there are hundreds of different presentations for that complex, it can prove confusing in many cases.

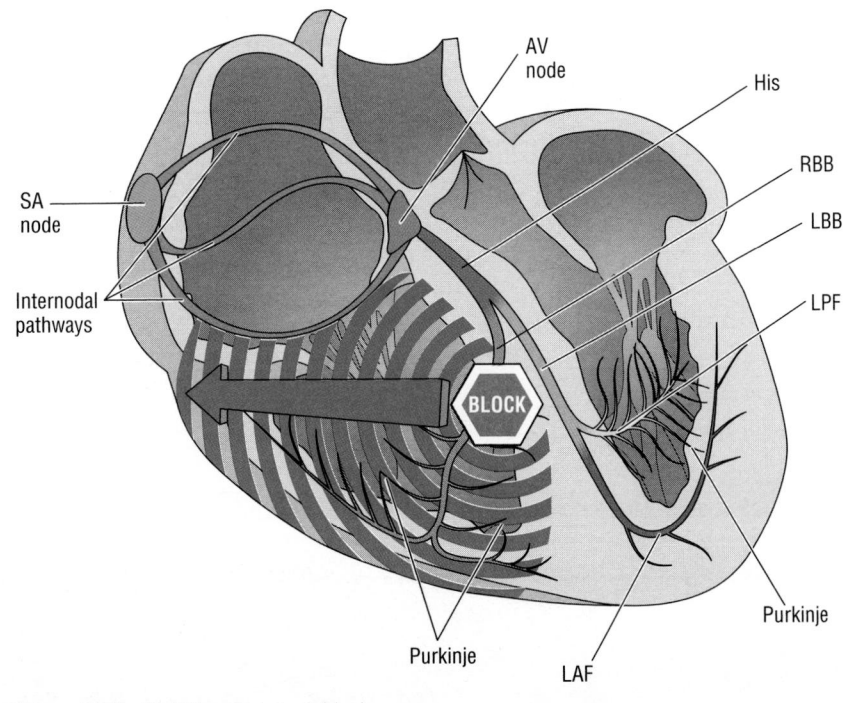

Figure 13-2: Right bundle branch block.

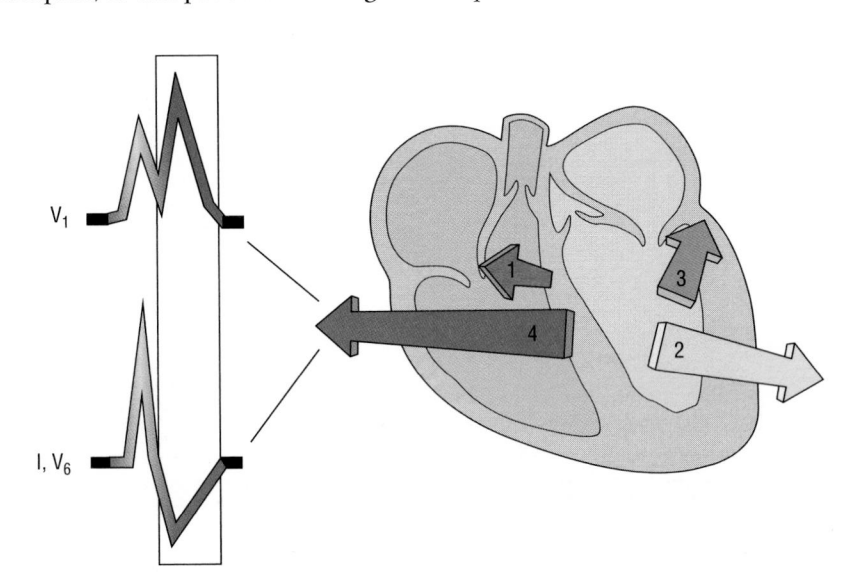

Figure 13-3: RBBB's effect on the ECG.

ECG Findings in Right Bundle Branch Blocks

The three major criteria for RBBB are:

1. *QRS ≥ 0.12 seconds*

Remember, if you are able to find one lead with a QRS complex of 0.12 seconds or more, you have a wide complex. Why? *Because all intervals are the same throughout the ECG!* This is a key point that you should always remember.

2. *Slurred S wave in leads I and V_6*

This is the major criterion that we will look at when we are evaluating for the presence of RBBB. The slurred S can have various morphologies as shown in Figure 13-4, but they are all prolonged and slow.

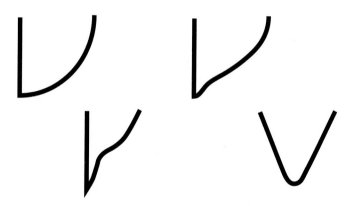

Figure 13-4: The various looks of a slurred S wave.

3. *RSR' pattern in V_1*

Just as there were many different types of slurred S waves, so too are there many presentations of the RSR' complexes. Some may not even look like RSR' complexes, especially if there has been a previous infarct of the anteroseptal area that gives rise to a QR' complex. A lot of folks call these "rabbit ears" (Figure 13-5). This is a good analogy because there are many different types of rabbits — floppy-eared, hairy,

cartoon, and so on. *The key point to remember about them is that they are all predominantly positive in lead V_1.* If you see an ECG with wide QRS complexes, slurred S waves, and a positive complex in lead V_1 (especially if it matches an RSR' complex or one of its possible variations), you have made the diagnosis of RBBB. Easy isn't it?

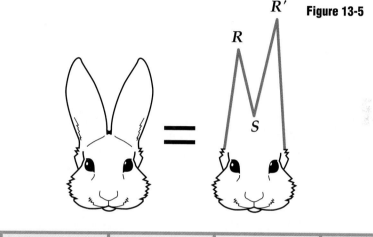

Figure 13-5

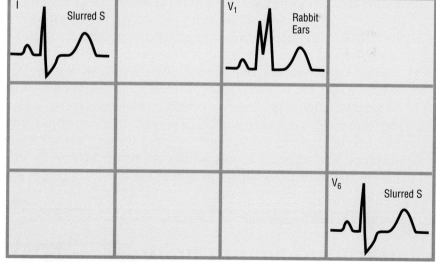

Figure 13-6: The ECG and RBBB.

244

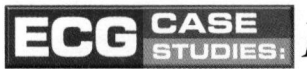

The QR′ Wave

There are a million examples of rabbit ears. One type, however, deserves special mention: the QR′, or qR′, wave. This occurs when an ECG shows the characteristic changes of an anteroseptal myocardial infarction (ASMI) — Q waves in leads V_1, *and* an RBBB. In these patients, the ECG will show a Q or *q* wave in place of the initial R wave of the RSR′ pattern. Think of it this way: Suppose the bunny had one of his ears shot and the ear could no longer stand upright (Figure 13-7). It would flop over and hang down. In other words, the R wave, which would be the first upright ear, is now dead and hangs down to become a Q wave. Because the Q wave takes the place of the R wave, the next positive wave is in reality an R′ wave; hence, the term QR′.

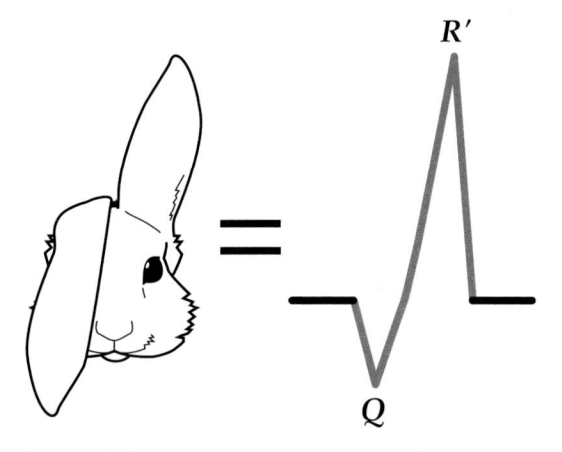

Figure 13-7: If you see a Q wave in lead V_1 in the presence of RBBB, the first positive deflection is called an R′ wave instead of an R wave.

ECG 13-1 This is a classic example of RBBB. When you look at leads V_1 and V_6, you see the classic slurred S wave with the slow downstroke and upstroke. This slurred S is caused by the vector representing the slow cell-to-cell transmission through part of the septum and the right ventricular myocardium (Figure 13-3, *vector 4*). Looking at lead V_1, we see the classic rSR′ complex that is typical of the rabbit-ear pattern. Lead III also shows some rSr′ pattern that is caused by the same vectors. This sometimes occurs without any bundle block because of an isolated, regional intraventricular conduction delay.

Notice that an RBBB will cause an increased R:S ratio in leads V_1 and V_2. This happens because the block causes the slow conduction through the right ventricular myocardium. Remember, because V_1 through V_3 are the right precordial leads, they will show the greatest change.

Start getting used to diagnosing RBBB by looking at the slurred S wave in leads I and V_6. Don't make the fatal, rookie mistake of looking for the rabbit ears. You will get fooled quite often if you look at V_1 initially. If your complex is 0.12 seconds wide or more, look for the slurred S wave; then, and only then, look at V_1. Leads V_1 and V_2 should have an increased R:S ratio and some semblance of an RSR′ or QR′ complex.

> **REMINDER:**
> A qR′ wave is a sign of an old or new infarct in a patient with RBBB. It is found in V_1.

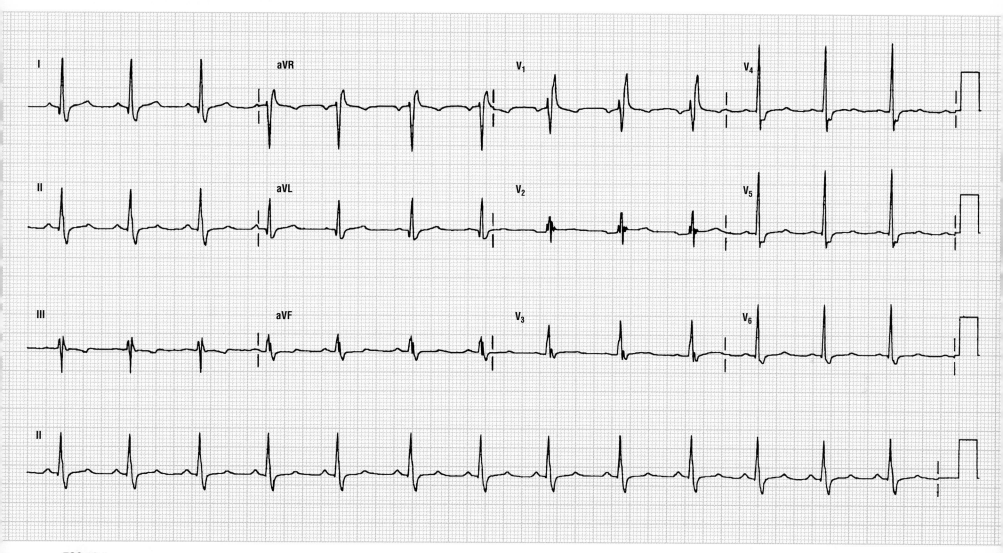

ECG 13-1

ECG CASE STUDIES: **CONTINUED**

2

ECG 13-2 Look at the beautiful slurred S waves on this ECG. The diagnosis of RBBB should leap out at you when you look at them. However, look at the complexes in lead V_1; they are not as clear. When you look very closely, you will note that they are in reality rsR'R" pattern. There is a tiny *rs* complex at the beginning of the complex. It is so small as to be almost imperceptible. Then there is an R' wave that progresses on to the next, and tallest, peak — the R" (also see Figure 13-8). Notice that there really is no S wave between these two. As you can see, the rabbit ear pattern is present, but it belongs to a mutant rabbit with serious ear problems.

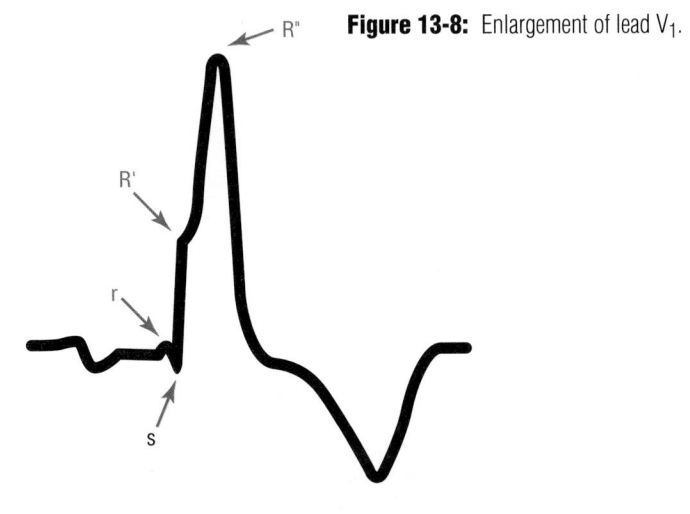

Figure 13-8: Enlargement of lead V_1.

3

ECG 13-2 Note that there is also evidence of a left anterior hemiblock (LAH), making this a bifascicular block. More on this later.

2

ECG 13-3 This one is similar to ECG 13-2. It also has very visible slurred S waves, and a bizarre complex in V_1. V_2 has more obvious notching and RSR' morphology than V_1.

An RBBB is usually associated with coronary artery disease. However, in many cases it is not due to an infarcted area of the heart. Many young people have the abnormality as a benign finding. Some folks with an incomplete RBBB pattern (an RSR' complex in V_1 or V_2 with no widening of the QRS complex) will progress on to complete RBBB as they age.

3

ECG 13-3 This ECG shows evidence of inferolateral ischemia. Leads III and aVF show concordance of the T waves with the terminal portion of the QRS complex. The lateral leads also show flattening that is consistent with ischemia.

In general, the ST segments should be on the baseline in patients with a normal RBBB pattern. However, ST depression is common in the right precordial leads. Remember, ST elevation in the right precordials in a patient with RBBB is consistent with AMI.

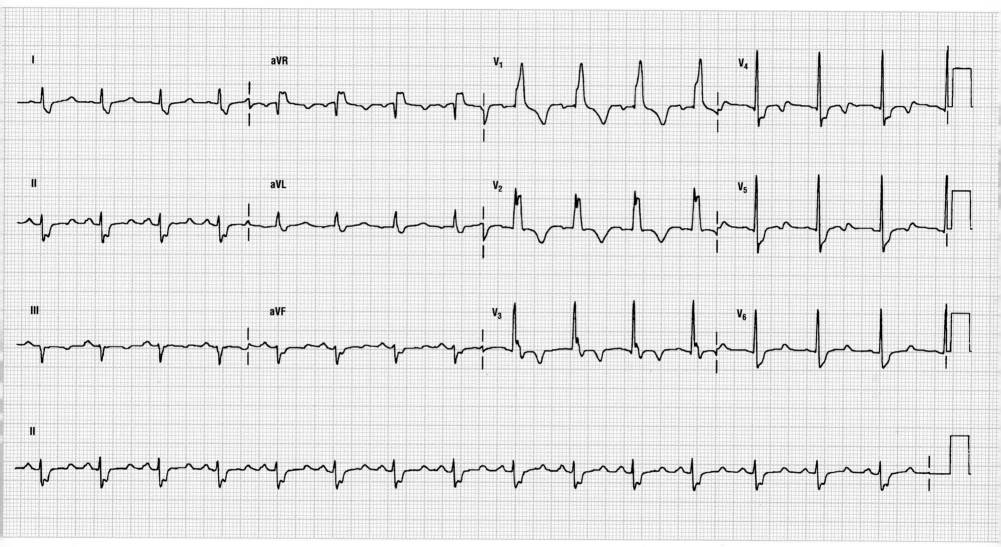

ECG 13-2

ECG CASE STUDIES: **CONTINUED**

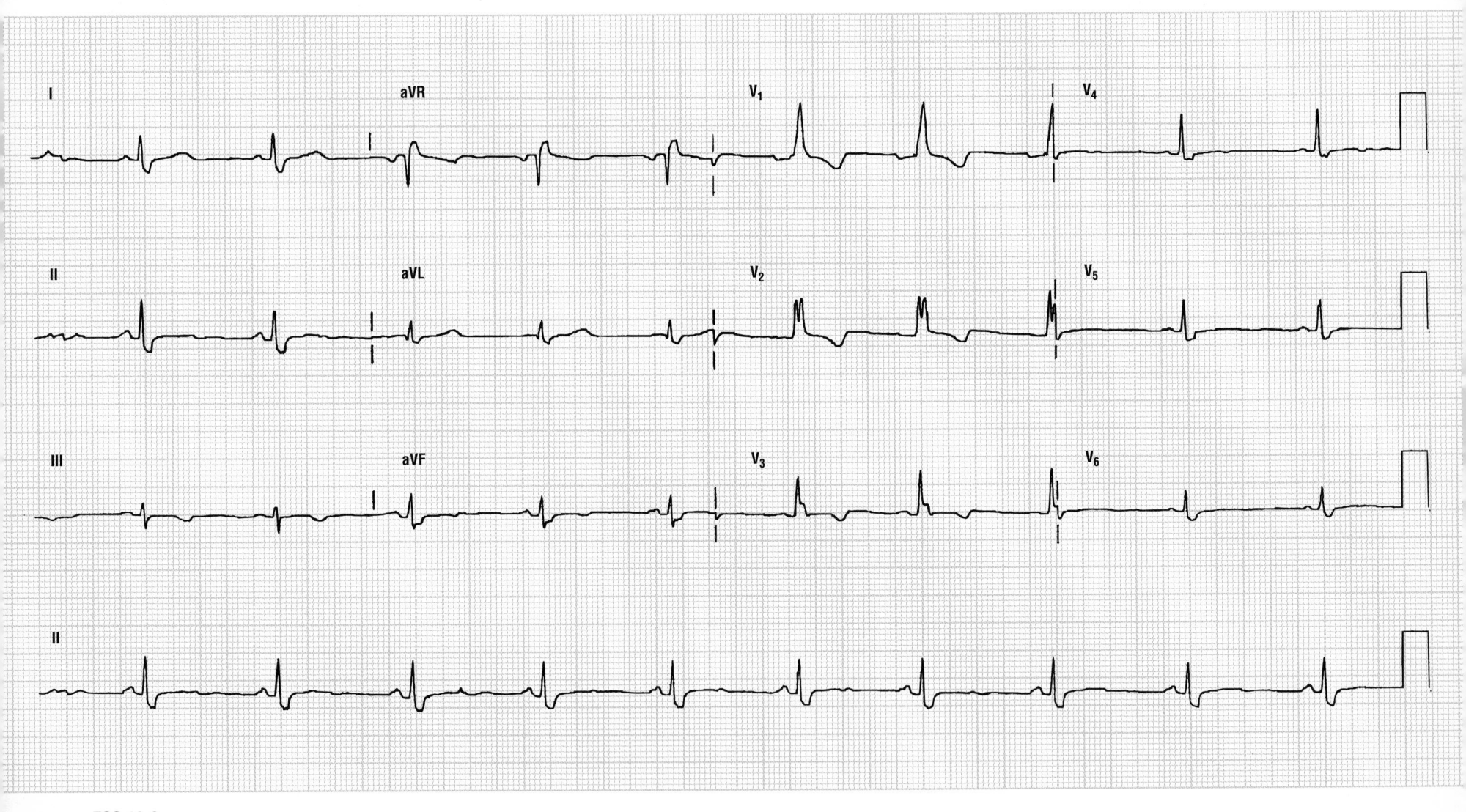

ECG 13-3

②

ECG 13-4 The complexes below easily measure more than 0.12 seconds, making this a block of some kind. Remember, your options are RBBB, LBBB, and intraventricular conduction delay. Once again, you could be in trouble if you look at only V_1. This is a qRR′ complex (also see Figure 13-9). Looking at the S waves in leads I and V_6, we see that they are slurred and consistent with an RBBB.

The differential diagnosis we mentioned above for a wide QRS complex is not complete. We could also have a VPC or an aberrantly conducted beat. However, remember that most VPCs exhibit either an RBBB or LBBB complex. This statement is also true for rhythms that have a ventricular origin — for example, ventricular tachycardia, idioventricular rhythms, and ventricular escape beats. You have to use "the company it keeps" to make the diagnosis.

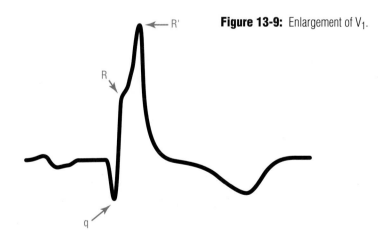

Figure 13-9: Enlargement of V_1.

②

ECG 13-5 What can you say about this ECG, except that it is an obvious RBBB? It meets all of the criteria for RBBB easily. Now, what about that little notch at the bottom of lead I? Is that anything to worry about? No, this is just a part of the complex. If you notice in lead III, there is a Qr complex. That little notch corresponds to the *r* wave. Use your straight edge to verify this. You do need to start looking at those little things in order not to miss important arrhythmias that could lie buried in the complex. If you see an abnormality, put on your Sherlock Holmes hat and go to work. The dividends that a search will pay are high indeed.

③

ECG 13-5 There is slight ST elevation in lead III, and the reciprocal and lateral leads show depressed ST segments. You need to be careful and use a straight edge and your calipers in many of these cases, because the width of the QRS complex can sometimes cause an "optical illusion." This can give you the impression that there are ST segments when there really are none. In this case, there is no illusion. The changes, although minimal, are troubling because they occur in reciprocal areas. You need some strong clinical correlation to interpret this ECG correctly.

REMINDER:

V_1 in a patient with RBBB can have many different looks.

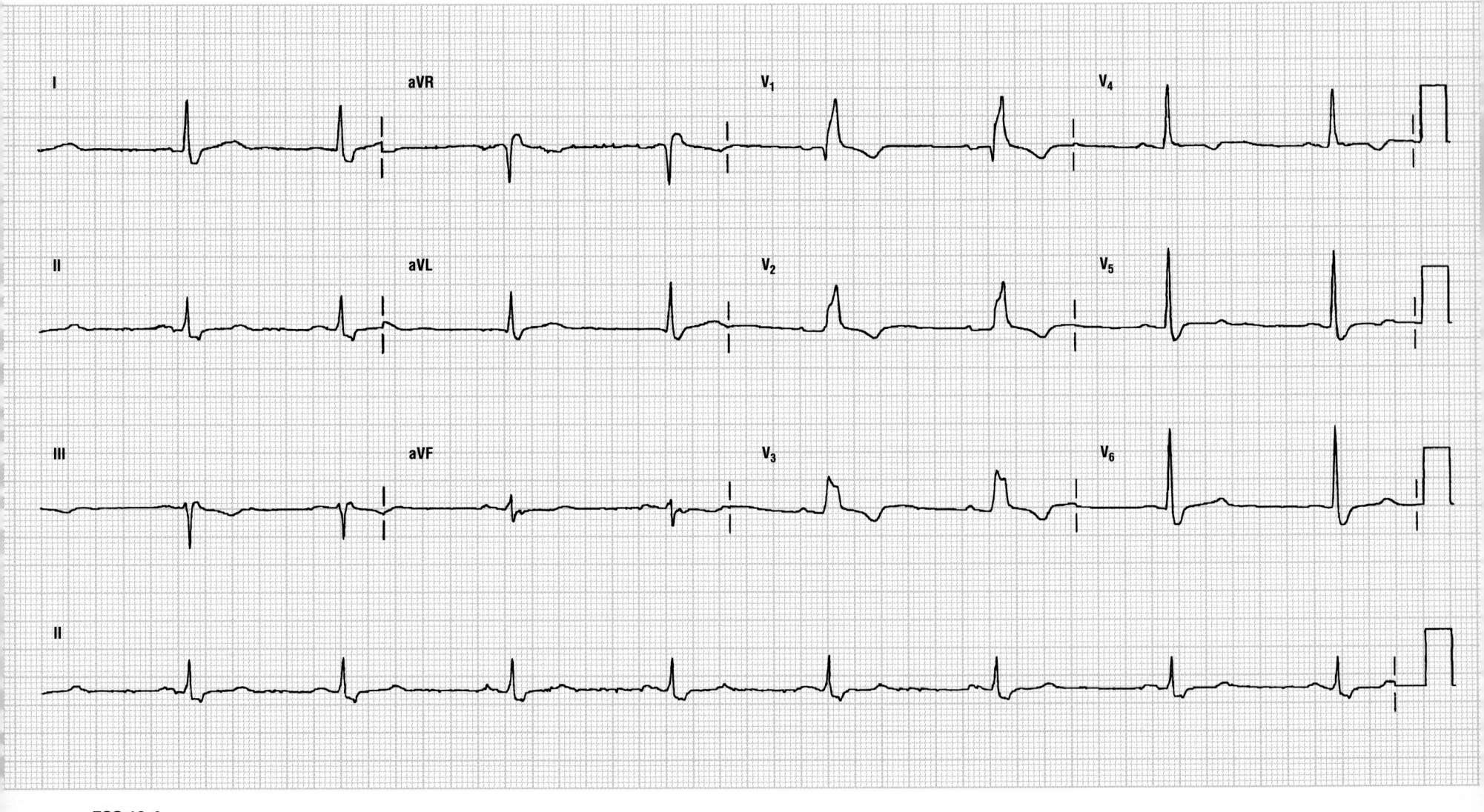

ECG 13-4

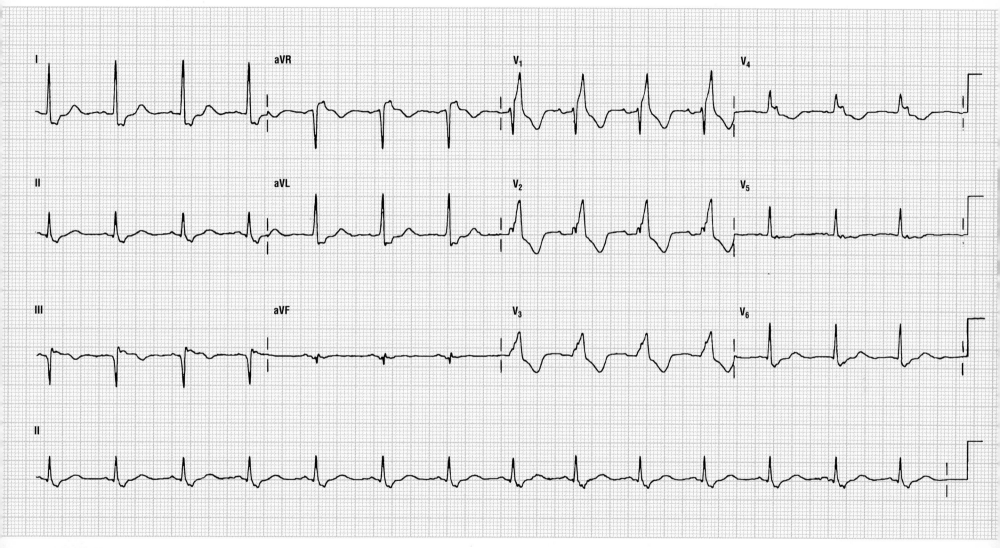

ECG 13-5

ECG CASE STUDIES: **C O N T I N U E D**

ECG 13-6 This is a little tougher to interpret, but let's break it down. Is it 0.12 seconds wide or more? Yes. Does it have slurred S waves in leads I and V_6? Yes. Is there an RSR' pattern in V_1? Yes; it is really an rSR' pattern, but who's counting? So, this is an RBBB.

What is different about this ECG? For starters, there is evidence of left ventricular hypertrophy (LVH): Lead aVL has an R wave taller than 11 mm. Can you make any comments about LVH in RBBB? Yes, you can. *In LBBB, you cannot make any statements about LVH, but in RBBB you can.* This is an important point. Finally, there is poor R-R progression.

ECG 13-6 This ECG shows a bifascicular block with RBBB and LAH patterns. In addition, there is strong evidence of left ventricular hypertrophy (LVH). Diagnosing LVH is not a problem in RBBB. Conversely, diagnosing right ventricular hypertrophy (RVH) is very difficult, if not impossible. (Some authors have suggested that an R wave more than 15 mm in lead V_1 is consistent with the diagnosis of RVH. However, this does not hold up with any certainty and should not be used.) Right atrial enlargement (RAE) can be diagnosed by the traditional criteria, and this may lead you to suspect RVH. If there are any questions about RVH, they can be answered with an echocardiogram.

REMINDER:

You cannot comment on LVH if LBBB is present, but in RBBB you can.

ECG 13-7 This ECG shows RBBB. Look at the complexes in lead V_1. Do you see the notching that occurs at the top of the QRS complexes? This is an RR' pattern that occurs commonly in RBBB. Do you see an S wave? No, the S wave is defined as the first negative deflection after the R wave, but it has to go below the baseline. So in these complexes, there really is no S wave. Many clinicians still call this an RSR' complex, although it is technically incorrect. This is all semantics and has no real clinical value. The main thing to keep in mind is that the notched, positive complex is in V_1. You will see similarly notched, positive complexes in LBBB. However, in LBBB they occur in leads V_5 or V_6. Don't get them confused.

REMINDER:

Remember, RBBB has to have a positive complex in V_1; LBBB must be primarily negative in V_1 and V_2.

ECG 13-7 While we are on the topic, the first R wave should be smaller than the R' wave. (The vector causing the R' wave is unopposed because of the block.) Remember, in RBBB, conduction is normal down the LBB, and the impulse depolarizes the left ventricle normally. The conduction to the right ventricle is then slowed by the need for direct cell-to-cell transmission. By the time that slow transmission takes place, the left ventricle has already depolarized. The vector is thus unopposed, giving rise to the slurred S wave and the higher R'.

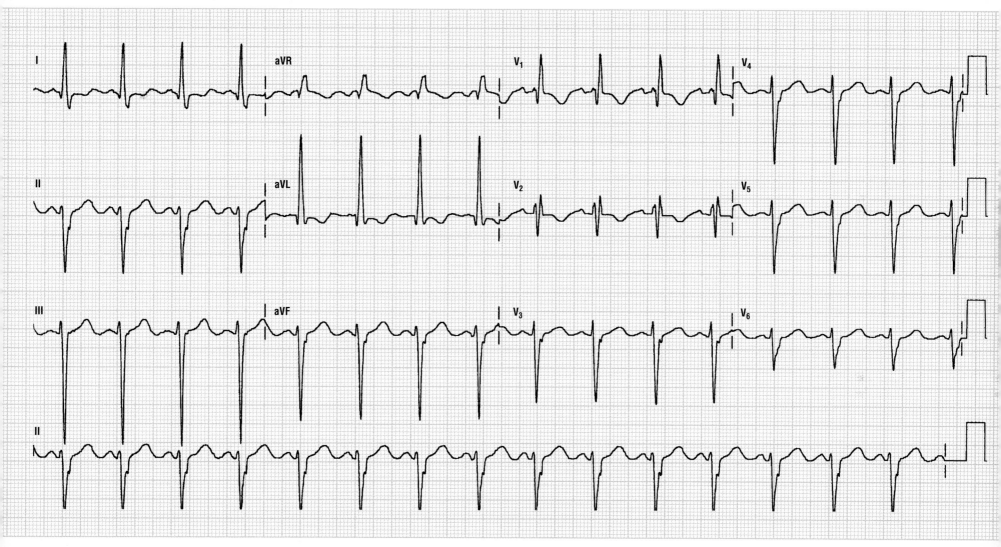

ECG 13-6

ECG CASE STUDIES: **CONTINUED**

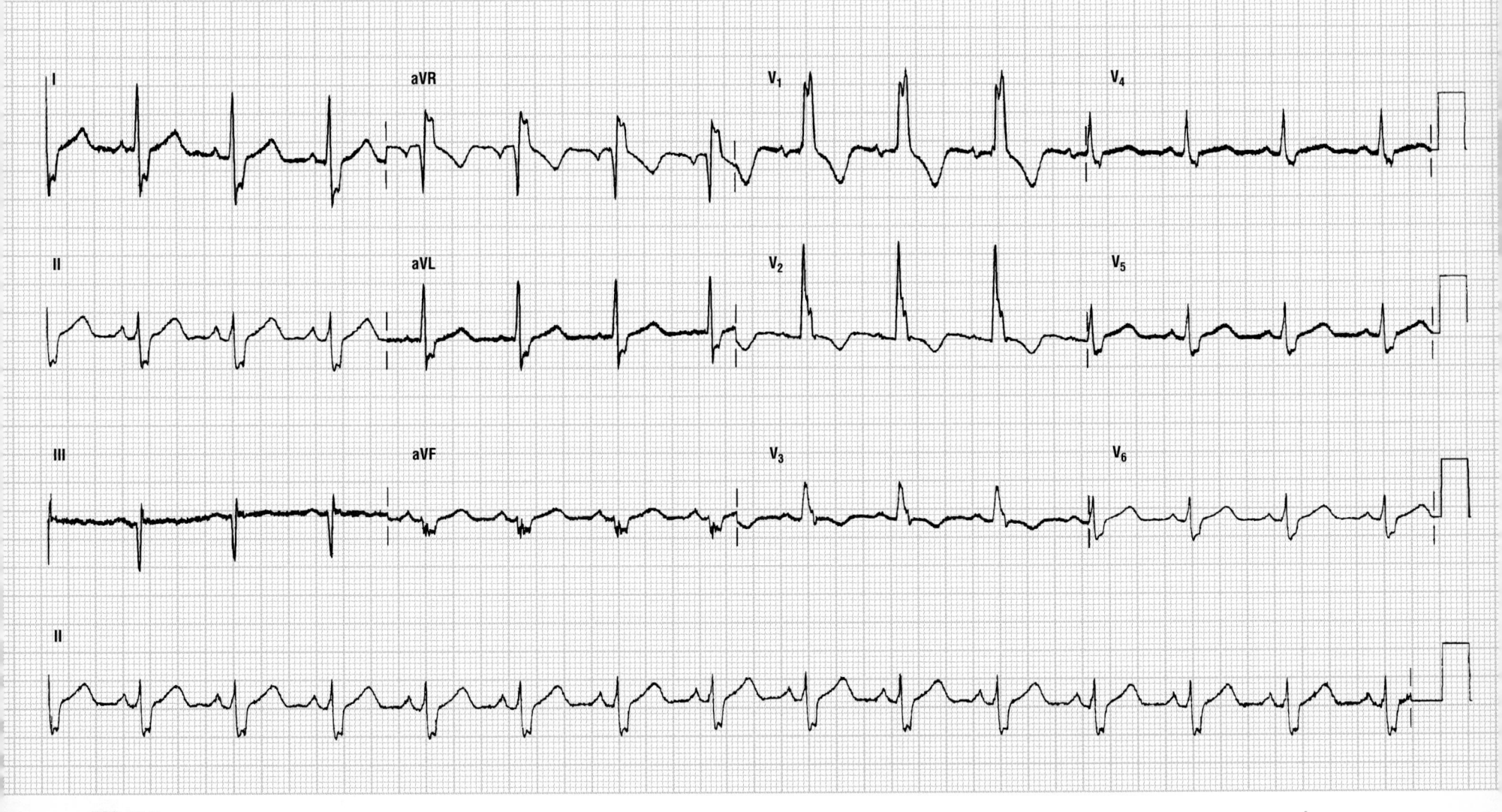

ECG 13-7

②

ECG 13-8 What an ugly looking ECG! This is because the complexes are so wide and small. As we can see, the rhythm is NSR and there is a P wave before each QRS complex. This is very reassuring because *complexes 0.16 seconds or more wide could represent a ventricular focus acting as the pacemaker, such as ventricular escape beats or ventricular tachycardia.* This is a clinical pearl that you should always keep in mind!

The ECG shows the traditional findings for RBBB, with slurred S waves and the rsR' complex.

②

ECG 13-9 Would you be able to diagnose RBBB by looking at lead V_1 in this ECG? Many textbooks state that the RSR' pattern in lead V_1 is the easiest way to diagnose RBBB. As you can see, it doesn't always work!

The slurred S waves in leads I and V_6 are present, and they help you make the diagnosis. This is clinched by the increased R:S ratio in lead V_1.

The beginning of the ECG shows a supraventricular bigeminy. The Level 3 material for this ECG explains the reasoning. If you feel comfortable, read that material; it is not very complicated. A U wave is present and visible in V_2 through V_6.

③

ECG 13-8 Did you notice the inferior infarct? Those Q waves are very classic and very wide. Is this a bifascicular block with RBBB and left posterior hemiblock (LPH)? No, because the Q wave is more consistent with an inferior wall myocardial infarction (IWMI) than with LPH. Remember, LPH is a diagnosis of exclusion. It is usually associated with a qR complex in lead III, not a QR complex. This is definitely a QR complex. Could there be a bifascicular block? We think anything could be hiding in there. The wide and slurred R' complex in lead V_1 that commonly occurs in LPH is present on this ECG. *We would clinically consider the diagnosis of bifascicular block, even though we can't officially make that diagnosis from the ECG.*

③

ECG 13-9 Is this a supraventricular bigeminy or a ventricular bigeminy? Well, let's look at the complexes that are aberrantly conducted. We see that they are wide, but not extremely wide. This could be caused by either of the scenarios above. Now, look at the first 0.03 seconds of both the aberrantly conducted complexes and the normal ones. They are identical. This similarity is due to the similar origins of the two complexes. They both travel down the AV node, then their paths split somewhere before the bundle branches. Because of this initial similarity, the aberrant beats have to originate from a supraventricular focus.

REMINDER:
When a complex originates in the ventricles, it will usually have either a LBBB or RBBB morphology.

ECG CASE STUDIES: **CONTINUED**

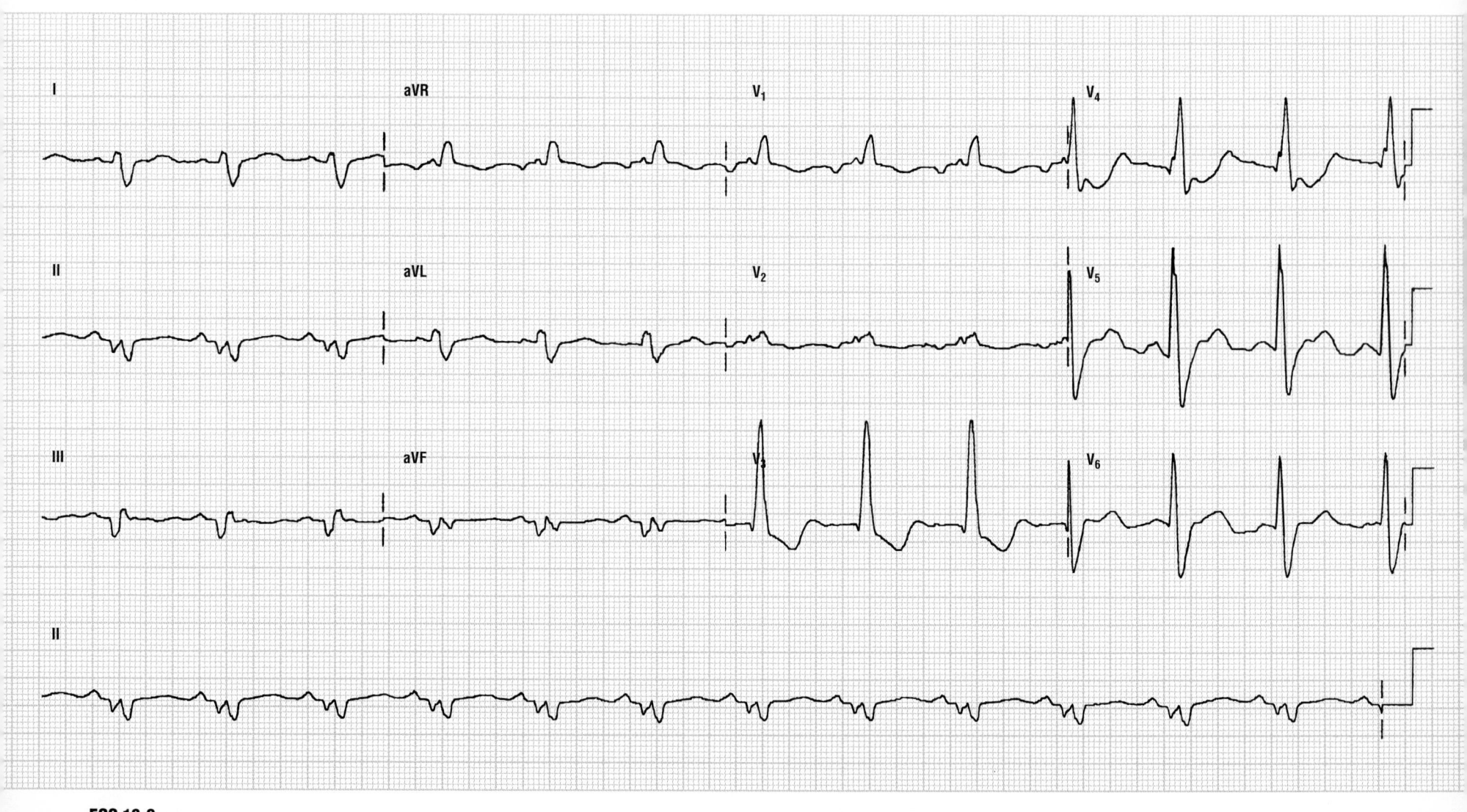

ECG 13-8

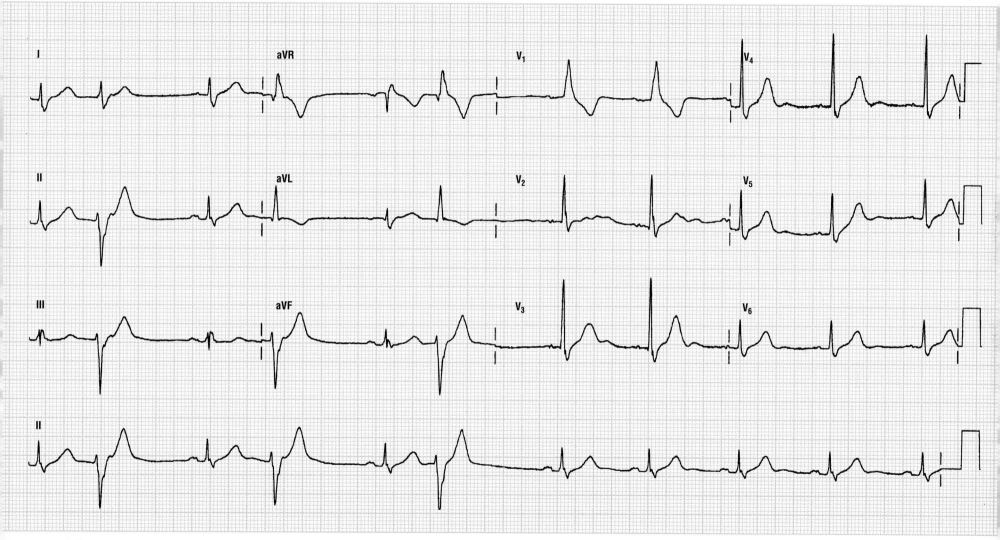

ECG 13-9

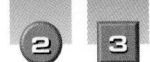

ECG CASE STUDIES: **CONTINUED**

②

ECG 13-10 This is another example of RBBB. You see the slurred S waves in leads I and V_6. They are small, but still they are slurred. There is also the classic rSR′ complex in lead V_1.

The rhythm is again interesting in the first part of the ECG. It is caused by atrial premature contractions. The rhythm is a supraventricular bigeminy caused by atrial premature contractions (APCs). Go down and use the rhythm strip to decide which are the normal complexes and which are the aberrantly conducted ones. This is yet another example of why that "real-time" rhythm strip at the bottom of the ECG is so helpful in making tough diagnoses.

③

ECG 13-10 Is this a supraventricular bigeminy or a ventricular bigeminy? We can use the same logic that we did with ECG 13-9. In addition, we see the premature P waves causing the complexes to fire. They are APCs, and this is once again superventricular bigeminy.

Did you notice the concordance problems? All of the complexes except for I, aVL, aVR, and V_2 are concordant. Is this abnormal? You bet it is! This could represent ischemia, central nervous system events, or some other cause of diffuse T-wave abnormality.

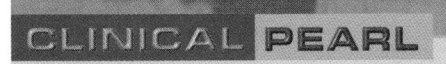

CLINICAL PEARL

Remember, RBBB is usually a stable pattern. However, you need to make sure that it is not a **new** RBBB pattern. Obtain an old ECG or the old medical records and review them closely. Leave no stone unturned in order to evaluate whether the RBBB is new or old. A new RBBB could be a harbinger of infarction or other impending problems!

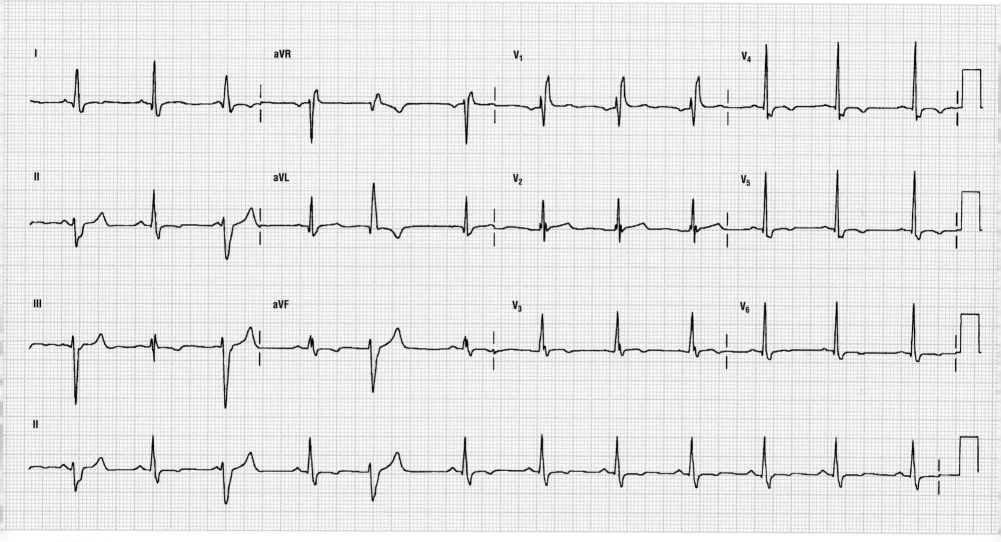

ECG 13-10

②

Left Bundle Branch Block

Remember these words of wisdom: Whenever you look at an ECG that has a regular rhythm and say, "Gee whiz, that's an ugly gram!" you are probably looking at LBBB. The left bundle is always 0.12 seconds wide or more. So what makes these ECGs so ugly? They are usually composed of *monomorphic complexes* (either all positive or all negative) and have ST depression or elevation, and broad T waves. Note that the T waves should be *concordant*. This means that the last part of the QRS complex and the T wave should both be either positive or negative. If they are opposite, it is called *discordant*; this is a sign of some pathologic process going on. (More on this in Chapter 14.) The result of all of these findings is a "hunchback of Notre Dame" ECG.

The pathology involved in LBBB is caused by a block of the left bundle *or* of both fascicles of the left bundle. This block causes the electrical potential to travel down the right bundle first. Then ventricular depolarization proceeds from right to left by direct cell-to-cell transmission (Figure 13-10). The left ventricle is so big that the transmission is delayed, hence the 0.12 seconds or more criterion, and the complexes are not initially sharp as they were in the RBBB pattern. This slowed transmission with no sharp vectors gives rise to the broad, monomorphic complexes classically seen in LBBB. Furthermore, because the vector is proceeding from right to left, those complexes are negative in leads V_1 to V_2, and positive in I and V_5 to V_6. In other words: *If you look at V_1 and V_6, you will note that the complexes are all positive or all negative, respectively* (Figure 13-10). (Note: V_1 and V_2 may have a small *r* wave due to the initial vector produced by innervation through the right bundle.)

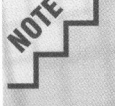 The left bundle branch block pattern is like a rock thrown up in the air; it goes either all up or all down!

Because the vector arising from the right bundle is small and canceled by the large vector from the left ventricle, the complexes are generally similar in different people. This makes the recognition of the LBBB pattern easier than that of RBBB. Just remember to look in V_1 and V_6; if the complexes are broad, monomorphic, and all up or down, you've identified LBBB!

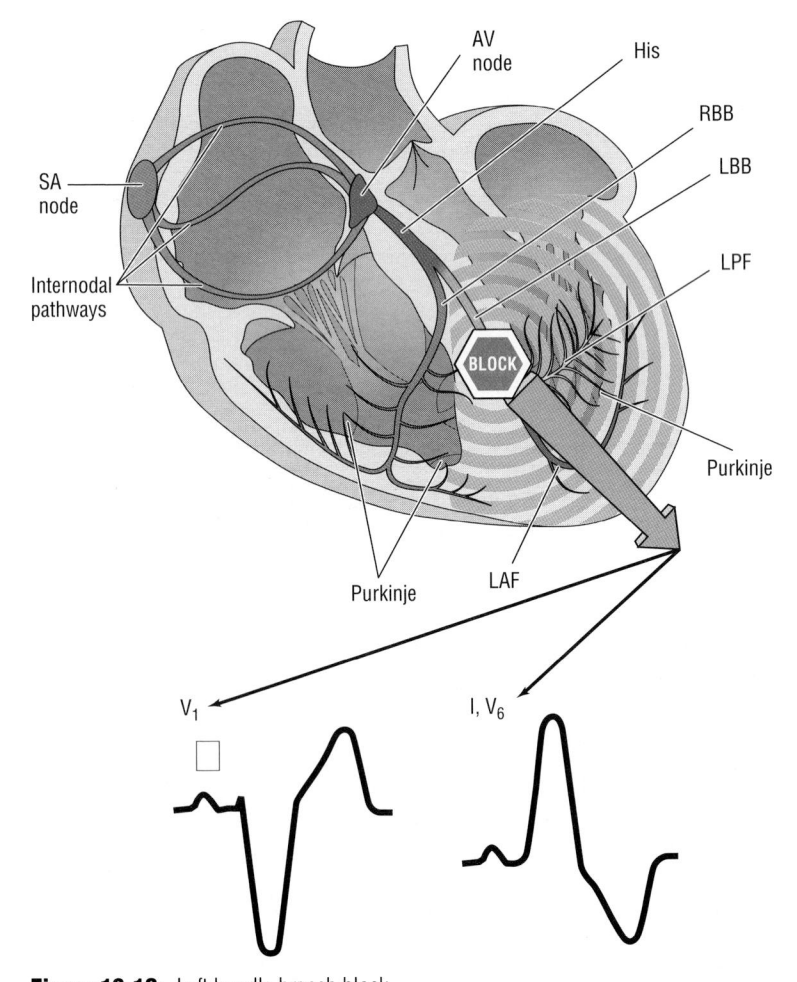

Figure 13-10: Left bundle branch block.

Criteria for Diagnosing LBBB

As with RBBB, there are three main criteria for diagnosing LBBB (Figure 13-11):

1. Duration ≥ 0.12 seconds
2. Broad, monomorphic R waves in I and V_6, with no Q waves
3. Broad, monomorphic S waves in V_1; may have a small r wave

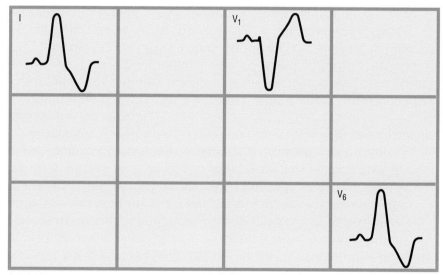

Figure 13-11: The ECG and LBBB.

Just as there are never any certainties in life, let us say that there are no certainties in the appearance of the complexes. In general, as mentioned earlier, all LBBBs are similar to each other — much more so than just about any other type of ECGs when it comes to the appearance of the complexes. However, having said this, some of the complexes may have various small differences; the R waves can be notched in V_6, for instance (Figure 13-12). This notching can rarely be mistaken for an RSR' pattern, but it is not RSR'! Remember that rabbit ears are associated with RBBB and are found in V_1, not V_6.

There can also be some variations in the size of the R wave in V_1. Note, for instance, that the R wave can be narrow — less than 0.03 seconds (Figure 13-12). Wider R waves can be a sign of a previous posterior AMI; more on this later.

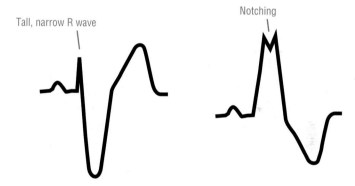

Figure 13-12: Here are some variations from the norm. Variations are not limited to the two examples shown in this illustration.

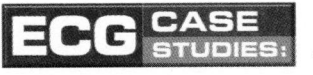 *Left Bundle Branch Block*

ECG 13-11 This is a classic example of an LBBB pattern. Notice how the complexes, which are wider than 0.12 seconds, are all up in lead V_6 and down in V_1. This is the classic finding: big, wide, monomorphic waves in those leads. Lead I follows the tradition of looking similar, if not identical, to lead V_6. We have discussed the similarities between lead I and V_6 before, but we should review them one more time. Lead I faces the left side of the body and is found in the fifth intercostal space in the mid-axillary line. The electrode for lead V_6 has an identical placement. Note that both have the same placement in 3-D space because they occur at the exact intersection of the two planes — the frontal and the Z. Therefore, the ECGs for leads I and V_6 should be identical, though there usually is some discrepancy in the appearances of the complexes because lead placement is not an exact science.

Remember the all-up-or-down criterion. It will help you greatly in making the diagnosis.

Notice that this ECG has a left axis. LBBB is either normal or left axis in most cases. In rare instances, it can even be a right axis. This occurs when there is a combination of RVH and an LBBB. The ECG will show the typical LBBB pattern on the precordial leads, but the frontal plane will be deviated to the right in the limb leads. This is very rare. You should just be aware that it can happen.

ECG 13-12 This is another example of LBBB. All of the criteria are met for the condition, beginning with the width of the QRS complex. The notching associated with the lateral leads of I, aVL, and V_5 to V_6 deserves mention. Notice how, compared with ECG 13-11, the notching causes an RR' pattern. The most important thing to observe is that it occurs in leads V_5 and V_6, but not in V_1, as you would expect in an RBBB pattern. This is a critical point. It is not just a set of rabbit ears that makes RBBB. It is also their location and their association with the slurred S waves.

Don't forget to look at the other interesting aspects found in this ECG. Make sure that you are going back and looking for all of the things you have reviewed to this point in the book. For example, look at the P waves. Is there anything unusual about them? Yes, there is definitely evidence of left atrial enlargement (LAE), with criteria present for both a P-mitrale and a large negative component in the last half of a biphasic P wave in lead V_1. Remember, those criteria? If you don't, go back to Chapter 9 and review them quickly.

Does the ECG show evidence of LVH? No one knows! You cannot make the diagnosis of LVH in LBBB because the size of the complexes is caused by an abnormal, unopposed vector depolarizing the left ventricle. It is not possible, therefore, to make any statements about the "true" height of the complexes.

CLINICAL PEARL

If an ECG looks wide, bizarre, and ugly, it is probably either a LBBB pattern or an IVCD associated with elevated potassium levels.

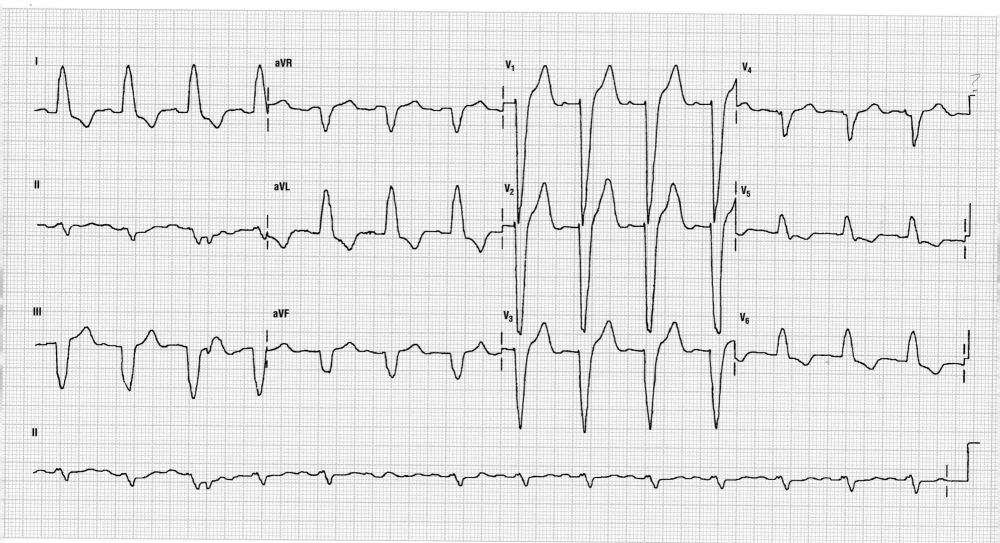

ECG 13-11

CHAPTER **13** • BUNDLE BRANCH BLOCKS AND HEMIBLOCKS

ECG CASE STUDIES: CONTINUED

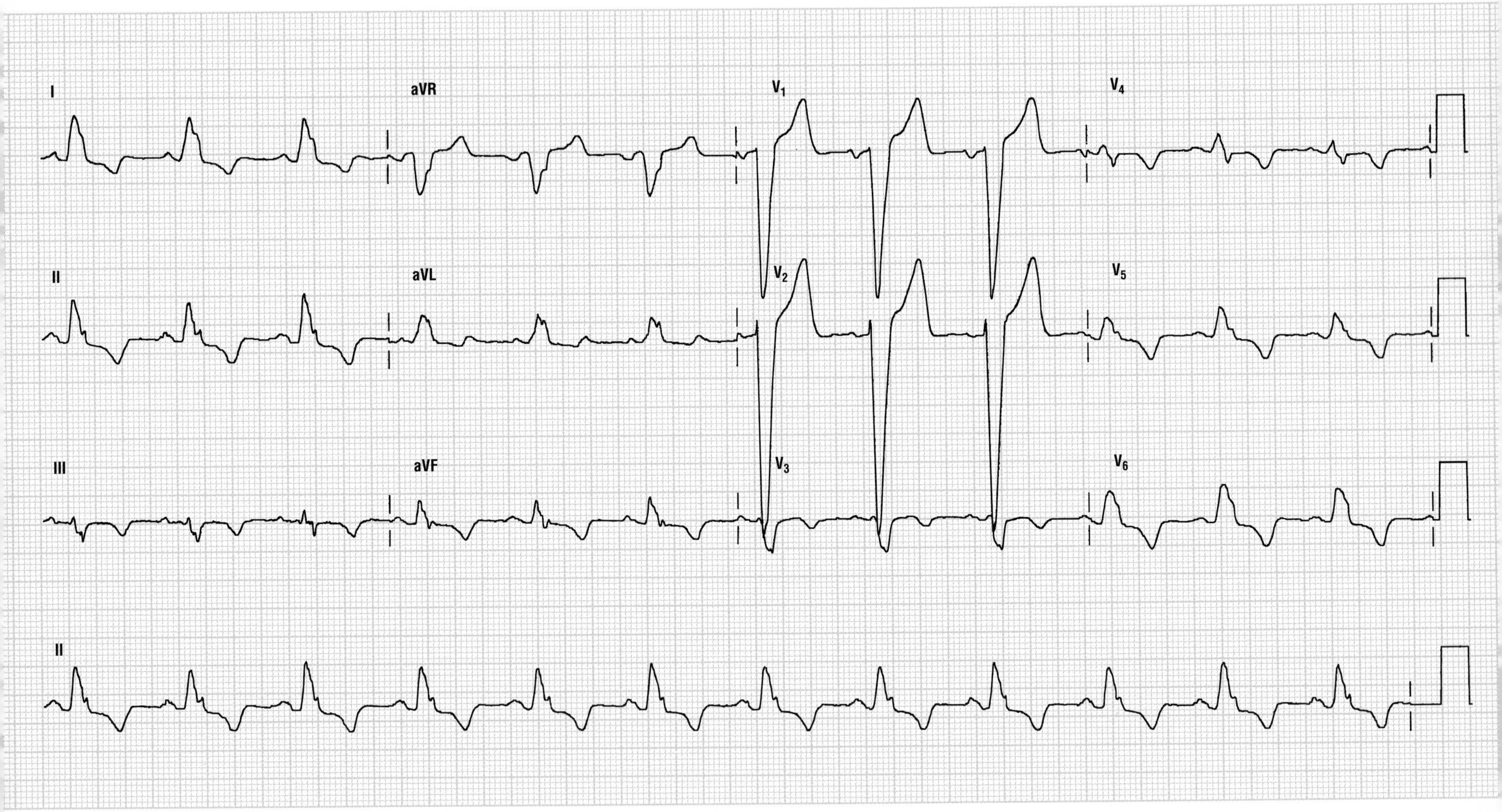

I   aVR   V₁   V₄

II   aVL   V₂   V₅

III   aVF   V₃   V₆

II

ECG 13-12

ECG 13-13 This example of LBBB is not as wide as the one in ECG 13-12. However, it is still greater than or equal to 0.12 seconds. In addition, it meets the all-up-or-down criterion with an rS complex in lead V_1, which is commonly seen in LBBB, and a monomorphic R wave in V_6. There is some notching present in leads I and V_5 to V_6.

Look at the complex in V_6 closely. Is that a delta wave? No, because the delta wave is not seen in any other leads. This is an example of the late intrinsicoid deflection that is common in LBBB, and also in LVH.

In addition to the LBBB, the frontal axis lies in the left quadrant and there is evidence of LAE.

ECG 13-14 Take a long, hard look at the ECG below. Now, go back to Chapter 11 and look at the ECGs that show LVH. What are some of the similarities and some of the differences? The precordial leads, V_1 to V_5, can be easily mistaken for LVH. The problem is that LVH should not be greater than or equal to 0.12 seconds wide. This ECG shows the wide complexes typical of LBBB, and also the notching in V_6. The limb leads are more typical of LBBB than of LVH, with easily identifiable wide complexes. Remember, the width of the intervals is the same throughout an ECG. If one lead shows a complex of 0.12 seconds wide or more, they are all 0.12 seconds wide or more. Be careful of snap judgments and look at every ECG carefully.

QUICK REVIEW

1. You can diagnose LVH in LBBB easily. The same criteria are used as in an ECG without LBBB. True or False.

2. LBBB can sometimes have some notching of the QRS complex in leads V_5 to V_6. True or False.

3. LBBB can have a normal, left, or right frontal axis. True or False.

1. False 2. True 3. True

QUICK REVIEW

1. LVH is typically _____ 0.12 seconds.

2. LBBB has either a _____ S wave or a small r wave with a deep S wave in lead V_1.

3. LBBB is either all _____ or all _____.

4. LAE (can/cannot) be diagnosed in LBBB.

1. Less than 2. Monomorphic 3. Up/down 4. Can

ECG CASE STUDIES: **CONTINUED**

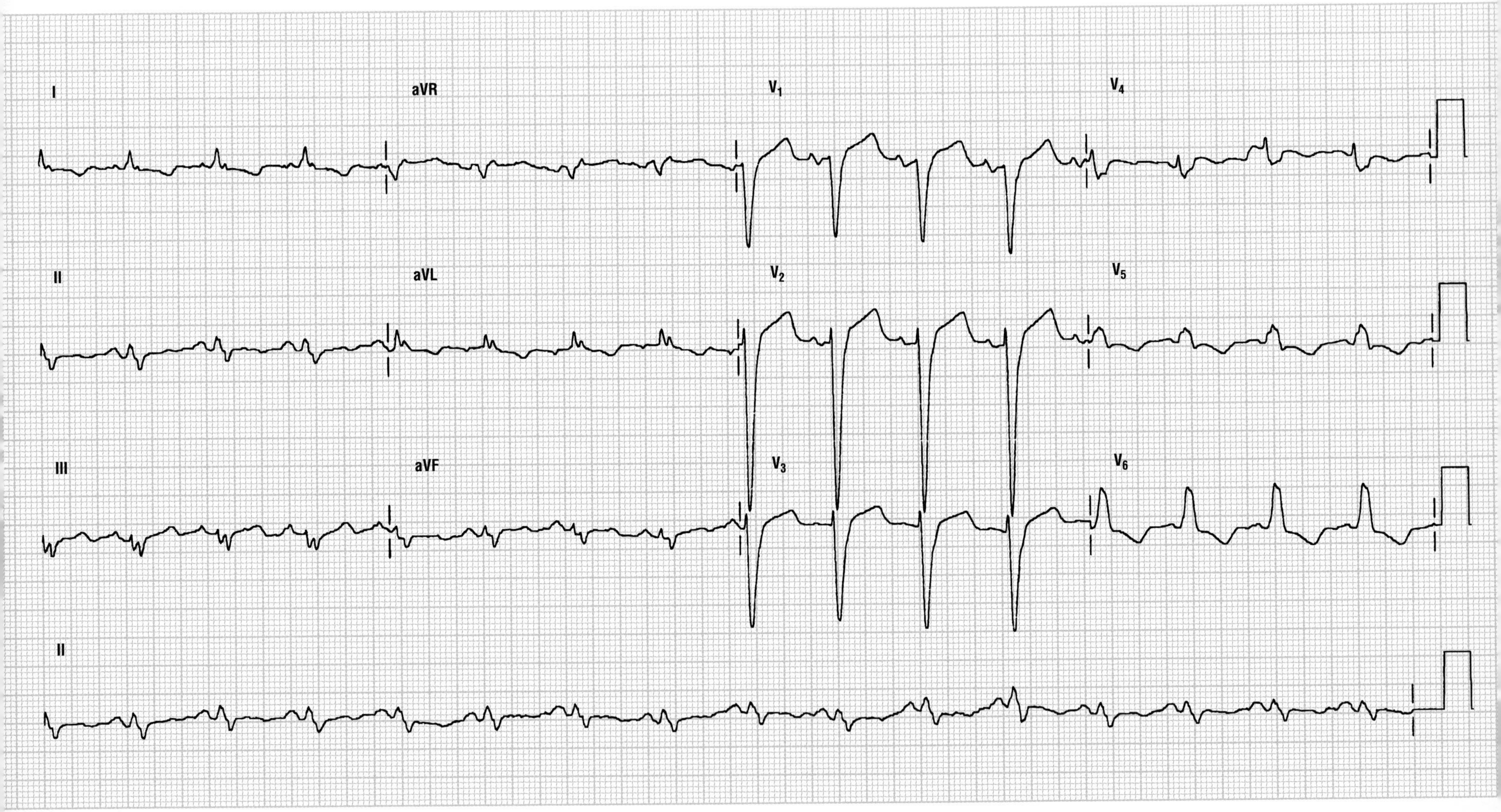

I aVR V₁ V₄

II aVL V₂ V₅

III aVF V₃ V₆

II

ECG 13-13

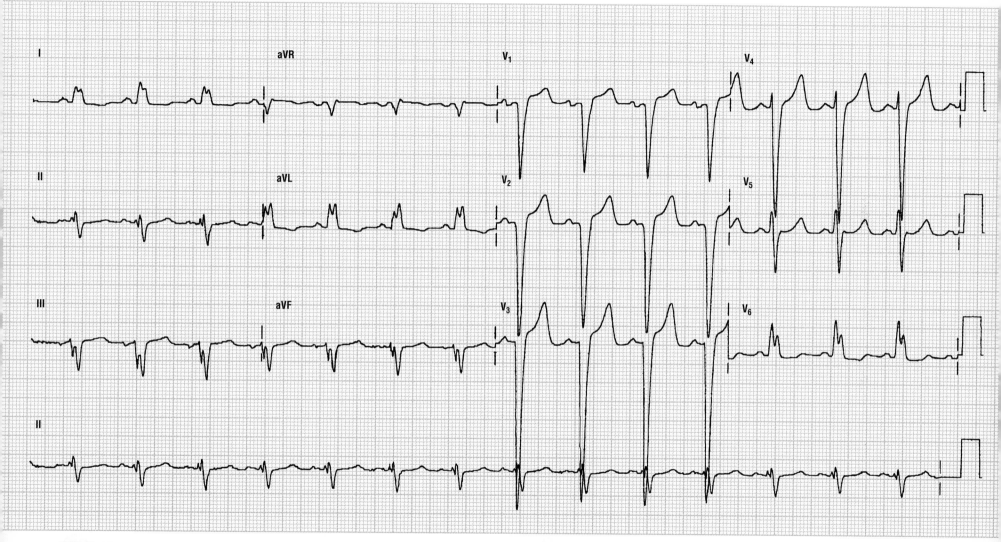

ECG 13-14

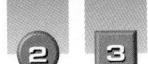

ECG CASE STUDIES: **CONTINUED**

2

ECG 13-15 This is more of the same. We are going to give you many examples of LBBB so that you can observe the different morphologies involved. As you can see, however, most of the ECGs resemble each other closely.

So what is unusual about this ECG, other than the LBBB pattern? This ECG shows evidence of P-pulmonale in lead II. There is also evidence of LAE in V_1, indicating biatrial enlargement.

What is the fourth complex from the end? Is it a VPC, or a junctional premature contraction (JPC) or APC with aberrancy? This is a tough one to diagnose! It looks like a JPC with aberrancy, but the axis of the complex is different from the normal one, and it has a differing terminal portion. This makes a JPC very unlikely. The most logical solution is that this complex is caused by a ventricular pacemaker in a portion of the ventricle not on the common depolarization path. Normally, the depolarization wave travels down the right bundle branch and then spreads by cell-to-cell transmission through the left ventricle. The path that the depolarization wave takes determines the shape of the complex. A focus that causes a depolarization wave to travel through the ventricle from a different direction will give rise to a different pattern. This concept is analogous to the appearance of a city when you approach it from various directions — the north, the south, the air, the water, and so on.

> **REMINDER:**
> At this point in your development, you should be reviewing each new ECG you encounter for all of the findings discussed so far. Remember to look for any differences between complexes or intervals and ask yourself, "Why are there differences?" Form good habits early.

2

ECG 13-16 This example shows an LBBB with all of the criteria: a wide QRS, an rS pattern in V_1, and a monomorphic R wave in V_6. The frontal axis is in the left quadrant. There is evidence of LAE in lead V_1. Finally, the rhythm is tachycardic.

Have you noticed that all of these complexes seem to have a long QT interval? This commonly occurs in BBBs, especially LBBB, because of the extended time that it takes to depolarize and repolarize the ventricle by direct cell-to-cell transmission. The extended time causes the QT prolongation. This prolonged QT interval does not carry the clinical significance that it does when present without a block, however.

3

ECG 13-16 What are the common causes of LBBB? The differential diagnosis includes:

1. Hypertension
2. Coronary artery disease (CAD)
3. Dilated cardiomyopathy
4. Rheumatic heart disease
5. Infiltrative diseases of the heart
6. Benign or idiopathic causes

The vast majority are due to hypertension, CAD, or both.

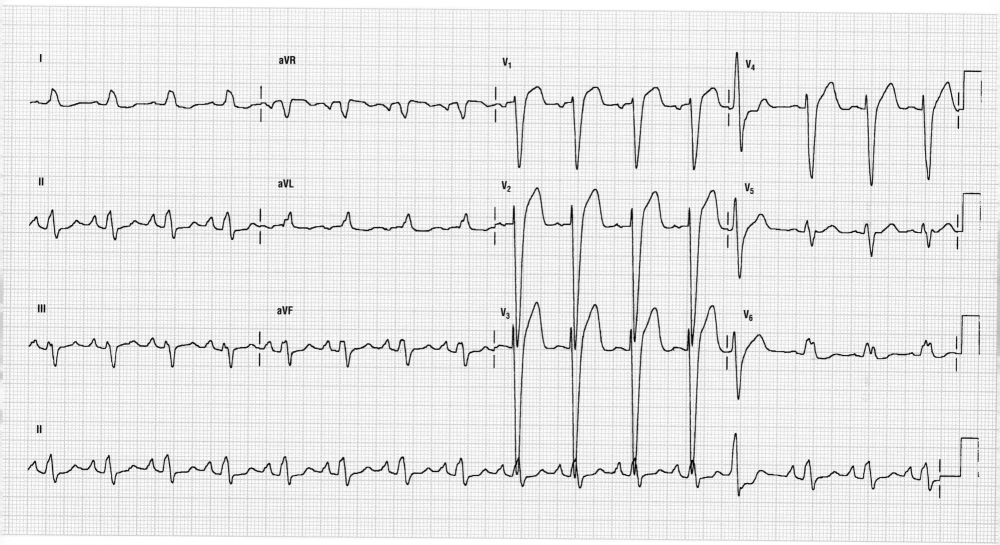

ECG 13-15

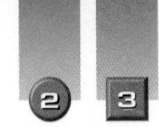

ECG CASE STUDIES: **CONTINUED**

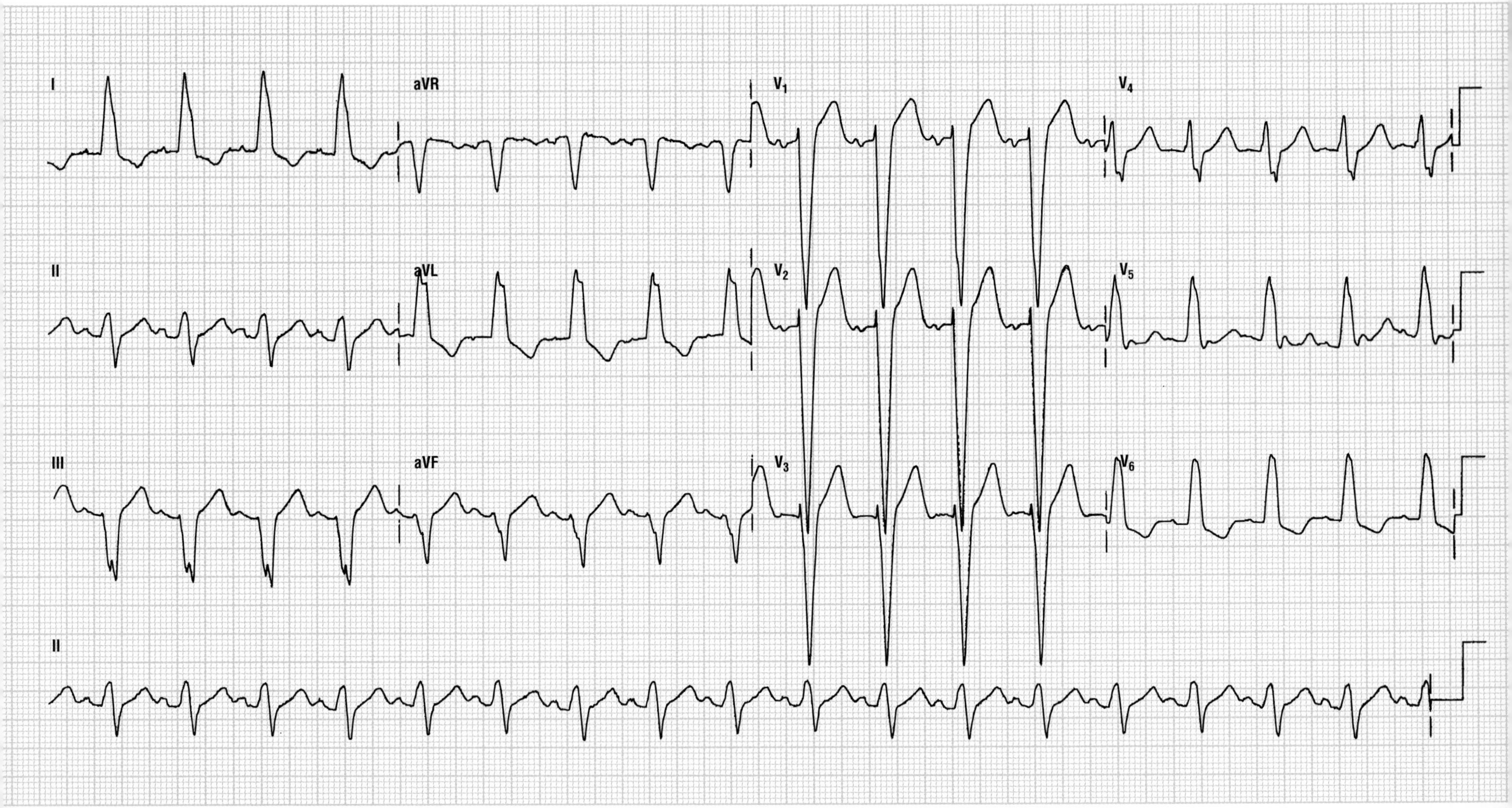

I aVR V₁ V₄

II aVL V₂ V₅

III aVF V₃ V₆

II

ECG 13-16

ECG 13-17 Well, this one is also an example of LBBB. We hope that you are getting the hang of making this diagnosis. Remember, the diagnosis of any BBB starts with the recognition that the complexes are 0.12 seconds wide or more. If you don't pick up this point, you will not make the right diagnosis. This is a pure and simple fact. Once you know that you are dealing with a wide complex, then you can focus on the location of the block.

ECG 13-18 This is, once again, obviously an LBBB. What is unusual about this ECG is the pattern of the QRS complex in the limb leads and V_5. The limb leads show multiple notches. The cause is unclear. The same holds for the complex in V_5, which has a small peak right after the P wave. Note that if you measure the intervals, all of the abnormalities in question occur within the QRS complex.

---

3 QUICK REVIEW

1. Abnormal Q waves are sometimes found in the inferior leads in many patients with LBBB. True or False.

1. True. Abnormal Q waves in the inferior leads may be due to the LBBB alone. However, you still need to consider the possibility of an old IWMI. Don't just assume it is due to block. Abnormal Q waves in the lateral or high lateral leads are pathologic and represent an old infarct.

---

2 QUICK REVIEW

Matching game (answers can be used more than once):

1. Slurred S wave
2. Wider than 0.12 sec.
3. rS complex in V_1
4. Increased R:S ratio in V_1
5. Frontal axis in right quadrant
6. Frontal axis in left quadrant
7. Able to leap tall buildings in a single bound

A. LBBB
B. RBBB
C. Both
D. Tom Garcia
E. Neil Holtz
F. None

1.B 2.C 3.A 4.B 5.C 6.C 7.F

ECG CASE STUDIES: **CONTINUED**

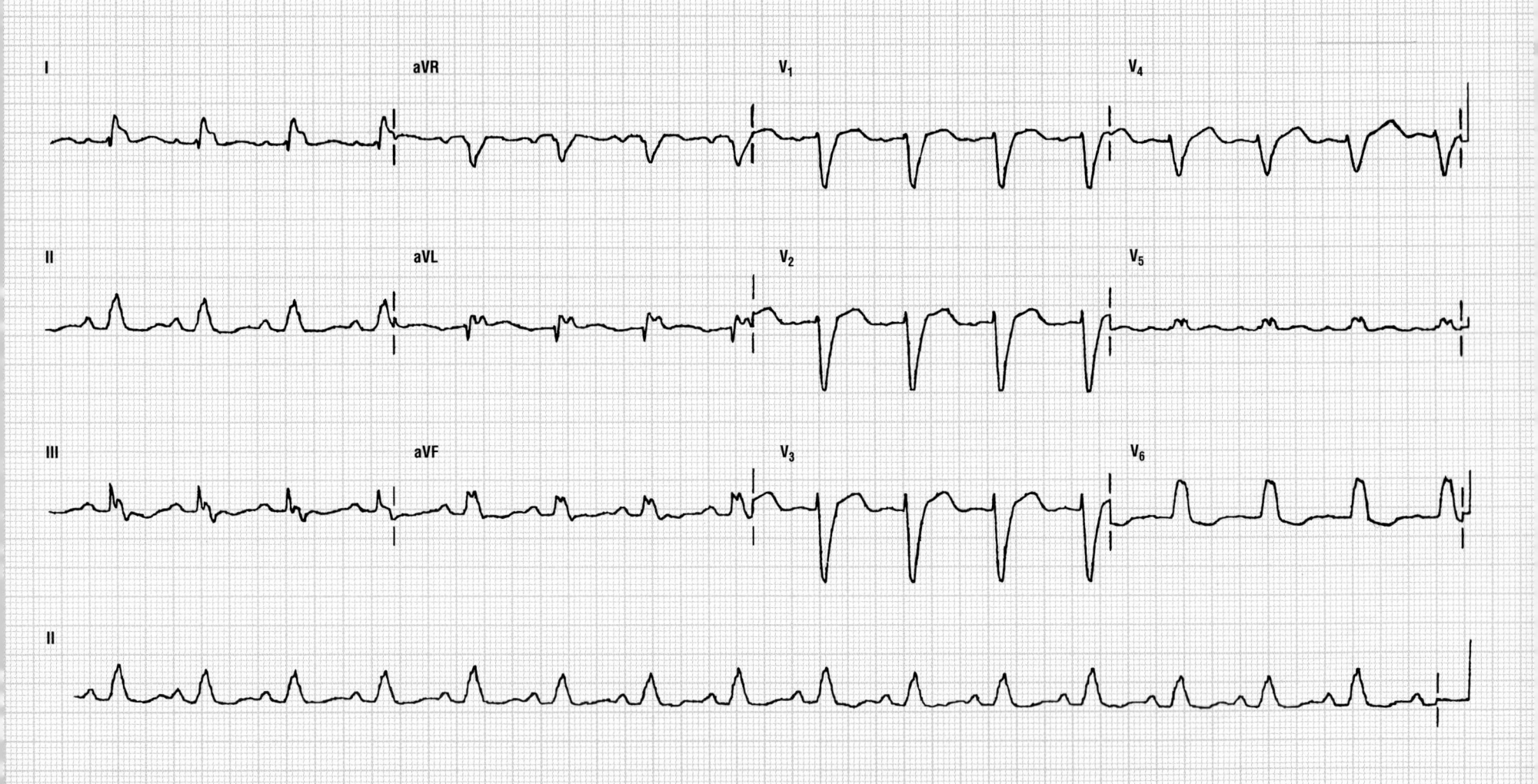

I   aVR   V₁   V₄

II   aVL   V₂   V₅

III   aVF   V₃   V₆

II

ECG 13-17

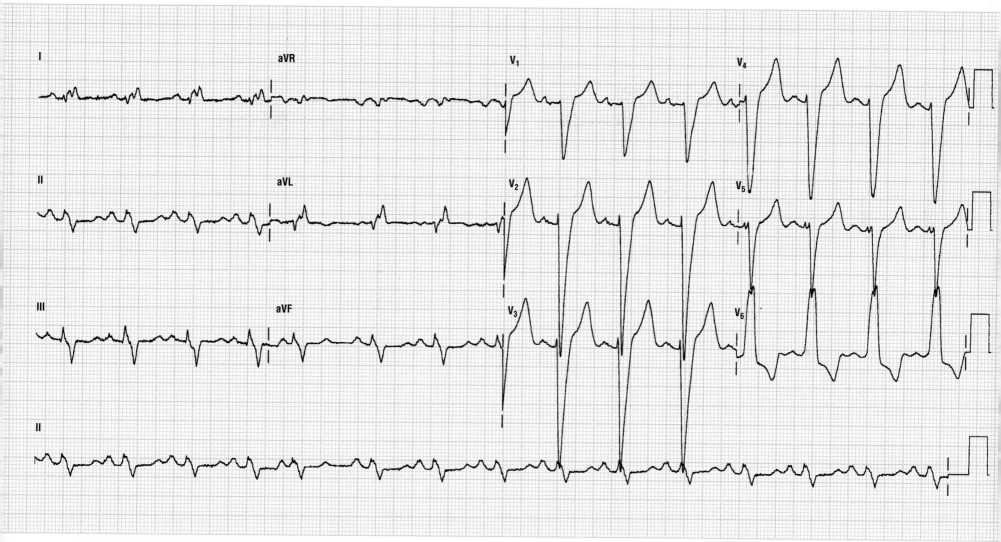

ECG 13-18

CHAPTER **13** • BUNDLE BRANCH BLOCKS AND HEMIBLOCKS

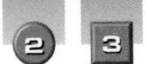

ECG CASE STUDIES: **C O N T I N U E D**

2

ECG 13-19 Because this is the section on LBBB, let's begin by looking at the QRS complexes. (Remember, you are really supposed to start with rhythm, rate, and so forth.) Are the complexes 0.12 seconds wide or more? Yes. Do we see any slurred S waves in I and V_6? No. Do we see monomorphic complexes that are either all up or all down in leads I, V_1, and V_6? Yes. Therefore, this is LBBB.

Do we see any P waves? There are some small ones in V_1 to V_3. But they are really small and wide, almost imperceptible. Look at lead III. Could that be a P wave with a first-degree heart block? No, because if you measure the waves, the hump is part of a biphasic T wave.

3

ECG 13-19 The frontal axis on this ECG is also in the left quadrant. This is commonly found in many patients with LBBB. There has been much controversy about the ability of an LBBB to cause a frontal axis shift, but the current belief is that an LBBB can do this all by itself. Part of the answer lies in where the initial depolarizing forces reach the ventricle. If the ventricle is initially innervated from the posterior wall, it will present similar to LAH and produce a leftward frontal axis. If the ventricle is initially innervated from the anterior wall or both walls simultaneously, it will create a normal or rightward axis.

2

ECG 13-20 OK, you hate us by now, but this is the last one. All of this repetition will pay off for you. The more you see, the more you'll remember. That is why we keep repeating the criteria. What are the criteria for LBBB? QRS $\geq$ 0.12 seconds wide, monomorphic S wave or rS complex in lead V_1, and monomorphic R wave in leads I and V_6.

So what is going on with all the weird beats? The P waves all map out without any problems. The PR intervals also are the same for the majority of the beats — the ones that are similar in morphology. There are other beats, such as the second, fourth, and fifth ones from the left, that are aberrant (compared with the native QRS complex). These appear to be VPCs, or JPCs with some aberrant component. The fifth beat appears to be from a different focus.

3

ECG 13-20 Why is this not ventricular tachycardia? Well, there is no AV dissociation, which is a mandatory criterion for that diagnosis. Could the aberrant beats be ventricular in origin? Sure they could, especially because there appear to be at least two ventricular foci giving rise to the abnormal complexes. Why don't the VPCs reset the sinus node, as usually happens with VPCs, and create a compensatory pause? The most logical explanation is that, because the AV node is diseased (note the first-degree heart block), there is no retrograde conduction through the AV node, and the atria and the sinus node are not affected.

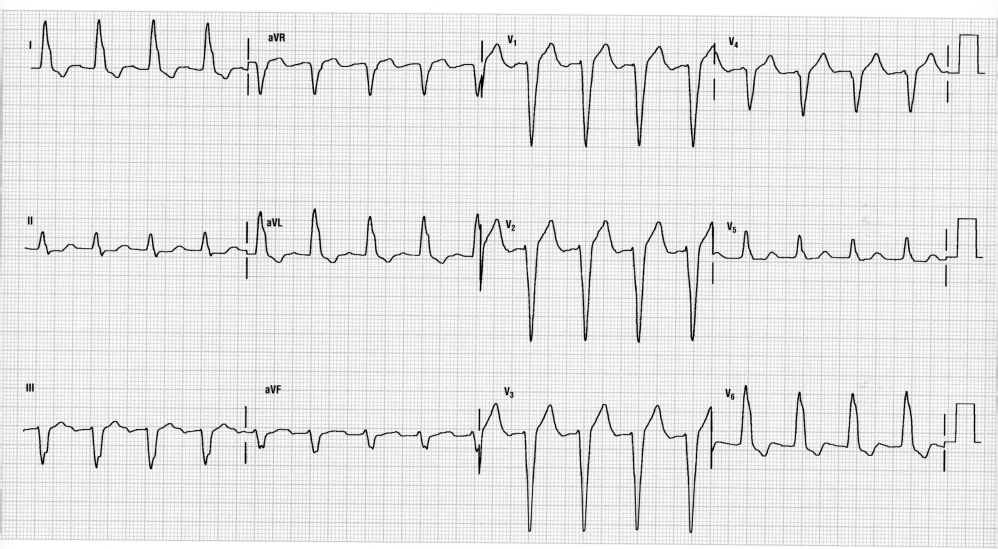

ECG 13-19

ECG CASE STUDIES: **CONTINUED**

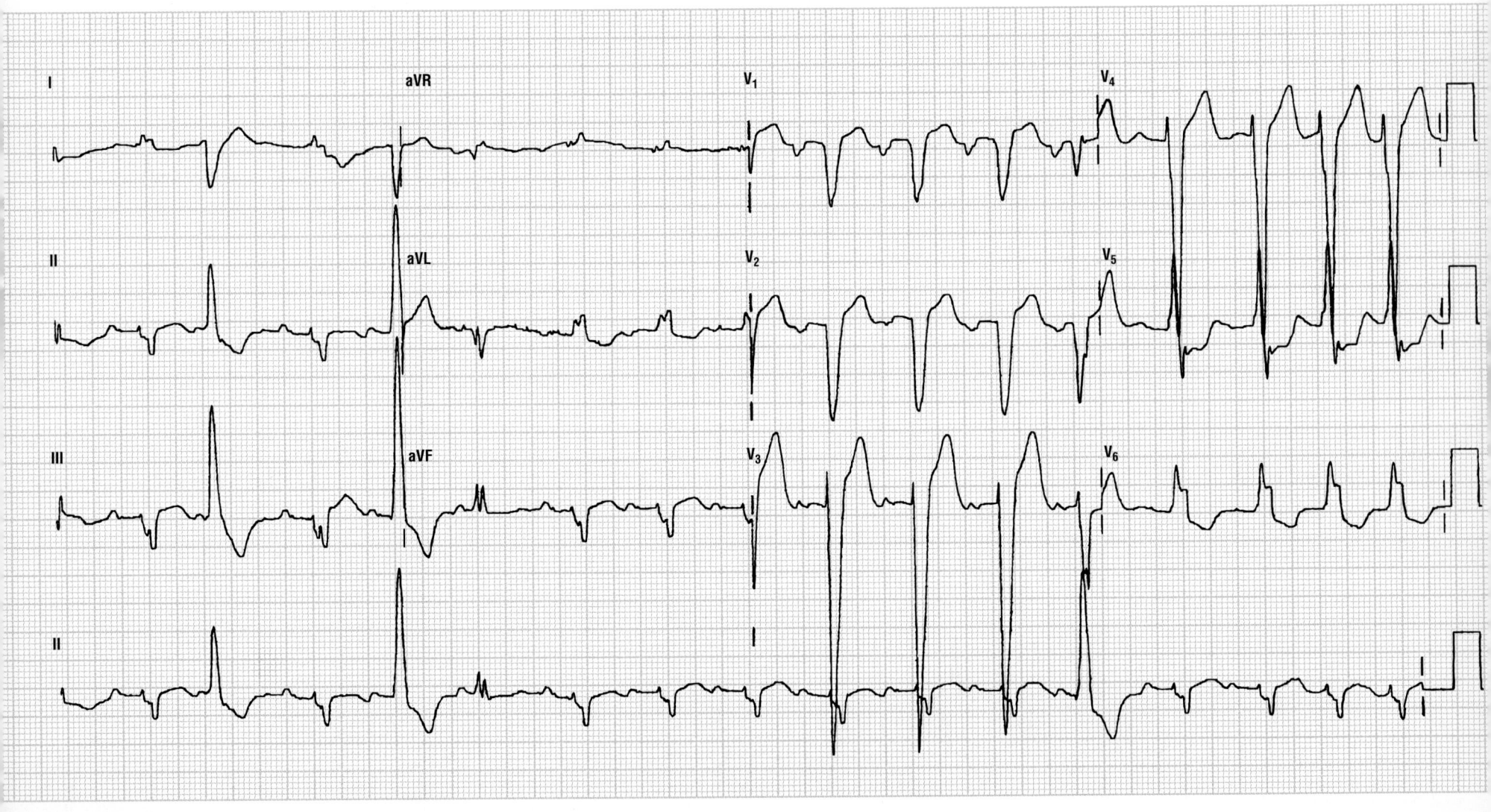

ECG 13-20

Intraventricular Conduction Delay (IVCD)

Intraventricular conduction delays (IVCDs) can either be localized to one lead or found throughout the ECG. First, let's talk about the localized ones. Localized IVCDs occur quite frequently and look like a QRS complex that has many peaks, kind of like an RSR' pattern but not wider than the normal beat. The key: *A localized IVCD is not greater than or equal to 0.12 seconds wide*. They occur very commonly in lead III.

An IVCD that is found throughout the ECG is one in which the QRS complexes are 0.12 seconds wide or more but do not have all of the characteristics of either LBBB or RBBB. In the typical presentation, the QRS complexes in V_1 have an LBBB pattern, whereas those in V_6

appear to have a RBBB pattern. Whenever you see a generalized IVCD, your first thought should be an electrolyte abnormality, especially hyperkalemia. Hyperkalemia is the deadliest cause of IVCD and should be treated immediately when found.

Summary Comments on Bundle Branch Blocks

In LBBB, it is not possible to diagnose LVH or RVH. This is because the complexes are conducted aberrantly for the most part; the true size of the complexes, if the block were not present, cannot be calculated. Most LBBBs have a normal axis. A left axis is also common. Infarction can be diagnosed in an LBBB, and we'll cover that briefly in Chapter 15. To evaluate pathology, remember the concept of concordance. Atrial enlargement can be diagnosed by the usual criteria.

RBBB, on the other hand, has a normal origin and is only delayed in the terminal portion of the complexes. You can therefore diagnose LVH by the normal criteria. RVH, however, cannot be diagnosed. Infarcts can be diagnosed using the normal criteria, as if there were no block present. To evaluate ischemia, remember the concept of concordance. Atrial enlargement also can be diagnosed by the usual criteria.

Take a few minutes to review the indications for pacemaker placement in your advanced cardiac life support (ACLS) book. Most of the indications refer to BBBs and bifascicular blocks.

Do not be overwhelmed when you look at an ECG that has a block. Once again, break it down. Figure out which type of bundle block is evident. *It is very beneficial to commit to memory the appearance of the normal LBBB and RBBB patterns.* When you look at the "normal" blocks, notice which leads show ST elevation and depression, what the Ts and QRS complexes should look like, what the axis should be, the regularity of the complexes, and so on. Knowing the appearance of the normal blocks will make any abnormality not caused by the block itself stand out like a sore thumb. This is the only way to really feel comfortable with the blocks.

CLINICAL PEARL

Thoughts About Wide QRS Complexes

When you see that the QRS complexes are 0.12 seconds wide or more, think of four possibilities:

1. LBBB

2. RBBB

3. IVCD

4. Ventricular or aberrantly conducted beats

Your next thoughts should be:

A. If the ECG appears to be an IVCD, focus immediately on hyperkalemia and its treatment.

B. If the ECG appears to be ventricular tachycardia, initiate treatment immediately.

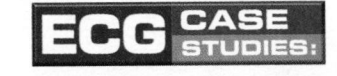 *Intraventricular Conduction Delay*

②

ECG 13-21 The ECG below has QRS complexes that are wider than 0.12 seconds. This makes it a block of some kind. Does it have a slurred S wave in leads I and V_6? Yes, it does. Does it have an increased R:S ratio in lead V_1? No! There is no evidence of an RBBB in lead V_1. So what is it? This is an intraventricular conduction delay. Now for the most important point: What is the most common cause of an IVCD? Hyperkalemia! As you will see in Chapter 16, when the patient gets to the point of having an IVCD, you've only got minutes to react. This patient was in cardiac arrest less than 5 minutes after this ECG was taken. Hard to believe, but true!

③

ECG 13-21 Some other findings for hyperkalemia are present on this ECG. Notice the PR prolongation. In addition, we see tall, broad T waves. This is due to the widening of the entire complex caused by the potassium effects. The QRS is also widened.

As we'll also see in Chapter 16, many patients with hyperkalemia (including this one) have QT prolongation because of an associated hypocalcemia. The combination of hyperkalemia and hypocalcemia is very common in end-stage renal disease patients on dialysis. Rapid treatment is critical before progression to sine waves (see Chapter 16) or asystole occurs.

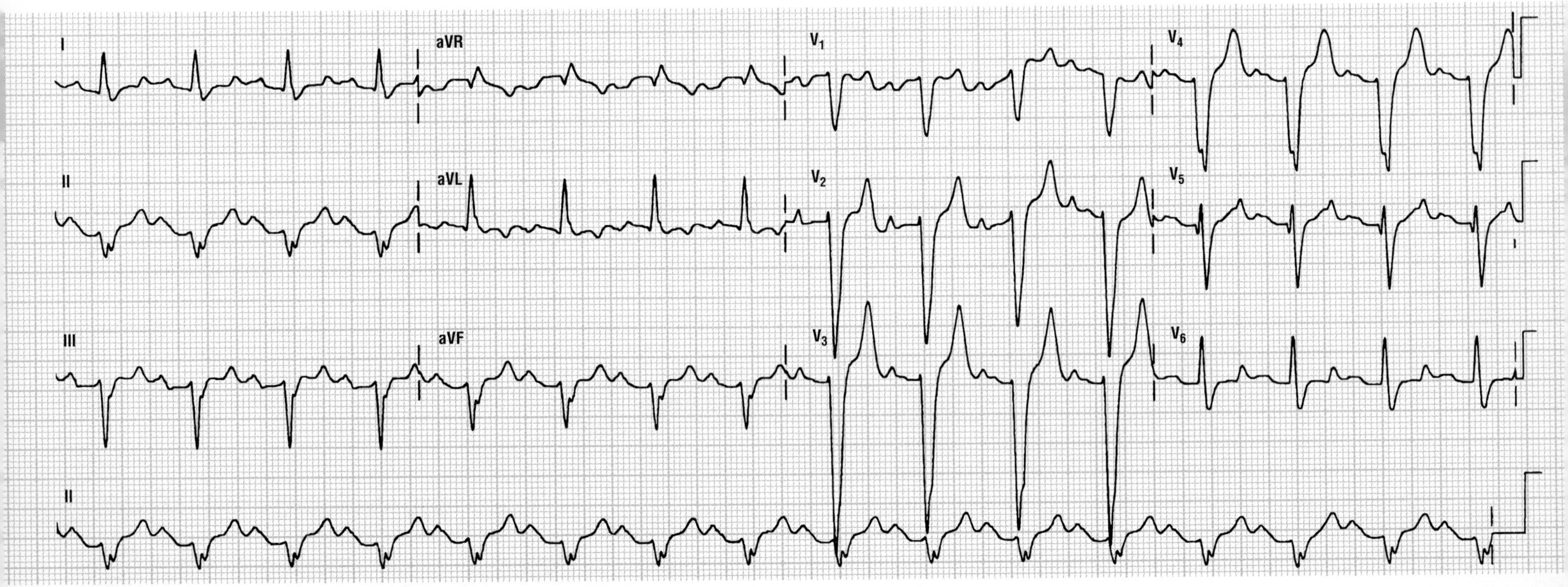

ECG 13-21

②

ECG 13-22 This ECG is really concerning. To begin with, no P waves precede any of the complexes. You see some areas of baseline wavering that make you think there is a P wave, but these are not consistent even within the same lead. This is simply a small amount of baseline artifact. It is really difficult to obtain a totally straight line on an ECG unless the lead falls off (see page 377, ECG 14-43B, for an example). The broad QRS complexes are much wider than 0.12 seconds and do not match either RBBB or LBBB pattern; this is consistent with an IVCD. So, what is the first thing you think of? Hyperkalemia. If you don't think about it, you can't make the diagnosis!

③

ECG 13-22 This ECG shows evidence of IVCD. In addition, the QRS intervals are very wide and there are no associated P waves. This is an example of severe hyperkalemia. It borders on a sine wave pattern. Luckily, the patient was treated and the ECG findings reversed. Notice that there is no prolongation of the QT interval. This is a unique finding with this level of potassium, which usually produces QT prolongation.

Differential diagnosis must include an accelerated idioventricular rhythm with various possible causes. However, you would also expect an associated QT prolongation in those cases.

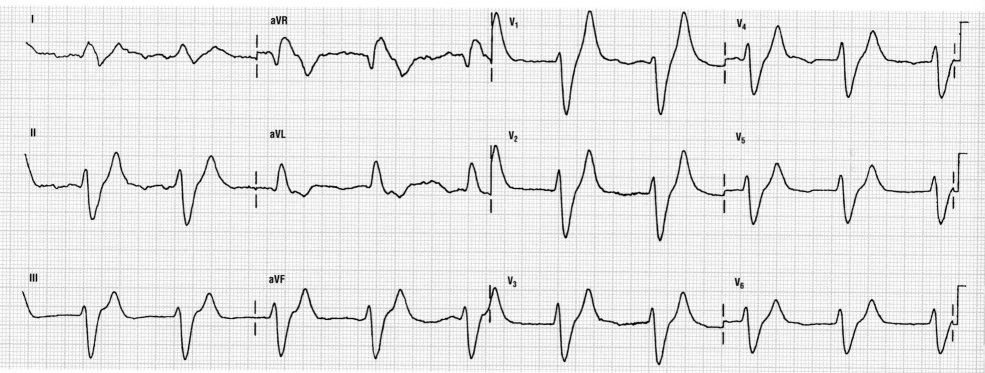

ECG 13-22

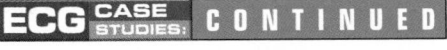

CASE STUDIES: **CONTINUED**

ECG 13-23 This really ugly ECG is actually quite simple. Do you see those small lines before each of the QRS complexes? Those are spikes from a pacemaker. This is an ECG taken from a patient with a ventricularly paced rhythm. The tip of the pacemaker is touching the interventricular septum and acting as the pacing source (Figure 13-13). This gives you a picture very similar to an ectopic ventricular focus in which some cell in the ventricle is doing the pacing. The initial pacing spike gives rise to a depolarization wave that spreads by direct cell-to-cell contact, producing the wide, bizarre complex. Many times these complexes take the form of LBBB, RBBB, or IVCD patterns.

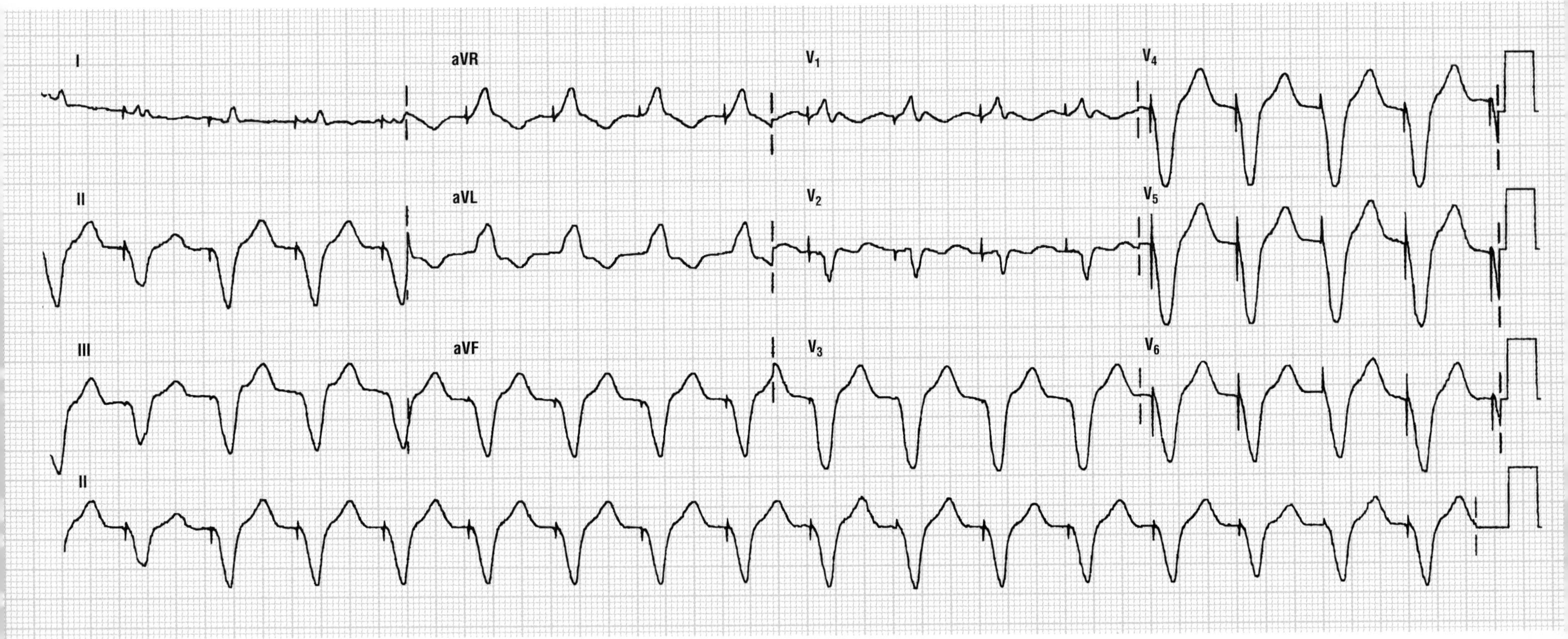

ECG 13-23

Hemiblocks

Hemiblock refers to a block of "half" of the left bundle branch after it splits into the left anterior and left posterior fascicles. (This classification is really incorrect because it does not follow the anatomical names of the structures involved. It is not really a block of half of the left bundle, but rather of an entire fascicle. However, this traditional classification is the one everyone uses.) A blocked left anterior fascicle is a *left anterior hemiblock,* or a left anterior fascicular block. Likewise, a blocked left posterior fascicle is a *left posterior hemiblock,* or a left posterior fascicular block.

The left anterior fascicle is an organized, thin bundle of fibers coming off of the left bundle that will give rise to the Purkinje fibers, which in turn innervate the anterior and lateral walls of the left ventricle (Figure 13-14). The left posterior fascicle also originates from the left bundle. However, the fibers are not organized into a tight fascicle; instead they disperse loosely and fan out. The left posterior fascicle is the origin of the fibers that innervate the inferior and posterior walls of the left ventricle. You can review this in Chapter 1.

Figure 13-13: Heart with pacemaker wire.

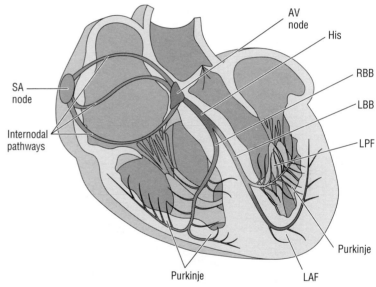

Figure 13-14: The heart and the electrical conduction system.

Hemiblocks cause the ventricles to be innervated asynchronously and aberrantly. They will, therefore, alter the vectors produced by the left ventricle. The different vectors will give rise to differing ECG patterns, which we will discuss presently.

Left Anterior Hemiblock

When the left anterior fascicle is blocked, the depolarization of the left ventricle has to progress from the interventricular septum, the inferior wall, and the posterior wall toward the anterior and lateral walls. This gives rise to an unopposed vector that is pointed superior and leftward (Figure 13-15). This will change the net axis of the ventricles toward the left, producing a left axis deviation. The electrical axis of the ventricles will be found in the left quadrant of the hexaxial system, specifically between -30 and $-90°$.

The other changes associated with LAH are a qR complex or a large R wave in lead I, and an rS complex in III. The small *q* and *r* waves are caused by the unopposed interventricular depolarization vector.

Criteria for diagnosing LAH:

1. Left axis deviation with the axis at -30 to $-90°$

2. Either a qR complex or an R wave in lead I

3. An rS complex in lead III, and probably also in II and aVF

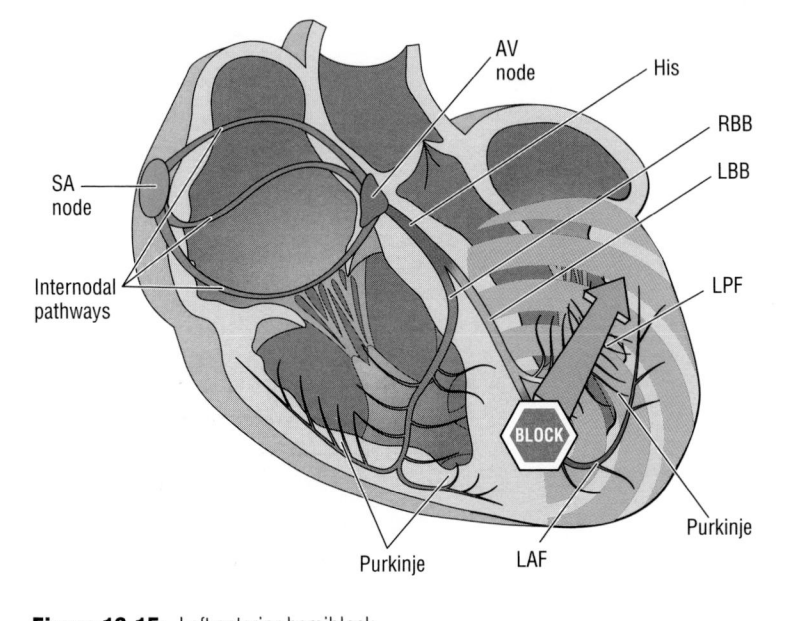

Figure 13-15: Left anterior hemiblock.

Shortcut to Recognizing LAH

The main criterion for diagnosing LAH is to have an abnormal left axis deviation between −30 and −90°. There is a really easy way to diagnose LAH based on the hexaxial system. See if you can figure it out if we give you a hint. Remember when we were isolating the quadrants and we used leads I and aVF? What leads would you need in order to isolate the area down to −30 to −90°? Well, you would use leads I, aVF, and II. You want the QRS complex to be positive in lead I, negative in aVF, and negative in II (Figure 13-16). Easy isn't it? On the ECG, look at I and aVF; if they are positive and negative, respectively, the axis is in the left quadrant. Now, look at lead II. If it is negative, you have LAH. With this method, you can diagnose LAH in less than 2 seconds. This will really impress your friends!

Many people state that you cannot make the diagnosis of LAH in patients with an inferior AMI. It is the Q wave in leads II, III, and aVF — they say — that causes an *initial* deflection of the vector rather than a *terminal* deflection of the vector, as in LAH. Our argument to these folks: Prove to us that LAH is not present! An abnormal left axis deviation (LAD) at −30 to −90° signifies pathology; the ECG is not normal. A small *r* wave in leads II, III, and aVF — if present — is even more proof of an LAH, but the main criterion is still LAD in the −30 to −90° range. A significant Q wave from an AMI could hide the small *r* wave. When we study bifascicular blocks, you will see that the presence of a bifascicular block in a patient with an AMI carries the possibility of developing a third-degree heart block. We would rather err on the side of calling a few extra LAHs than missing a few of them. If we miss the diagnosis, the patient may die; if we overcall it, the ECG is still abnormal and we haven't hurt anyone. Understand the reasoning of the purist and don't be too strict.

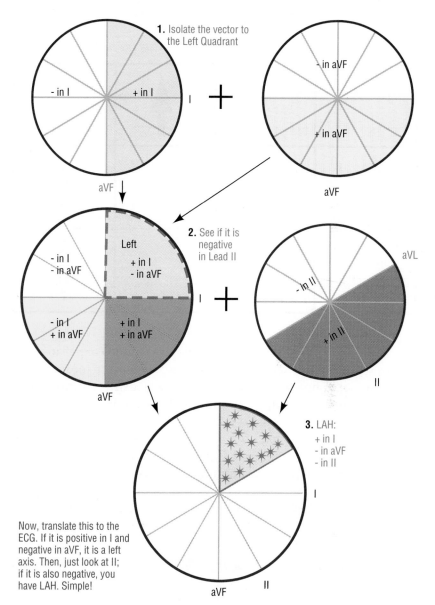

Now, translate this to the ECG. If it is positive in I and negative in aVF, it is a left axis. Then, just look at II; if it is also negative, you have LAH. Simple!

Figure 13-16: Isolating the axis in -30° to -90°.

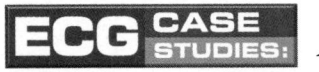 *Left Anterior Hemiblock*

②

ECG 13-24 What quadrant holds the frontal axis of the heart? Well, the complexes are positive in lead I and negative in aVF. That puts the axis in the left quadrant. Now, the left quadrant is made up of 90° — 0° to −90°, to be exact. We need to know if this is benign axis deviation from 0 to −29°, or pathological deviation due to LAH. In order to differentiate quickly between these two possibilities, we just look at lead II. If it has positive complexes, the axis must lie between leads 0 and −29°, because anything over −30° would make the complexes appear negative. If the complexes in lead II are negative, therefore, the axis must be between −30 and −90°. In this ECG, the complexes in lead II are negative. By using the logic above, we know that the axis must lie in the left quadrant, between −30 and −90°. That is the only slice of the "frontal" pie that matches all three conditions: positive in I, negative in aVF, and negative in II.

The additional criteria for LAH, either a qR complex or an R wave in lead I and an rS complex in III, are also present. Yes, there is a tiny *r* wave at the beginning of the QRS complex in III. If you don't believe us, use a magnifying glass. We are not being sarcastic in saying this, but rather introducing you to another tool that is helpful in ECG interpretation. Sometimes the waves are very small, but they are present nonetheless.

REMINDER:

Use the shortcut method to establish a quick diagnostic possibility of LAH.

ECG 13-25 This ECG also shows all the evidence of LAH. First, let's look at the axis. Is it in the left quadrant? Yes, we see positive complexes in lead I and negative ones in aVF. Is lead II positive or negative? Negative. This meets LAH criterion number one (Figure 13-17). Next, a qR wave is present in lead I. Finally, you notice the typical rS pattern in lead III. It is a little bit easier to see the *r* wave in this ECG, isn't it? Remember, it doesn't matter how big a wave is, just that it is there.

The ECG also shows evidence of LAE. Where is the transition in the precordials? Between V_5 and V_6! Remember, you're looking for the transition from a negative complex to a positive one. Leads V_2 to V_5 are still negative complexes. Use your calipers!

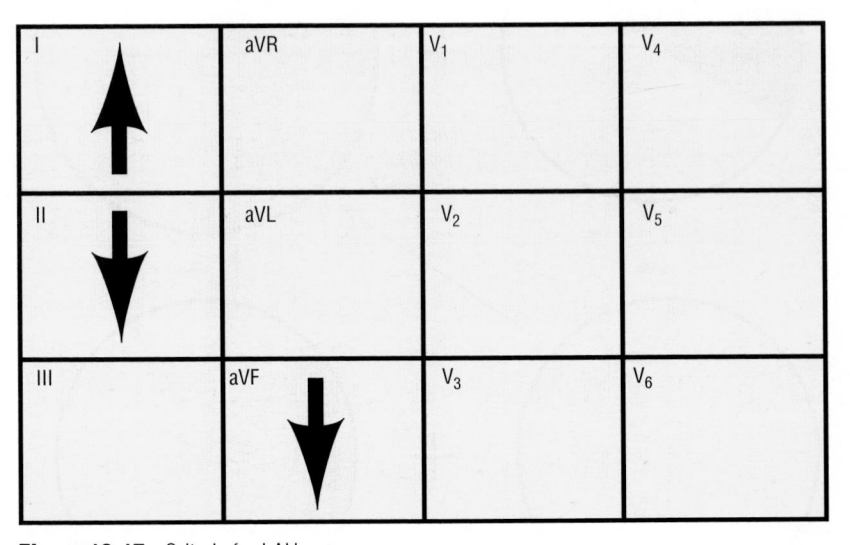

Figure 13-17: Criteria for LAH.

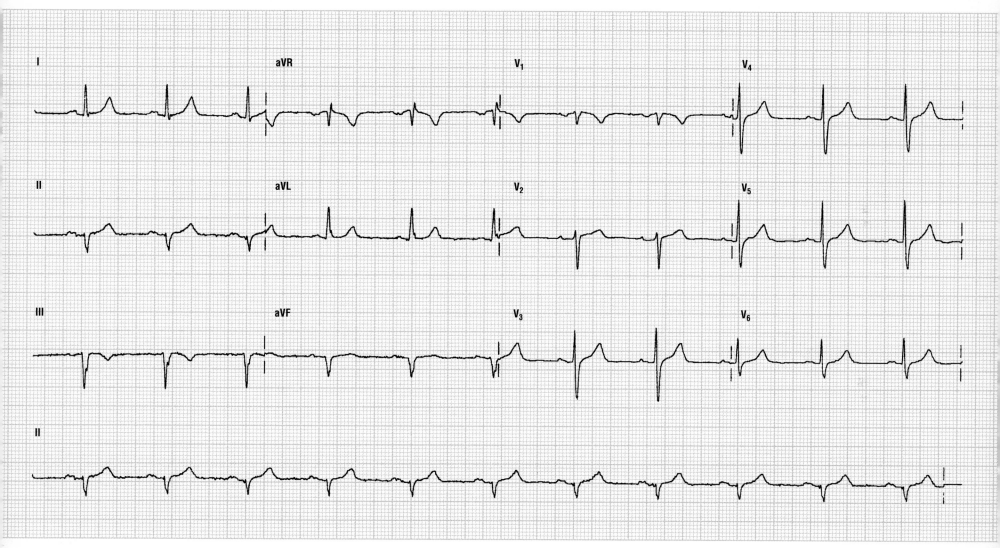

ECG 13-24

CHAPTER **13** • BUNDLE BRANCH BLOCKS AND HEMIBLOCKS

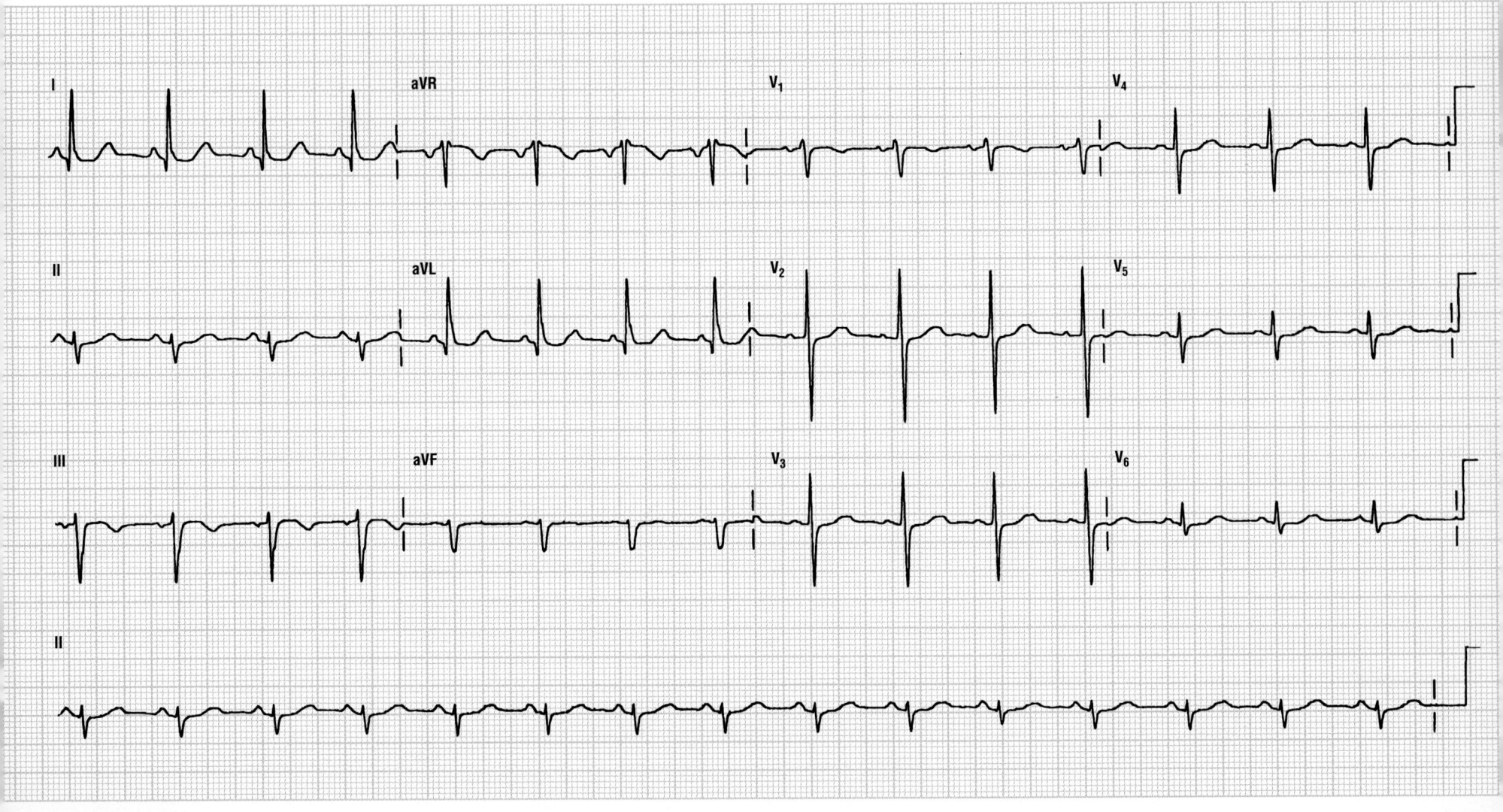

ECG 13-25

ECG 13-26 This is another example of LAH. It meets all of the criteria for the diagnosis. What are the criteria? If you've forgotten, go back and review them. The ECG also shows very low voltage. As a matter of fact, it misses the pericardial effusion criterion by only a millimeter. In some of the complexes in lead II, it is only 5 mm, and in others it is 6. Why the variation? Well, remember the respiratory variation we went over in the QRS chapter? Here it is again. As the patient breathes, the axis shifts just a small amount, causing a change in the height or depth of the complexes. This ECG probably belonged to a patient with a large body habitus — an obese patient. These patients typically have small complexes and a noticeable respiratory variation because their hearts are more horizontal.

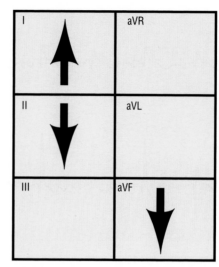

"It only takes a few seconds."

Note: LAH is so common that we will not be giving you a lot of examples here. Look around. You'll see them throughout the book.

Figure 13-18: Criteria for LAH, abbreviated version.

ECG CASE STUDIES: **CONTINUED**

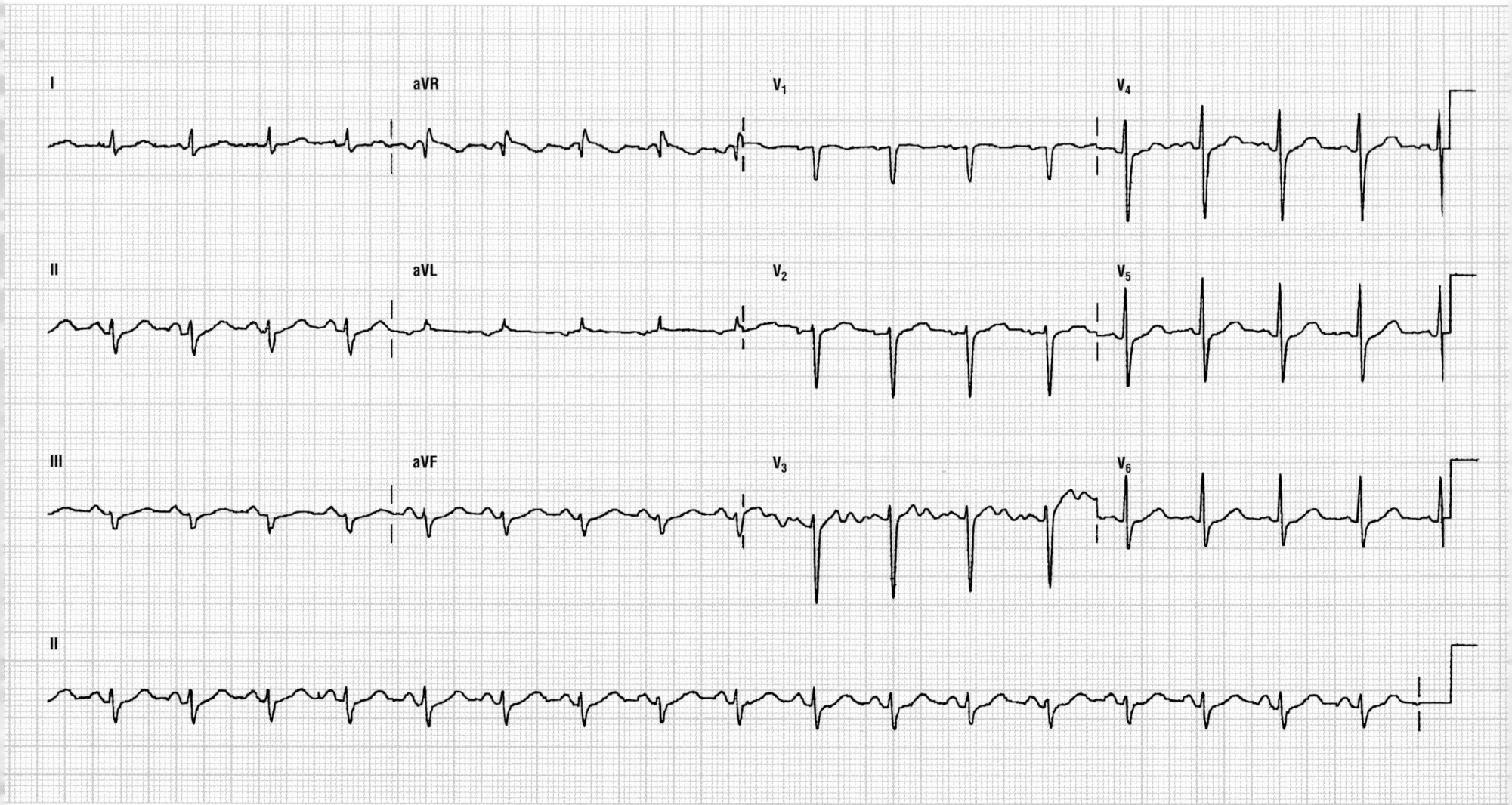

ECG 13-26

Left Posterior Hemiblock

The left posterior fascicle is difficult to block because the fibers are not organized as a discrete bundle, but instead are spread throughout the posterior and inferior walls of the left ventricle. Because of this spread, the lesion that could cause this type of block would have to be quite large. These hemiblocks are therefore rare. They are also difficult to diagnose. You could read 2,000 to 3,000 ECGs and be lucky to find one LPH. That is why we are going to give you more examples of this type of hemiblock. LAHs are very common and easy to diagnose in comparison.

When the left posterior fascicle is blocked, the depolarization of the inferior and posterior aspects of the left ventricle is delayed. The resulting unopposed vector is directed inferior and to the right (Figure 13-19). The net result of the vector is a rightward deflection of the ventricular axis into the right quadrant — right axis deviation. The original vectors that depolarize the interventricular septum and the superior-anterior walls are unopposed. This produces a small *r* wave in lead I and a small *q* in aVF.

Criteria for Diagnosing LPH:

1. An axis of 90 to 180° (the right quadrant)
2. An *s* wave in lead I and a *q* in III
3. Exclusion of RAE and/or RVH

The difficulty in diagnosing LPH lies in excluding other causes of a right axis. You need to understand clearly the criteria for RAH and P-pulmonale. You also need to understand RVH (Chapter 11) and the RVH with strain pattern, which will be further discussed in Chapter 14. *Remember, the most common cause of a right axis is RVH. You therefore need to exclude its presence in order to diagnose LPH.* Because the most common cause of right atrial enlargement is RVH, this should also be excluded. There are, if you notice, no criteria that can effectively "rule in" LPH. Instead, LPH is a diagnosis of exclusion; once you have excluded other causes for a right axis and you match all of the criteria above, you can call it LPH.

The key in diagnosing LPH is to think about it! When you are reading an ECG and you notice that you have an axis in the right quadrant — a negative QRS in lead I and a positive QRS in lead aVF, for example — your next thought should be: *Is this LPH?* If there is an *s* wave in I and a *q* in III, and no other evidence of RAE or RVH, then you have diagnosed LPH. If you don't think about it, you'll miss it!

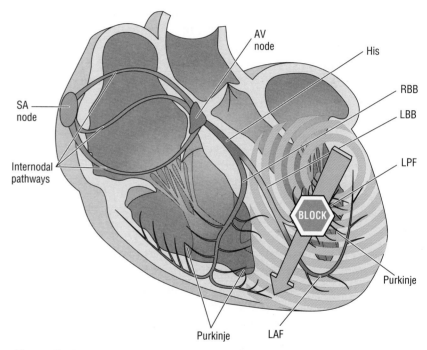

Figure 13-19: Left posterior hemiblock.

REMINDER:

If you have a right axis deviation, ask yourself: Is this a left posterior hemiblock?

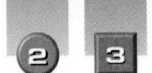

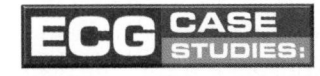 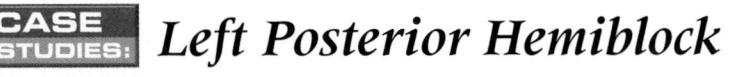 **Left Posterior Hemiblock**

ECG 13-27 This ECG is a typical example of LPH. To begin with, the axis is in the right quadrant; *not the extreme right quadrant,* just the plain old right quadrant. There is an S wave in lead I and a small Q in III, and no evidence of either RAE or RVH. Extensive lateral wall myocardial infarctions can also produce an abnormal right axis because of all the dead myocardium in the lateral wall. This causes a vector shift that creates the right axis deviation. Therefore, all of the criteria are met and we can call this LPH.

The problem arises in differentiating the $S_1Q_3T_3$ pattern from LPH. An $S_1Q_3T_3$ pattern includes an S wave in lead I, a Q or q wave in lead III, and a flipped T wave in lead III. You hear about the $S_1Q_3T_3$ pattern being found in patients with pulmonary emboli, and this occurs in about 15 to 30% of the cases. This is caused by an acute right ventricular strain. There is literally no one way to distinguish between LPH and this pattern in many cases. It is critically important to obtain a clinical history from the patient to distinguish between the two. We've said it before and we'll say it again: You can't interpret ECGs with any degree of certainty in a vacuum. You need to know some history or physical exam findings. The patient from whom we obtained the ECG below had no evidence of pulmonary embolus, and the history was not consistent with it in any way. So, you can say with certainty that it is LPH. The $S_1Q_3T_3$ is also discussed in Chapter 14 on page 346.

ECG 13-28 This ECG also shows a deviation of the frontal axis in the right quadrant between 90 and 180°. There is an S wave in lead I and a small *q* in III. This time, however, there is no flipped T wave to complete the $S_1Q_3T_3$ pattern for acute RVH strain. There is, however, pretty severe tachycardia. This tachycardia may be caused by a pulmonary embolism, or there could be some other source. You need to correlate the history to the ECG to make the diagnosis. There is no evidence of RAE, and the only criterion for RVH is a right axis. None of the other RVH criteria are present: increased R:S ratio in V_1, presence of RAE, and so on.

ECG 13-28 A few things about this ECG are troubling. To begin with, there's the LPH, with coronary artery disease (CAD) as the most common causative culprit. Next is the obvious QT prolongation. Finally, there are the tall and nearly symmetrical T waves in many leads. Many things can give you these exact findings: ischemia, hemorrhagic shock with associated hypocalcemia after massive transfusion, pulmonary embolus, congestive heart failure (CHF) in an end stage renal disease (ESRD) patient, and others. Clinical correlation is required to make the diagnosis. They are all life-threatening events and all will need immediate intervention.

REMINDER:
Remember, you cannot call a LPH if the electrical axis falls in the extreme right quadrant or if you have met any of the exclusion criteria.

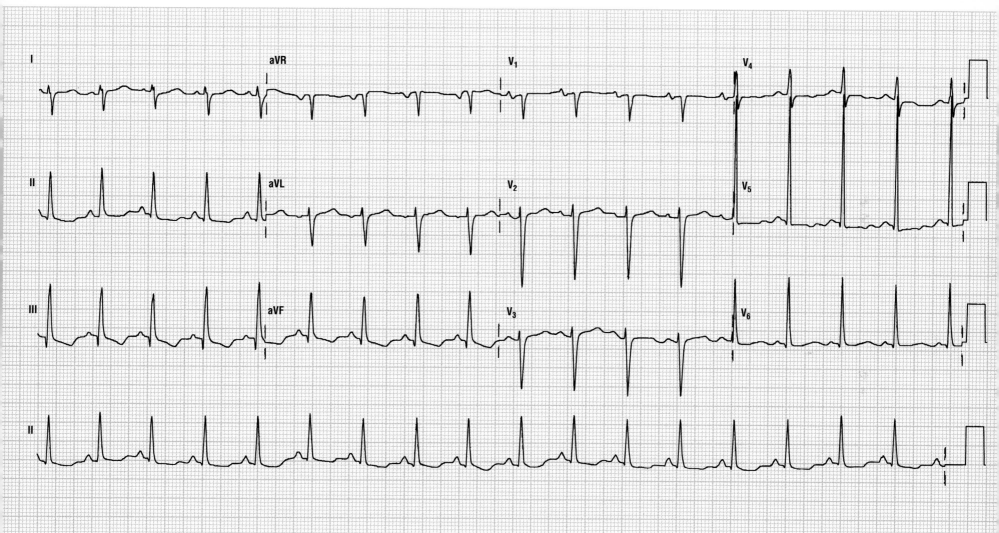

ECG 13-27

ECG CASE STUDIES: **CONTINUED**

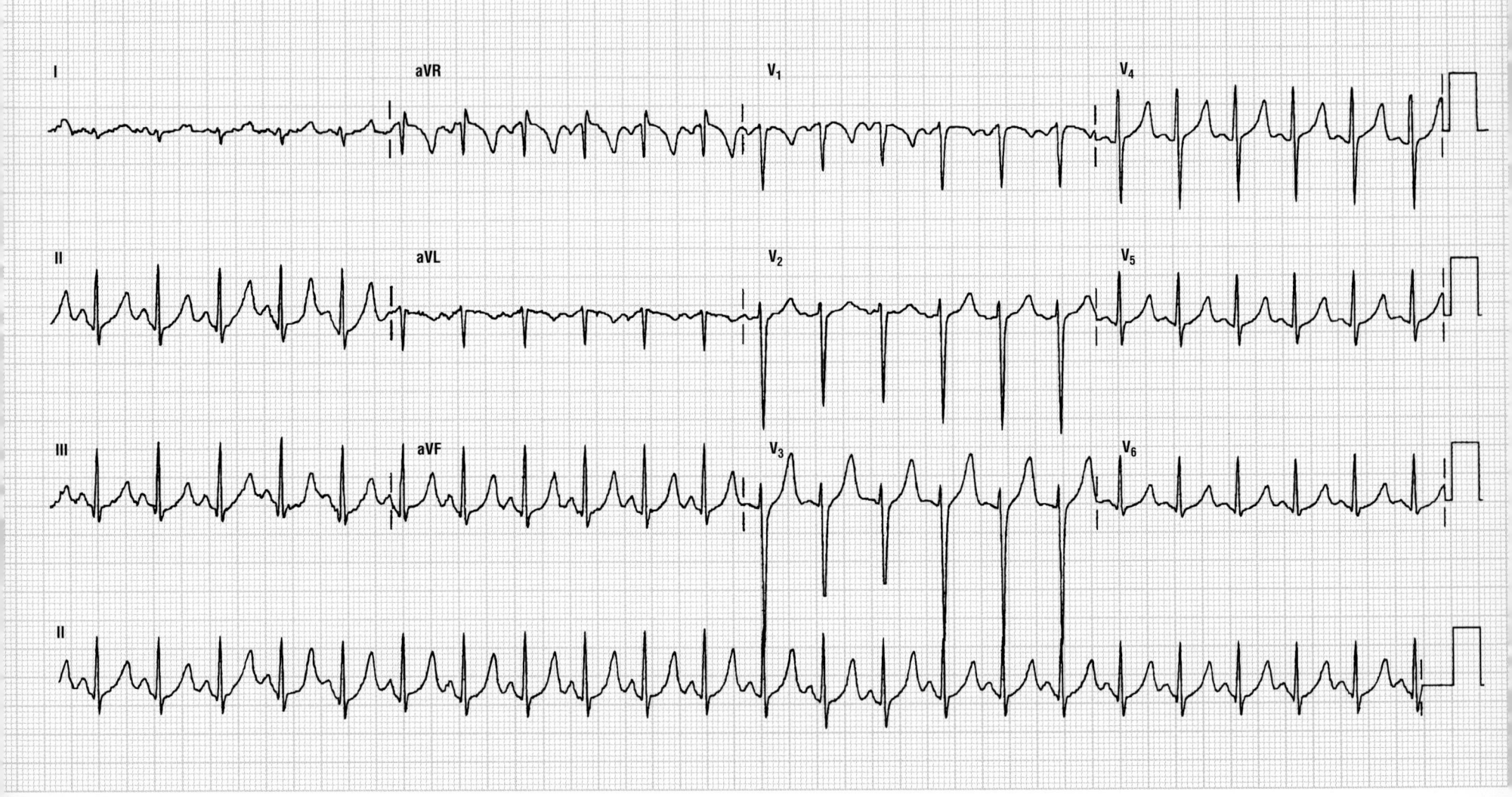

ECG 13-28

②

ECG 13-29 What about this one? Do you see the criteria for LPH, or is there something that prevents you from making the diagnosis? Actually, there is nothing there to prevent you from making it. There is a tall P wave, but it is not 2.5 mm wide or more, which is the criterion for P-pulmonale. There is a late clockwise transition, but no Q waves are present to indicate a lateral infarct in the past. There is no evidence for RVH. There is an $S_1Q_3T_3$ pattern that needs to be addressed clinically, but it is not associated with the tachycardia you would expect in a pulmonary embolus. The criteria for LPH, however, are met: an S in lead I, a small q in III, and a frontal axis deviation to the right quadrant.

 An $S_1Q_3T_3$ pattern is *not* pathognomonic for a pulmonary embolus! It is suggestive of one. Don't let anyone tell you otherwise.

ECG 13-30 Does this ECG show an LPH pattern? There is an S wave in lead I and a q wave in III, and the frontal axis is in the right quadrant. This meets all of the criteria for an LPH. Or does it? Don't forget that LPH is a diagnosis of exclusion! You must exclude other causes of an abnormal right axis in order to make the diagnosis. Is there evidence of RAE? There sure is: a P wave that is 2.5 mm tall or more in lead II. This meets criteria for P-pulmonale, and so eliminates the possibility of LPH. In addition, there is a very early counter-clockwise transition with a significantly increased R:S ratio in lead V_1. This is consistent with RVH. This also excludes LPH. The $S_1Q_3T_3$ pattern, therefore, arises from RVH in this patient, not LPH.

② 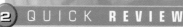QUICK **REVIEW**

Matching game:

1. Axis between −30 and −90°
2. Axis between 90 and 180°
3. Increased R:S ratio in lead V_1 is *not* an exclusionary criterion
4. q wave in lead I
5. q wave in lead III
6. A diagnosis of exclusion

A. LPH
B. LAH
C. None
D. Both

1. B 2. A 3. A 4. B 5. A 6. A

ECG CASE STUDIES: CONTINUED

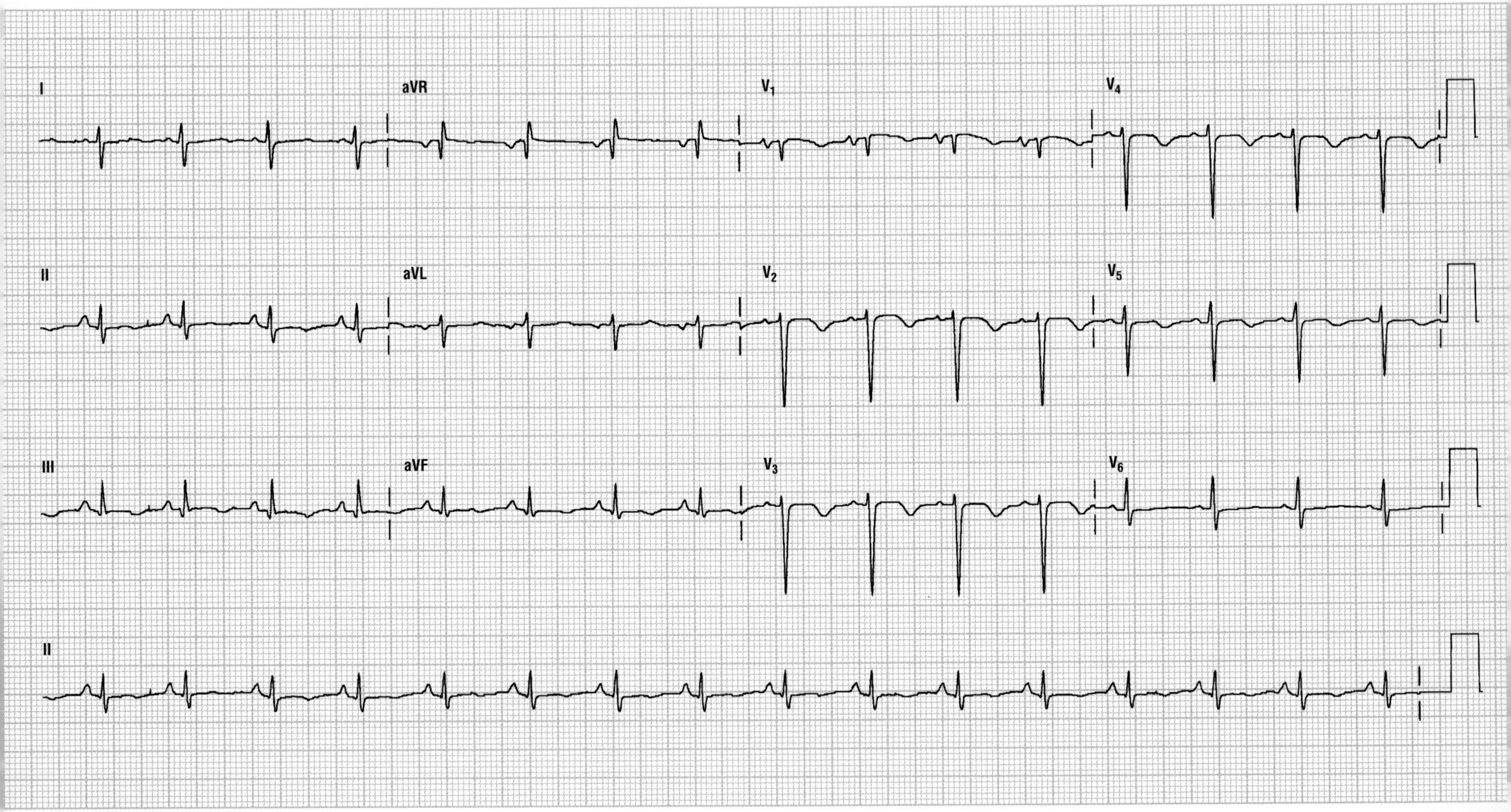

I   aVR   V₁   V₄

II   aVL   V₂   V₅

III aVF   V₃   V₆

II

ECG 13-29

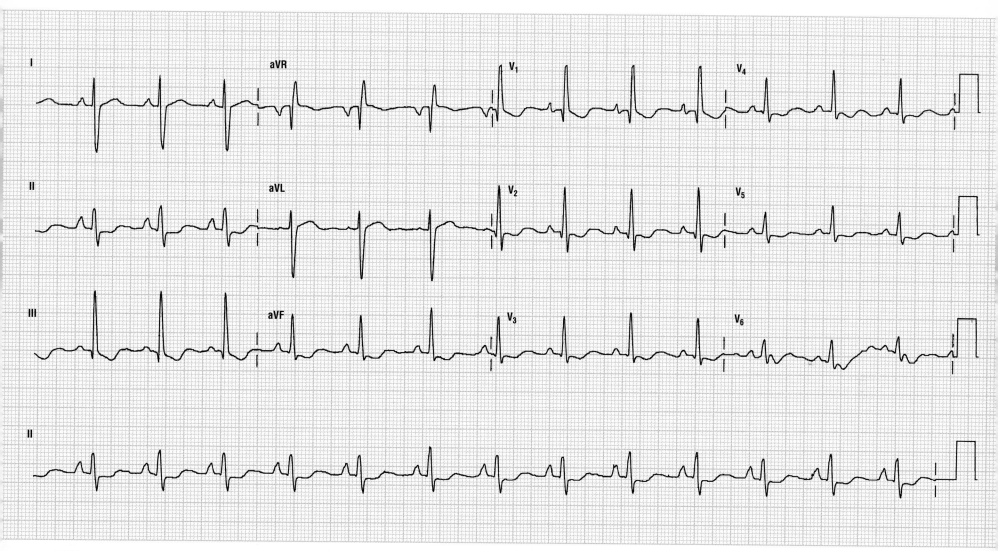

ECG 13-30

CHAPTER **13** • BUNDLE BRANCH BLOCKS AND HEMIBLOCKS

ECG CASE STUDIES: CONTINUED

2

ECG 13-31 This is another example of LPH. It meets all the criteria, and there are no exclusionary problems evident on close examination.

As mentioned, LPH is very rare by itself. It is consistently missed, even by advanced clinicians, because it is so rare. You cannot make the diagnosis unless you think about it. Whenever you see a rightward axis in the 90 to 180° range, immediately ask yourself, "Is it an LPH?" We know we keep repeating these points, but in our experience, this is a recurrent problem with advanced interpreters.

3

ECG 13-31 This ECG shows a very probable cause for the LPH: an IWMI. There is ST elevation in the inferior leads with reciprocal changes in the high lateral leads. The lateral precordial leads also show a minimal elevation, but this is difficult to call. The "company it keeps," however, makes you think that these are pathological (or they will be in another 10 minutes!).

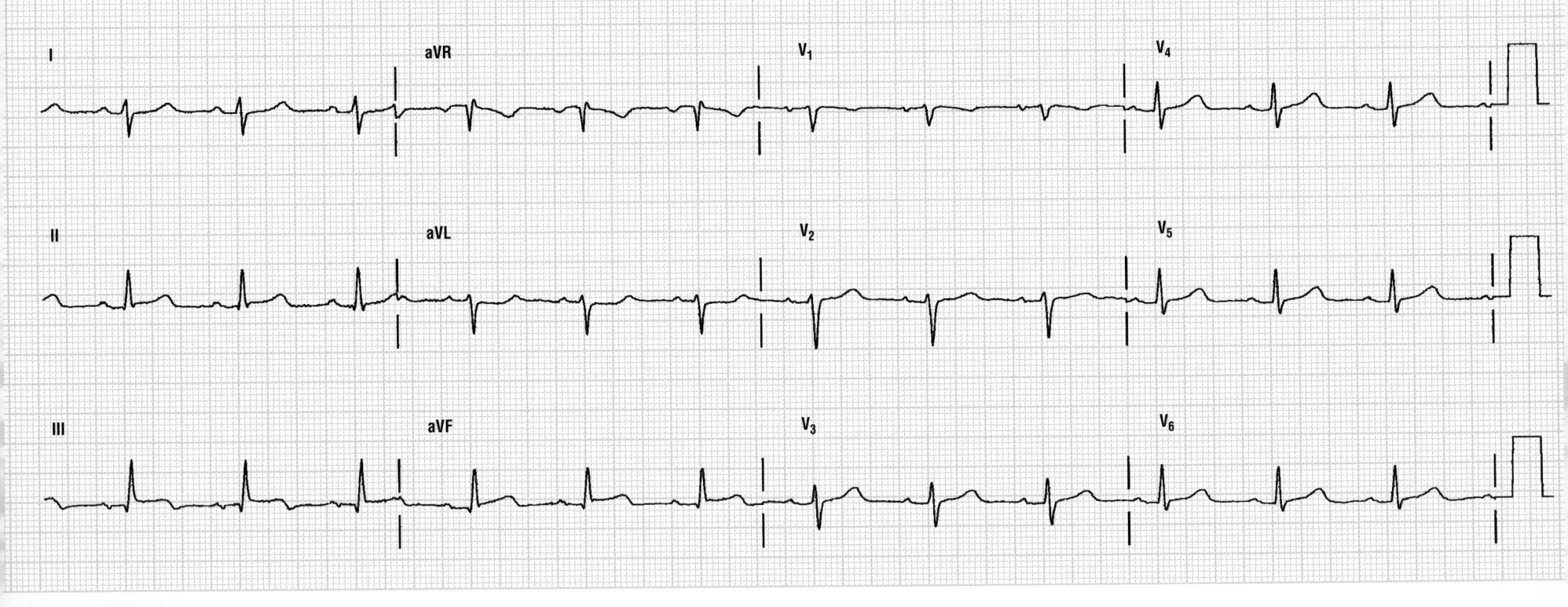

ECG 13-31

Bifascicular Blocks

By now you should be really good at picking up the blocks and hemi-blocks. Now, just to make things more interesting, we are going to combine them. There are three fascicles innervating the ventricles: the right bundle, the left anterior fascicle, and the left posterior fascicle. When we discuss *bifascicular block,* we are going to be talking about concurrent findings of RBBB combined with either LAH or LPH. Some authors make a distinction between a left bundle block and a bifascicular block involving the LAF and LPF. Because this combination presents essentially the same as an LBBB, however, we are going to disregard it here.

A combination of RBBB and LAH is a common presentation on many ECGs. It is a stable pattern except in cases of new-onset bifascic-ular block with ischemia. The typical ECG will show the slurred S wave in leads I and V_6, a rabbit-ear pattern in V_1 of an RBBB with a delayed QRS complex 0.12 seconds or more, and the left axis deviation and rS waves in lead III that are typical of LAH.

A combination of RBBB and LPH is more common than just LPH by itself. (The amount of tissue that needs to be affected to cause an LPH is extensive because of the fanning of the fibers.) Tissue damage that extensive is usually associated with damage to the other tracts of the ventricles, in particular the right bundle branch. RBBB with LPH is not a very stable pattern; it deteriorates into complete heart block in many cases, especially in the setting of acute AMI, because it takes only a small amount of additional damage to injure the left anterior fascicle. The ECG shows an RBBB pattern, along with right axis deviation and a small *q* wave in lead III.

Figure 13-20 shows the two common bifascicular block patterns: RBBB (*black*) combined with either LAH (*blue*) or LPH (*green*). Study these patterns and proceed on to the ECGs that follow.

> **REMINDER:**
> When we discuss bifascicular blocks, we are talking about an underlying RBBB with either a LAH or a LPH.

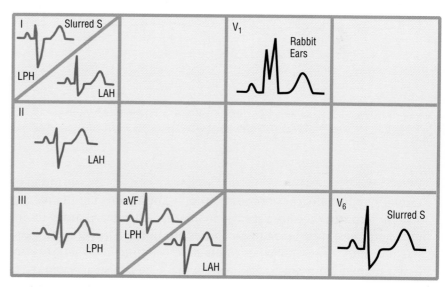

Figure 13-20: Bifascicular block.

ECG CASE STUDIES: *Bifascicular Block*

ECG 13-32 To approach an ECG with a bifascicular block like the one below, you need to start by answering some simple questions. Are the complexes 0.12 seconds wide or more? Yes, they are. Is there a slurred S wave in leads I and V_6? Yes. An increased R:S ratio in V_1 or an RSR′ pattern in V_1 or V_2? Yes. You now know that you are dealing with a RBBB.

Next, using the quadrant method of isolating the frontal axis, you calculate that — because the complexes are up in lead I and down in lead aVF — you are dealing with an axis found in the left quadrant. Now you look at lead II. It is negative, which means that the axis must lie between −30 and −90°. You now further know that LAH is present.

Bifascicular blocks composed of an RBBB-LAH pattern are very stable and usually do not break down into a complete heart block. The exception is an AMI in progress. This could cause ischemia or death of the remaining left posterior fascicle, leading to a complete heart block. This can be a real disaster, especially if the patient having an AMI has poor cardiovascular status to begin with. A bifascicular block with RBBB-LAH in the setting of an acute AMI is an indication for an acute pacemaker placement. This is critical to institute *before* the patient decompensates and the procedure becomes much harder to perform.

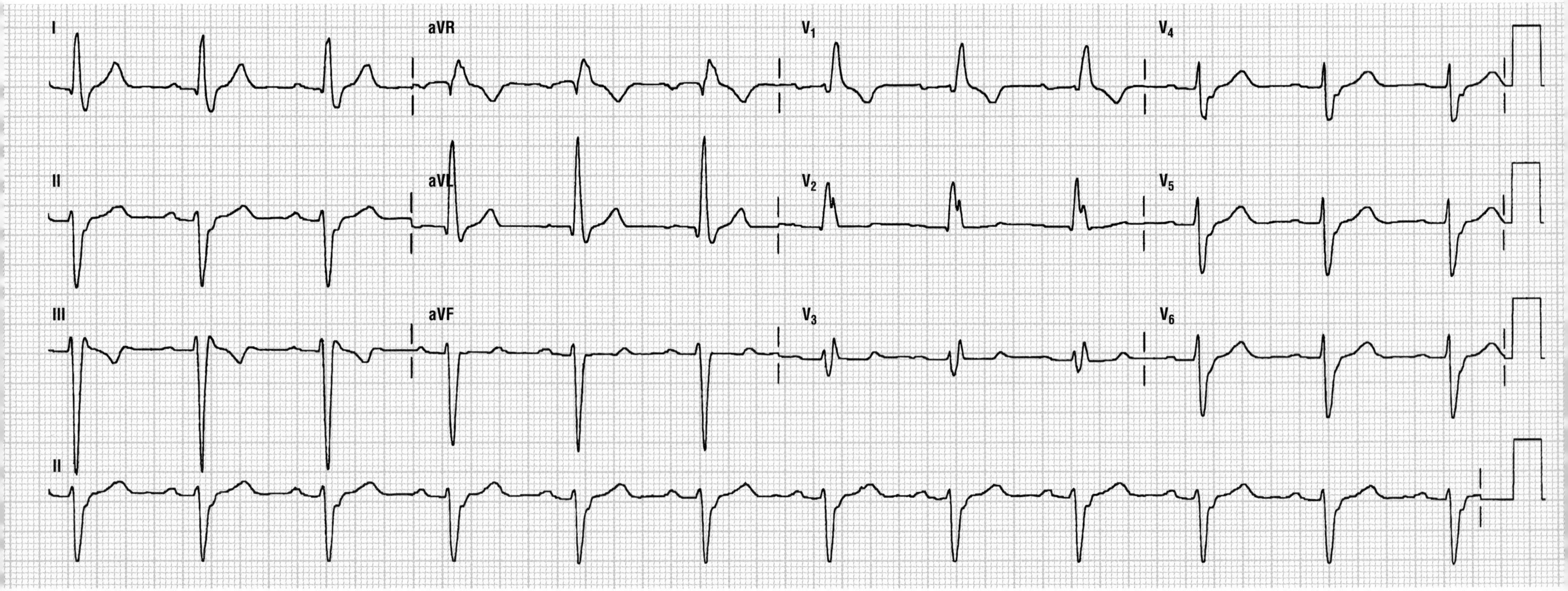

ECG 13-32

②

ECG 13-33 This ECG also has the morphology of a bifascicular block. Signs are present to suggest an RBBB-LAH pattern. Let's go through the same process as in ECG 13-32: Are the complexes 0.12 seconds wide or more? Yes. Is there a slurred S wave in leads I and V_6? Yes. An increased R:S ratio in V_1 or an RSR' pattern in V_1 or V_2? Yes. You now know that you are dealing with an RBBB.

Next, use the quadrant method of isolating the frontal axis. Because the complexes are up in lead I and down in aVF, the axis is in the left quadrant. Lead II is negative, so the axis must lie between -30 and $-90°$. This is LAH.

CLINICAL PEARL

If the QRS is positive in lead I and there is a slurred S wave, you're looking at one of two possible conditions:

1. RBBB with a normal axis

2. A bifascicular block with RBBB-LAH

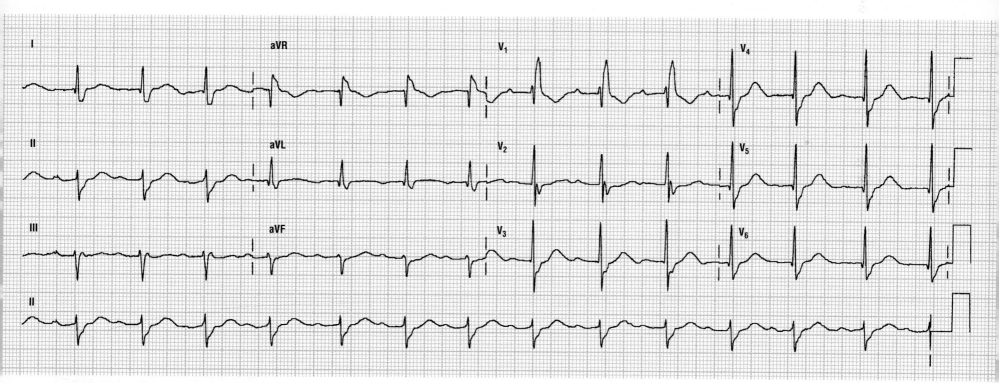

ECG 13-33

CHAPTER **13** • BUNDLE BRANCH BLOCKS AND HEMIBLOCKS

ECG CASE STUDIES: CONTINUED

②

ECG 13-34 Here is another example of RBBB-LAH, but with a different twist. The twist is the arrhythmia. It is an irregularly irregular rhythm with no P waves. That's right. It's atrial fibrillation. When they were handing out bifascicular blocks, they didn't want to discriminate, so even patients with arrhythmias, AMIs old or new, LVH, atrial abnormalities, and so on, received their share. Isn't life wonderful! As we mentioned before, these blocks are very stable and do not present any real problem unless there is an acute ischemic event taking place.

This is as good a time as any to point out the differences between AV blocks and bundle blocks. We are basically talking about different parts of the conduction system. AV blocks are caused by a diseased or malfunctioning AV node. This malfunction causes a slowdown of the conduction through the node, which in turn produces a first-, second-, or third-degree heart block. Bundle branch blocks, on the other hand, are caused by a block of the conduction through a bundle branch or a fascicle. They are totally separate animals, and, thus, can coexist in the same patient. You can see a first-degree heart block with a bifascicular block, or a second- or third-degree heart block with an LBBB. The word "block" leads to this potential confusion, so you need to be straight on what the two entities entail and the pathology associated with each. Review them as many times as you need to.

ECG 13-35 Take a look at the ECG below and go through the complete interpretation of the sections we have covered so far. This is a normal sinus rythm (NSR) at about 80 BPM. Measure the intervals in order to be complete. When you measure the QRS complex, you see that the complexes are wider than 0.12 seconds. Immediately, your razor-sharp mind asks the question: What kind of block am I dealing with? You look for slurred S waves in I and V_6, and you assume that it is an RBBB. You then look at lead V_1, which shows an rsR' pattern, and you confirm the RBBB pattern.

The next thing to evaluate is the frontal axis. You use the quadrant system and note that the complexes are positive in lead I and negative in aVF. This places the axis in the left quadrant. Now, to further isolate the axis and determine possible pathology, you look at lead II. Because the complexes are negative there, you identify an axis between $-30°$ and $-90°$. You observe an Rs complex in lead I and an rS complex in III, which further confirms your diagnosis of LAH. You are, therefore, dealing with a bifascicular block: RBBB-LAH.

The precordial leads show a counter-clockwise transition due to the RBBB. There is also increased voltage in aVL, which is greater than 11 mm and meets LVH criteria. The S wave is around 19 mm, so it just misses qualifying for LVH in aVF.

② QUICK REVIEW

1. Can an AV block and a bundle branch block occur simultaneously?

Yes. Remember, these two possibilities occur because of different patho-physiologic mechanisms and can therefore occur simultaneously.

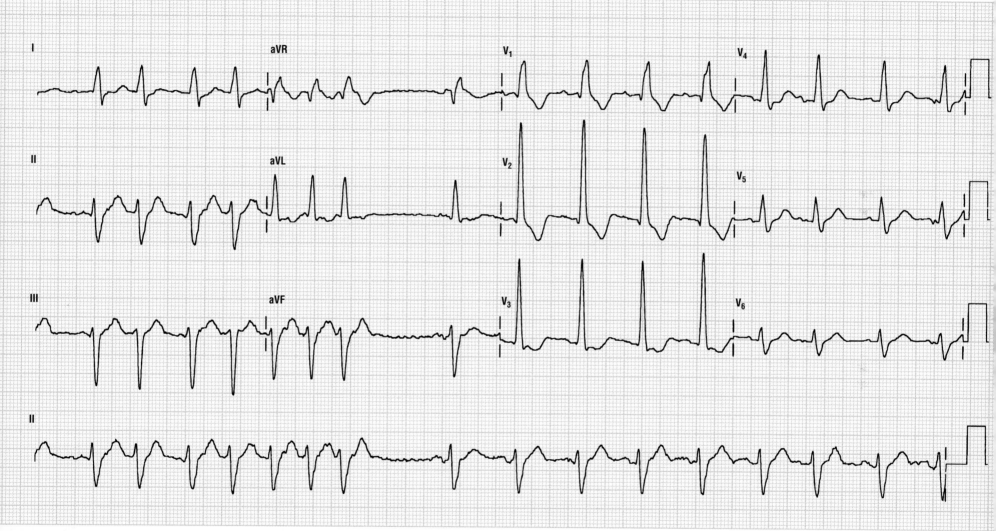

ECG 13-34

CHAPTER **13** • BUNDLE BRANCH BLOCKS AND HEMIBLOCKS

ECG CASE STUDIES: **CONTINUED**

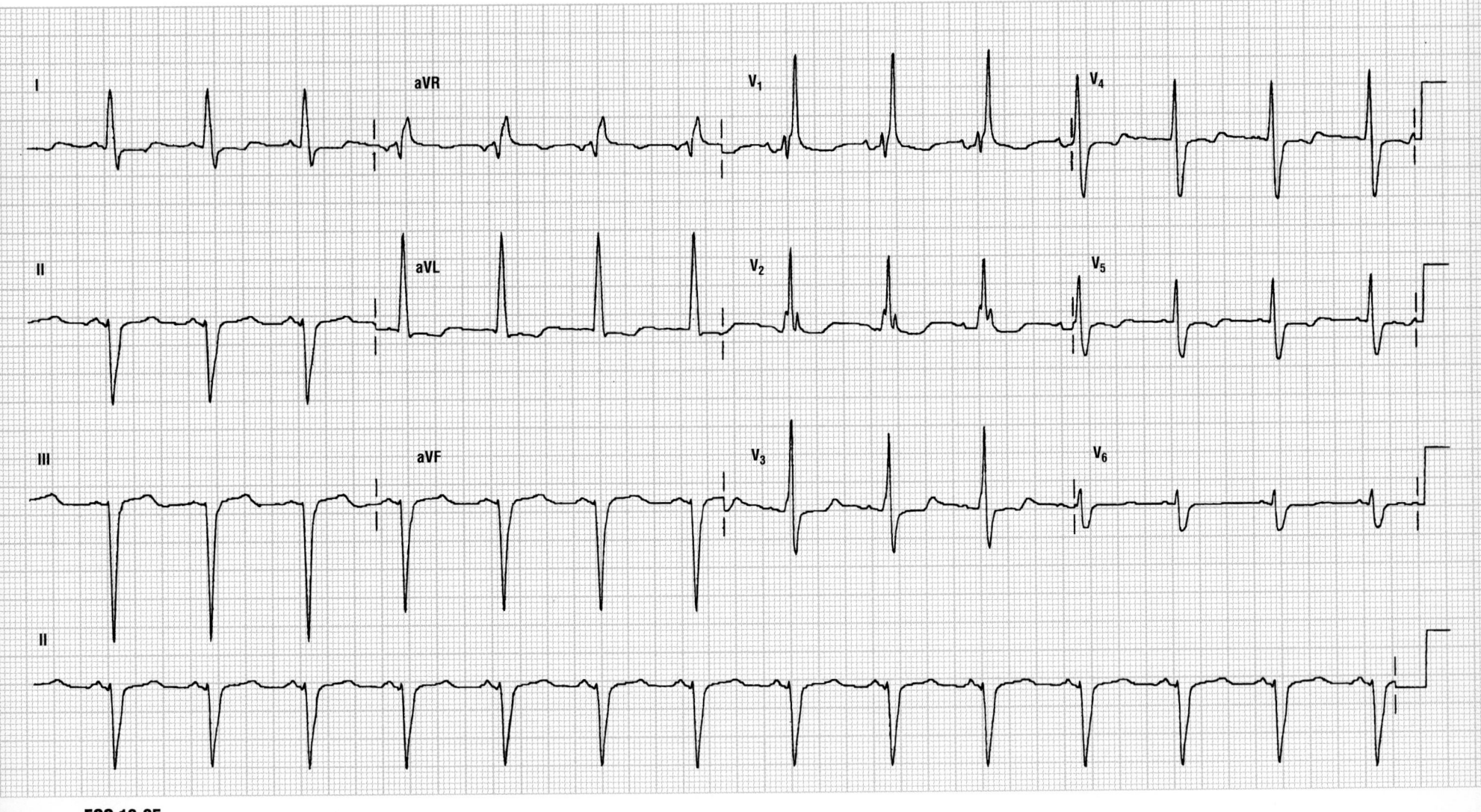

ECG 13-35

ECG 13-36 Go through the same process you used on ECG 13-35. You will find that you have the exact same interpretation. The main difference between this ECG and 13-35 is the tachycardia. In addition, the R wave progression—normal here—was abnormal in the previous one.

Remember, there are certain questions that should immediately pop up as you go through your interpretation process. When the QRS is wide: Is there a bundle branch block? When you are evaluating the frontal axis and you find a left axis deviation: Is LAH present? We have given you many examples of these questions, and there are more coming. If you answer them and write the answers down, you'll arrive at a correct diagnosis.

QUICK REVIEW

Matching game (answers may be used more than once):

1. RVH	**A.** Is it all up or all down?
2. LVH	**B.** I note increased R:S ratio in V_1. Why?
3. LBBB	**C.** I see PR depressions. Why?
4. RBBB	**D.** I note S waves ≥ 20 mm deep in aVF. Why?
5. Pericarditis	

1. B 2. D 3. A 4. B 5. C

ECG 13-37 Take a look at the ECG below and interpret the findings, then come back and see if you were right. (Remember, this is what you are supposed to be doing with every ECG to get the most out of the book.)

The first thing you notice is the rate and rhythm: It is NSR at about 75 BPM. Now, if you measured the intervals, you noticed that the QRS complexes were 0.12 seconds wide or more. You looked for slurred S waves and found them only in lead I, not V_6. Is this normal for a RBBB? No, but sometimes the complexes just don't appear to change like they do in this ECG from lead V_2 to lead V_6. The reason for the similarity is incorrect placement of the leads on the patient's chest. If you place the precordial leads too tightly on the chest and don't follow the appropriate placement pattern, you get an ECG like the one below. All of the precordial leads were placed very tightly on the chest wall, so there is no variation. V_6, if the lead was placed properly, should have a slurred S wave. V_1 has a qR' complex with an increased R:S ratio. This is RBBB.

The frontal axis is in the right quadrant. You immediately ask yourself, "Is this LPH?" Your answer is no, because there is a P-pulmonale in lead II. This is an exclusionary criterion for LPH. We have to throw in an ECG to keep you on your toes every once in a while.

ECG CASE STUDIES: CONTINUED

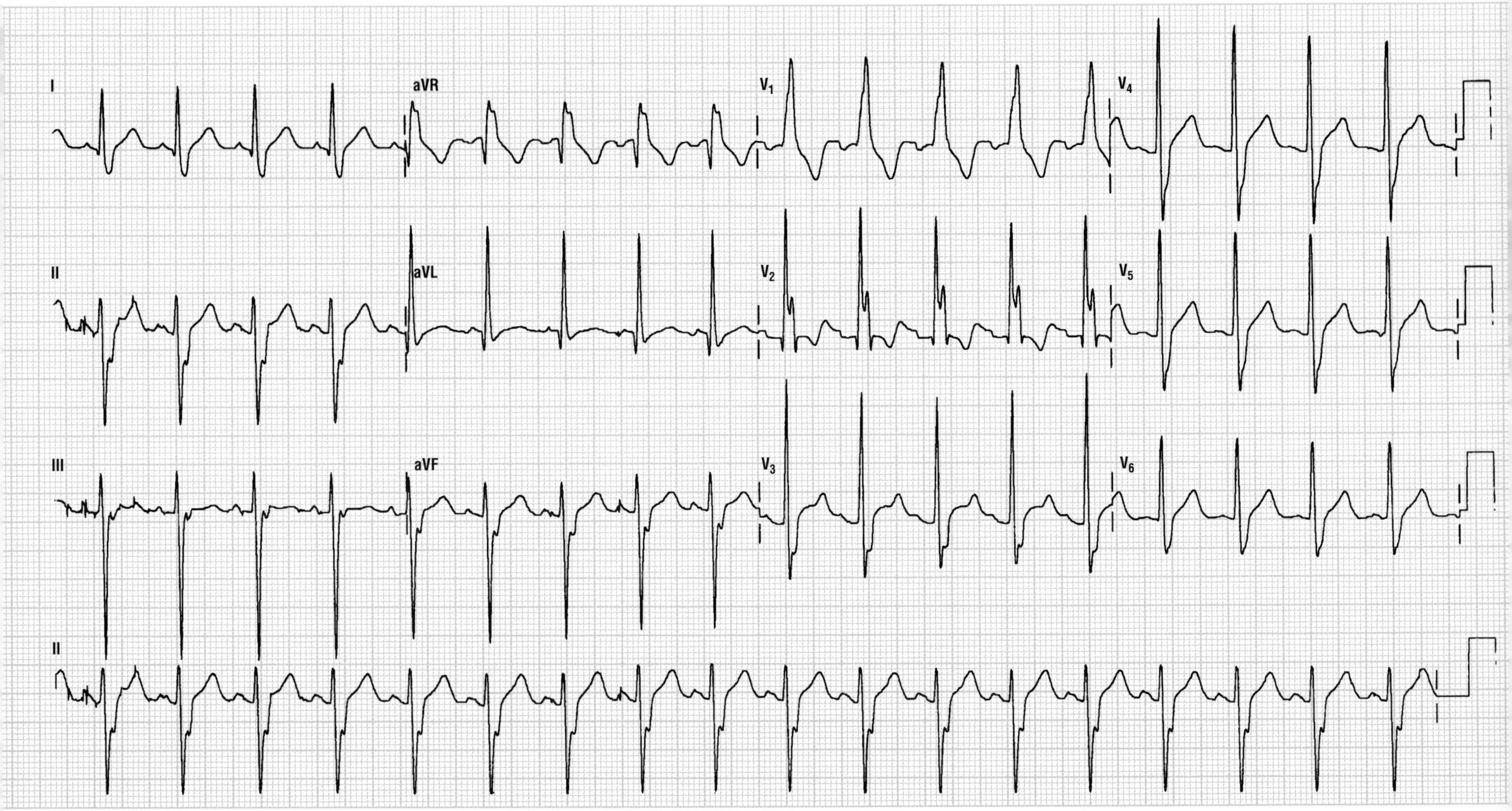

I aVR V₁ V₄

II aVL V₂ V₅

III aVF V₃ V₆

II

ECG 13-36

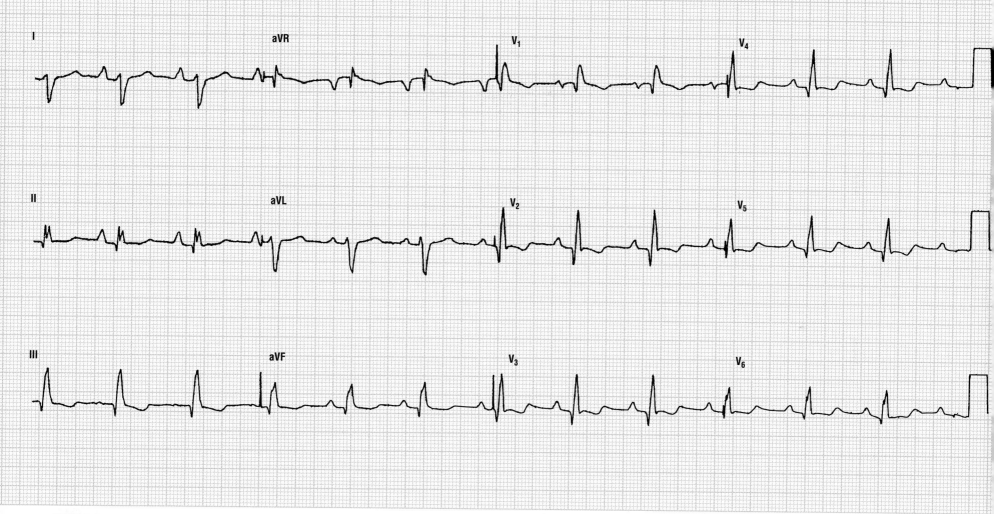

ECG 13-37

I aVR V₁ V₄

II aVL V₂ V₅

III aVF V₃ V₆

CHAPTER **13** • BUNDLE BRANCH BLOCKS AND HEMIBLOCKS

ECG CASE STUDIES: CONTINUED

ECG 13-38 The ECG below demonstrates criteria for both RBBB and LPH. There are slurred S waves in both leads I and V_6, and an RR′ complex in V_1 consistent with RBBB. The frontal axis is in the right quadrant, and there is an S wave in lead I and a qS complex in III consistent with LPH. There are no exclusionary criteria present. Finally, there is a first-degree heart block.

The bifascicular combination of RBBB and LPH is, as mentioned previously, more common than just LPH by itself. Why? Because damage extensive enough to cause an LPH usually blocks another fascicle as well. This gives rise to either a bifascicular block involving both left fascicles, or to an RBBB-LPH pattern.

Is RBBB-LPH more unstable than RBBB-LAH? Well, if you think about it anatomically, you will see that the RBBB-LPH is much more unstable. Remember we mentioned that the left anterior fascicle is a thin, cordlike structure? Any small infarct or infiltrative process involving that area would block the anterior fascicle. On the other hand, you have to work hard to block the entire fanlike left posterior fascicle. Because the most common cause of LPH is CAD and ischemia, any little additional insult to the heart will block either the right bundle or the left anterior fascicle, or both, leading to a bifascicular block. RBBB-LPH is unstable, especially in the face of an AMI.

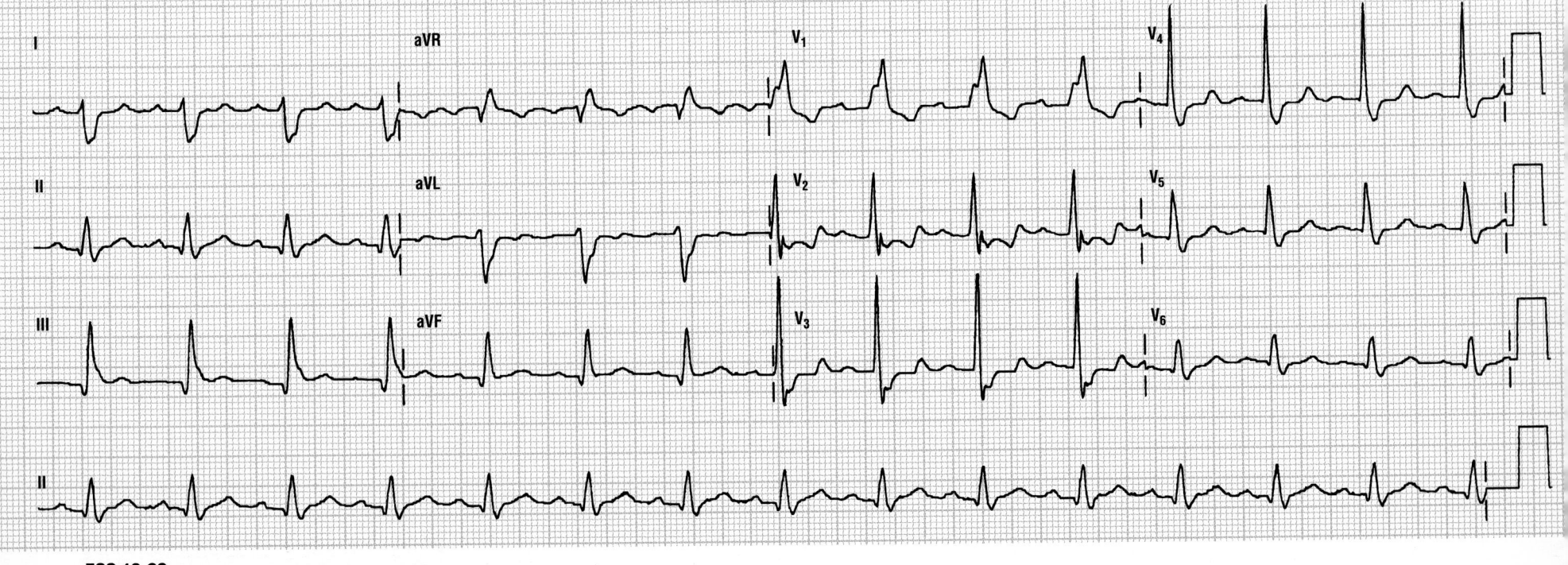

ECG 13-38

②

ECG 13-39 This ECG also demonstrates criteria for both RBBB and LPH. There are slurred S waves in both leads I and V₆, and an rsR′ complex (the *r* wave is miniscule but present!) in V₁ consistent with RBBB. The frontal axis is in the right quadrant, and there is an S wave in lead I and a qS complex in III consistent with LPH. There are no exclusionary criteria present.

This is the last ECG of the chapter. We would like to take this time to offer some friendly advice. Make sure you understand the concepts presented in this chapter, and in Chapter 14 on ST segments and T waves. These two chapters cover the main things that cause confusion and missed interpretations. That is why we have tried to show you many examples of actual ECGs, and why the chapters are so long. When you get done with Chapter 14, come back and review both 13 and 14 a few times before you go on to AMIs. We understand you want to get to the fun stuff, but if you don't have a firm mastery of these two chapters, you are bound to make mistakes. Mistakes in diagnosing AMIs are life-threatening. You need to be very clear on what an AMI is, and what is benign or caused by other, less life-threatening pathology. Sometimes the path to this distinction is full of potholes. The ability to steer clear of potholes is what separates the intermediate from the advanced clinician.

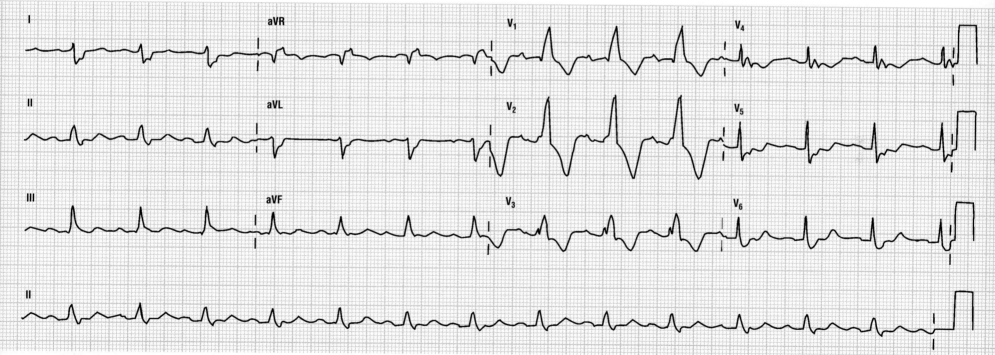

ECG 13-39

CHAPTER **13** • BUNDLE BRANCH BLOCKS AND HEMIBLOCKS

CHAPTER IN **REVIEW**

1. Because all RSR' complexes are close in appearance, all you need to diagnose RBBB is to identify their presence in V_1. True or False.

2. The three major criteria for diagnosing RBBB include:
   A. QRS ≥ 0.12 seconds
   B. Slurred S wave in leads I and V_6
   C. RSR' pattern in V_1
   D. All of the above
   E. None of the above

3. Rabbit ears always begin with an R wave in V_1. True or False.

4. In LBBB, you cannot make the diagnosis of LVH, but in RBBB you can. True or False.

5. In RBBB, there can be a negative complex in V_1 or V_2. True or False.

6. The major criteria for diagnosing LBBB include:
   A. QRS ≥ 0.12 seconds
   B. Broad, monomorphic S wave in leads I and V_6
   C. Broad, monomorphic R wave in V_1
   D. All of the above
   E. None of the above

7. In LBBB, there can be some notching of the QRS complex in leads V_5 to V_6. True or False.

8. The most common cause of IVCD is hyperkalemia. True or False.

9. The criteria for LAH include:
   A. Left axis deviation with the axis at −30 to −90°
   B. Either a qR complex or an R wave in lead I
   C. An rS complex in III, and probably II and aVF
   D. All of the above
   E. None of the above

10. The criteria for LPH include:
    A. An axis in the right quadrant
    B. An *s* wave in lead I and a *q* in III
    C. Exclusion of RAE and RVH
    D. All of the above
    E. None of the above

11. In LPH, the axis is in the extreme right quadrant. True or False.

12. Which bifascicular blocks are stable if present chronically?
    A. RBBB and LAH
    B. RBBB and LPH
    C. Both A and B
    D. None of the above

13. Which bifascicular blocks are stable if present acutely?
    A. RBBB and LAH
    B. RBBB and LPH
    C. Both A and B
    D. None of the above

14. The presence of a monomorphic rS complex in V_1 and a slurred S in leads I and V_6 is consistent with what type of bundle branch block or bifascicular block?
    A. RBBB
    B. LBBB
    C. IVCD
    D. RBBB and LAH
    E. RBBB and LPH

15. VPCs are always:
    A. RBBB
    B. LBBB
    C. Either A or B
    D. None of the above

1. False 2. D 3. False 4. True 5. False 6. A 7. True 8. True 9. D 10. D 11. False 12. A 13. A 14. D 15. C

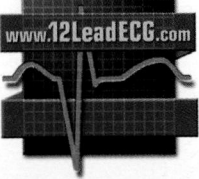

Basics

It would be very difficult to discuss the ST segment and T wave separately. In this chapter, we will move back and forth between them, and occasionally talk about them together depending on the section and the topic involved. Chapter 15 covers the areas related to infarction and injury of the myocardium, but the topic is introduced in this chapter.

Electrically, the ST segment represents that section of the complex in which the ventricles are between electrical depolarization and repolarization. The segment is measured from the *J point*, where the QRS complex and the ST segment meet, to the beginning of the T wave (Figure 14-1). In most instances, the measurement is an approximation, either because the J point is not sharp or because the beginning of the T wave is not clearly visible. The J point can be sharp and clearly identifiable, or it can be diffuse (shown in Figure 14-2).

Considered together, the ST segment and T wave are one of the most important aspects of the ECG for you to master, because this is the area that reflects ischemic insult or injury to the myocardium. *In general, ST depression and T waves in the opposite direction from what is normal are a sign of ischemia. ST elevation, with or without T wave changes, is a sign of myocardial injury.*

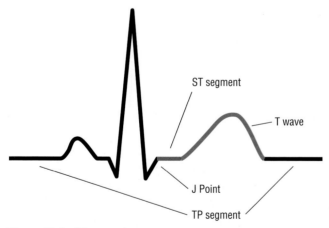

Figure 14-1: ST segment.

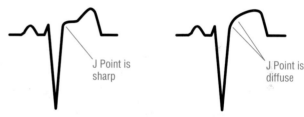

Figure 14-2: Sharp and diffuse J points.

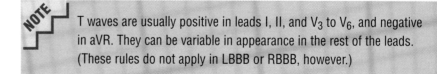

NOTE

T waves are usually positive in leads I, II, and V_3 to V_6, and negative in aVR. They can be variable in appearance in the rest of the leads. (These rules do not apply in LBBB or RBBB, however.)

Where Is the J Point?

You can clearly identify the J point in Figure 14-3. There is a definite spot where the transition occurs between the QRS complex and the ST segment. You will easily be able to identify the J point on most ECGs.

Figure 14-4 presents more of a problem. Where is the exact J point? As you can see, it is very difficult to take your caliper leg and place it on one spot and state definitively that you have it on the J point. Because it is a slowly curving segment, you can only isolate an *area* where the J point should be found. We have labeled that area with a red rectangle. Narrowing it down any closer is guesswork.

Diffuse J points are associated with early repolarization, LVH with strain, and pericarditis. AMIs sometimes have a diffuse J point, especially when there is tombstoning. We will be discussing these conditions shortly.

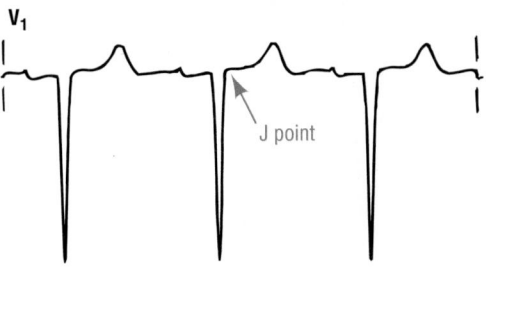

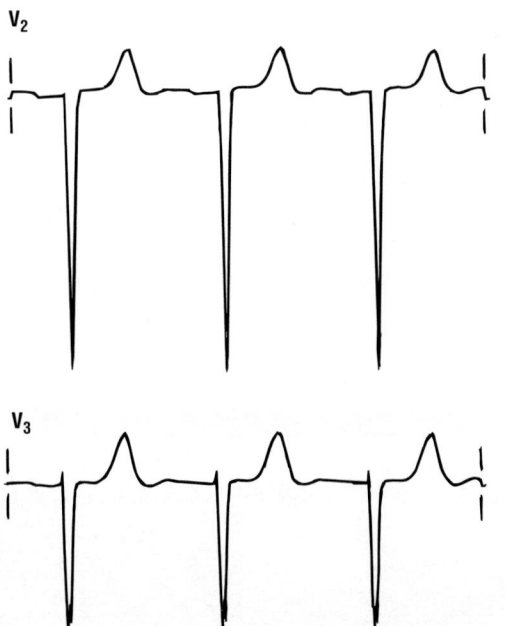

Figure 14-3: Sharp J point.

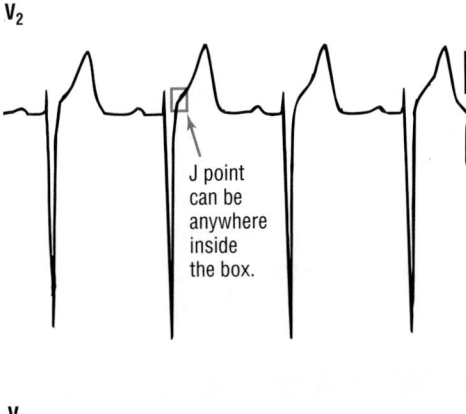

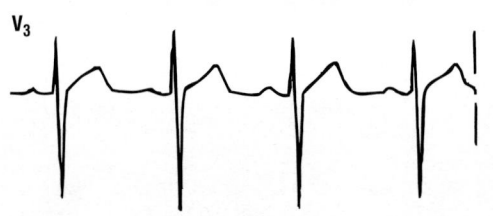

Figure 14-4: Diffuse J point.

ST Elevation or Depression

The key thing to identify when examining an ST segment is its relationship to the baseline. This will determine the presence of *ST elevation or depression*, examples of which are shown in Figure 14-5. If you remember, the baseline is measured from TP segment to TP segment. This is a critical determination. Using a clear ruler with hairline rules will help you greatly in identifying the baseline. In certain cases, especially tachycardias, the TP segment is difficult to identify because the T and P waves overlap. When this occurs, you have to use your best judgment and the PR interval to determine the baseline.

ST elevation of less than 1 mm is considered normal in the limb leads. In the precordials, V_1 to V_3 can show elevation of up to 2 to 3 mm in LVH with strain, which we will cover soon. *You must be very careful, however, because any elevation is important if it was not there on a previous ECG, or if the history matches the presence of ischemia.* Remember "the company it keeps." If there are other signs of ischemia, any elevation can be pathological.

ST Segment Shapes

The shape of the ST segment can be quite variable. However, certain shapes are more common than others. Because some of these shapes are found in specific conditions, they are helpful in making the diagnosis. Other shapes are just a different "normal" presentation. We'll diagram some of these shapes for you, and list possible causes underneath each one in Figure 14-6. Each can occur with positive or negative QRS complexes. Don't worry if you don't know what the terms mean. You will when you finish the Level 2 sections in this chapter.

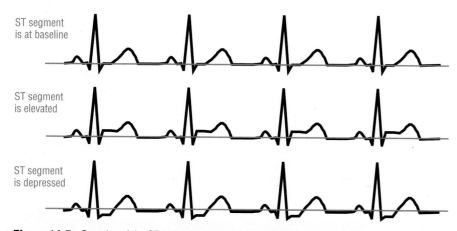

Figure 14-5: Samples of the ST segment at baseline, elevated, and depressed.

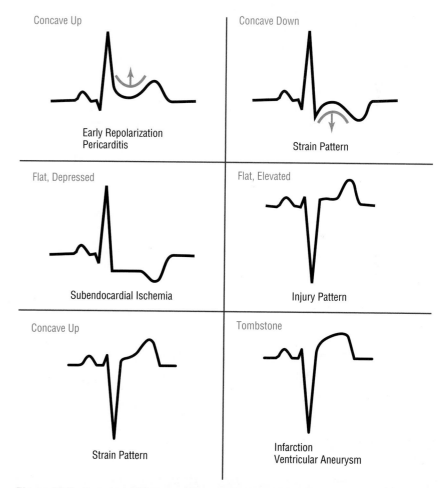

Figure 14-6: Examples of ST segment shapes and possible causes.

CHAPTER **14** • ST SEGMENT AND T WAVES

The T Wave

We have already covered T wave basics in Chapter 6 (The T Wave, page 44) and — as they relate to the blocks — in Chapter 13 (see page 260). Take a few minutes to review those two passages. In this chapter, we will begin to explore the differing morphologies associated with T waves. They can be tall or short, broad or narrow, symmetrical or asymmetrical, and positive, negative, or biphasic. These are the three things we want you to concentrate on: shape, polarity, and height or depth.

T Wave Shape *Asymmetry is the normal presentation of the T wave.* Symmetrical T waves are found in pathological states including ischemia, electrolyte abnormalities, and CNS problems. Asymmetrical and symmetrical T waves are shown in Figure 14-7. T waves can also be normally symmetrical in some people, but they should be considered pathological until proven otherwise. "The company it keeps" will be your motto from now on. You must rule out the conditions listed above before you can call symmetrical Ts normal. It's hard to believe, but we have picked up many AMIs early on by spotting symmetrical T waves. Tall, narrow Ts are common in hyperkalemia. Very broad T waves have been found in CNS events, especially intracranial hemorrhage.

To determine symmetry, place your hairline ruler vertically on the peak of the T wave as shown in Figure 14-8. If the two sides separated by the dividing line are mirror images, the T wave is symmetrical. If they are not, it is asymmetrical.

Many times, the ST segment causes difficulty in evaluating for symmetry. When this occurs, as in Figure 14-8, extend the two legs of the T wave as a straight line down to the baseline. This simple technique will make it easy to evaluate symmetry.

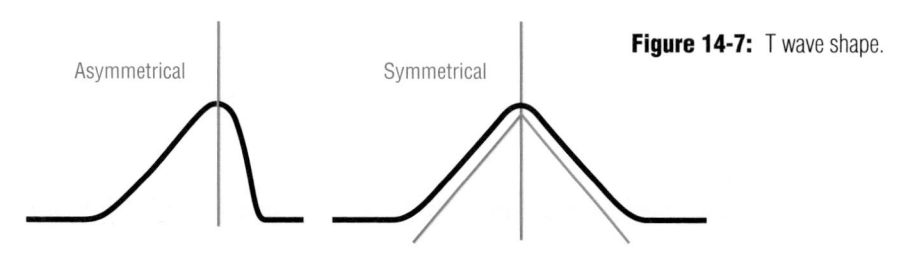

Figure 14-7: T wave shape.

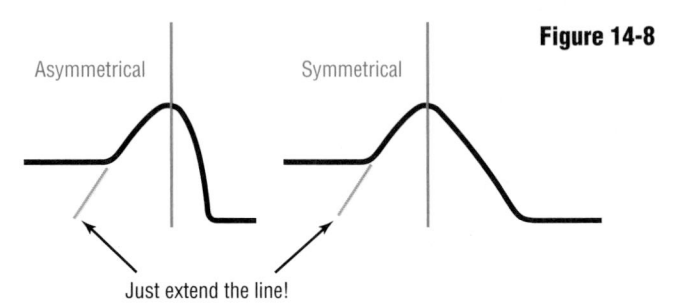

Figure 14-8

Just extend the line!

Here are some additional examples:

Figure 14-9: Additional examples of T wave shapes.

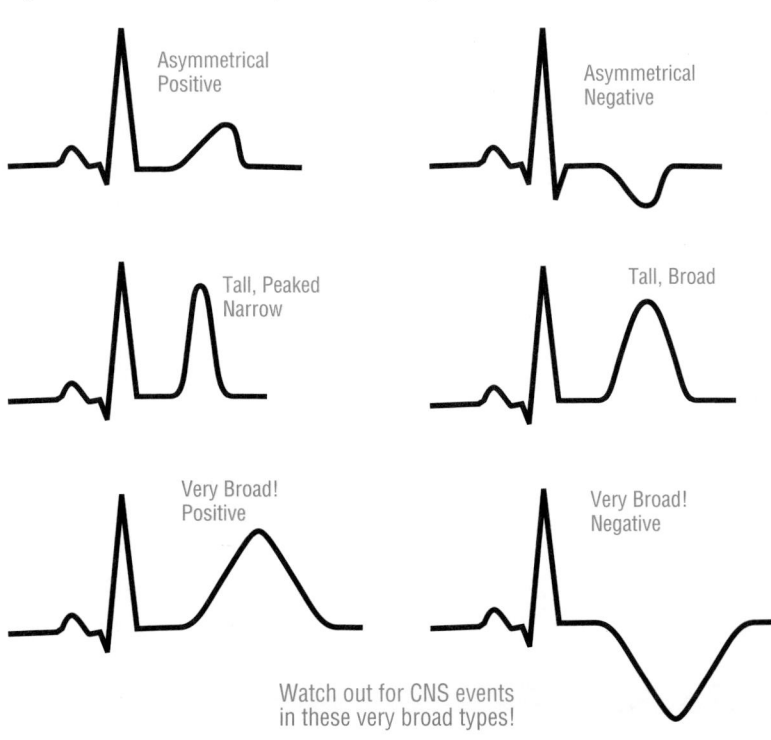

Watch out for CNS events in these very broad types!

Biphasic T Waves Biphasic T waves can occur in any lead, but especially the leads transitioning between a positive and a negative T wave. If the first part of the T wave is negative, the cause is more likely to be pathological. When you look at the examples in Figure 14-10, remember that there is a spectrum of positivity to negativity.

T Wave Polarity Because repolarization is associated with its own vector, T waves can be positive, negative, or anywhere in between. The orientation of this vector in three-dimensional space will determine T wave appearance in each lead. T waves are usually positive in leads I, II, and V_3 to V_6, and negative in aVR. In the rest of the leads, the T wave is variable. You will see later on that there are some variations in these rules — in the BBBs, for instance.

If the T wave is negative where it should be positive, such as lead II, we say that the T wave is *flipped*. Flipped T waves are sometimes indicative of ischemia. They can also be found in severe ventricular hypertrophy. *Remember, in bundle branch blocks, all bets are off!*

T Wave Height or Depth In general, T waves should not be more than 6 mm high in the limb leads and 12 mm in the precordials. *A good rule to remember is that if the T wave is more than 2/3 the height of the R wave, it is definitely abnormal.* Tall T waves are associated with ischemia and infarction, CNS events, and high potassium levels.

A Few Last Words on T Waves Remember, the T wave does not live in a vacuum. Its appearance can be altered by the ST segment before it. When you are looking at the T waves, remember the old adage, "Intervals are always the same in all leads." Measure where the T waves begin and end in a lead that clearly shows the whole wave, and transfer that distance to the lead with the bizarre appearance. This will help you isolate the T wave.

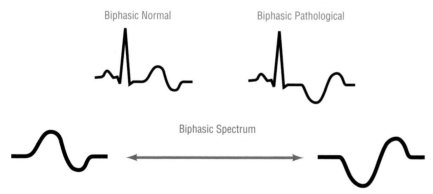

Figure 14-10: Biphasic T waves.

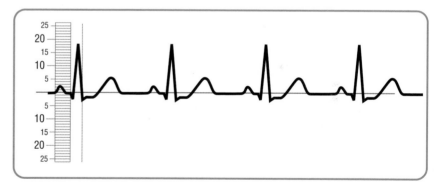

Use your tools! A hairline on a clear ruler is a great help in evaluating ST segments and T waves.

Figure 14-11: ECG ruler with ECG strip.

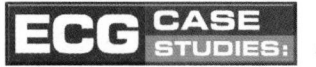 *ST Segments and T Waves*

ECG 14-1 As we have said, it is very difficult to separate ST segments and T waves in most discussions. So, in this chapter we are going to be discussing both in most ECGs.

The format of this chapter is very ECG-intensive. This is because the ST segments (and sometimes the T waves) are the most confusing parts of the ECG for most students. The distinction between normal and pathological is minor in many cases; it requires a well-trained eye. We sat down and tried to figure out how most experts develop that "eye" for pathology. We came up with a simple answer. They have seen so many thousands of ECGs that they simply know there is an abnormality present. We are going to start you down that path by showing you many examples of different kinds of abnormalities. After you finish the chapter, it will benefit you to go back and review all the ECGs covered to this point in the book.

This ECG shows scooped ST segments and tall, asymmetrical T waves. The T waves are tall but they are not pathologically tall. They need to be taller than 2/3 the height of the R wave to be considered pathological. However, if the T waves were this tall *but symmetrical*, they would be pathologic. Hyperkalemia, ischemia, and CNS events present with this type of symmetrical T waves in many cases. Remember, you need to put the ECG together with the patient.

ECG 14-2 This ECG also shows scooped ST segments and asymmetrical T waves. If you notice, the T waves are not as tall as in ECG 14-1. The T waves are close to symmetrical but, as the old saying goes, close only counts in horseshoes and hand grenades. These are not pathological T waves by any criteria. They are upright in leads I, II, and V_3 to V_6, and negative in aVR, which represents a normal T wave vector.

The ST segments are scooped out in appearance with some slight elevation, and are concave upward in most cases. The ST segment in V_1 is flat and concave downward, which is troubling. This is not normal. However, when you look at the surrounding leads, there is no continuation of the pathological process. In general, *one* isolated lead with obvious pathology is not very clinically significant. However, we once again must invoke the principle of "the company it keeps." Look at the patient and evaluate her as well as her complaints. If she is young and is seeing you because she fractured a finger, you need go no further. The ECG would be an example of early repolarization, which we will review later this chapter. If she is visiting for chest pain, you need to evaluate further. If you take another look, there is minimal PR depression and some notching at the end of the QRS complex. This ECG could be compatible with early pericarditis. The history and physical exam are crucial in making the definitive diagnosis.

REMINDER:
Look at and evaluate as many ECGs as possible. Experience is your best teacher for ST and T wave issues.

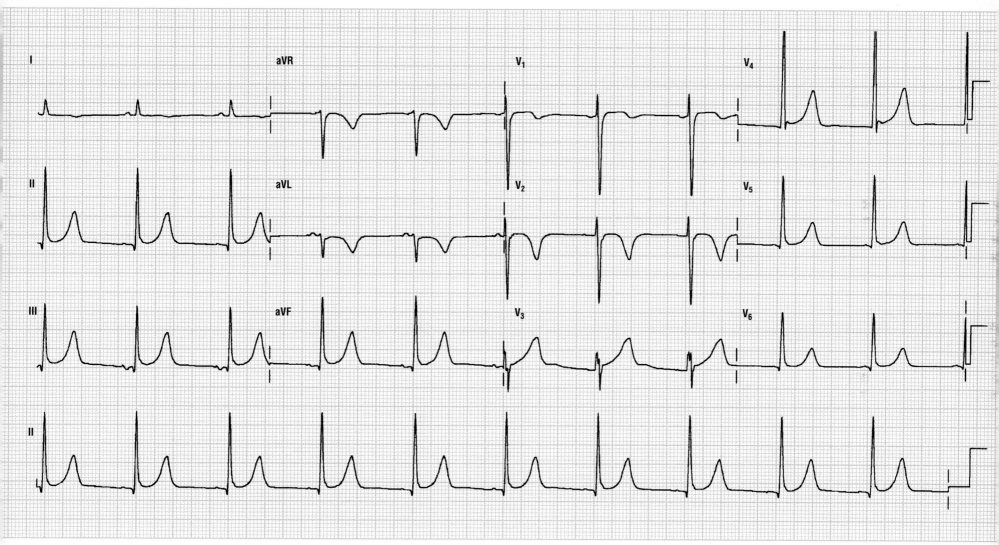

ECG 14-1

ECG CASE STUDIES: **CONTINUED**

I	aVR	V₁	V₄
II	aVL	V₂	V₅
III	aVF	V₃	V₆
II			

ECG 14-2

ECG 14-3 Let's look at the ECG below and focus on the T waves. Can you see anything abnormal about them? They are upright in leads I and II, which is normal, right? But what about V_3 to V_6? They are flipped and symmetrical, as shown close-up in Figure 14-12. This is an example of abnormal T waves indicative of ischemia.

When you look at V_2 to V_4, it is difficult to see that the T waves are symmetrical because of slight ST elevation that is distorting the T wave. Remember to draw the extending lines from the T wave itself to see the symmetrical qualities in these waves.

In addition, notice that the T waves in the limb leads are kind of flat. This is also a sign of pathology. We would call this abnormality a nonspecific ST-T wave change (NSSTTWΔ, in abbreviated form).

ECG 14-4 It doesn't take an expert to notice that the T waves in the precordials of this ECG are *ugly*! They are flipped, and greater than $2/3$ of the R or S wave with which they are associated, as shown in close-up in Figure 14-13. In addition, they are definitely symmetrical. Get used to using a clear straight edge to evaluate symmetry.

The T waves in the limb leads also show abnormalities in leads I and aVL. They, too, are symmetrical and flipped.

Do you notice anything unusual about the rhythm? Can you figure out what it is? It is an irregularly irregular rhythm with varying P waves and PR intervals. Yes, it is a wandering atrial pacemaker. This case is not associated with any obvious COPD pathology, but it may be due to ischemia, represented by the flipped, symmetrical T waves.

As you can see, they really are symmetrical. Beware of optical illusions!

Figure 14-12: Enlargement of lead V_5.

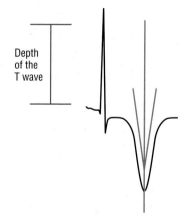

Depth of the T wave

The T wave is symmetrical and more than $2/3$ of the height of the R wave of the same complex.

Figure 14-13

CHAPTER **14** • ST SEGMENT AND T WAVES

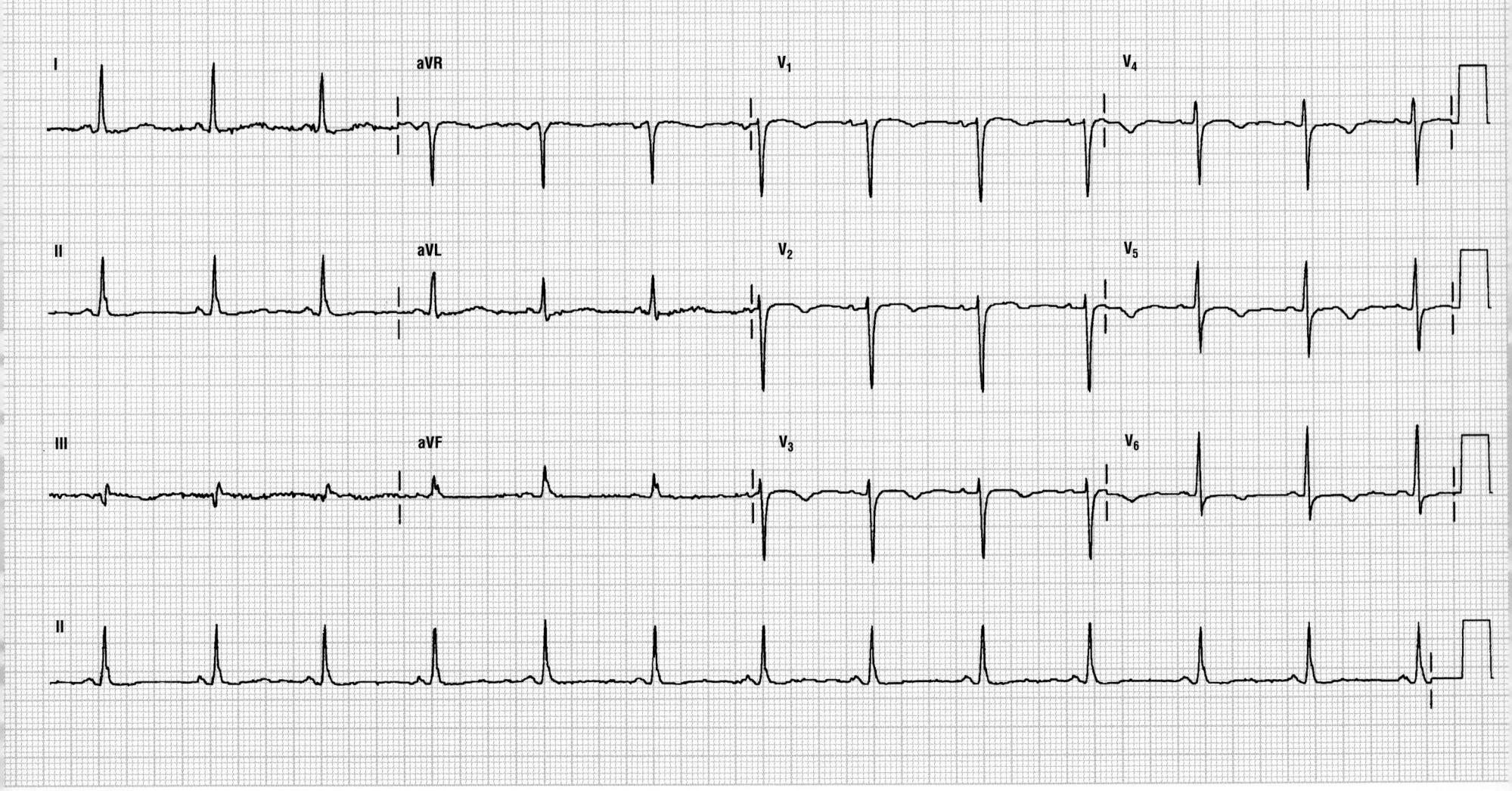

ECG 14-3

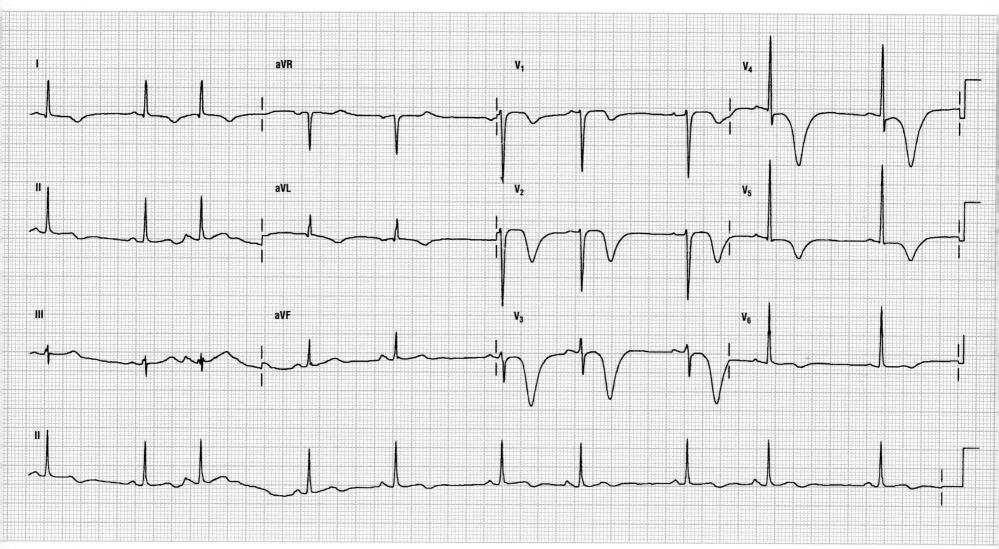

ECG 14-4

ECG CASE STUDIES: **CONTINUED**

②

ECG 14-5 This is very similar to ECG 14-4 except that the T wave abnormalities are more diffuse. Note that there are abnormalities in leads II and aVF. (The T waves are markedly flattened in aVF.)

What other abnormalities are found in this ECG? Well, there are left atrial enlargement criteria in V_1. In addition, the Q waves in leads II, III, and aVF are pathological. They meet both criteria: width more than 0.03 seconds, and height more than $^1/_3$ the R wave height.

③

ECG 14-5 There are definitely signs of an old IWMI in this patient. The diffuse quality of the flipped, symmetrical T waves poses a list of possible differential diagnoses: ischemia, CNS event, electrolyte abnormality, and resolving pericarditis (especially post-infarct pericarditis because of the presence of the old IWMI). Clinical correlation is needed to completely interpret this ECG.

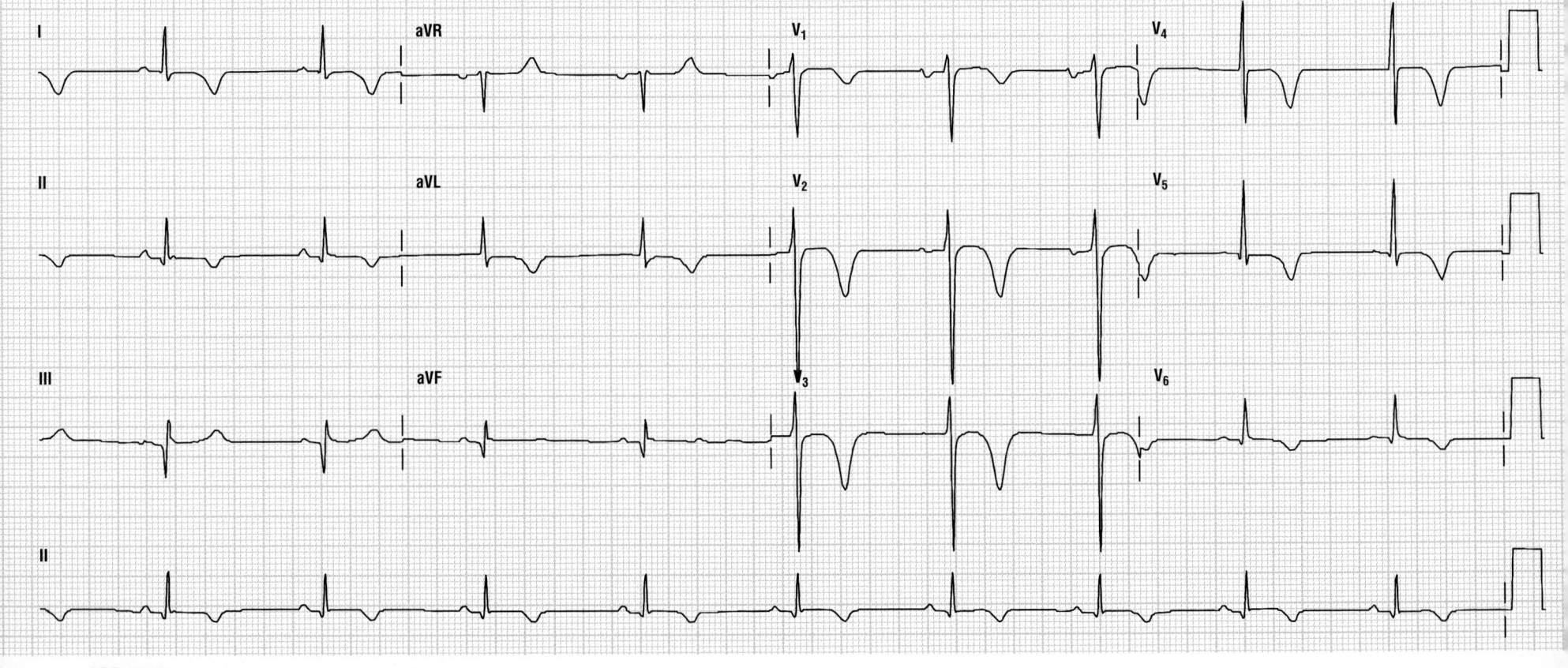

ECG 14-5

②

ECG 14-6 Are these normal T waves? Of course not! They are flipped in leads I, II, and V₃ to V₆. As a matter of fact, they are upright only in aVL and aVR. (Remember, they should be flipped in aVR.) They are symmetrical. Finally, they are more than $2/3$ the height of the associated R waves in many leads.

The ECG also has an abnormal R:S ratio in V₂ and shows evidence of an early clockwise transition in the precordial leads. Could this be due to a large right ventricle? Probably. Are the T wave abnormalities associated with the RVH? No, they are too diffuse and symmetrical. RVH, as we will see later in the chapter, is associated with asymmetrical

T waves. There is evidence for an intraatrial conduction delay (IACD), but the criteria for RAE are not met.

Lastly, there is obvious evidence of QT prolongation: The QT interval is more than $1/2$ the R-R interval.

What are some of the clinical scenarios that could give rise to such an ECG? Electrolyte abnormalities are certainly a possibility. Diffuse ischemia and a CNS event are also very high on the list of differential diagnoses. You will need to obtain an old ECG, if possible, and rule these things out (or rule them in) to come up with the final answer. Remember always to put the ECG and the patient together in your mind.

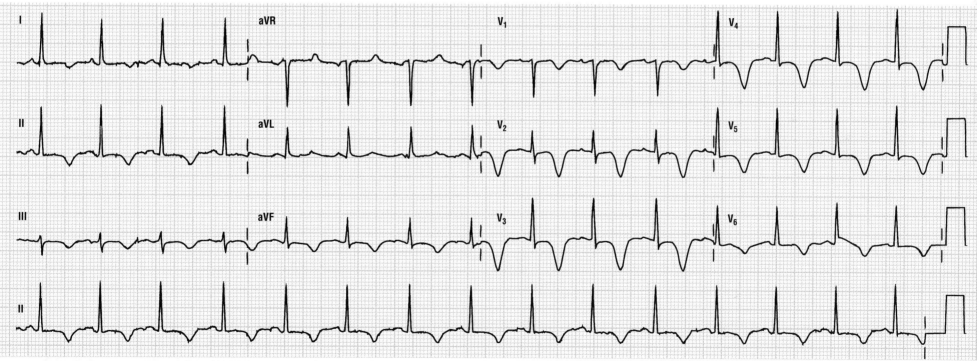

ECG 14-6

ECG CASE STUDIES: **CONTINUED**

②

ECG 14-7 Now let's go from deep T waves to tall ones. Look at the T waves in the mid-precordial leads. They are tall and symmetrical. We're going to spend much more time on this topic in Chapter 16, but this is as good a time as any to introduce you to hyperkalemia. When you see tall, symmetrical T waves, especially in the mid-precordials, you should always think of hyperkalemia. It is critical that you make this association, because in many cases you will not have a great deal of time to initiate therapy before complications such as arrhythmias set in. Sometimes you have just a few minutes, sometimes hours; you just can't tell which patient will give you the luxury of time.

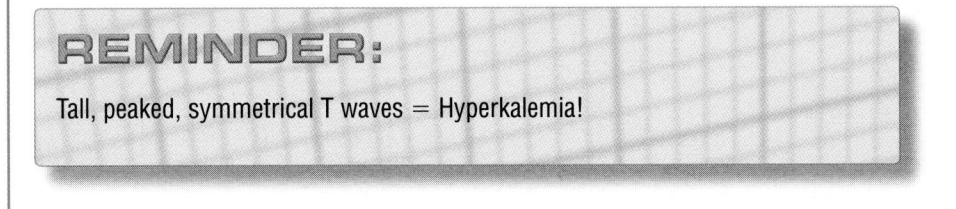

REMINDER:

Tall, peaked, symmetrical T waves = Hyperkalemia!

Is hyperkalemia the definitive diagnosis in this case? No, a few other things are possible, such as ischemia. However, being the astute ECG expert that you are, some other things here make you suspicious. For example, even though none of the limb leads are less than 5 mm tall, the small complexes in the limb leads may signify a small pericardial effusion. Do renal failure patients develop pericardial effusions? Yes! You also notice a prolonged QT interval that could indicate hypocalcemia. This, too, commonly appears in renal failure patients. See how experts start to put things together?

ECG 14-8 After the discussion of ECG 14-7, what should your next question be? What is the potassium level?! These T waves are more classic for hyperkalemia in that they are very tall, narrow, and pointed. (Figure 14-14)

Are the QRS complexes more than 0.12 seconds wide? Sure are. Does it match left or right bundle criteria? Neither one actually fits this ECG. This is therefore an IVCD. One of the most common causes of an IVCD is hyperkalemia.

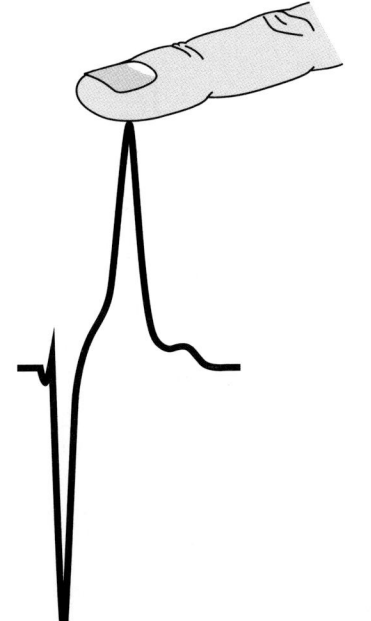

Figure 14-14: Sharp T wave.

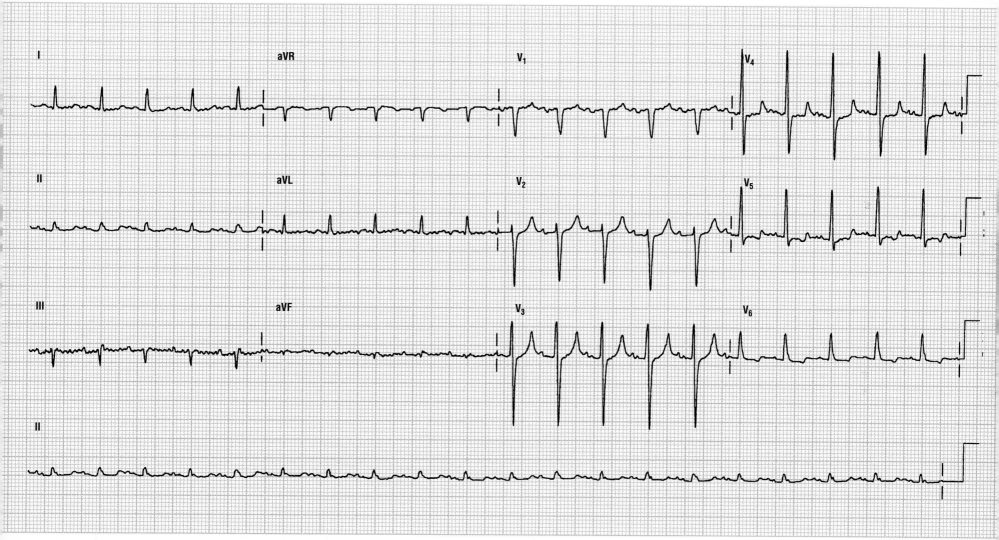

I aVR V₁ V₄

II aVL V₂ V₅

III aVF V₃ V₆

II

ECG 14-7

CHAPTER **14** • ST SEGMENT AND T WAVES

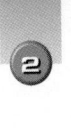

ECG CASE STUDIES: **C O N T I N U E D**

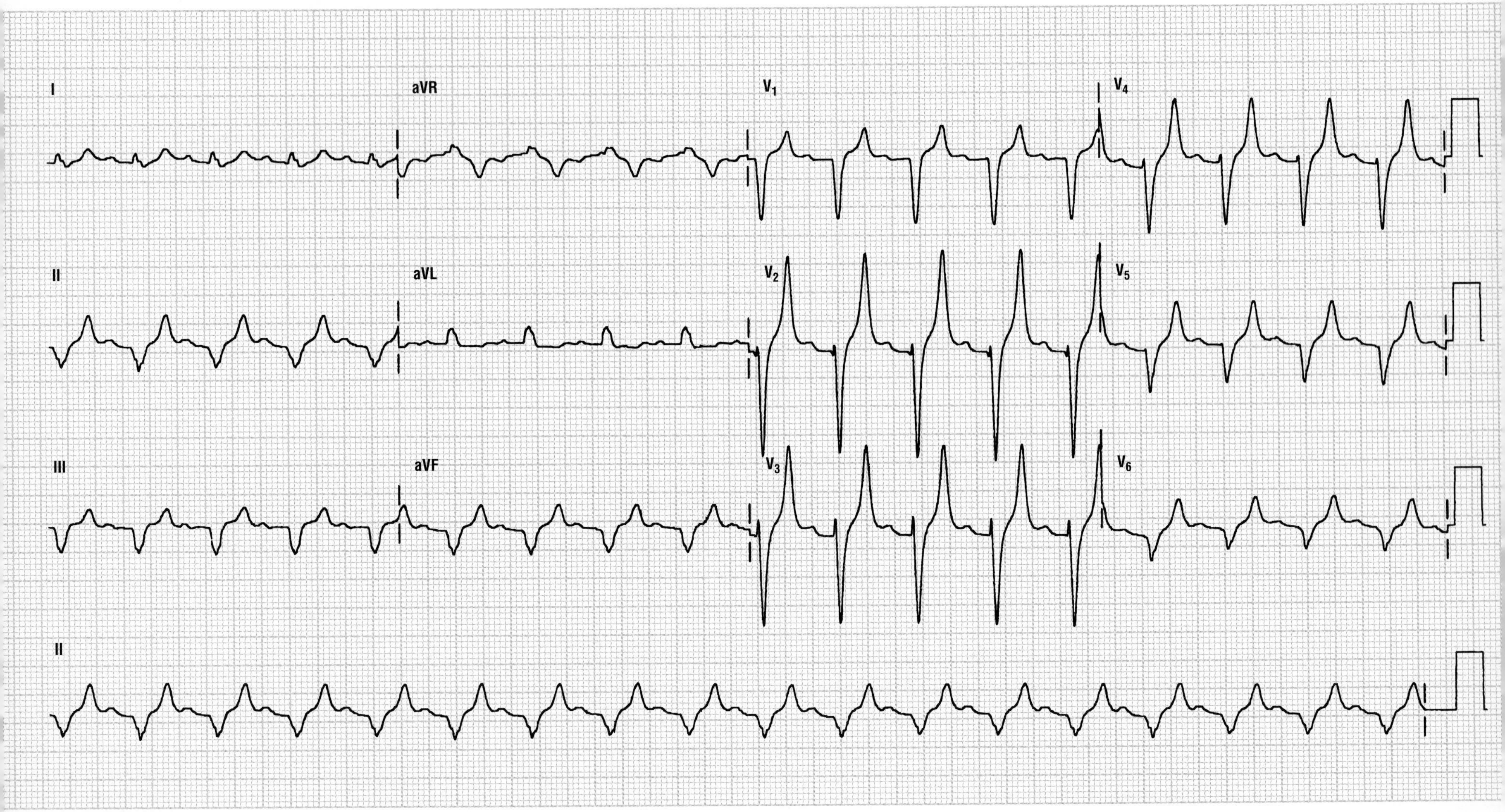

I   aVR   V₁   V₄

II   aVL   V₂   V₅

III   aVF   V₃   V₆

II

ECG 14-8

ECG 14-9 The T waves in this ECG, too, are peaked and symmetrical. They are also wide, and they end with some aberrancy. Notice that the T wave begins to descend and then flares out toward the next complex. This is an abnormal pattern that is rarely seen. It may be due to the main problem with the ECG, the rhythm abnormality. This ECG is extremely difficult to sort out, but let's give it a try. Is it fast or slow? Fast; it is a tachycardia. Are the QRS complexes wider than 0.12 seconds? Yes. So, this is a wide-complex tachycardia. Are there P waves? Yes. Are they associated with the QRS complexes? Not really. Look at leads II and V_1 specifically. In lead II, do you see that the P waves seem to be moving toward the QRS complexes, and actually disappear into the complexes?

This is an example of AV dissociation. It is not third-degree heart block because the P waves are not much faster than the QRS complexes. In other words, the ratio of P waves to QRS complexes is 1:1. Now, putting it together, we have a wide-complex tachycardia with AV dissociation, which by definition is ventricular tachycardia! If you have problems picking these findings up, don't worry — you're in good company. Experts pick them up only with very concentrated effort. This is a really tough ECG. It is a great one, though, to show you how to break down the problems into manageable chunks.

ECG 14-10 Okay, so what is the potassium level here? Once again we are faced with tall, somewhat wide T waves that are definitely pathological in appearance. The first thought that should come to mind is hyperkalemia. The rest of the differential is the same as previously mentioned: CNS event, ischemia, and other electrolyte problems. Ischemia is doubtful because the changes are quite global in nature. The most probable culprits are CNS events and electrolyte abnormalities.

The rest of the ECG shows an early counterclockwise transition with the change from negative to positive occurring slightly before V_2. The axis is in the normal quadrant. There is no evidence of atrial hypertrophy.

QUICK REVIEW

1. ST and T wave abnormalities isolated to one lead are a sign of significant pathology. True or False.

2. Diffuse J points are associated with a benign process in most cases. True or False.

3. T waves are normally upright in aVR. True or False.

1. False 2. True 3. False

ECG CASE STUDIES: **CONTINUED**

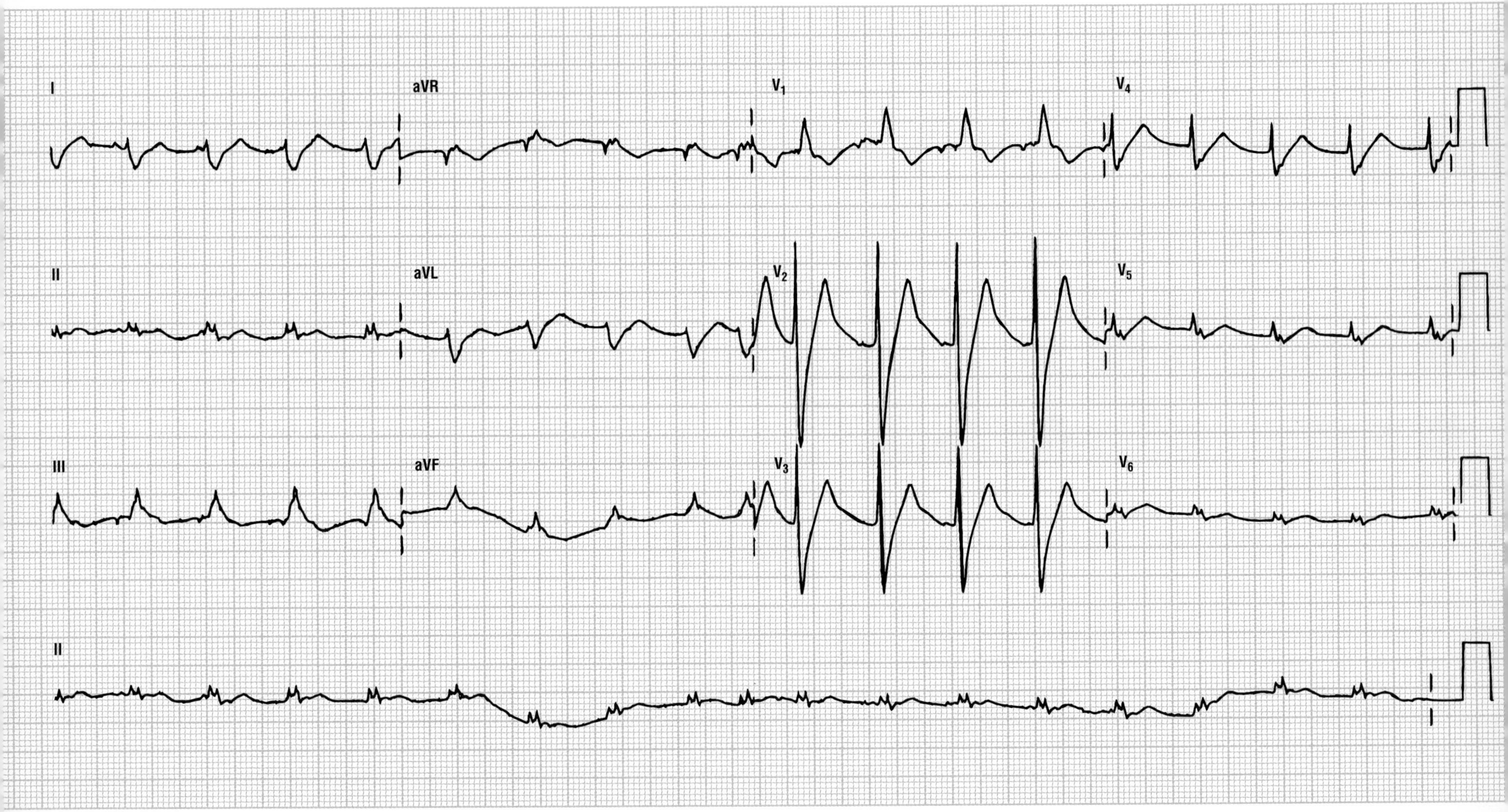

I aVR V₁ V₄

II aVL V₂ V₅

III aVF V₃ V₆

II

ECG 14-9

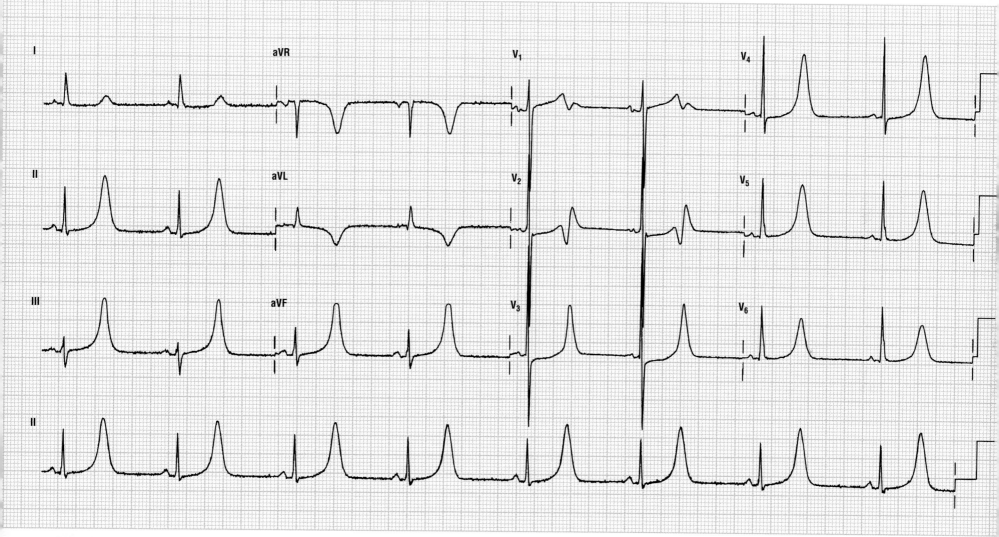

ECG 14-10

ECG CASE STUDIES: CONTINUED

ECG 14-11 Boy, this ECG is really chock full of pathology! The T waves are extremely tall. Should you think about potassium abnormalities? First and always! Let's look at the rate, which is the first thing we examine in any ECG. The atrial rate is fast, compatible with an atrial tachycardia. The QRS rate, however, is very slow at about 40 BPM. The P waves are not associated with the QRS complexes; because the atrial rate is much faster than the ventricular rate, this indicates third-degree heart block.

Now, let's turn our attention to the QRS complexes. The complexes are wide and bizarre. The pattern of a monomorphic S wave in V_1 and a monomorphic R in leads I and V_6 is compatible with a left bundle branch block. The person may have an underlying LBBB or, because the QRS complexes are so bizarre, the complexes may come from an aberrant pacemaker somewhere in the ventricles (the right ventricle, to be exact, because the pattern is that of LBBB). The second option is more likely: This ECG demonstrates a third-degree heart block with atrial tachycardia and a ventricular escape rhythm.

When you are faced with a very bizarre ECG, don't panic! Instead, break it down into its components by going through it in an organized fashion. This will make it much easier to figure out the pathology involved.

ECG 14-12 The T waves in this ECG are pretty impressive, especially in the precordials. The ST and T waves abnormalities are indicative of a hyperacute AMI (one that is very recent in onset). It is rare to capture this finding because most patients with chest pain present late to the emergency department, after this hyperacute period. In what leads are the ST segments elevated? If you are like most people, you immediately noticed the precordials. However, there is also significant elevation in leads II, III, and aVF. There is also ST depression in I and aVL. In Chapter 15, we will see that these indicate an IWMI.

ECG 14-12 This is a textbook example of a hyperacute infarct. Is the infarct in the anterior or inferior wall? Most people state that the infarct is in the anterior wall. However, this ECG shows the classic changes of an IWMI with an associated hyperacute right ventricular infarct. The criteria that are present include: (1) an IWMI; (2) ST elevation in lead III greater than lead II; and (3) ST elevation in V_1 (which can extend to V_6 in some cases). Echocardiography revealed a functioning anterior wall, but also motion abnormalities of the inferior wall and changes consistent with an RV infarct.

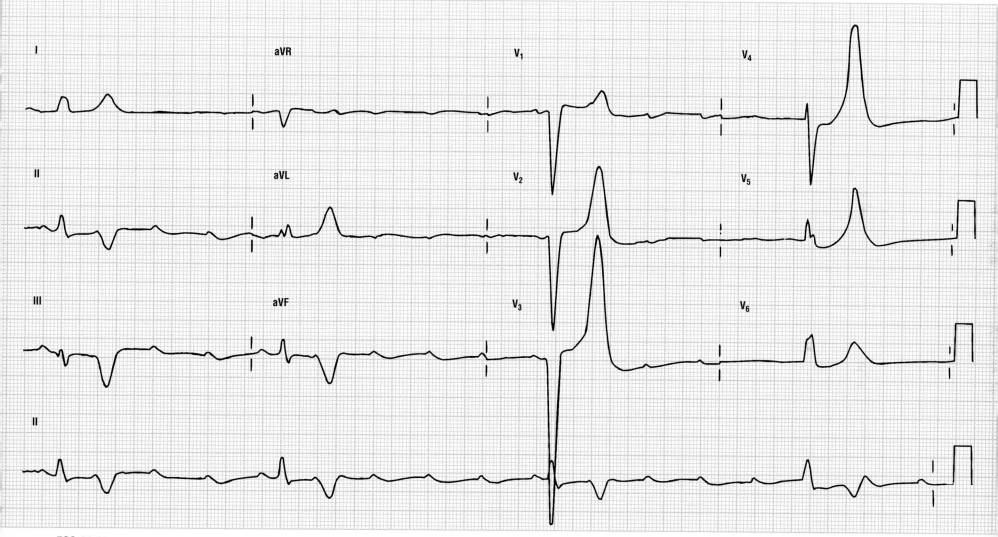

ECG 14-11

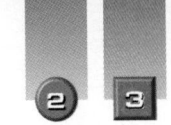

ECG CASE STUDIES: **CONTINUED**

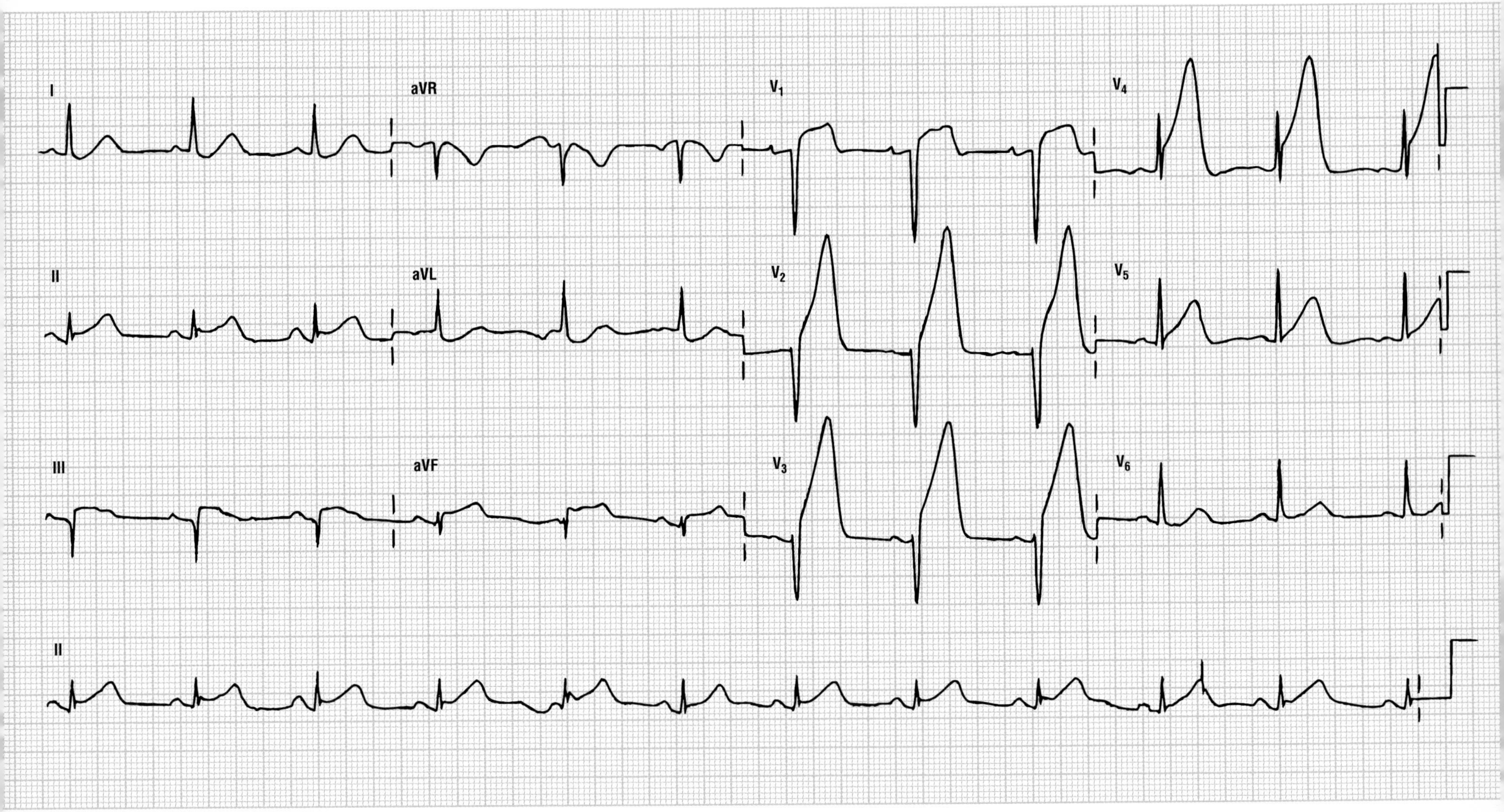

I aVR V₁ V₄

II aVL V₂ V₅

III aVF V₃ V₆

II

ECG 14-12

ECG 14-13 We are now moving away from tall T waves to broad ones. Notice that the ST segments in this case are diffuse and nebulous. The T wave in V_1 is slightly asymmetrical, but in the other leads they are either symmetrical or flattened. These are not normal T waves; we should approach them with caution. The presence of an old ECG would be extremely helpful, but if one is not available we have to assume the worst. The worst-case scenarios are ischemia and CNS events with electrolyte abnormalities — a distant possibility as there is a very small U wave in some leads, especially V_2 to V_3.

QUICK REVIEW

1. Flipped Ts are always a sign of pathology. True or False.

2. If a BBB is present, the T waves can be flipped and still be normal. True or False.

3. Flat ST segments that are elevated or depressed are always secondary to benign causes. True or False.

1. False: review the criteria. They are normally flipped in aVR; they *can be* flipped and still be normal in III, aVL, aVF, and V_1 to V_2, but always be *careful!* 2. True 3. False

CLINICAL PEARL

Always compare your interpretation of the ECG with your patient. Use the ECG to help guide your thought process in establishing the diagnosis.

ECG 14-14 This is another tough ECG. It appears fairly normal at first glance, but start going through it in an organized fashion and you'll see the problem. Do you see any P waves? Yes. Are they associated with the QRS complexes? No, they are not. If you look at the rhythm strip, you notice that some P waves are easy to spot, such as the one marked by the fourth star. Some of the other P waves are less obvious because they are buried inside the QRS complexes, ST segments, or T waves. When you map out the Ps using calipers, you'll note that they are almost always the same distance apart, give or take a small amount. This is consistent with AV dissociation, which is present in this ECG. This is a normal sinus rhythm with AV dissociation and junctional escape beats.

This chapter, however, is about T waves and ST segments. We note that there are some slightly elevated ST segments in the right precordial leads of V_1 to V_3. These are associated with some concave, upward scooping of the segments, which appears fairly benign. The T waves, though, are wide and slightly asymmetrical. Remember to use your clear ruler to evaluate the symmetry of the wave. The asymmetry eases some of your concern about the width of the T waves. Because AV dissociation is present, you should still correlate your findings to the patient — as always — to be completely sure of the benign quality of the segments.

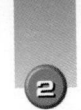

ECG CASE STUDIES: CONTINUED

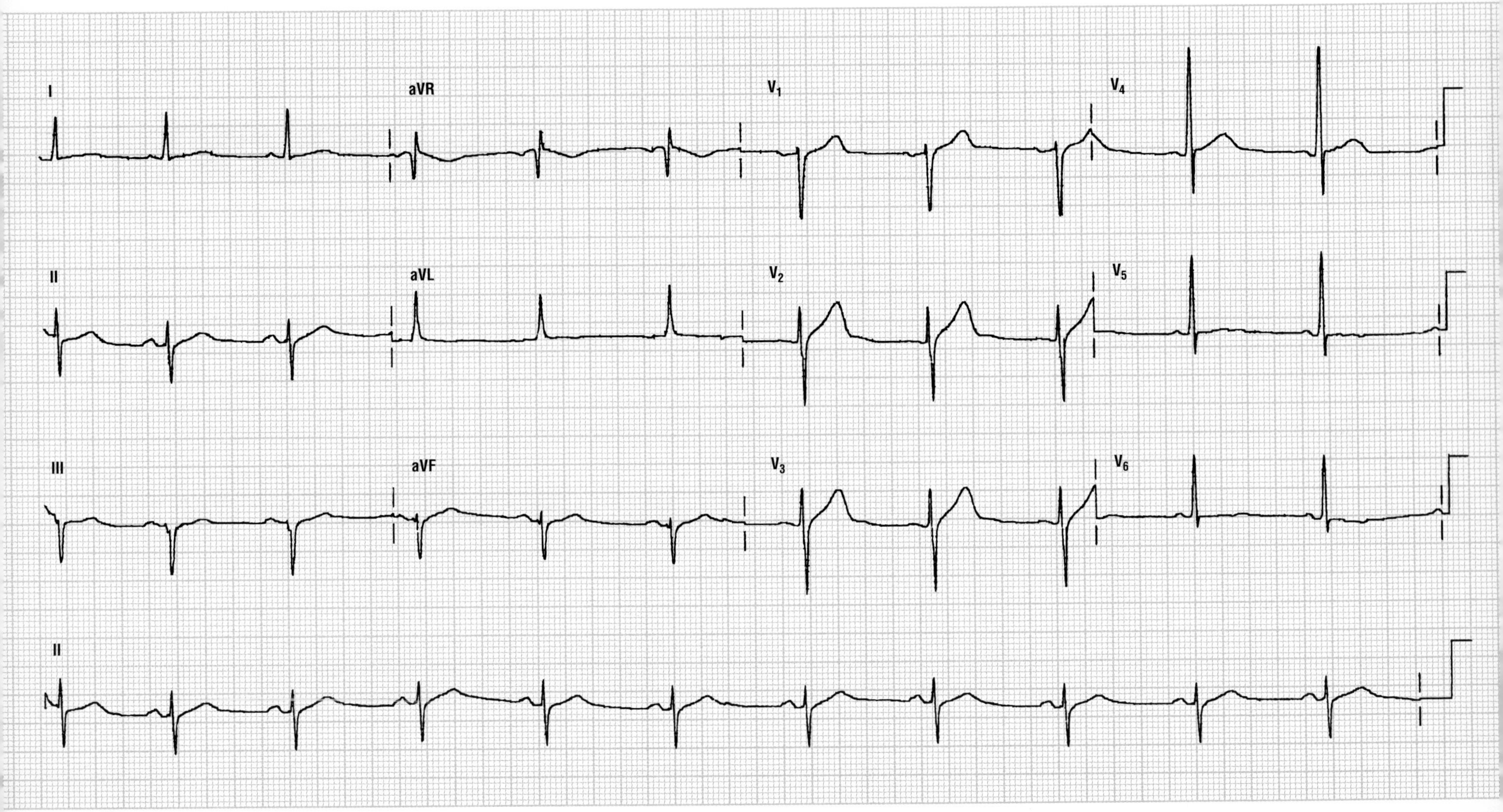

I aVR V₁ V₄

II aVL V₂ V₅

III aVF V₃ V₆

II

ECG 14-13

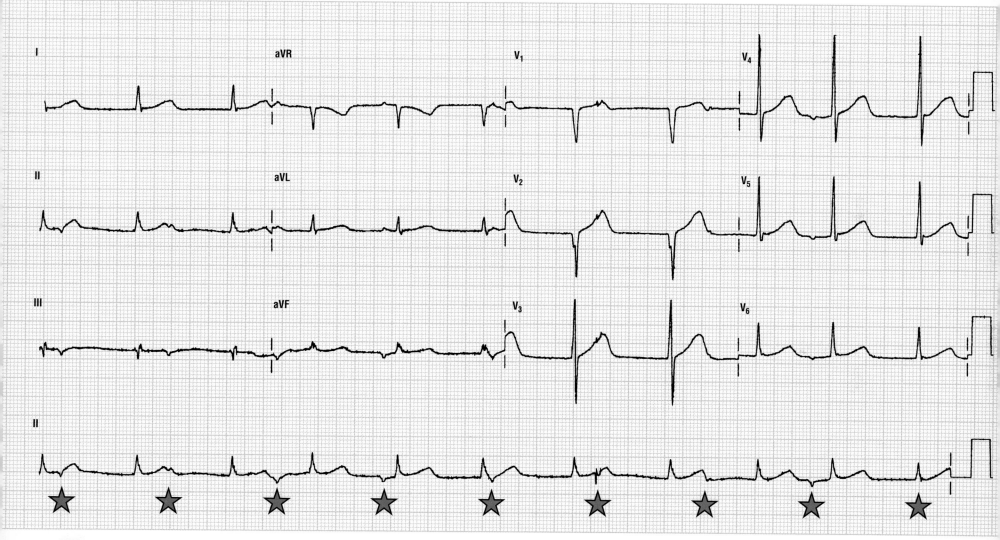

ECG 14-14

ECG CASE STUDIES: **CONTINUED**

ECG 14-15 This ECG has some pretty wide ST segments and broad T waves that are grossly abnormal. This patient was having an intracranial hemorrhage and had very high intracranial pressures. This is the classic, but very rare, electrocardiographic finding for this disorder. You need to commit it to memory because the patient with this ECG will be in coma, unable to give you a history.

What is that little spike pattern in leads I, III, and aVL? Is it a pacemaker? No, pacemakers will never fire that fast. The rate is well over 300 BPM. This is artifact caused by interference from some electrical device. Don't worry about it.

ECG 14-16 This ECG also has some pretty wide ST segments and broad T waves that are grossly abnormal. This is another example of a patient with an intracranial hemorrhage. This time the T waves are not as impressive, but they are still quite wide.

Note that in leads V_1 to V_3, there is a second hump after the initial T wave. Is this indicative of a U wave? Well, remember we have said that intervals are always the same throughout the ECG. In comparing the QT interval in V_5 to V_6, we see that the second hump falls well within the QT interval and is not a U wave. Could it be the missing P wave, buried in the T wave because of first-degree heart block? Could be, and it probably is the P wave. P waves are usually best seen in V_1 or V_2.

REMINDER:
Very broad, symmetrical T waves are classic for major intracranial bleeds or strokes.

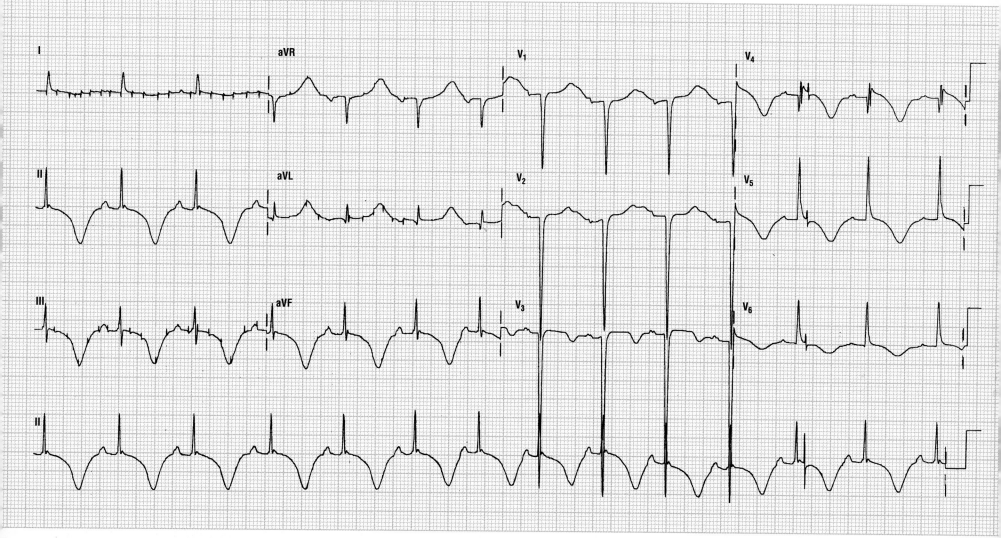

ECG 14-15

ECG CASE STUDIES: CONTINUED

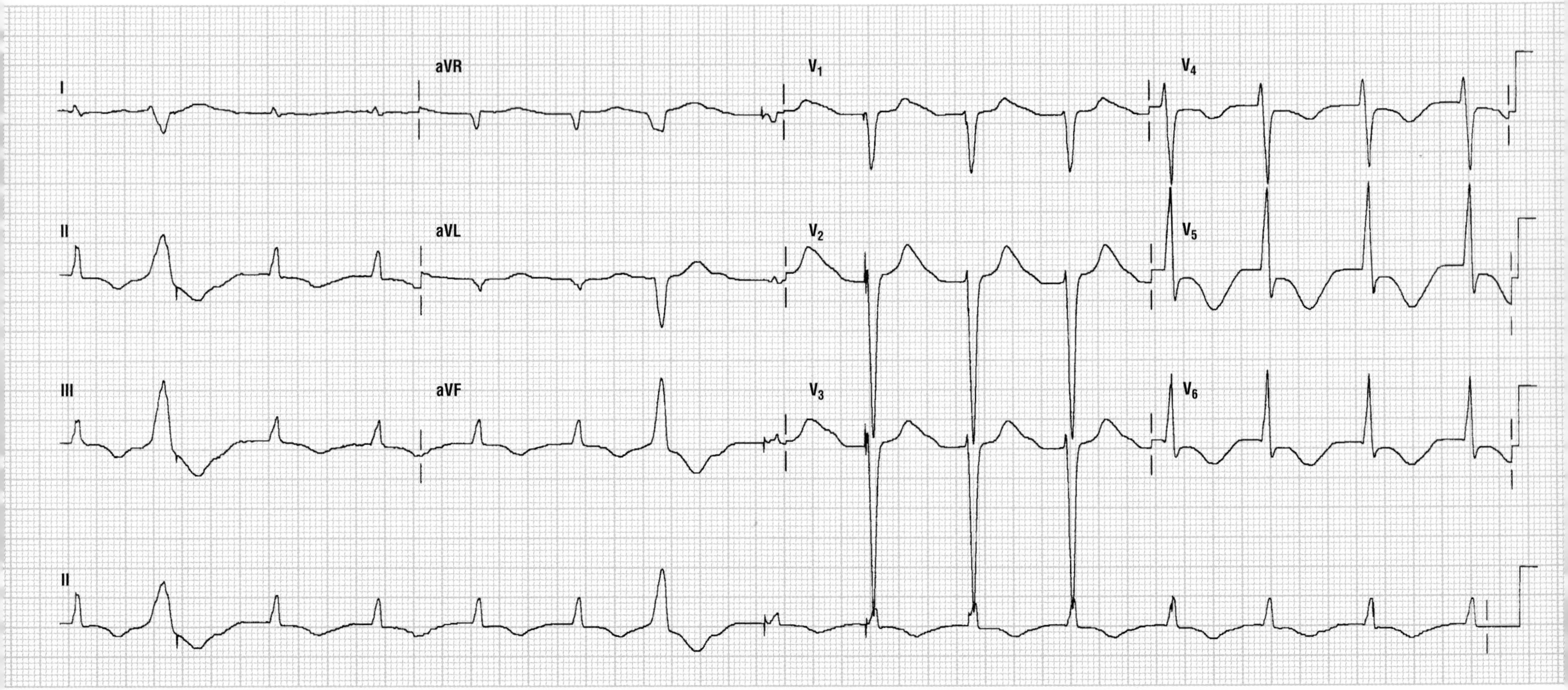

I aVR V₁ V₄

II aVL V₂ V₅

III aVF V₃ V₆

II

ECG 14-16

ECG 14-17 The ST segments are markedly elevated in this patient's precordial leads. The T waves are flipped and symmetrical in leads I, aVL, and V_2 to V_6. What do you think they call this kind of ST segment, and can you imagine why? If you are having any doubts, look at Figure 14-15. These are classic tombstones. They indicate a large myocardial infarction. We have often asked you to obtain an old ECG for comparison before making a definitive diagnosis, but when you see these, you already have the definitive diagnosis. You don't need any additional information. Can you have these changes with little or no chest pain? Yes. Patients who have altered pain sensation secondary to nerve damage or neuropathies can have silent AMIs. This occurs in normal folks sometimes, as well.

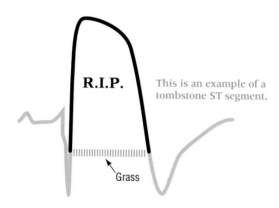

R.I.P.

This is an example of a tombstone ST segment.

Grass

Figure 14-15: Tombstone segment.

ECG 14-18 This is an example of a biphasic T wave that is pathological. Look at lead V_2 and you will notice that it is negative and then positive. Normally, T waves are inverted first positive and then negative — the opposite of the one in the example.

The T wave accompanies a slightly elevated ST segment that is associated with some QRS complex notching in the lateral precordials. When you see notching, you can usually state with some certainty that the ST elevation is benign. In this case, though, you need to be careful because of the pathologic T wave. You will need an old ECG and some corroboration with the patient's condition to make the definitive diagnosis.

NOTE

Pretend that the T wave is a roller coaster. You need to travel up the mountain first so that the fall will make you gain speed. This is normal. This is good. You don't start off by going down in order to gain speed to climb the mountain. That is against the laws of theme parks. That is bad.

ECG CASE STUDIES: **CONTINUED**

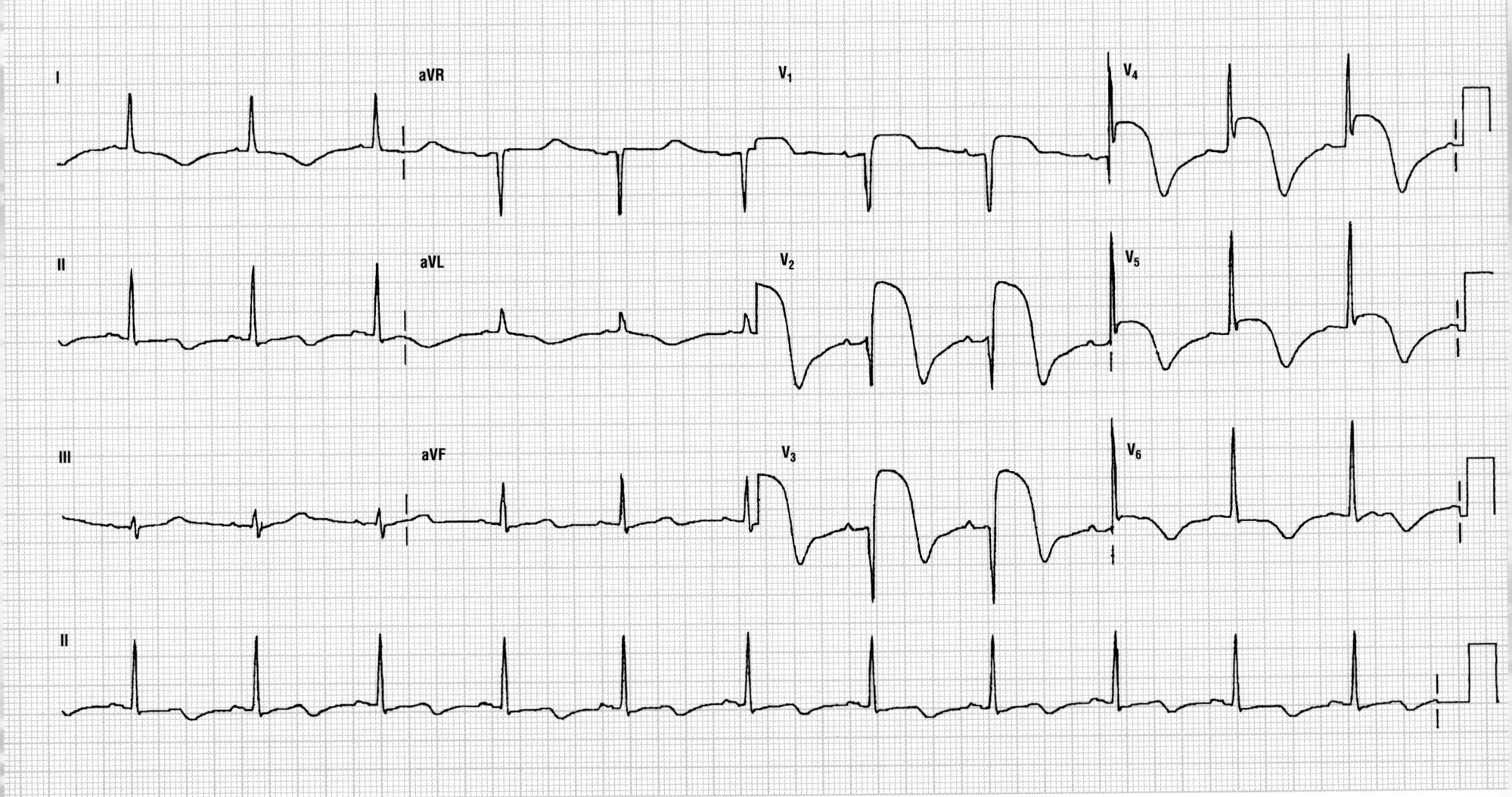

ECG 14-17

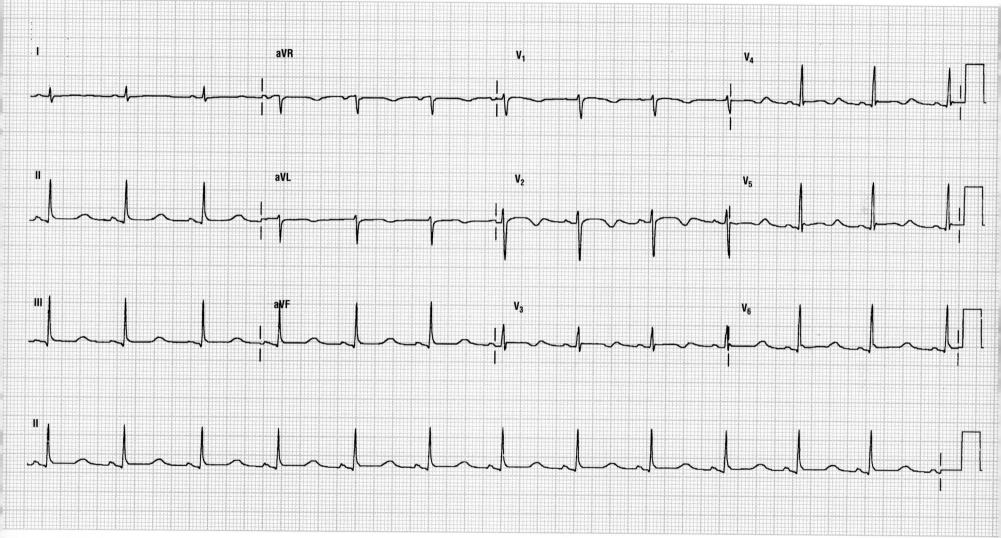

ECG 14-18

Ischemia and Injury

The most important diagnosis made with the ST segment and the
T wave is that of ischemia and injury. We will spend more time on
this in Chapter 15. However, we cannot complete this chapter without
raising the issue.

It is not only the presence of ST elevation or depression that makes
the ECG ischemic. Various other things must be present. The ST segment should be flat and/or downward sloping (Figure 14-16). The
T wave needs to be symmetrical or, if biphasic, it should start with
a negative deflection (Figure 14-16). In addition, you should see a
regional distribution of ST elevation or depression affecting these leads.
Remember when we were discussing vectors and we touched on the
concept of regional ECG sectors (Chapter 3, Localizing an Area: Inferior
Wall)? To review briefly, the ECG is divided into various sectors corresponding to the septum and the inferior, anterior, lateral, and posterior
walls. We will be spending much more time on this in Chapter 15. For
now, just remember that the changes have to be in a regional distribution.

ST depression is indicative of ischemia or a non-Q-wave infarction.
(The infarction is not transmural, and is therefore not associated with
a Q wave.) ST elevation, which suggests injury, is usually present in
infarction (Figure 14-17). More in Chapter 15.

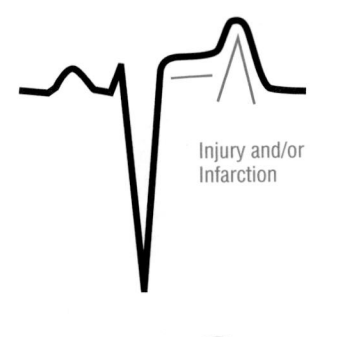

Figure 14-17: Injury and/or infarction.

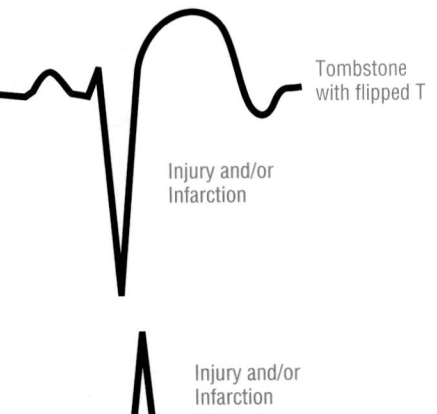

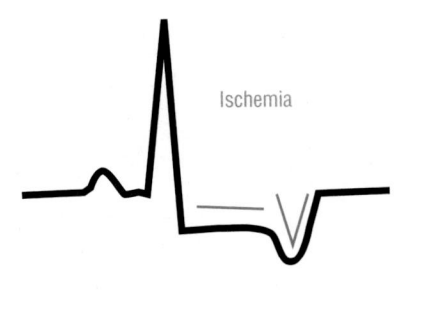

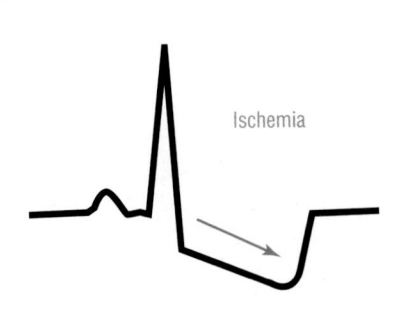

Figure 14-16: Ischemia.

ECG 14-19 Look at the ST segments below and you will see quite a few leads with ST depression. The depression is definitely flat and therefore represents ischemia. Now, let's try to figure out the location. (We will cover this in greater detail in Chapter 15; this is just an exercise.) In the limb leads, the ST is depressed in II, III, and aVF. If you remember, these are the leads that face the inferior wall. In the precordials, we have ST depression in V_2 to V_6. Leads V_5 to V_6 represent the lateral wall, and these are also ischemic. V_2 to V_4 are an extension of the ischemic episode through additional areas. This patient, therefore, has severe inferolateral ischemia involving quite a large portion of the heart.

Why does aVR have ST elevation? Going back to the hexaxial system of the limb leads, aVR is always opposite the rest of the leads. Therefore, if the others have ST depression, then aVR — nonconformist that it is — will show ST elevation. Think of aVR kind of like your kids or your baby sibling. They will always do the opposite just for spite!

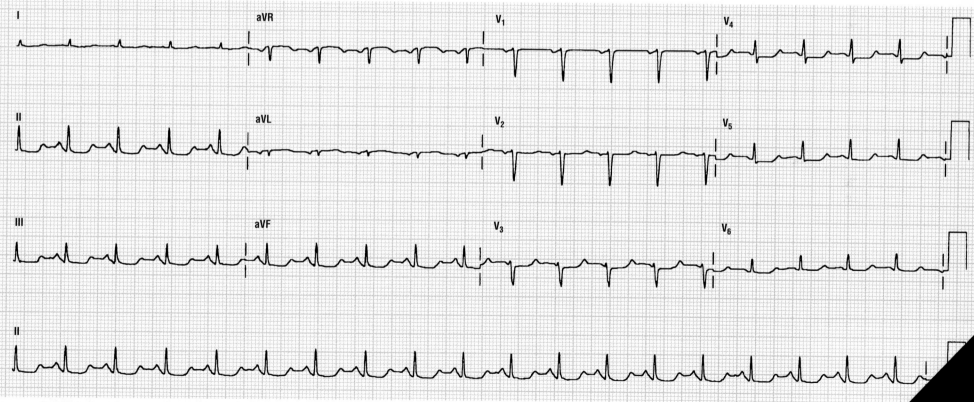

ECG 14-19

ECG CASE STUDIES: **CONTINUED**

②

ECG 14-20 This is a classic ECG for an AMI. Notice the ST segments in leads II, III, and aVF. They are flat, elevated, and associated with flipped T waves. Looking at the QRS complexes, take notice of the Q waves in III and aVF. These changes are all consistent with an inferior wall AMI.

There is ST depression in leads I, aVL, and V₂ to V₆ (and some minimal depression in V₁, as well) that is consistent with ischemia.

The ECG is also significant for LVH and a first-degree heart block.

③

ECG 14-20 Once again, there is evidence of an IWMI with right ventricular involvement.

LVH is present by multiple criteria, but the ST depression in the lateral leads is not consistent with LVH with strain. This is a continuation of the lateral wall ischemia associated with the infarct. The first-degree heart block may be acutely due to increased vagal stimulation caused by the inferior MI, or it may have been present for an indeterminate amount of time.

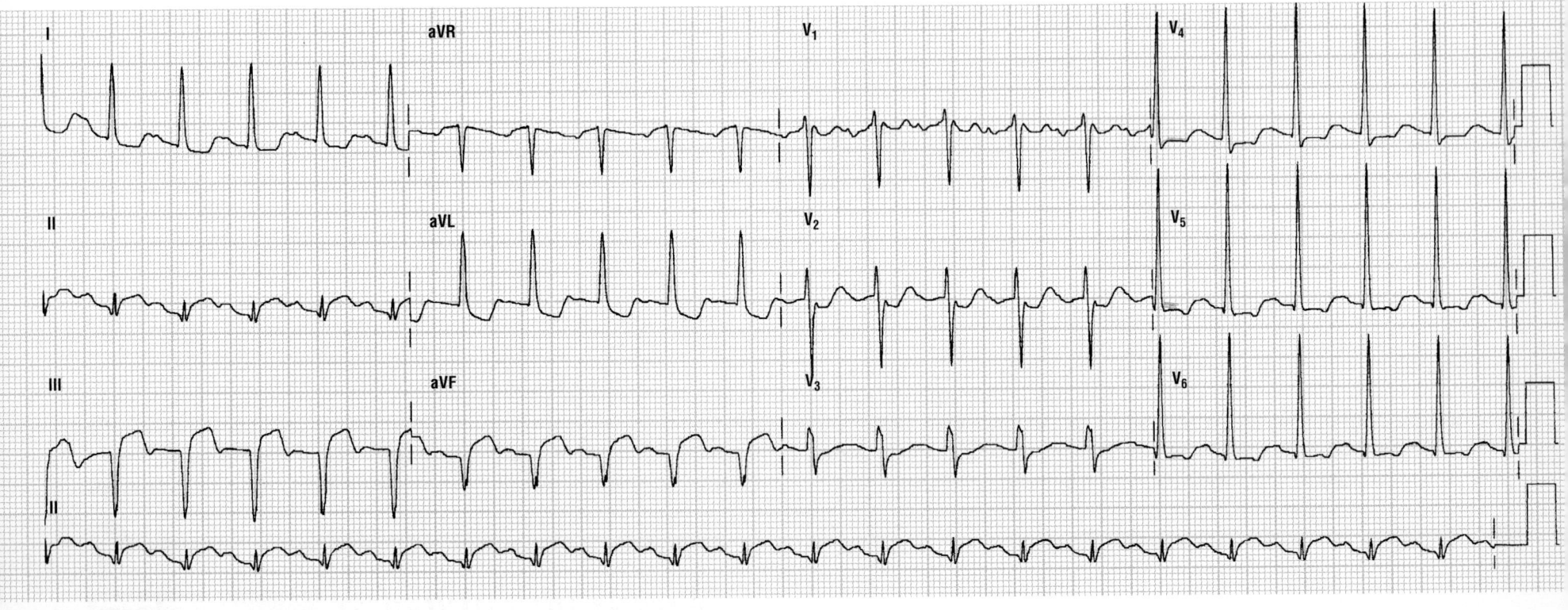

ECG 14-20

②

ECG 14-21 This ECG is a veritable smorgasbord of ST segment changes. There is marked elevation in leads II, III, aVF, and all of the precordials. The STs in V_1 to V_4 are definitely tombstones.

The Q waves in II, III, and aVF are quite significant. There is also a QS wave in V_1. Leads V_2 to V_5 have a very small *r* wave at the beginning of the complex so they are not truly QS waves. There is, in addition, a late clockwise transition present that could be the result of a significant loss of myocardium in the anterior wall.

③

ECG 14-21 This is one of those ECGs that you just don't want to go near without some clinical correlation. There is evidence of an AMI of indeterminate origin in the inferior leads — significant Q waves. Minimal ST elevation is also present in the inferior leads, but without reciprocal changes in I and aVL. The ST segments in leads V_1 to V_6 are markedly elevated, consistent with an AMI or a ventricular aneurysm. (Changes with an aneurysm usually do not extend through V_5 to V_6, so this is less likely.) The patient was having active pain. The only entity that can produce an AMI of both the right and left coronary arterial systems simultaneously is an aortic aneurysm, which you need to rule out aggressively in this patient.

②

ECG 14-22 This ECG has some tombstone changes in leads V_1 to V_4 associated with flipped T waves. The Ts are symmetrical in all of the precordials, and in leads I and aVL. However, they are asymmetrical in the inferior leads of II, III, and aVF.

This is an example of an electrocardiographic pattern that develops when a patient has had a previous anteroseptal AMI that killed off enough tissue to cause a ventricular aneurysm. It is impossible, electrocardiographically, to distinguish this from an acute myocardial infarction. The only way to distinguish between the two is to be lucky enough to have an old ECG with the same findings and, naturally, to talk to the patient and find out about current complaints. There are also some physical examination findings that will help in your differential; you can consult a physical diagnosis book to search them out. Our personal experience is that the tombstoning in a ventricular aneurysm is minimal, but the QS waves cover at least V_1 to V_3, as in this case. The QT interval also appears normal to slightly decreased. We wish there were some magic rule to give you but, unfortunately, none exists to our knowledge. Whenever you see this pattern, assume the worst until proven otherwise. If the patient is asymptomatic, get an old ECG and contact a cardiologist right away. *Remember never to give thrombolytics to an asymptomatic patient unless approved by a cardiologist!*

CLINICAL PEARL

Advanced clinicians: Always compare your ECG findings to your patient's complaints. Administration of thrombolytics for a ventricular aneurysmal pattern is not an uncommon scenario.

ECG CASE STUDIES: CONTINUED

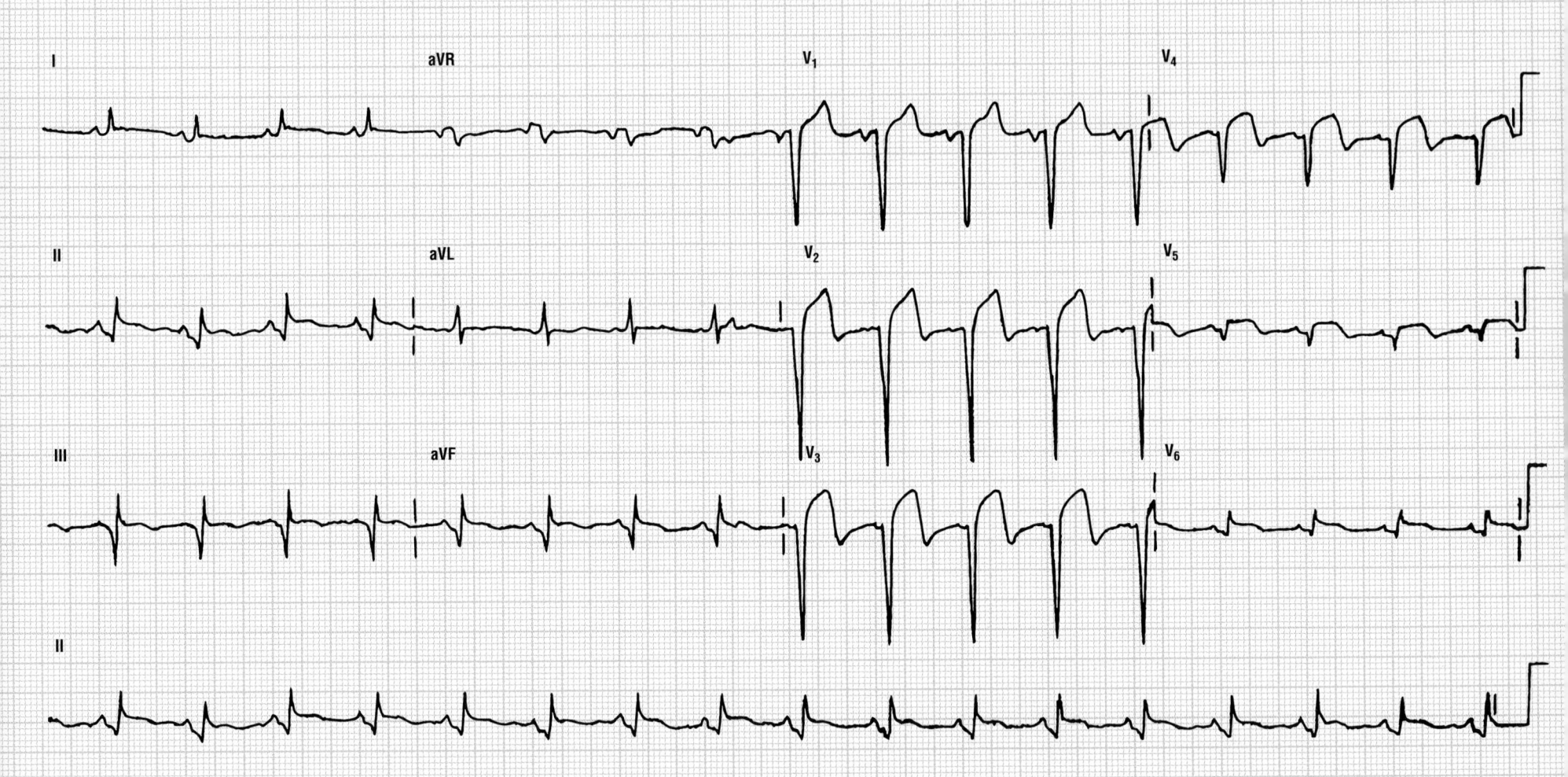

ECG 14-21

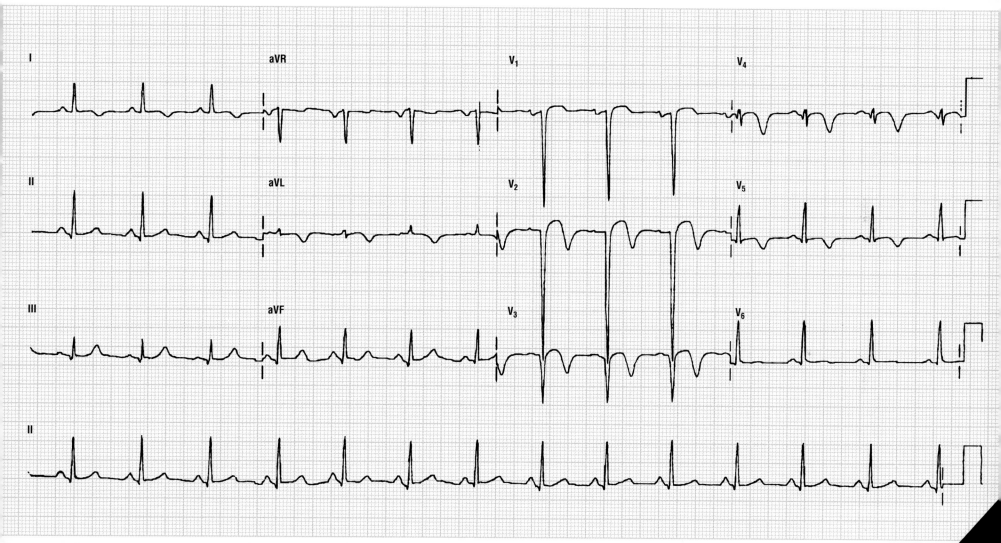

ECG 14-22

Strain Pattern

Strain pattern refers to the ST and T wave configurations that arise from repolarization abnormalities found in either RVH or LVH.

Right Ventricular Strain Pattern

The vector in RVH is anterior and to the right. This gives rise to an increased R wave component in the right precordial leads of V_1 and V_2, as we saw in the axis material in Chapter 12. This increased R:S ratio would be found in RVH alone. There are, however, some other characteristics that add the "strain" to the strain pattern. These are a concave, downward ST segment that is depressed, and a flipped, asymmetric T wave, as seen in Figure 14-18.

If the T wave is biphasic instead of inverted, the first part will usually be negative and the second part positive in RVH (and, as we shall see, in a posterior wall AMI). If the first part of the biphasic T wave is positive, it does not necessarily signal pathology.

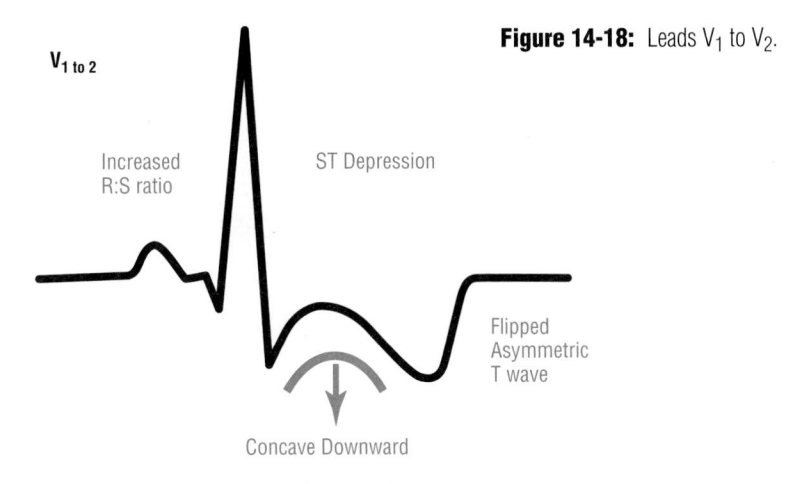

$V_{1 \text{ to } 2}$

Increased R:S ratio

ST Depression

Concave Downward

Flipped Asymmetric T wave

Figure 14-18: Leads V_1 to V_2.

Acute right ventricular strain, as occurs du[...]lus, can cause a rotation of the heart and the axis. This will give rise to a particular pattern on the ECG known as the $S_1Q_3T_3$ pattern. What this means is that there is an S wave in lead I, a Q or q wave in III, and a flipped T in III. This is not, however, pathognomonic of a pulmonary embolus; it can occur in other states. However, if you suspect a pulmonary embolus in the presence of an $S_1Q_3T_3$ pattern, you do have some additional support for your diagnosis.

Let's quickly review the criteria for RVH that we have covered so far. You do not need all of the criteria in order to make the diagnosis, but you should have more than one.

1. P-pulmonale (RAE)
2. Right axis deviation
3. Increased R:S ratio in V_1 and V_2
4. RVH strain pattern
5. $S_1Q_3T_3$ pattern

The most important of these criteria is the increased R:S ratio. Rather than burden you with a large number of facts, we prefer to discuss the concepts. As you progress, you will be able to remember more information and criteria. When you review the book again as an advanced practitioner, which is not too far away, you will remember more of these minor criteria. Just to mention a few more now, they include an incomplete RBBB pattern, an R wave in V_1 that is 7 mm or more, S wave in V_1 that is 2mm or more, and a qR pattern in V_1.

Have you noticed that there are fewer Level 3 boxes in this part of the book? You are approaching that fine line that separates intermediate from advanced ECG readers. Congratulate yourself. You deserve it!

2

ECG 14-23 This is the most picture-perfect ECG for RVH that we have ever seen. It almost looks as if it were computer generated, but it actually came from a young woman with pulmonary hypertension. All five criteria are present in this ECG: P-pulmonale (RAE), right axis deviation, increased R:S ratio in V_1 to V_2, RVH strain pattern, and $S_1Q_3T_3$ pattern.

It is very important to remember the differential diagnosis points for an increased R:S ratio in V_1 or V_2. It will greatly assist with your interpretation of the ECG. Carry a flash card until you've committed these to memory.

1. Right ventricular hypertrophy
2. Right bundle branch block
3. Posterior wall AMI
4. WPW type A
5. Young kids and adolescents

When you see an increased R:S ratio in V_1 or V_2, run through the list and see which one fits the bill.

ECG 14-24 Let's try a little experiment. Does this ECG demonstrate RVH with strain? Go ahead and take a close look before you come back.

The answer is no. The ECG shows right axis deviation and a RBBB. If you measure the QRS complexes in V_4 to V_6, you will see that they are just at or slightly above 0.12 seconds. This makes it a block of some sort. There is also a slurred S in leads I and V_6. Why the increased R:S ratio? Go through the differentials offered with ECG 14-23. You will see that this fits into one of the categories: RBBB. This is a tough one.

3

ECG 14-24 This ECG shows RBBB with an R wave instead of a full RSR′ complex. Because it is an RBBB, the T waves in the inferior leads and precordials are abnormal. They are strongly concordant, which could indicate ischemia. An old ECG would be very helpful for comparison, and you need clinical correlation to completely interpret the ECG.

2

ECG 14-25 This ECG shows a right axis deviation, P-pulmonale, and an $S_1Q_3T_3$ pattern, but no increased R:S ratio in V_1 to V_2. The pattern is still one of RVH-with-strain. There is also some pretty significant LVH present, which may account for the absence of the increased R wave in V_1 to V_2. There is strong evidence of LAE, as well. So putting it all together, you have enlargement of all four chambers of the heart. This could signify cardiomyopathy.

The second beat is a VPC. There is also a borderline first-degree heart block.

 QUICK REVIEW

1. You cannot diagnose RVH accurately in the presence of RBBB. True or False.
2. You can diagnose LVH in the presence of RVH. True or False.
3. $S_1Q_3T_3$ pattern is indicative of right-sided strain. True or False.

1. True 2. True 3. True

ECG CASE STUDIES: **CONTINUED**

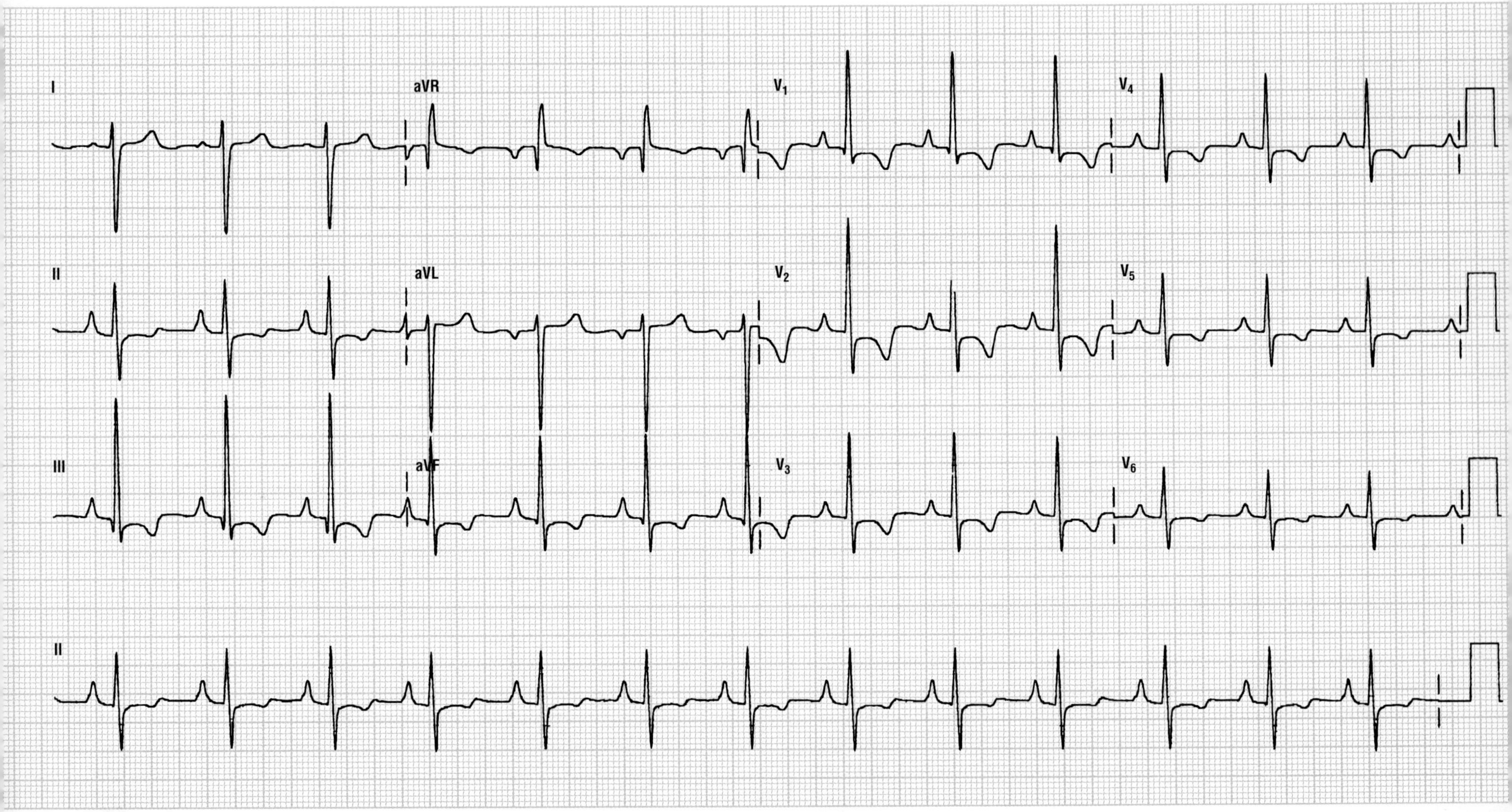

I   aVR   V₁   V₄

II   aVL   V₂   V₅

III   aVF   V₃   V₆

II

ECG 14-23

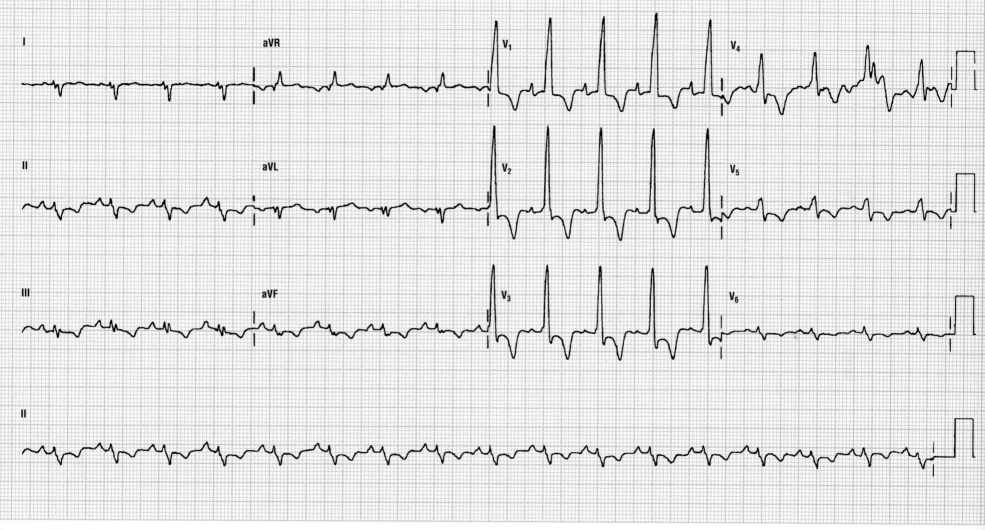

ECG 14-24

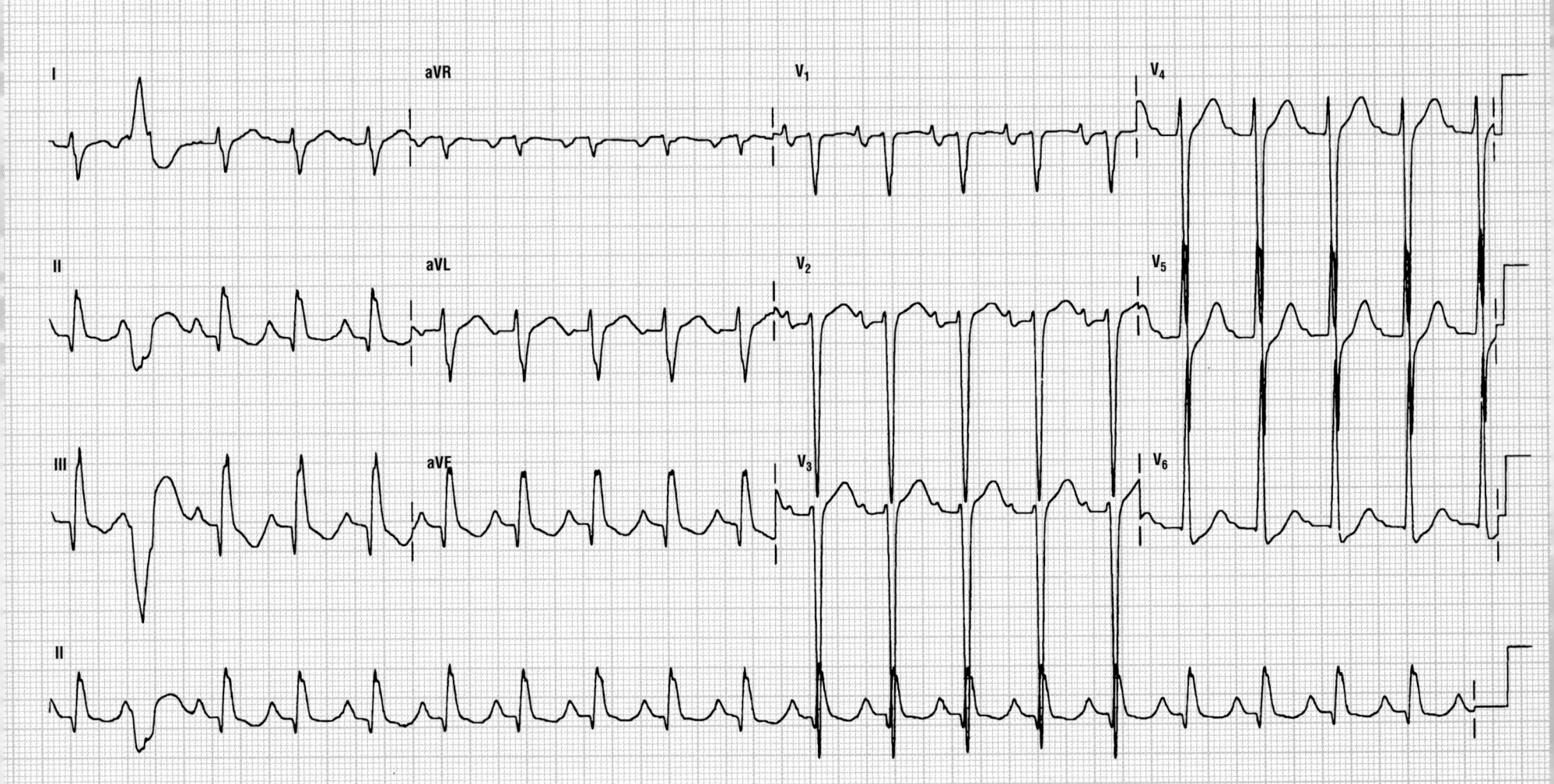

ECG 14-25

Left Ventricular Strain Pattern

The left ventricle can also develop a strain pattern if there is significant hypertrophy. Once again, the strain pattern is caused by repolarization abnormalities of the hypertrophied ventricle. The pattern is different from that found in RVH, however, as you would expect. In LVH with strain, we see a pattern of ST depression with downward concavity, and a flipped and asymmetric T wave in the left precordial leads of V_4 to V_6 (Figure 14-19). In the right precordials, there is a reciprocal change, so to speak, of the left ventricular pattern: ST elevation with upward concavity, and an upright, asymmetric T wave (Figure 14-20). The ST elevation can be 1 to 3 mm in V_2 to V_3, and in some cases more than that.

A key point to remember: *The strain pattern is the greatest in the lead with the tallest and deepest QRS pattern.* In other words, if the S wave in V_2 is 15 mm and the S wave in V_3 is 20, you would expect V_3 to have the highest ST elevation (Figure 14-21). Conversely, if V_5 has an R wave that is 20 mm tall and the R in V_6 is 15 mm, V_5 should have the most depression. Think of it this way: the taller or deeper the wave, the bigger the strain.

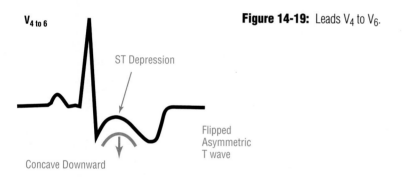

Figure 14-19: Leads V_4 to V_6.

$V_{4 \text{ to } 6}$

ST Depression

Concave Downward

Flipped Asymmetric T wave

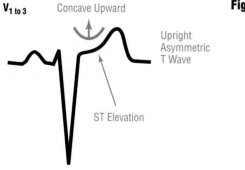

Figure 14-20: Leads V_1 to V_3.

$V_{1 \text{ to } 3}$

Concave Upward

Upright Asymmetric T Wave

ST Elevation

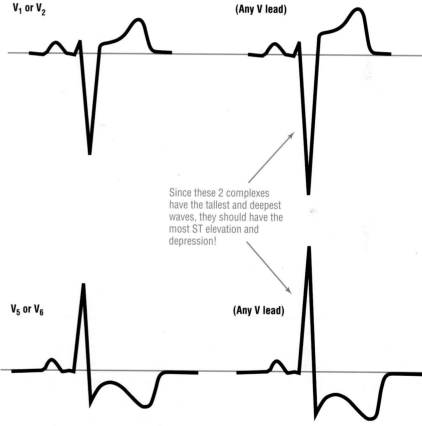

V_1 or V_2 (Any V lead)

Since these 2 complexes have the tallest and deepest waves, they should have the most ST elevation and depression!

V_5 or V_6 (Any V lead)

Figure 14-21: ST elevation and depression.

More on LVH with Strain LVH with strain is one of the most problematic interpretations in electrocardiography. This is because you must distinguish it from ischemia and infarction, a potentially life-threatening distinction. As we saw in the ischemia section, *ST elevation or depression that is ischemic in nature is usually flat rather than concave, and the T wave is symmetrical, not asymmetrical* (Figure 14-22)! This interpretation is easy in some ECGs, but not so easy in others.

A sharp J point is also more indicative of ischemia or infarction. LVH with strain usually has a more diffuse J point in the right precordials, V_1 to V_3.

The strain pattern in V_5 to V_6 may become flat or downwardly depressed. The key thing to note is that somewhere in the V_4 to V_5 area, the complexes will look identical to what you would expect,

with concavity downward and an asymmetric T wave (Figure 14-23). Remember, symmetric T waves are bad!

Last but not least, remember the "company it keeps." If your patient is visiting you because he stubbed his toe, it is more likely strain pattern. If he comes in diaphoretic and complaining of chest pain, with a blood pressure of 60 palpable and looking like he's going to die, it may be LVH with strain — but you'd better also be treating him for the AMI he is probably having. If you are unsure of your decision, contact a cardiologist. There is nothing wrong in asking for help. Nothing is worse, in our opinion, than to let someone die because of the clinician's vanity.

Figure 14-23

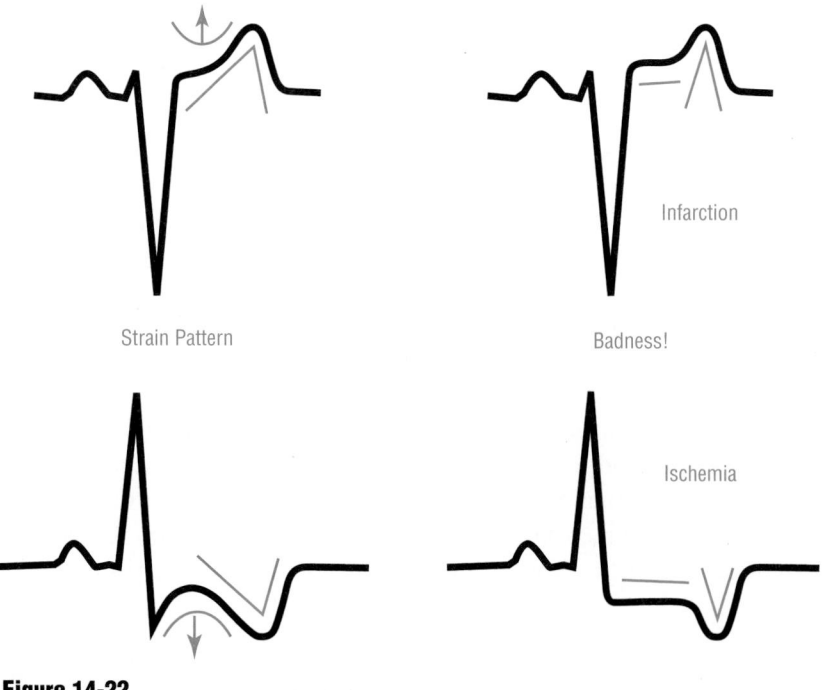

Infarction

Badness!

Ischemia

Strain Pattern

Figure 14-22

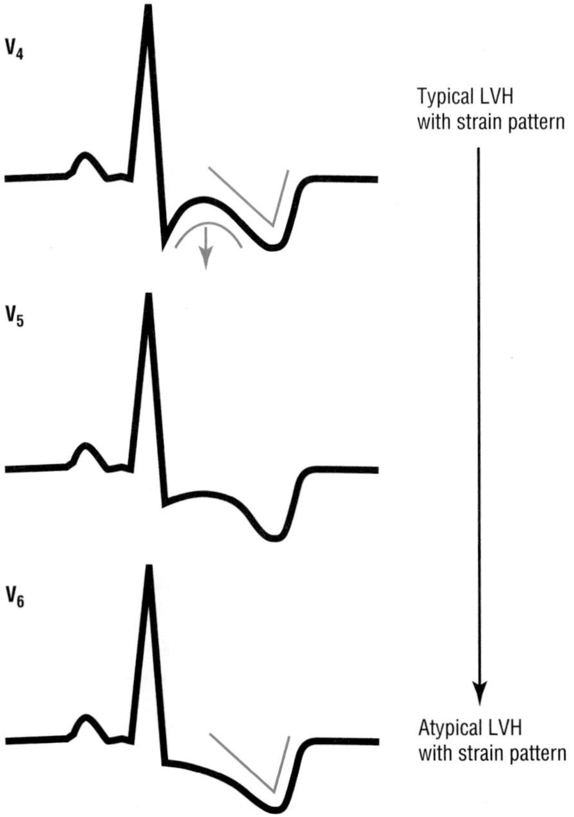

V_4

V_5

V_6

Typical LVH
with strain pattern

Atypical LVH
with strain pattern

ECG 14-26 This is a typical LVH-with-strain pattern. LVH is present by multiple criteria including S in V_1 to V_2 plus R in V_5 to V_6 that is more than 35 mm, R in aVL that is 11 mm or more, and R in I that is 12 mm or more. When you first look at the ECG, you see many ST segment and T wave abnormalities. You see downwardly concave ST segment depression in V_5 to V_6 associated with a flipped, asymmetric T wave consistent with LVH with strain. Notice that the lead with the tallest R wave has the deepest ST depression. In addition, ST elevation in V_1 to V_2 is upwardly concave. Once again, the highest ST segment elevation occurs in the lead with the deepest S wave. The LVH with strain pattern is carried over to leads I and aVL, the high lateral leads. In addition, there is evidence of LAE, which occurs commonly.

ST depression is always a sign of pathology. The main problem is to decide what pathological condition is involved. Is it ischemia? Is it a strain pattern? BBB? WPW? Is it resolving pericarditis? A CNS event? When you see the abnormality, you must begin the hunt to find the definitive answer. Sometimes there are other clues on the ECG, or on an old one. Sometimes the clues come from the patient. Put on your Sherlock Holmes hat and go to work!

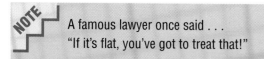

NOTE

A famous lawyer once said . . .
"If it's flat, you've got to treat that!"

ECG 14-27 So what do you think is causing the ST segment and T wave changes on this ECG? It meets many criteria for LVH, and also shows the changes necessary to diagnose the strain pattern. We want you to notice that the ST segments in V_6, I, and aVL are flat. They are not indicative of ischemia because of the company they keep. The leads immediately preceding them show concavity downward, and the flat segments are merely a continuation of the process. Also, are the T waves symmetrical or asymmetrical? They are asymmetrical, and this pattern is not indicative of ischemia. Go back and take a look at some of the ischemic ECGs, and you will see the difference. We will be spending a lot more time on this later in the chapter.

One good thing to remember is that the greatest deviation in the ST segment is always found in the leads with the tallest or deepest complexes. Can you identify ischemic pathology in LVH-with-strain? Definitely. The ST segments will not transition through the concave pattern that we are showing you on these ECGs. Recall that the ST elevation of LVH with strain is concave upward in V_1 to V_3, and the ST depression is concave downward in I, aVL, and V_4 to V_6. You will occasionally see upwardly concave ST segment elevation in V_5 to V_6 associated with a small Q wave in LVH. We will show you an example soon.

ECG CASE STUDIES: **CONTINUED**

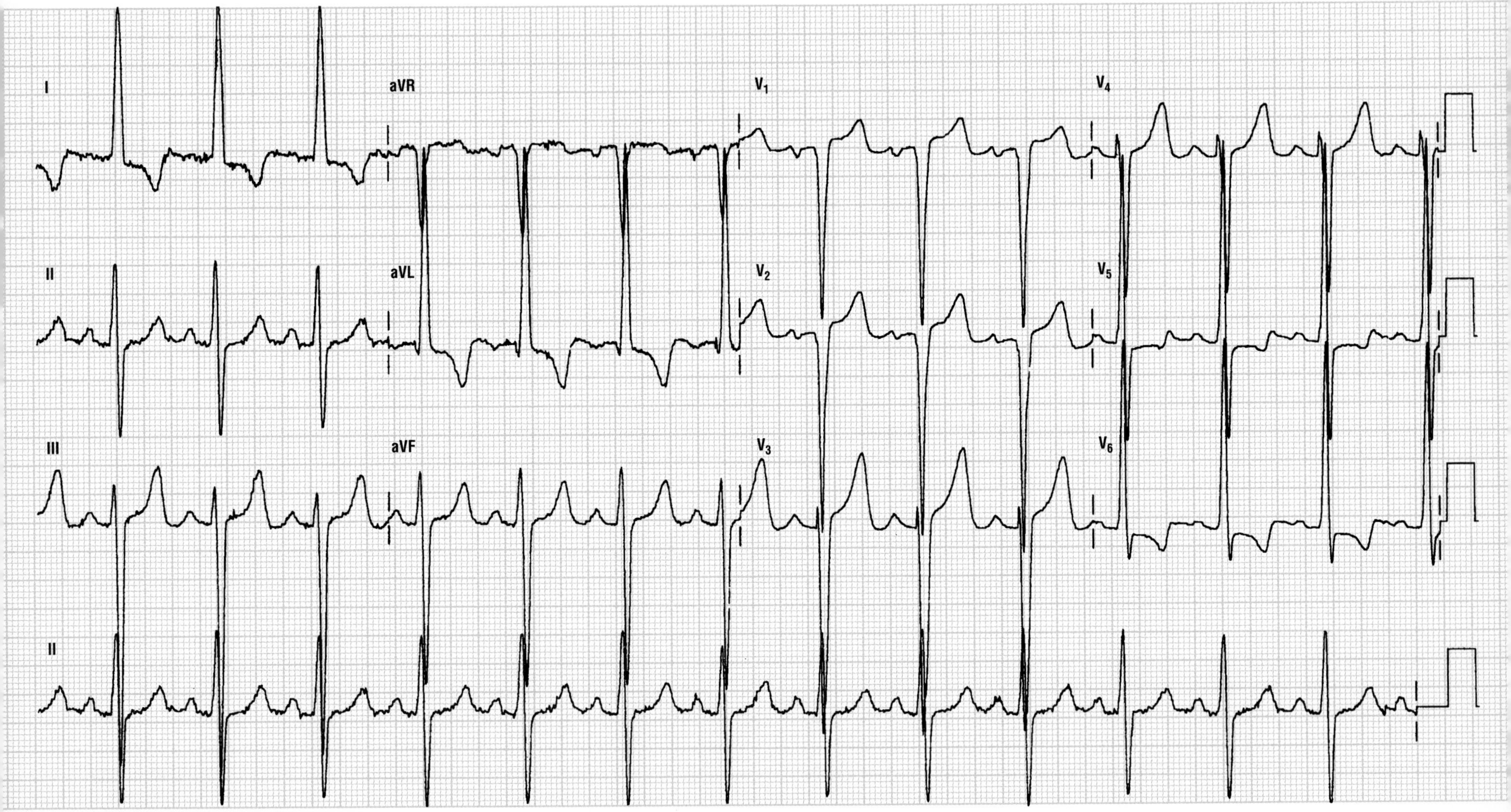

I   aVR   V₁   V₄

II   aVL   V₂   V₅

III   aVF   V₃   V₆

II

ECG 14-26

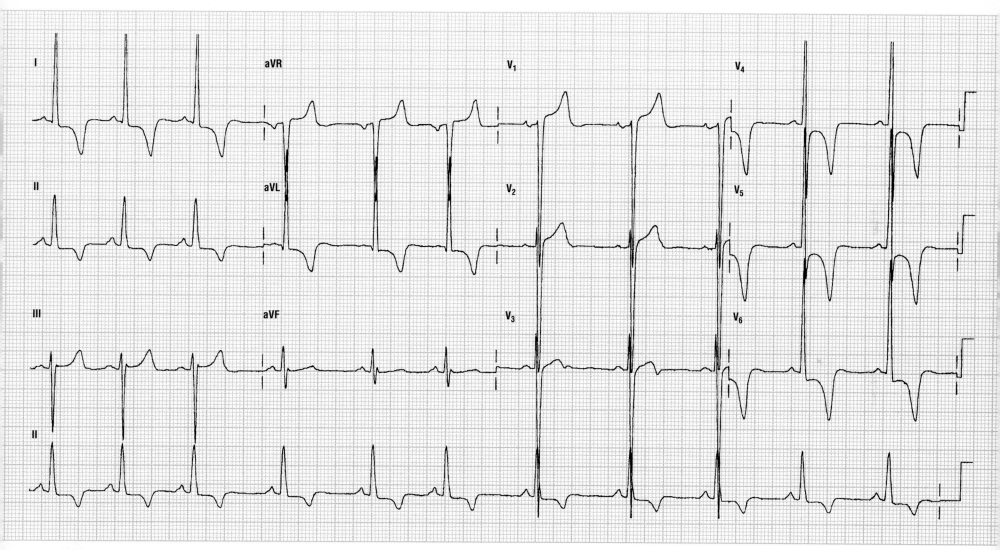

ECG 14-27

ECG CASE STUDIES: **CONTINUED**

ECG 14-28 Now we are going to show you a few more examples of how the ST segment progresses from concave downward to flat in the lateral precordial leads. Look at V_1 to V_6 in this ECG. We see the ST segment changing from one that is concave upward to flat in V_3, to concave downward in V_4 to V_5, and finally to depressed, downward sloping, and flat in V_6. Figure 14-24 gives a simplified look at this progression. This represents a benign transition in a patient with obvious LVH. Note the last statement: *in a patient with obvious LVH*. If the patient does not have obvious LVH, then all bets are off and this could represent ischemia. That is a key point. The strain pattern is only present in obvious LVH. *If you cannot diagnose LVH, you cannot diagnose LVH with strain.*

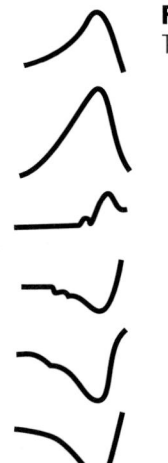

Figure 14-24: Transition of the ST segments and T waves of the precordial leads in ECG 14-28.

ECG 14-29 This is another example of LVH with strain. As in ECG 14-28, the ST segments progress to a flatter presentation in V_6. The flipped, asymmetric T waves in the inferior leads are also caused by LVH. Once again, notice that they are asymmetric and the ST segments are slightly concave downward. You still need to consider other possibilities, however, such as ischemia secondary to tachycardia or CAD.

The rest of the ECG is remarkable for sinus tachycardia and LAE. The QT interval is prolonged.

QUICK REVIEW

1. If a large pericardial effusion is present in a patient with LVH with strain, the voltage criteria may not be obvious. True or False.

2. You cannot diagnose AMI in LVH. True or False.

3. You cannot diagnose LVH in LBBB. True or False.

1. True 2. False 3. True

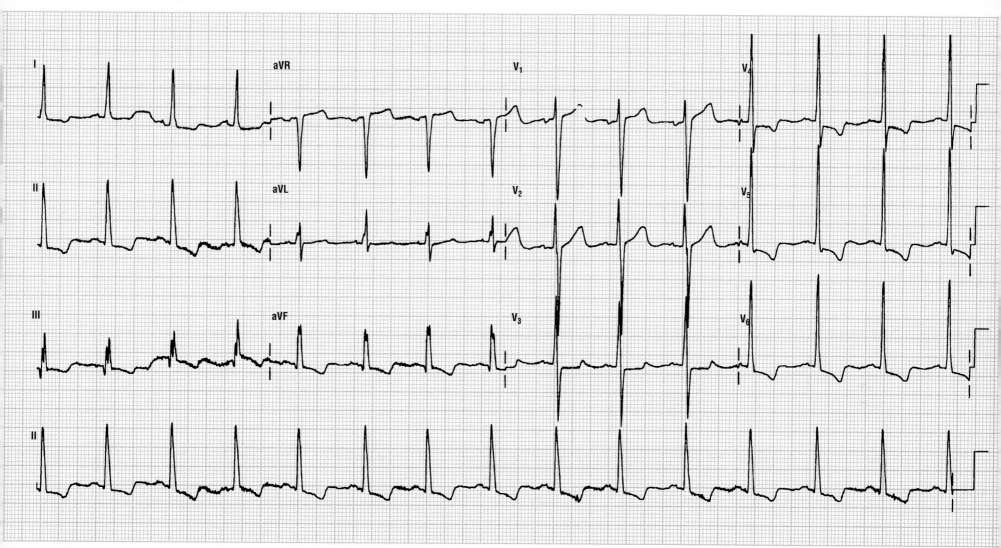

ECG 14-28

ECG CASE STUDIES: CONTINUED

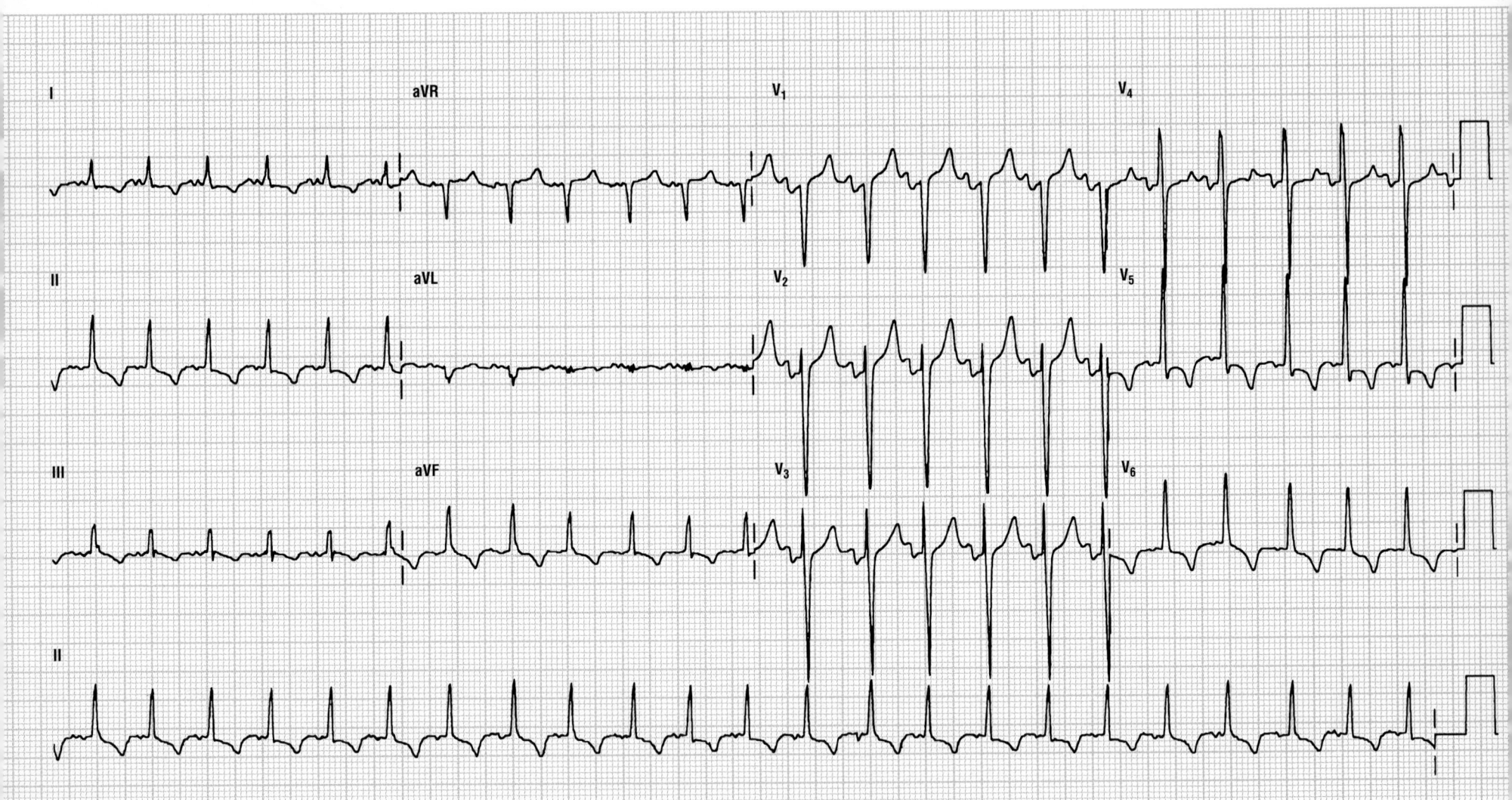

ECG 14-29

ECG CASE STUDIES: CONTINUED

②

ECG 14-30 This is another example of LVH with strain. This time we have added a few other goodies to the mix by giving you one with atrial fibrillation and a VPC. It is atrial fibrillation because of the irregularly irregular rhythm with no obvious P waves. The undulating baseline in V_1 is a coarse atrial fibrillation pattern. It is coarse because the undulation is very obvious (see also Figure 14-25, top). Compare that with the artifact at the beginning and the end of the ECG, which shows very fine, narrow spikes (Figure 14-25, bottom). It is important to be able to distinguish between artifact and real pathology on ECGs. That is why we have not removed artifact from the ECGs in this book.

Coarse atrial fibrillation

Figure 14-25

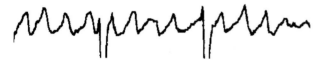

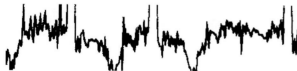

Artifact

②

ECG 14-31 A few ECGs ago, we mentioned that some examples of LVH present with small q waves in V_6 and are associated with a concave, upward scooping of the ST segments. This is just such a case. The LVH is obvious in this case, but the typical strain pattern is not present. This is a type of strain pattern found in patients with large, dilated left ventricles. It is caused by volume problems (aortic regurgitation, severe mitral regurgitation, and so on), not afterload pressure problems (systolic hypertension). This is an advanced concept, just mentioned here so that you will not be shocked when you see it in a real patient.

③

ECG 14-31 Dr. J. Willis Hurst describes two types of LVH patterns. The first is caused by systolic pressure overload as occurs in systolic hypertension or an outflow problem at the aortic valve. This type gives rise to the concave, downward ST depression and flipped T wave that we have already discussed. He also describes a second type, produced by diastolic pressure overload problems in ventricular hypertrophy with high volume (severe mitral or aortic regurgitation). That pattern is similar to the one below, with a small q wave and a concave, upward deflection of the ST segment. (See the Additional Readings section for further information.)

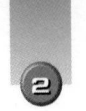

ECG CASE STUDIES: **CONTINUED**

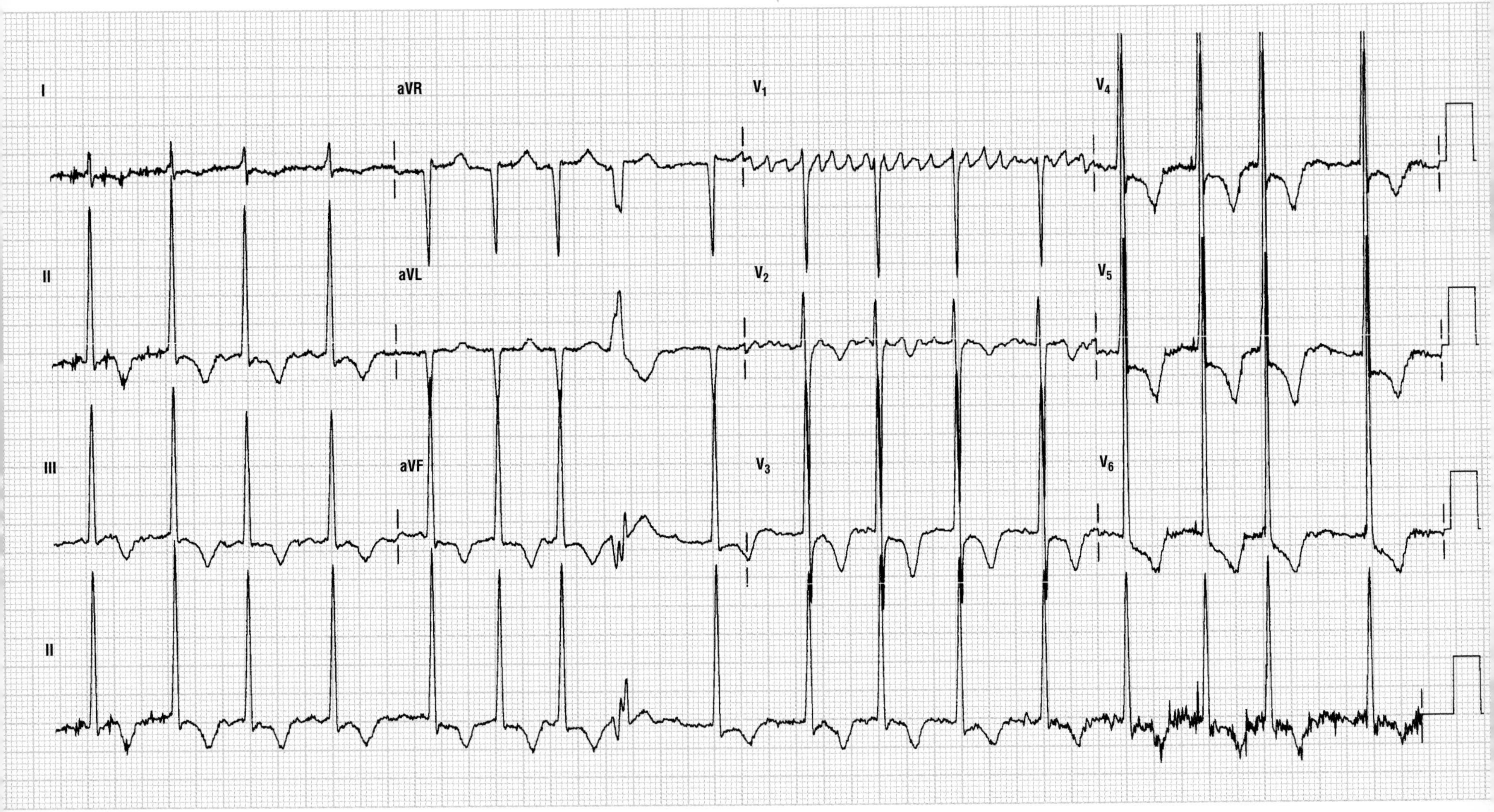

I aVR V_1 V_4

II aVL V_2 V_5

III aVF V_3 V_6

II

ECG 14-30

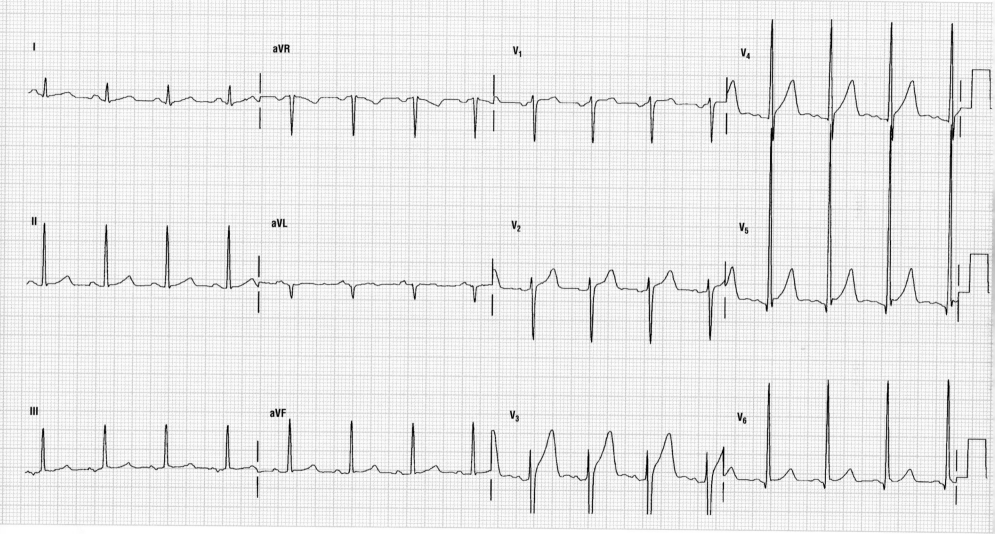

ECG 14-31

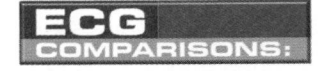 *Benign Changes Versus Infarct*

The toughest thing for any intermediate student is to decide if ST and T wave changes reflect infarct or a more benign form of pathology. We are going to give you 20 examples of each, side by side, to compare. Note that, by saying "good," we don't mean normal, but rather the lesser of two evils when compared with an infarct. Let's get started.

Good: ECG 14-32A These ST segments show the typical changes for LVH with strain. Note the asymmetrical T waves throughout.

Bad: ECG 14-32B These ST segments, in comparison, are flat and either elevated or depressed. Note that they are elevated in the inferior leads of II, III, and aVF, and depressed in the reciprocal areas of I and aVL. We will spend more time on reciprocal changes in Chapter 15. For now, just understand that I and aVL should show changes opposite to those in II, III, and aVF, if there is an AMI present. Note the presence of a pathological Q wave starting in lead III.

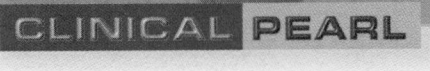

Always remember that ECGs, just as most medical tests, cannot be interpreted in a vacuum. What we mean is that you have to use all of the information available to you at the time of interpretation to make your diagnosis. "The company it keeps" is our motto. If an ECG looks pathological but the patient does not, question the diagnosis. Could this be a ventricular aneurysm? Could it be someone else's ECG that was given to you by mistake? Could it be silent ischemia? Could it be an electrolyte problem? Always put your ECG and what you know about the patient together in your mind. If something does not match, there is always a reason.

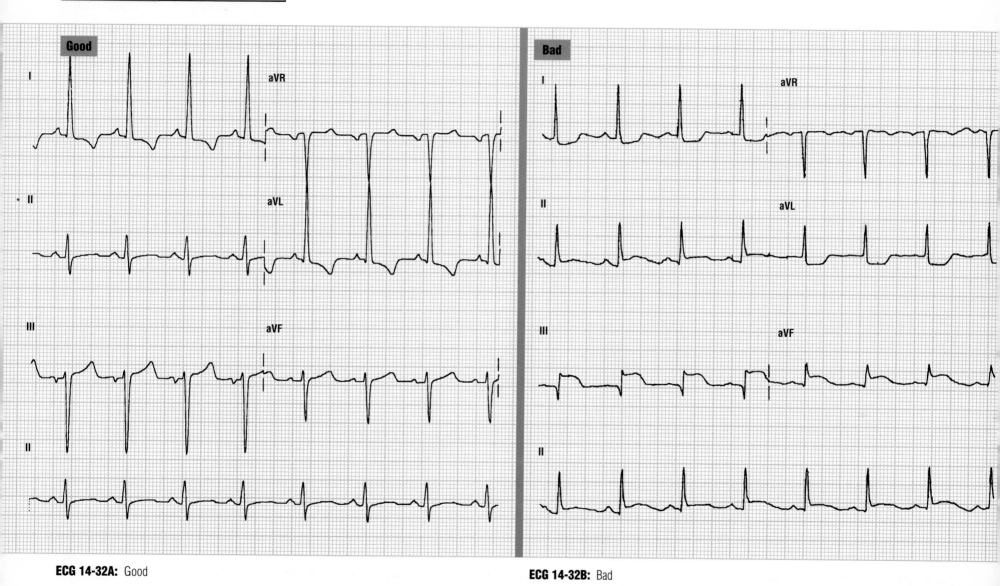

Good

Bad

ECG 14-32A: Good

ECG 14-32B: Bad

ECG COMPARISONS: CONTINUED

Good: ECG 14-33A This is another example of LVH with strain. Notice the quality of the strain changes in A and compare them to the "bad" example in B. Also note that the flipped Ts are asymmetrical in both I and aVL and II and aVF, which could represent pathology.

Hopefully you are picking up on what we are trying to do in this section. We want you to begin to get a feel for life-threatening ST changes. This is a critical step in your development, and you should be sure you understand the differences.

Bad: ECG 14-33B These ST segments are, once again, flat in the reciprocal leads. There is no concavity, or very little, in their slopes. Nor is there any gradual transition to flat. They are just flat to start with. Notice the symmetrical quality of the Ts; they almost blend with the ST segments. This is an IWMI.

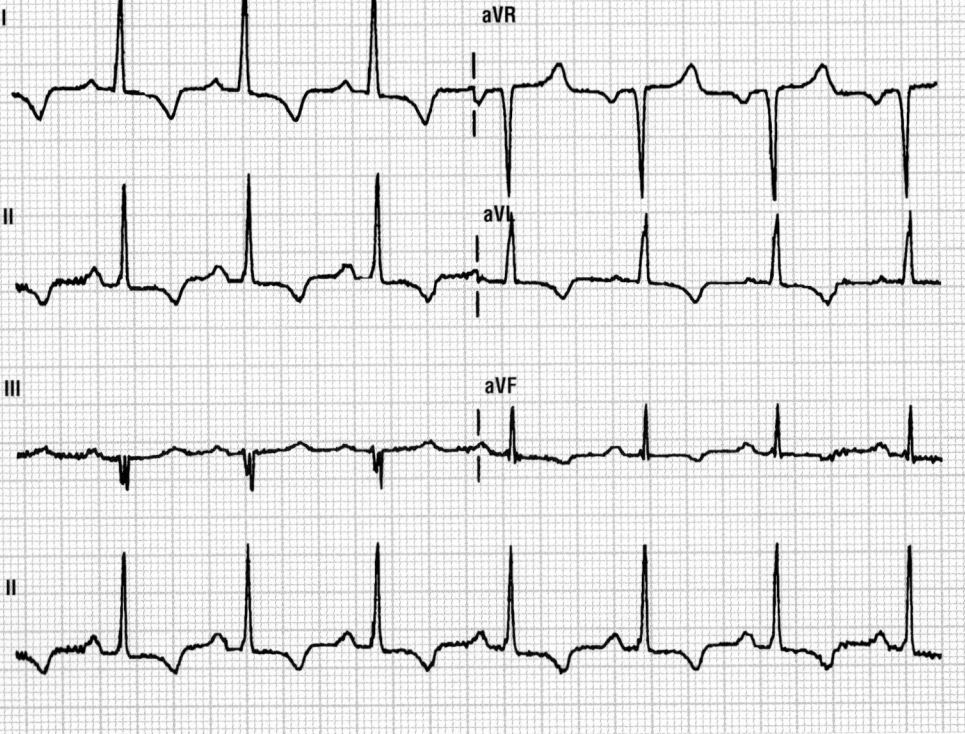

ECG 14-33A: Good

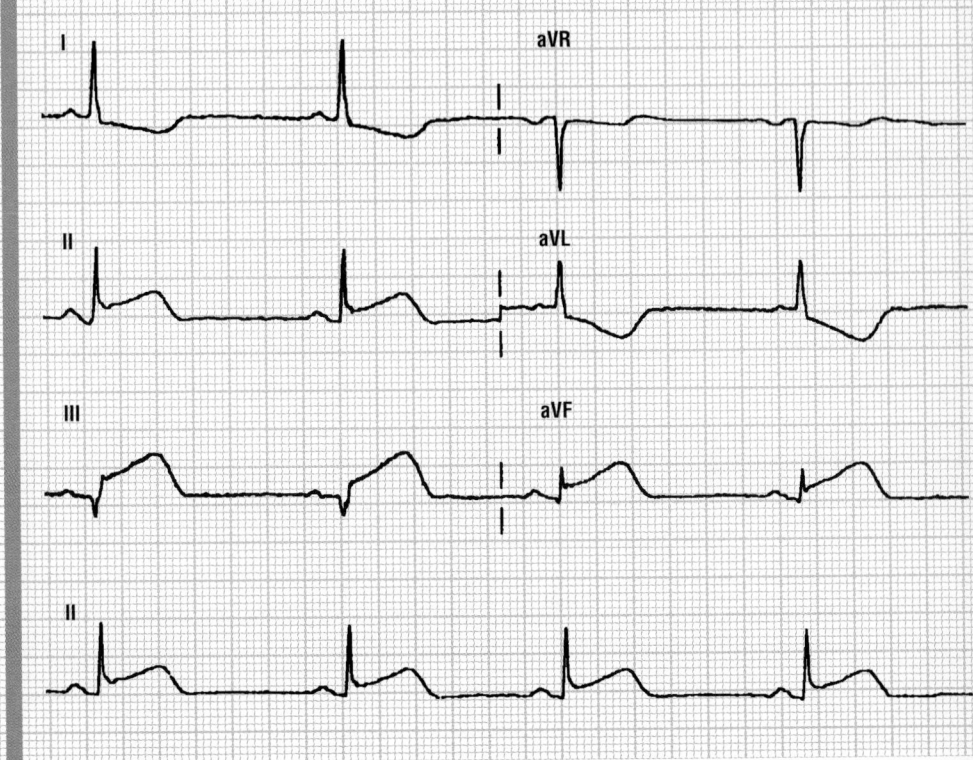

ECG 14-33B: Bad

Good: ECG 14-34A This is RVH with strain. The ST segments have a definite concavity. The T waves are also asymmetrical, and there is a smooth transition from the ST segment.

Bad: ECG 14-34B This is an example of a posterior wall AMI. The ST depression is obvious and the slope is negative. Notice how the ST segments transition to horizontal and flat without going through any concave phase. Finally, look at the rhythm strip, which is lead II. The ST elevation suggests an inferior wall MI, as well. Don't worry about the regions for now; just concentrate on the differences in appearances.

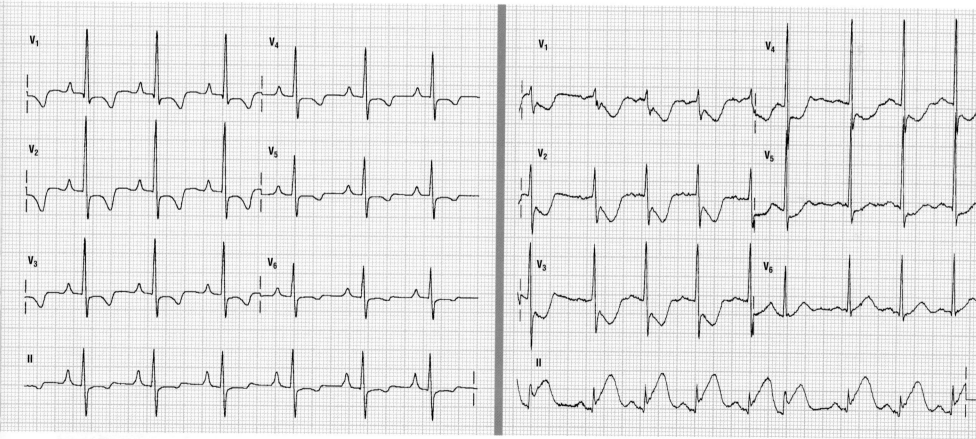

ECG 14-34A: Good

ECG 14-34B: Bad

CHAPTER **14** • ST SEGMENT AND T WAVES

ECG COMPARISONS: CONTINUED

Good: ECG 14-35A Remember this ECG? It was the strange RBBB with no RSR' wave in V_1. There are diffuse ST segment changes, all concave. Notice the width of the R wave in V_1 to V_2. It is very wide because of the RBBB; this is an RSR' pattern.

Bad: ECG 14-35B This ECG also has a wide R wave, greater than 0.03 seconds. There is an increased R:S ratio in V_2, although it does not approach 1:1. This time it is not due to an RBBB because there is not an increased R:S ratio in V_1, or a slurred S wave in V_6. The ST depression in V_2 to V_6 is pathological. What was the differential diagnosis for increased R:S ratio in lead V_1 or V_2? If you review the criteria, you will note that this is another posterior wall AMI.

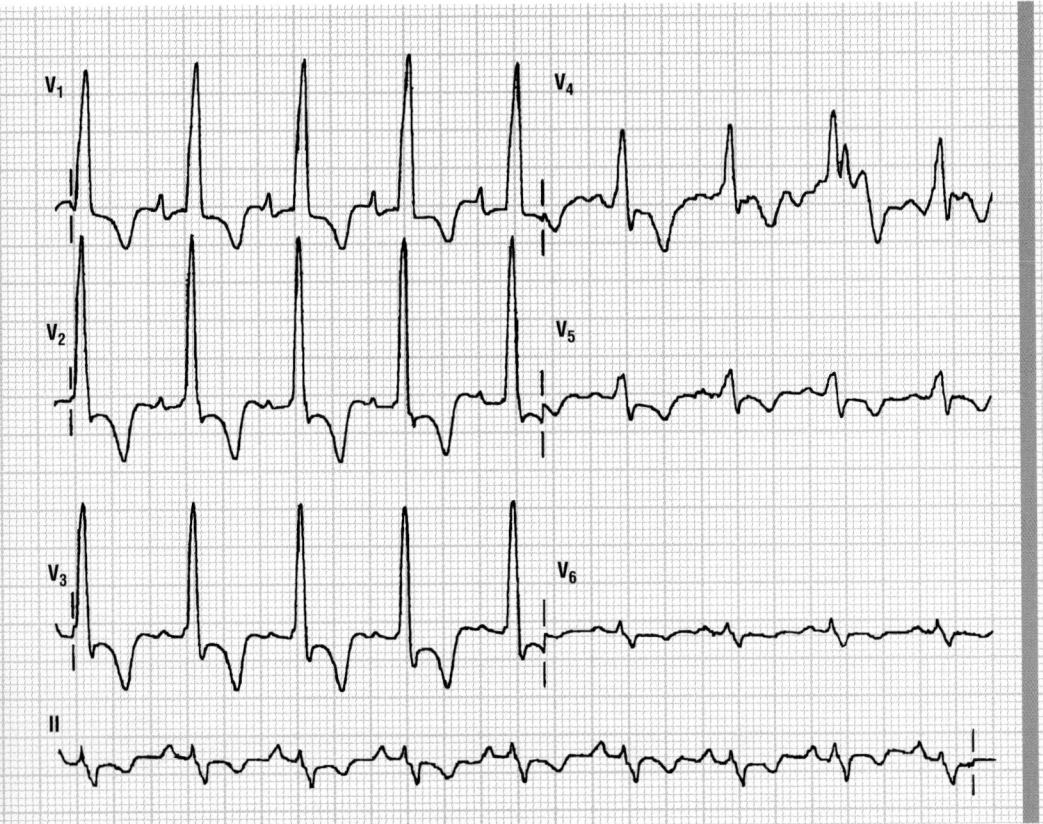

ECG 14-35A: Good

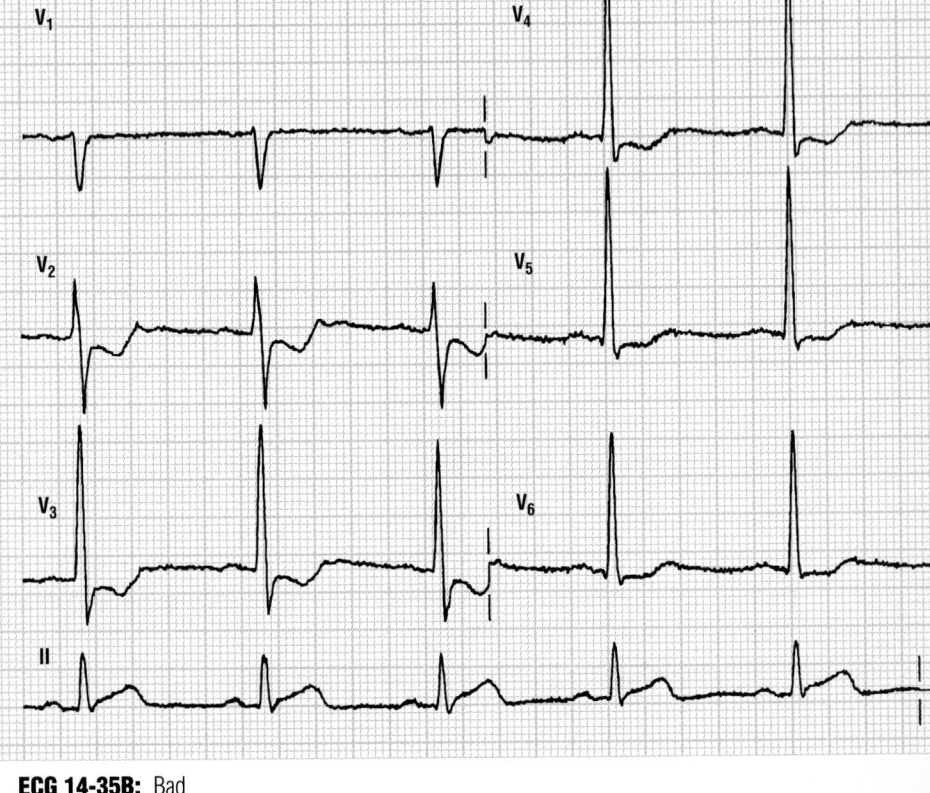

ECG 14-35B: Bad

Good: ECG 14-36A This could be minimal pericarditis, or a variant of normal known as early repolarization. Notice how the waves are benign in appearance. The QRS complexes have some notching in the lateral leads, so the ST segment elevation is therefore associated with a benign cause. There is minimal PR depression, but it is within normal limits. All of the ST segments are concave upward, except for V_1. Also note that the lead with the tallest R wave has the most ST elevation.

Bad: ECG 14-36B This ECG has a transition from ST depression to elevation, but the ST segments are always flat. The T waves are symmetrical and broad. Note the increased R:S ratio in V_2. Go through your differentials for this finding. What is the most likely culprit? Posterior wall AMI. The ST elevation along the lateral leads is consistent with a lateral wall infarction. Lateral wall MIs are associated with posterior wall MIs. Don't worry about the exact diagnoses for now; just note the MIs.

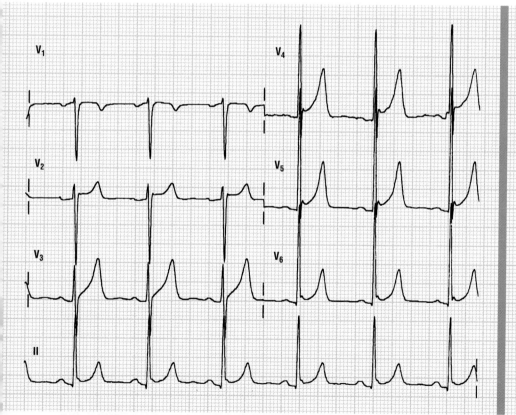

ECG 14-36A: Good

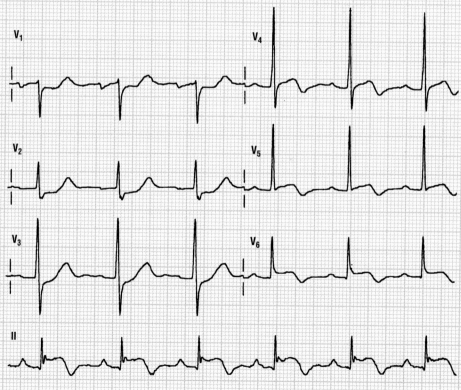

ECG 14-36B: Bad

CHAPTER **14** • ST SEGMENT AND T WAVES

Good: ECG 14-37A This is similar to ECG 14-36A, and is due to one of the same two causes. The notching is a bit more obvious, and the ST elevation a little more prominent.

Bad: ECG 14-37B The ST elevation in this ECG starts off flat, with an upward slope in lead V_4. This is a sign of an injury/infarct pattern. It affects the lateral leads, and so represents a lateral infarct. Did you notice the rhythm strip at the bottom? The ST elevation in II also leads one to believe that the inferior wall is involved. Make sure you note the differences between the ST segments of the lateral leads in these two ECGs. They're dramatic.

REMINDER:

Notching is usually benign. It can, however, also occur in pericarditis and hypothermia. Once again, remember the motto, "the company it keeps." If the person is having chest pain that is worse when lying back and eases when sitting up, it is probably pericarditis. If the person has no symptoms and is young, it is probably early repolarization. If the person is cold, has an altered mental status, and the temperature outside is 20° below zero, it is probably hypothermia.

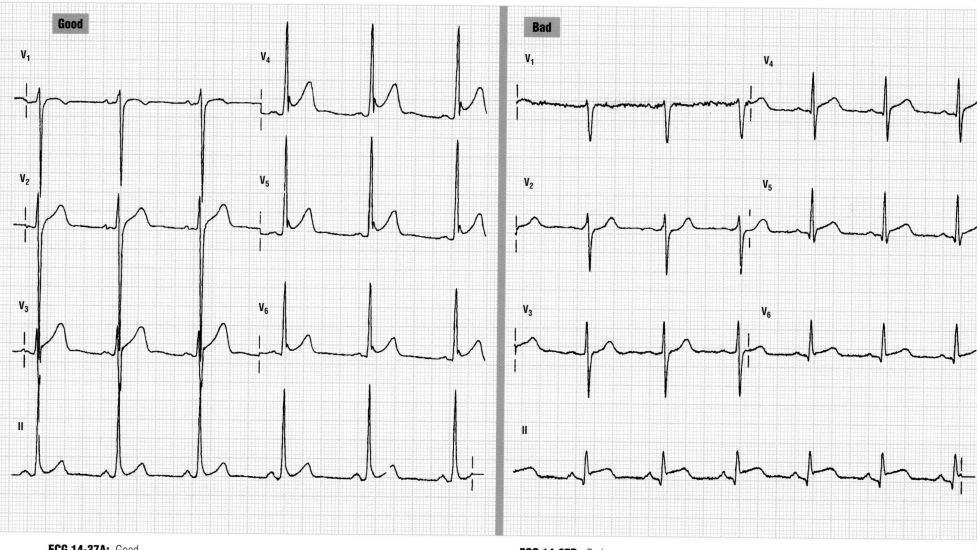

Good

V₁

V₂

V₃

II

V₄

V₅

V₆

Bad

V₁

V₂

V₃

II

V₄

V₅

V₆

ECG 14-37A: Good

ECG 14-37B: Bad

CHAPTER **14** • ST SEGMENT AND T WAVES

ECG COMPARISONS: C O N T I N U E D

Good: ECG 14-38A The lateral leads definitely show LVH with strain. The anterior leads are also consistent with the strain pattern, but are a little flat for our taste. We would still be very concerned about this pattern except that the patient also had this on an old ECG, and was asymptomatic. There is still some concavity to the ST segment, and the one with the tallest ST elevation is V_1, which has the deepest S wave. With these findings and correlations, we can state that this is LVH with strain.

Bad: ECG 14-38B The main focus of this ECG is the lateral leads. Notice how the ST segments there are deep and flat? This is definitely lateral ischemia and not LVH with strain. LVH is present, but the depression is not indicative of strain. V_1 is troublesome but, because it appears in one lead only, it is not highly significant for infarct.

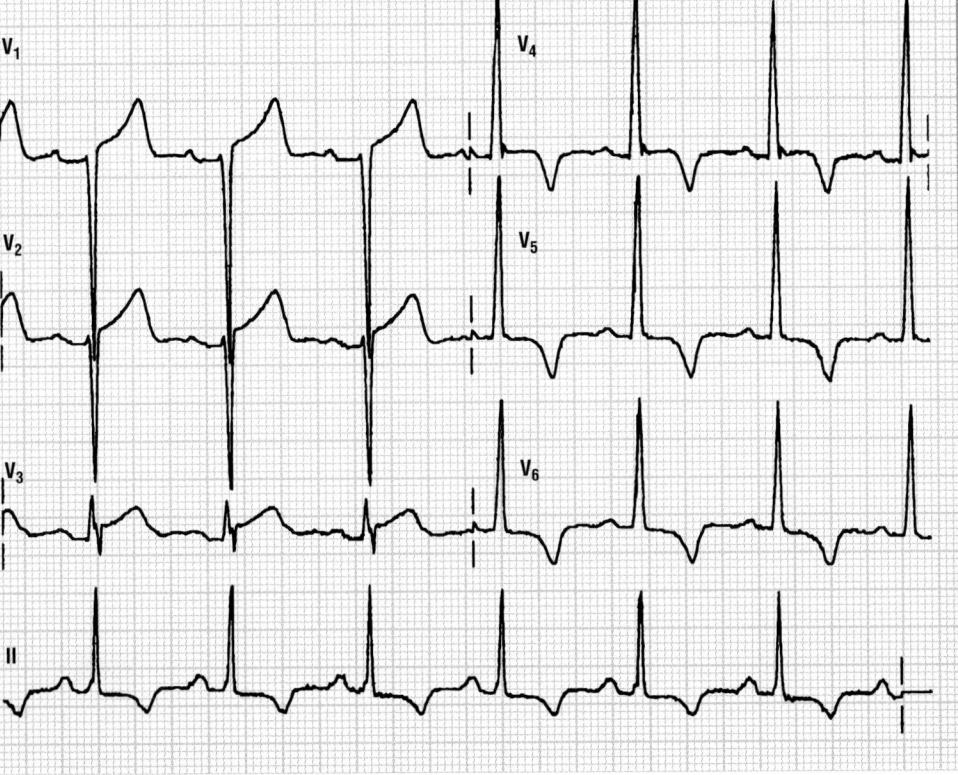

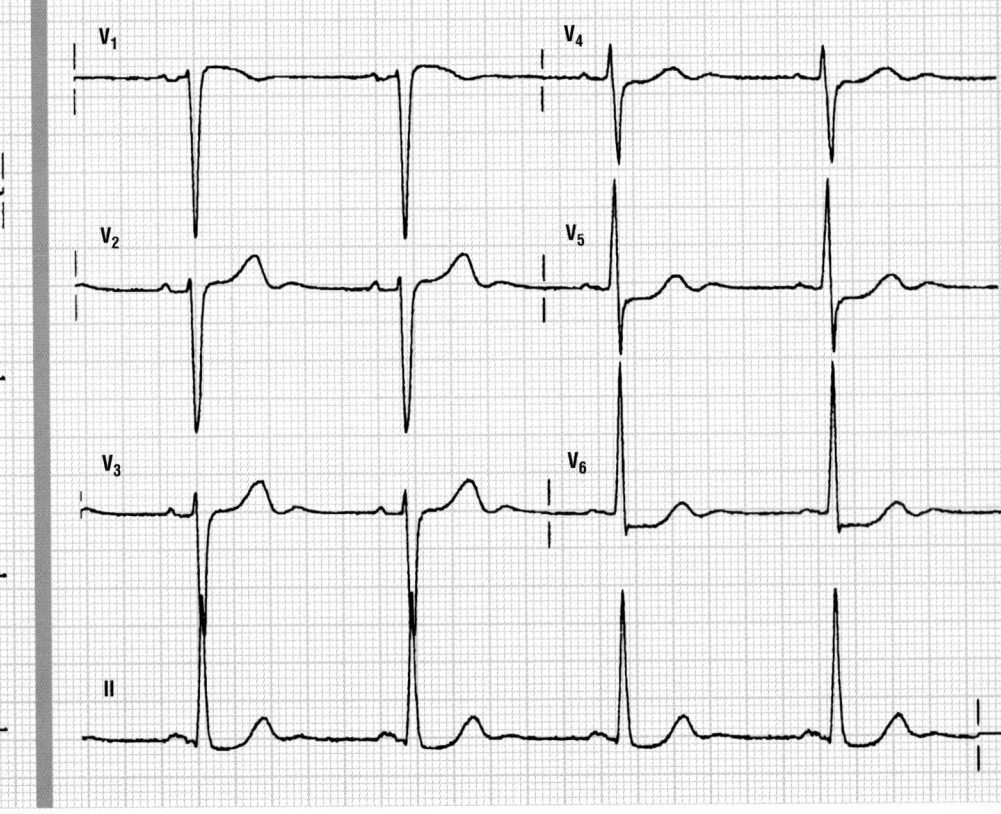

ECG 14-38A: Good

ECG 14-38B: Bad

Good: ECG 14-39A This is another example of a strain or early repolarization pattern. The criterion for LVH is met by adding the S wave in V_2 to the R wave in V_6. Once again, there is concavity of the ST segments, and the lead with the deepest S wave has the highest ST segment. The J point is quite diffuse in V_2, and even in V_1.

Bad: ECG 14-39B Badness, badness everywhere. . . . The ST segments are elevated through all of the precordial leads. The QT interval is short, so it gives the complexes a bizarre appearance. The Q waves in the lateral leads are not significant.

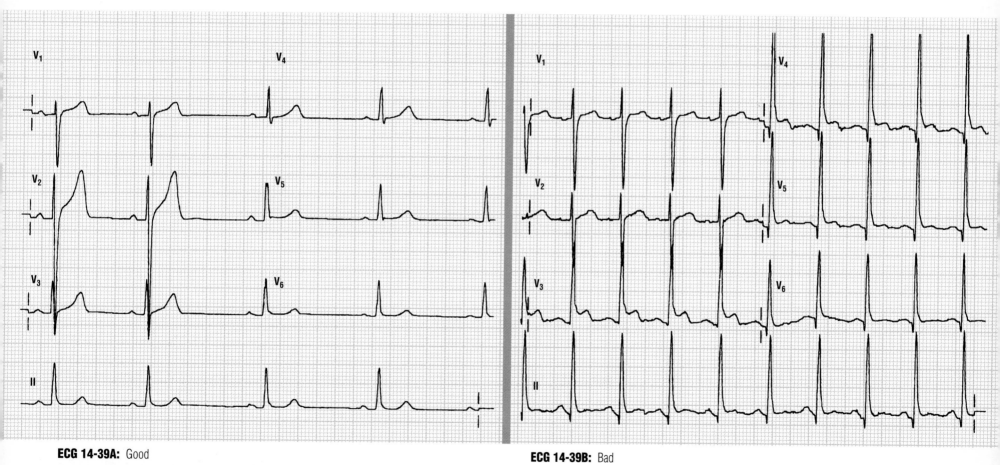

ECG 14-39A: Good

ECG 14-39B: Bad

CHAPTER **14** • ST SEGMENT AND T WAVES

ECG COMPARISONS: **CONTINUED**

Good: ECG 14-40A This ECG meets multiple criteria for LVH with strain. LAE is also present. We don't want to bore you with repetition, but repetition is the only way you can understand the comparison between good and bad. Only after seeing hundreds of ECGs with these changes will you feel comfortable making the call.

Bad: ECG 14-40B The ST segment changes are again indicative of ischemia. The ECG suggests a posterior wall AMI because of the increased R:S ratio, the flat ST segments, and the final positive deflection of the T wave. This time, however, there is no associated infarct in the inferior leads. Lead II also shows ST depression suggestive of ischemia. These diffuse ST depressions are sometimes seen in global subendocardial ischemia (ischemia of the myocardium lining the ventricles).

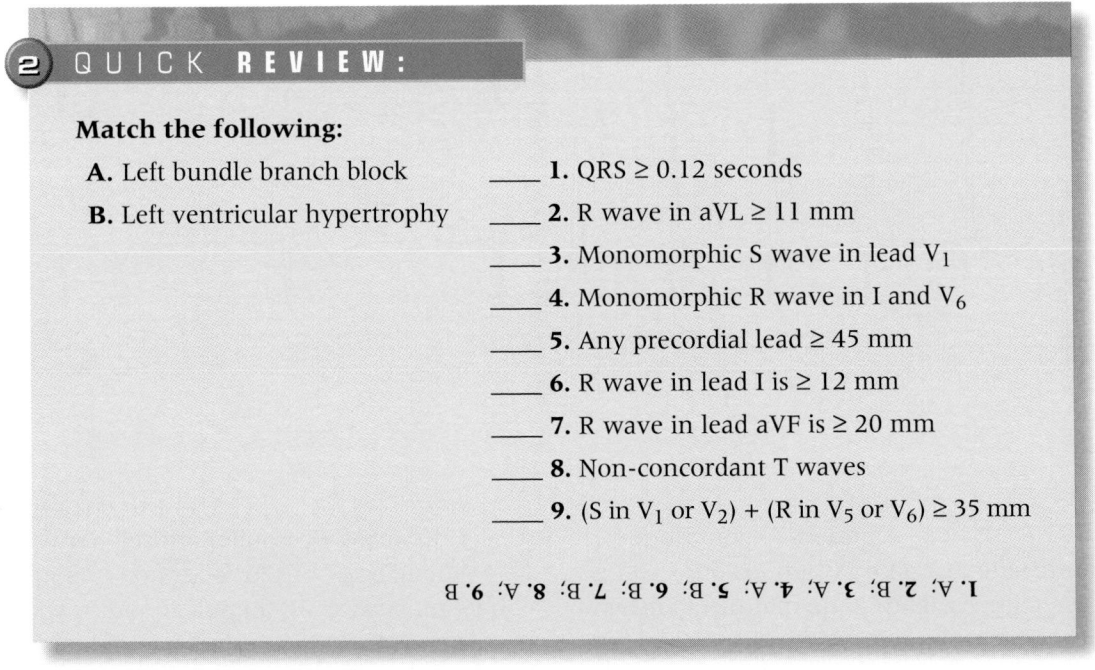

QUICK REVIEW:

Match the following:

A. Left bundle branch block

B. Left ventricular hypertrophy

_____ **1.** QRS ≥ 0.12 seconds

_____ **2.** R wave in aVL ≥ 11 mm

_____ **3.** Monomorphic S wave in lead V_1

_____ **4.** Monomorphic R wave in I and V_6

_____ **5.** Any precordial lead ≥ 45 mm

_____ **6.** R wave in lead I is ≥ 12 mm

_____ **7.** R wave in lead aVF is ≥ 20 mm

_____ **8.** Non-concordant T waves

_____ **9.** (S in V_1 or V_2) + (R in V_5 or V_6) ≥ 35 mm

1. A; 2. B; 3. A; 4. A; 5. B; 6. B; 7. B; 8. A; 9. B

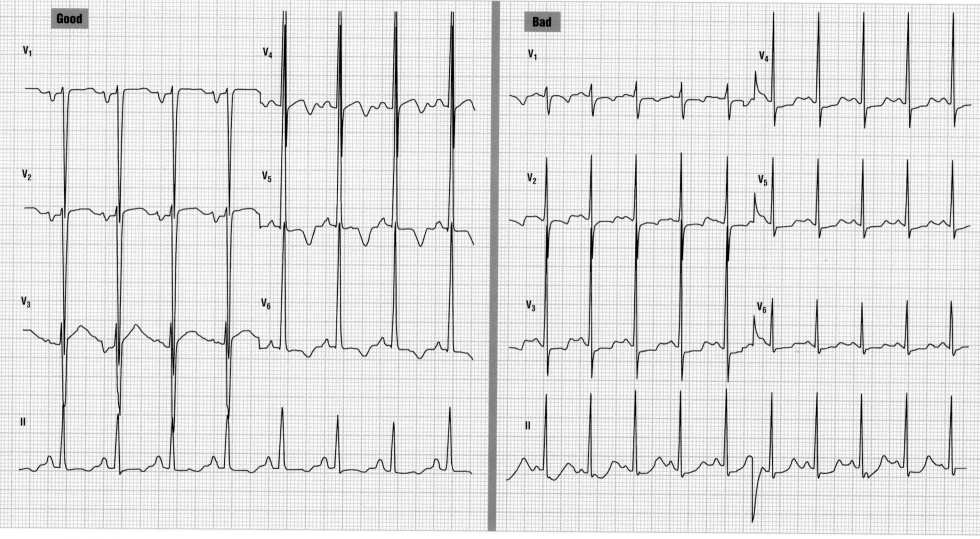

Good

V₁

V₂

V₃

II

V₄

V₅

V₆

Bad

V₁

V₂

V₃

II

V₄

V₅

V₆

ECG 14-40A: Good

ECG 14-40B: Bad

CHAPTER **14** • ST SEGMENT AND T WAVES

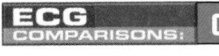
Good: ECG 14-41A This is another beautifully clear example of LVH with strain. You should be getting familiar with this pattern by now. Are you starting to feel comfortable with the difference? You should be starting to, but remembering the differences when you are faced with an ECG that doesn't have a bad one standing next to it is a bit tougher.

Bad: ECG 14-41B This ECG was taken from a patient who had markedly elevated blood pressure and diffuse subendocardial ischemia, similar to ECG 14-40B. However, look at how pronounced the changes are in comparison. The ST elevation in lead V_1 is also indicative of injury or infarction.

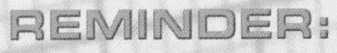

REMINDER:

ST depression in leads V_1 and V_2 is always pathological in adults. It can be due to right ventricular hypertrophy, a right bundle branch block, a posterior wall MI, or WPW. Think of the differential diagnosis of the problem and see which one of the differentials best matches your patient and the ECG.

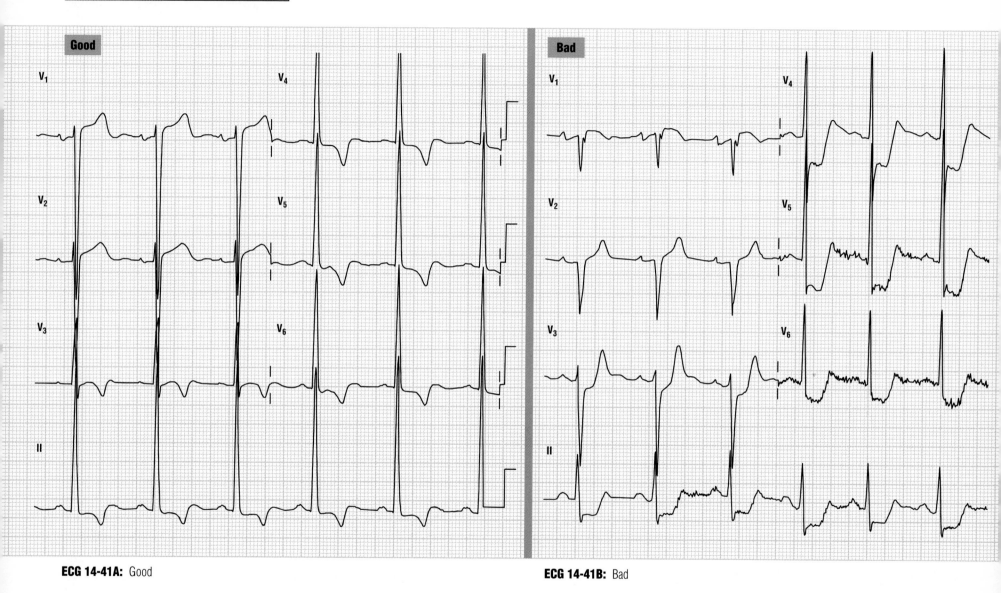

Good

V₁ V₄

V₂ V₅

V₃ V₆

II

Bad

V₁ V₄

V₂ V₅

V₃ V₆

II

ECG 14-41A: Good

ECG 14-41B: Bad

CHAPTER **14** • ST SEGMENT AND T WAVES

ECG
COMPARISONS: **CONTINUED**

Good: ECG 14-42A Is this one an LBBB pattern? Go ahead and measure the QRS complexes out with your calipers. They don't quite make it to 0.12 seconds, so it is just a really wide LVH with strain. The amplitude of the QRS complexes is impressive, more than meeting the 45 mm criterion.

Bad: ECG 14-42B This ECG shows the obvious ST deformities characteristic of ischemia. Once again, notice the flat, downward-sloping ST segments.

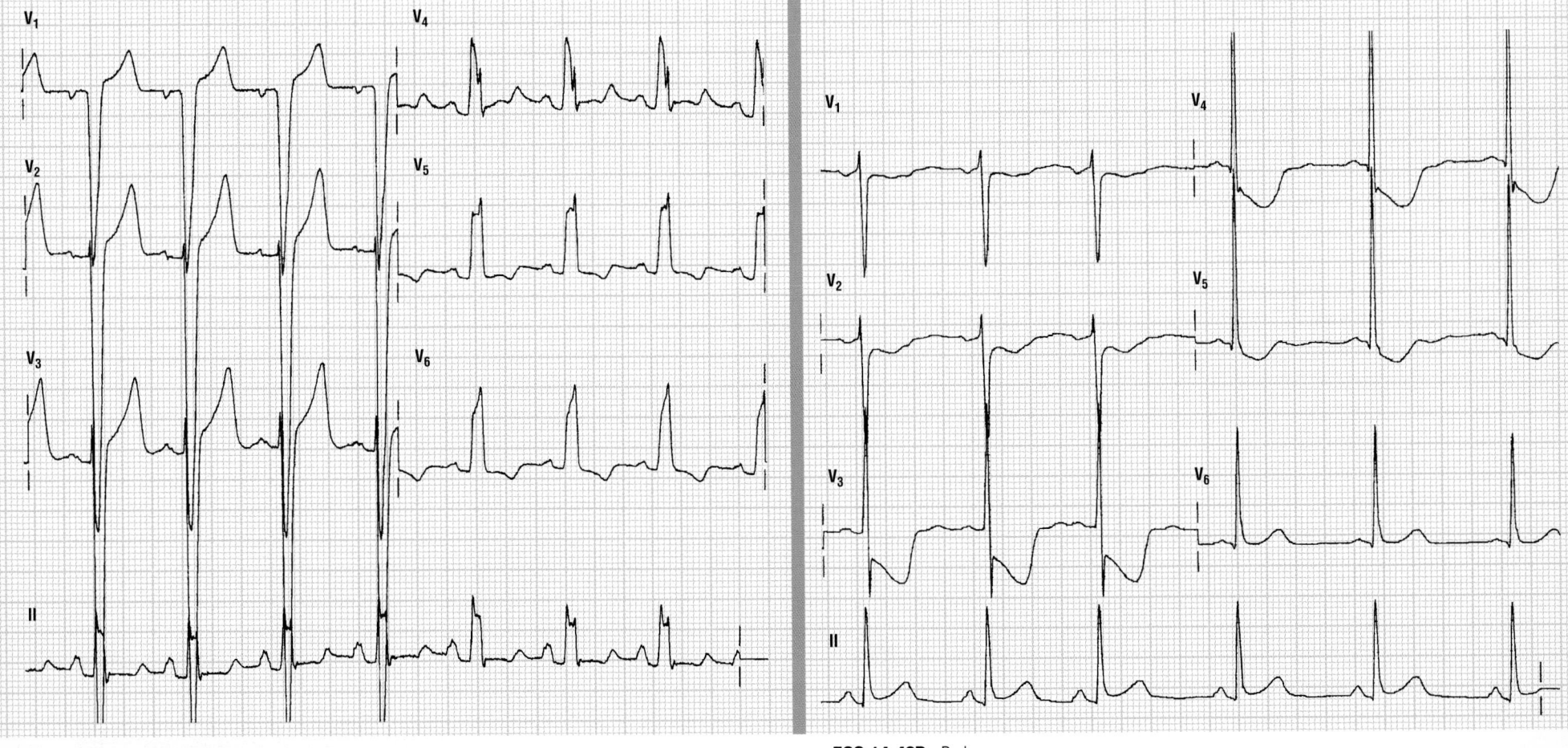

ECG 14-42A: Good

ECG 14-42B: Bad

Good: ECG 14-43A Even though this ECG is obviously LVH with strain, notice how similar B at right is to leads V_1 to V_3. The upward concavity is a great tip-off, but this can be deceptive. What can we use to help distinguish between the two ECGs? Remember "the company it keeps." The lateral leads show the typical changes of LVH with strain on A, but they are not present on B. In many cases, the lateral leads will help you sort out the right precordial leads.

Bad: ECG 14-43B This ECG came from a patient suffering an anteroseptal AMI. The J point is diffuse, but notice the flat ST segments, especially in V_1 and V_2. What appears to be concavity is actually the symmetrical, broad T wave starting off the ST segment. Draw the two legs of the T wave in V_2 down to the baseline to see what we mean. The ST elevation in V_4 is also very flat. (Did you notice V_6? This is what happens when a lead falls off.)

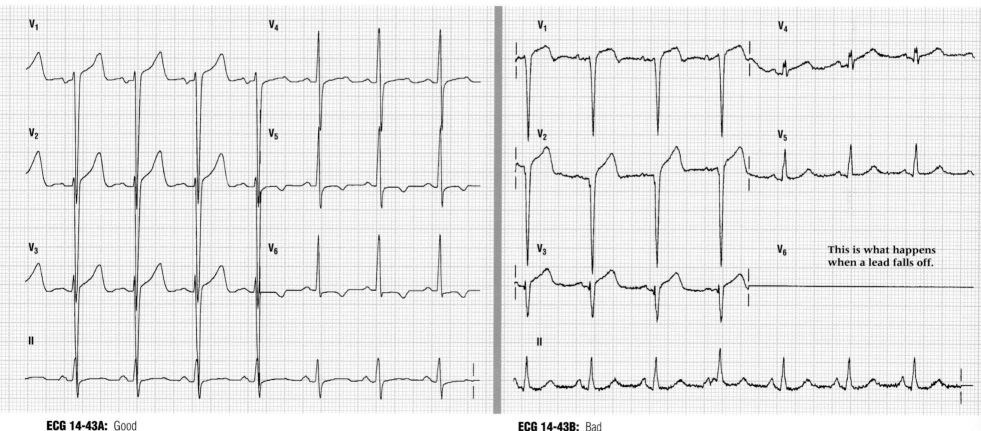

ECG 14-43A: Good

ECG 14-43B: Bad

ECG COMPARISONS: CONTINUED

Good: ECG 14-44A Are the ST segment changes caused by LVH with strain? Perhaps, but this time the strain pattern is not obvious. Could this ECG be from a young man with some early repolarization changes? Yes, the J point is diffuse and it would match the pattern. Whatever the source, we see some notching in V_4 to V_6 and definite asymmetry of the T waves, to make us feel comfortable in making the call that this is benign ST elevation. Clinical correlation is mandatory, however.

Bad: ECG 14-44B If you were to look just at V_1 and V_2, this would be a tough call because some LVH with strain looks just like these leads. However, once you get down to V_3, your answer is clear. Bad. This is an anteroseptal AMI with lateral extension.

Look at the similarity between V_6 on this ECG and on *A*. Scary, isn't it? Remember always to look at the company it keeps — and at the patient!

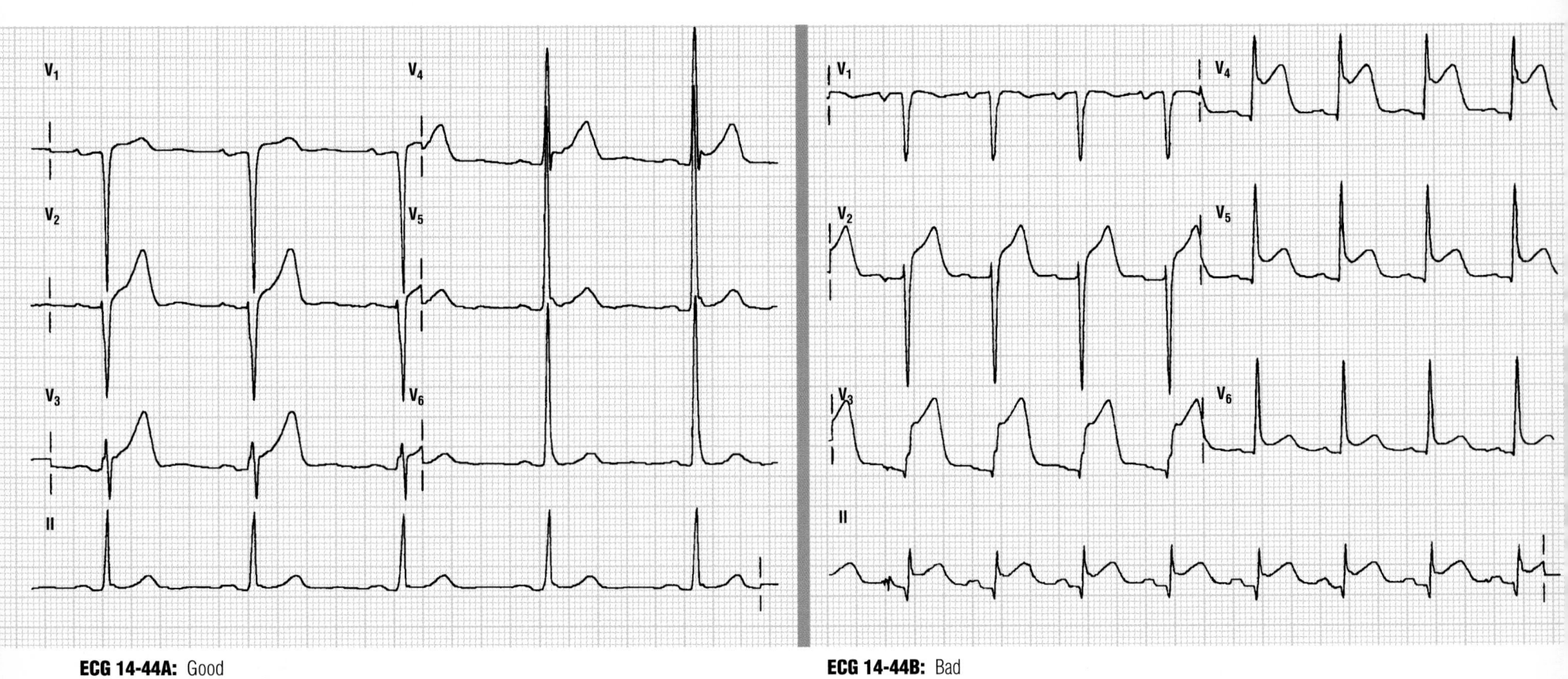

ECG 14-44A: Good

ECG 14-44B: Bad

Good: ECG 14-45A We are dealing with a wide LVH with strain once again, not an LBBB. There is a late intrinsicoid deflection. (Whoa, there's something we haven't discussed in awhile; go ahead and review it on page 43 to refresh your memory.) There is also a very pretty U wave present after the T in most leads, which is a benign finding.

Bad ECG 14-45B This is an ugly anteroseptal infarct with lateral extension right from V_1 through to V_6. The ST elevation is quite marked and the T waves are symmetrical.

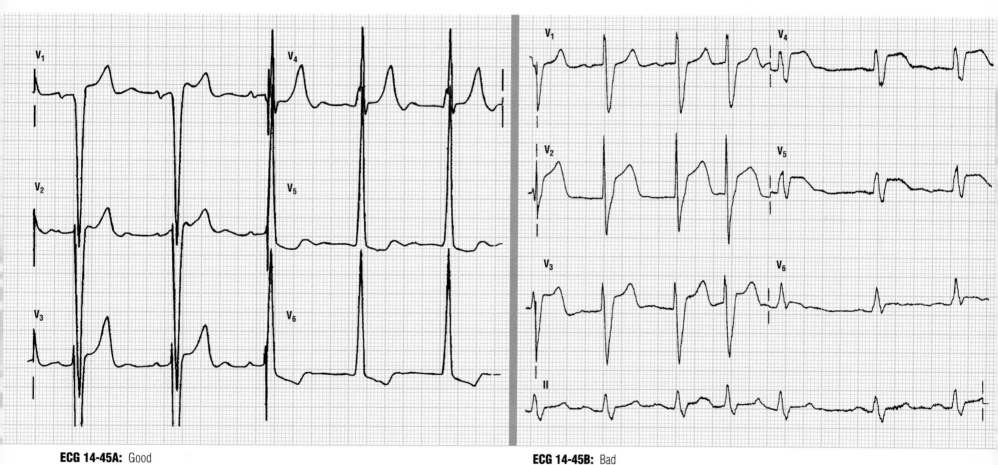

ECG 14-45A: Good

ECG 14-45B: Bad

1. False! If there is one thing you should always remember, it is that many times you cannot tell the difference between LVH with strain and an acute infarct. You always need to clinically correlate your ECG with your patient. You should also try to obtain an old ECG whenever possible to compare with the new one. I have known many unfortunate clinicians (who have many unfortunate patients!) who have given thrombolytics for LVH with strain in asymptomatic patients. I know many, many more who have not given thrombolytics to patients with AMI because they thought it was just LVH with strain. These are experienced clinicians that have been practicing for years. It is not always clear. Remember, always interpret an ECG in the company that it keeps! **2.** False. It is usually depressed in the left lateral leads of V_4 to V_6. **3.** False. The ST segment is usually depressed in leads V_1 and V_2 in patients with RVH with strain. **4.** False! This is another big fallacy. Remember, however, that many times an AMI patient may subsequently develop pericarditis either acutely or after a few weeks (Dressler's syndrome). Always interpret an ECG by the company it keeps! If you are unsure, get some help! Never assume that you are correct — always **make sure** that you are before you treat any patient. **5.** B.

2 QUICK REVIEW:

1. You can always tell the difference between LVH with strain and an AMI or ischemia. True or False.

2. The ST segment in LVH with strain is always elevated. True or False.

3. The ST segment in RVH with strain is always elevated in V_1 and V_2. True or False.

4. You can always distinguish the ST elevation of pericarditis from that of LVH with strain or AMI. True or False.

5. A famous lawyer once said: If it's flat . . .
   a. I'm OK with that!
   b. You gotta treat that!
   c. You gotta give a thrombolytic to that!
   d. You can ignore that!
   e. Who cares about that!

Bad: ECG 14-46A This ECG appears very benign but there are some things that make it troubling. Can you spot them? Well, for starters, the ST segment elevation in V_1 to V_2 is flat. Next, the T waves are symmetrical through the entire precordium. There is definitely LVH present, but there is no classic strain pattern. Beware of this benign ECG! It could spell big trouble if you don't get an old one or correlate it closely to the patient's symptoms.

Worse: ECG 14-46B Notice that there are QS waves all the way to V_4. These QS waves are associated with some tombstoning ST segments. This is an anteroseptal infarct that has been going on for some time and has already formed Q waves. By the way, did you notice the PR interval? Pretty wide.

2

ECG COMPARISONS: CONTINUED

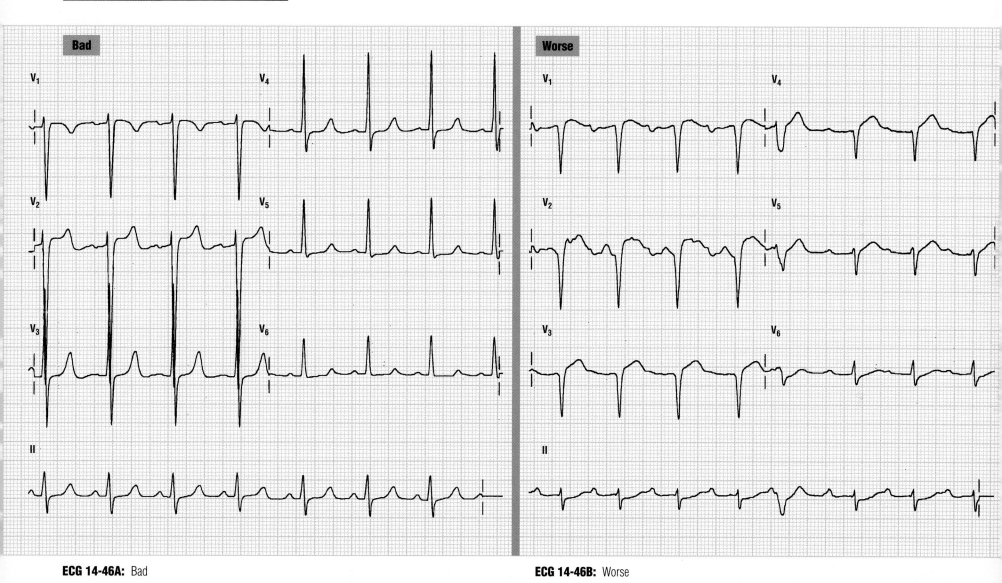

Bad

V₁

V₂

V₃

II

Worse

V₁

V₂

V₃

II

V₄

V₅

V₆

ECG 14-46A: Bad

ECG 14-46B: Worse

ECG COMPARISONS: CONTINUED

Good: ECG 14-47A Well, we're back to our benign pattern again. ECG 14-46 was just thrown in there to keep you awake. This ECG is either early repolarization pattern or LVH with some strain in the right precordial leads.

Bad: ECG 14-47B These ST segments are obviously pathological, with flat segments and a positive slope. The T waves in the lateral leads are also flipped and symmetrical. This is an anteroseptal AMI with lateral extension.

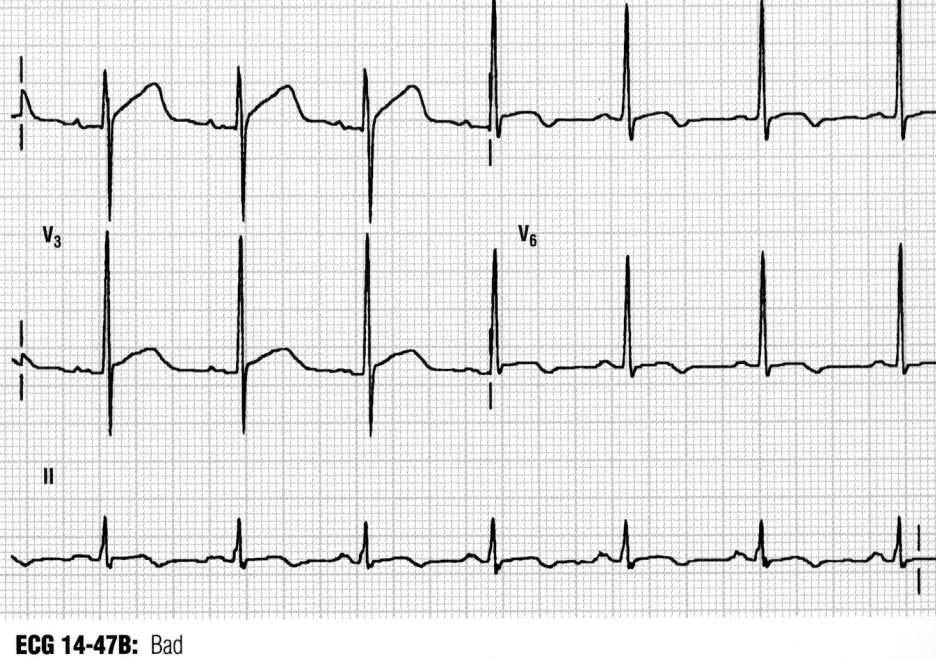

ECG 14-47A: Good

ECG 14-47B: Bad

Good: ECG 14-48A This also is benign elevation, due either to LVH or early repolarization pattern. Why do V₁ to V₂ look so strange? Because there is an incomplete RBBB pattern with an rSr′ pattern.

Bad: ECG 14-48B This ugly, flat ST elevation is associated with QS waves and a late transition, all markers for an anteroseptal AMI of indeterminate duration, but probably not brand new. It is at least a few hours old. There has to have been just enough time to kill off the anterior wall of the heart.

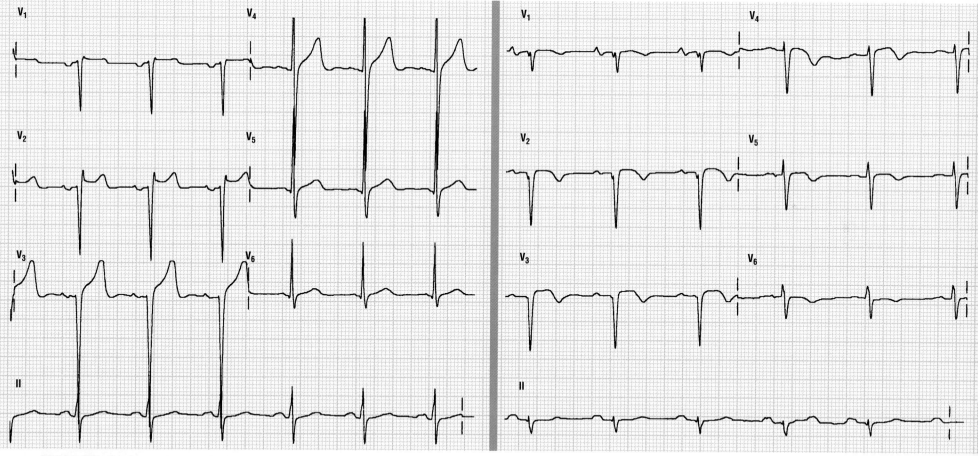

ECG 14-48A: Good

ECG 14-48B: Bad

ECG COMPARISONS: CONTINUED

Good: ECG 14-49A We're getting close to the end, so hang in there. Believe us, we wouldn't be spending this much time on this if it weren't a major problem area for most students.

This is a wide LVH-with-strain pattern with the typical features of the condition.

Bad: ECG 14-49B We have significant elevation in V_1 to V_2, which is consistent with injury or ischemia of the septal wall.

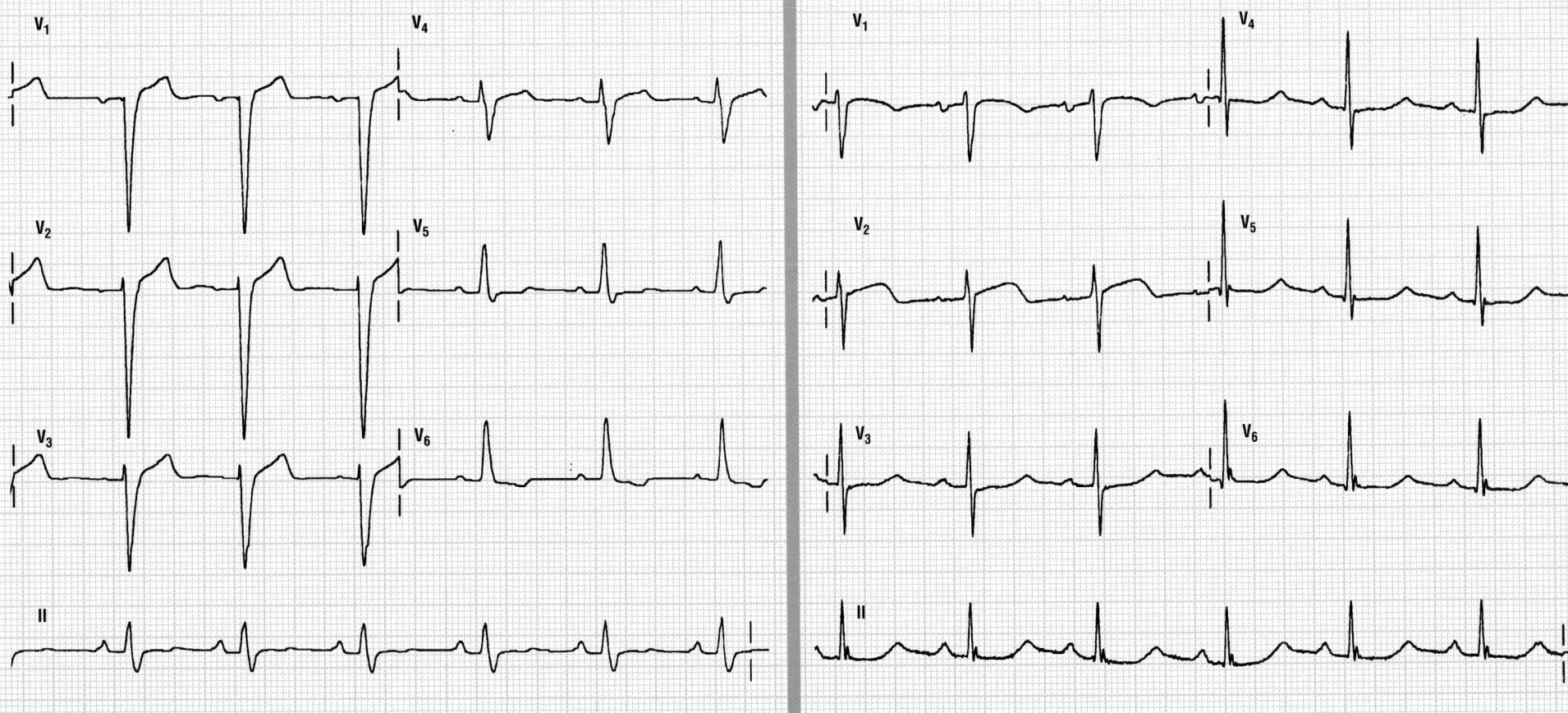

ECG 14-49A: Good

ECG 14-49B: Bad

Good: ECG 14-50A This is an obvious LVH pattern with the T waves not completely flipped by V_6. There is a late intrinsicoid deflection, best seen in V_5.

Bad: ECG 14-50A We see elevation in V_1 to V_4 that is associated with QS waves. This could be significant for AMI of indeterminate age versus ventricular aneurysm. Clinical correlation is required for definitive interpretation.

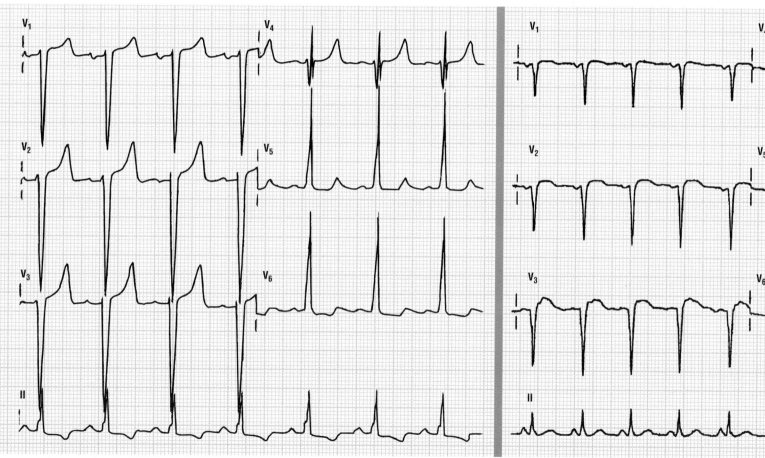

ECG 14-50A: Good

ECG 14-50B: Bad

ECG
COMPARISONS: **CONTINUED**

Good: ECG 14-51A This is a perfect example of LBBB. It has all of the criteria associated with the electrocardiographic presentation of the block: wide QRS, monomorphic S in V_1, monomorphic R in V_6. Compare these ST segments and the T waves to those in B. Try to remember the T waves and ST segments in this example. It will help you dramatically when you are trying to determine the extent of pathology in either another block or an AMI.

Bad: ECG 14-51B This ECG shows diffuse ST elevation and flipped T waves in V_1 to V_5. In addition, there are QS waves in these leads. The transition, therefore, is clockwise and very late. Notice the asymmetry of the T waves.

This ECG represents an age-indeterminate anteroseptal AMI with lateral extension, or a ventricular aneurysm, or both. In the case of an aneurysm, an AMI has always preceded the aneurysm. (Scar tissue from an AMI causes the aneurysm to develop because it is weaker and non-contractile compared with normal, viable myocardium. The force within the ventricle causes the scar tissue to bulge out giving rise to the aneurysmal outpouching of the wall.) An old ECG and clinical correlation are essential to make the distinction between a ventricular aneurysm and an age-indeterminate AMI in these cases.

REMINDER:

LBBB patients usually, but not always, have a small r wave at the beginning of the QRS complexes in lead V_1. Patients with LVH may or may not have a small r wave; a QS wave is present when there is no small r wave at the start of the complexes in leads V_1 and V_2 (some authors state that it needs to extend to V_3) and is a sign of an age-indeterminate anterior wall myocardial infarction. LBBB patients with no r waves in V_1 are easy to diagnose because of the presence of the wide QRS complex and the presence of the rest of the LBBB criteria throughout the rest of the ECG.

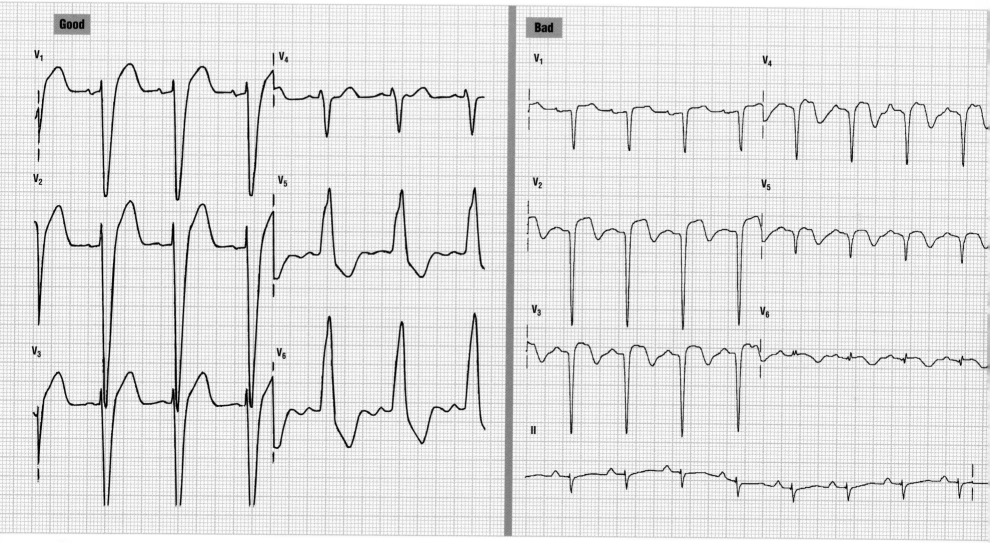

Good

V₁

V₂

V₃

V₄

V₅

V₆

Bad

V₁

V₂

V₃

V₄

V₅

V₆

II

ECG 14-51A: Good

ECG 14-51B: Bad

ECG COMPARISONS: CONTINUED

Bad: ECG 14-52A This ECG was obtained when a patient first arrived in the emergency department, complaining of episodes of substernal chest pain that came on at various times during the day and awakened the patient from sleep. There was no active chest pain at the time the ECG was done. Notice the late clockwise transition with QS waves in V_1 to V_2. The ST segments in V_5 to V_6 are slightly depressed and have flattened T waves. The decision was made to admit the patient for unstable angina.

Really Bad!: ECG 14-52B Suddenly, 20 minutes later, the patient began to complain of chest pain and ECG B was obtained. Notice how the ST segments and T waves in the lateral leads (and inferiorly — look at the rhythm strip) are now sloping downward and have much more depression than before. The T waves are now pronounced and flipped. This ECG and its brother (A) are classic for the changes that occur in unstable angina. The changes are caused by ischemia of the subendocardial tissue of the ventricles.

CLINICAL PEARL

ECGs and their findings are not static. The changes that are present on an ECG are only a 12-second movie clip of what is happening in the heart during any particular time period. A pathological process is a continuum of disease and you should not think of it as static. If the clinical history is highly suggestive of a pathological process but the ECG shows non-specific or minimal abnormalities, do not hesitate in obtaining a repeat ECG in a few minutes. We had one patient who went from a benign ECG to a hyperacute infarct pattern in a matter of 3 minutes. If we had only obtained the first one, we would have been lead into a false sense of security. Obtain an ECG when the story or the symptoms change or when you see a rhythm change on a monitor.

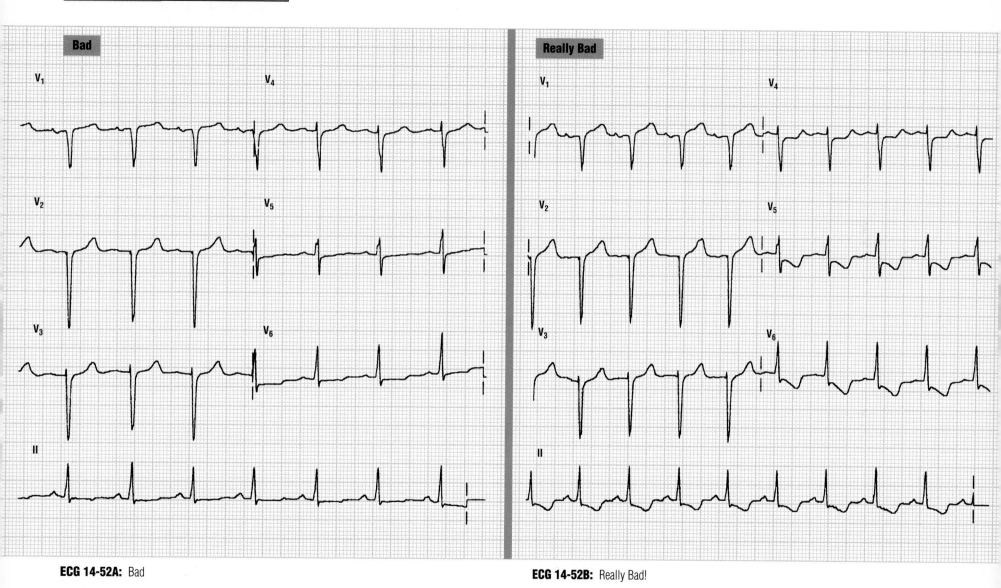

ECG 14-52A: Bad

ECG 14-52B: Really Bad!

Pericarditis Revisited

We began to introduce you to the concept of pericarditis in Chapter 10 when we reviewed the PR segment. If you remember, the PR segment is depressed in pericarditis. Here is the full list of criteria:

1. PR depression

2. Diffuse ST elevation

3. Scooping, upwardly concave ST segments

4. Notching of the end of the QRS

We have covered numbers 1 and 4 above. Let's look at the issues with the ST segments. In pericarditis, the ST segments are definitely elevated from the baseline. The amount of elevation is variable and can be quite high, up to 4 to 5 mm. The ST segments are scooped in an upwardly concave pattern; they may start at the end of the QRS notching. Tachycardia is frequently associated with these other findings.

Why are the ST segments elevated diffusely rather than just in certain leads? The entire pericardium is usually irritated. The irritation causes a net positivity of the epicardium, or outside surface of the heart, depicted in Figure 14-26. This net positivity is expressed as ST elevation.

When you first look at an ECG and see ST elevation in leads I and II (especially if the segments are scooped out and upwardly concave), your diagnosis of pericarditis is very likely. Next, look for the presence of PR depression and notching in these leads and in others, as shown in Figure 14-27. *These criteria do not have to be found in every lead, just a lot of them.* If you have all of the criteria, you will be about 80% of the way to the diagnosis. You still need one more critical aspect, however: a history and physical examination consistent with pericarditis. If they match the ECG findings, you can make the diagnosis. We suggest that you use a book on clinical medicine to review the findings in pericarditis.

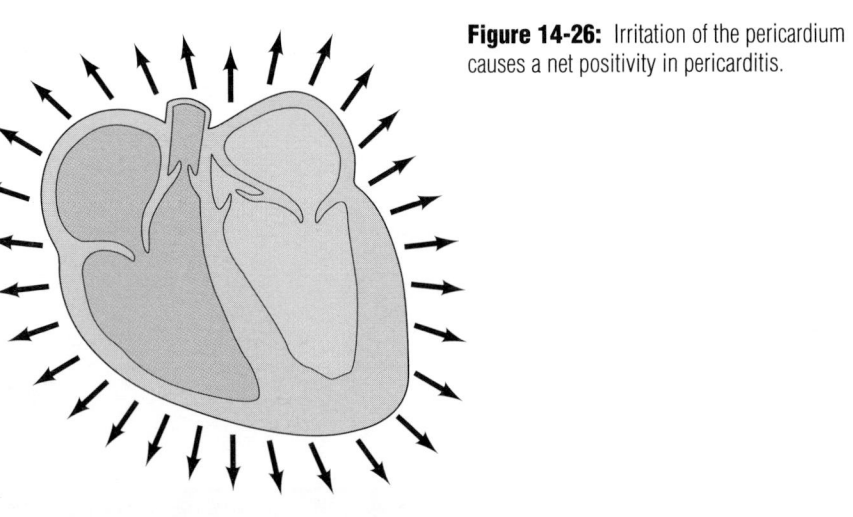

Figure 14-26: Irritation of the pericardium causes a net positivity in pericarditis.

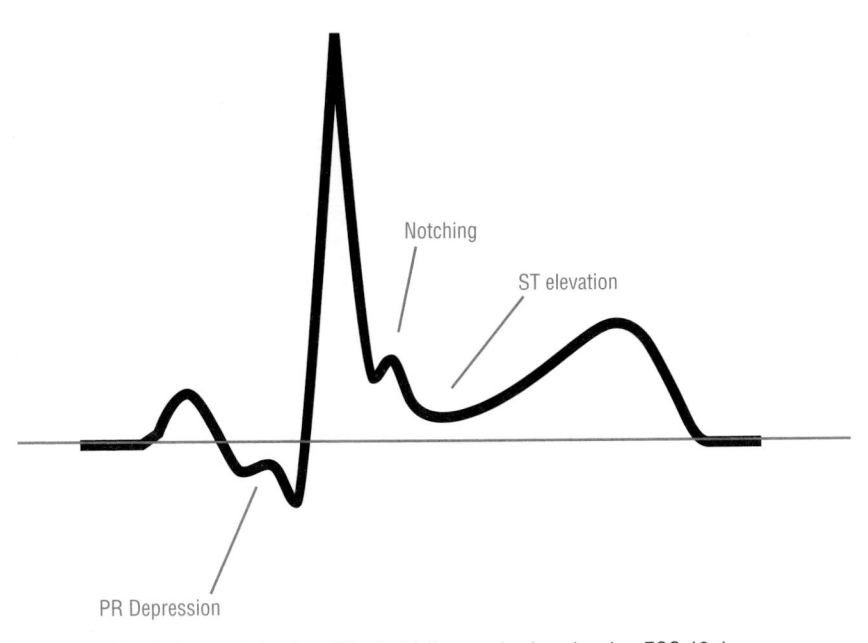

Notching

ST elevation

PR Depression

Figure 14-27: Before studying the ECGs that follow, go back and review ECG 10-1.

ECG 14-53 This is an example of pericarditis. The PR depression is not very impressive in this example. We urge you to review the other ECGs with pericarditis that we have presented thus far. The ST elevation is present in leads I, II, aVF, and V_1 to V_6. The QRS complexes have the notching indicative of benign ST elevation. The heart rate is technically not tachycardic, but it is in the 90 BPM range. The patient's history was consistent with pericarditis, and the ECG clinched the diagnosis.

Now, suppose the patient's history is not classic for pericarditis but he comes in for, say, a knee injury. Could these changes be seen in another entity? Yes, as long as the PR interval is not depressed greater than 0.8 mm (just under one small block deep), it could be associated with early repolarization. Early repolarization is a benign ST elevation, usually minimal and upwardly concave, that occurs in young people. Sometimes it can be found in middle-aged individuals, but you should get an old ECG to document its prior existence before concluding that it is early repolarization. Any PR depression deeper than 0.8 mm is pathological. When diagnosing pericarditis and early repolarization, we need to remember to look at the company it keeps. You should not make either diagnosis in a vacuum, but only after obtaining a history and carefully considering the differential.

ECG 14-54 This is another example of pericarditis. Can you tell why? Well, there is diffuse ST elevation in leads I, II, III, aVF, and V_1 to V_6 that is upwardly concave and scooping in nature. There is some notching in the lateral leads. The patient is not tachycardic. Why, then, can it not be early repolarization instead of pericarditis? For starters, the patient's history was consistent with the diagnosis. This is extremely important to your interpretation of the ECG. Secondly, the PR depression in lead II is 1 mm deep. This is pathological PR depression. Because the rest of the ECG and the history match the diagnosis, we have our answer.

ECG CASE STUDIES: **CONTINUED**

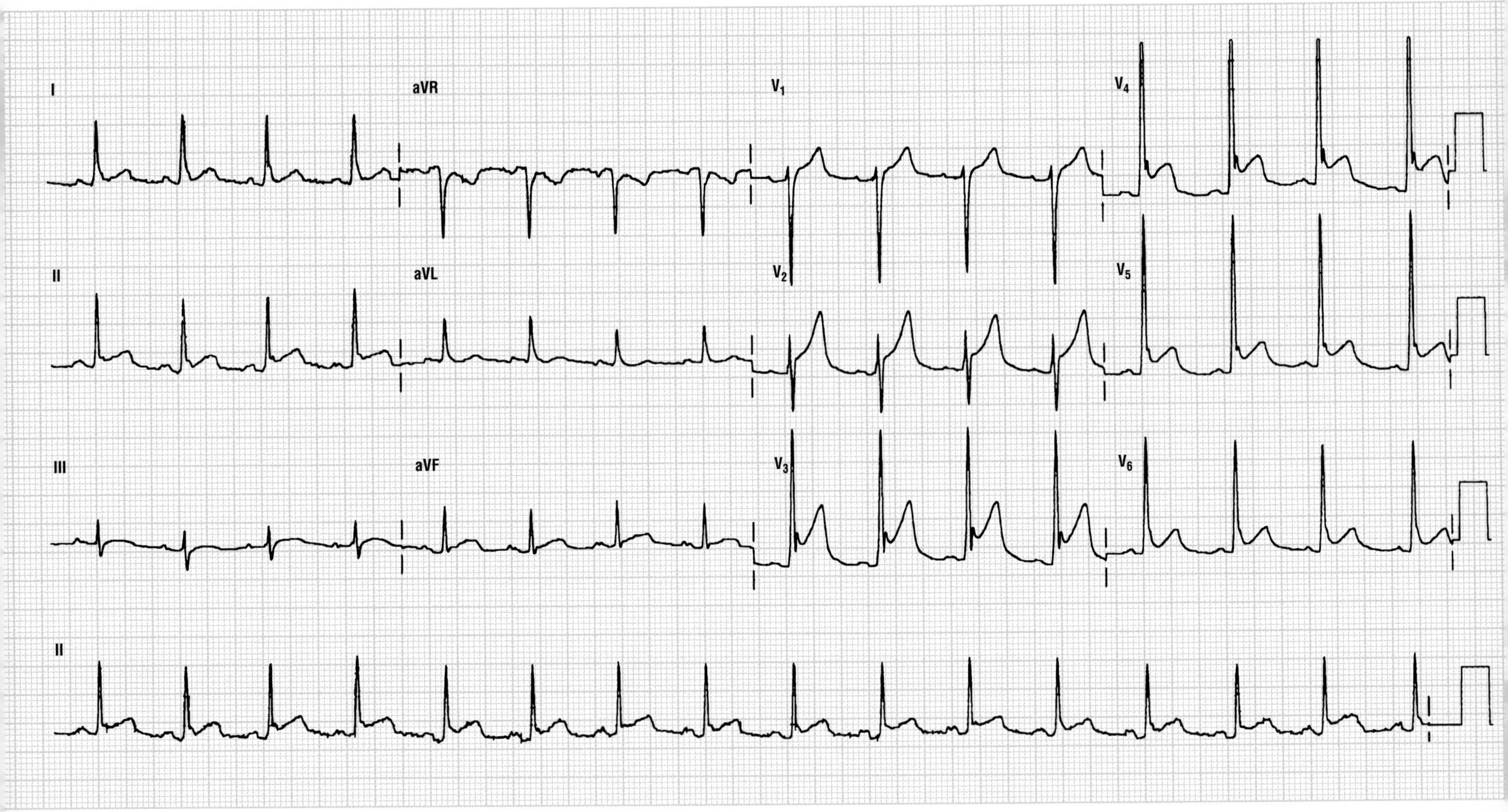

I	aVR	V₁	V₄
II	aVL	V₂	V₅
III	aVF	V₃	V₆
II			

ECG 14-53

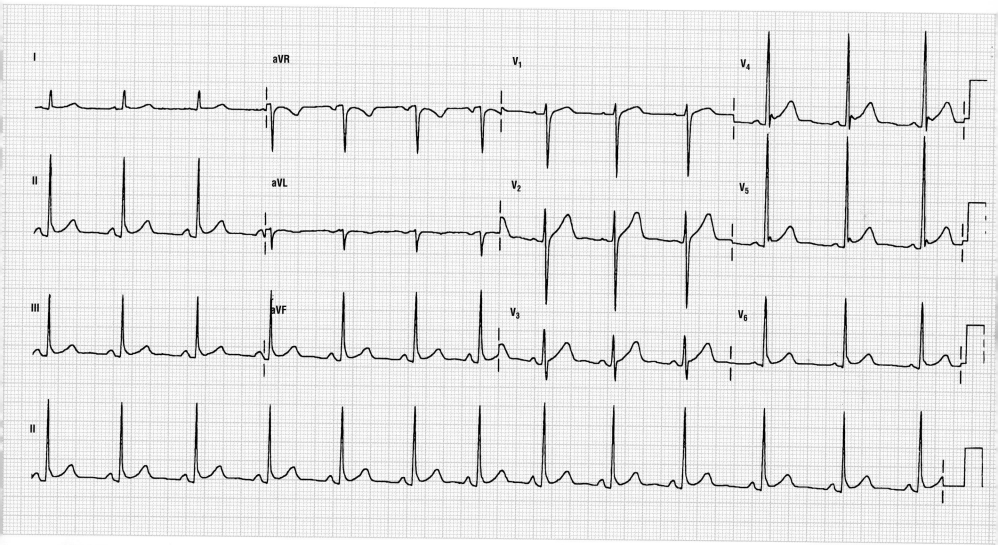

I   aVR   V₁   V₄

II   aVL   V₂   V₅

III   aVF   V₃   V₆

II

ECG 14-54

CHAPTER **14** • ST SEGMENT AND T WAVES

ECG CASE STUDIES: **CONTINUED**

ECG 14-55 This ECG was taken on a 24-year-old man who was being admitted to the hospital for a noncardiac problem. What do you think: Is it early repolarization (slang: early repol) or pericarditis? It's early repol. The patient had no symptoms consistent with cardiac involvement of any kind, and the ECG is consistent with the early repol pattern.

Q U I C K REVIEW

1. All ST elevation in young patients is due to an early repolarization pattern and is not pathological. True or False.

2. Pericarditis patients can have an underlying early repolarization pattern on an old ECG. True or False.

3. ST elevation from early repolarization is flat. True or False.

1. False 2. True 3. False

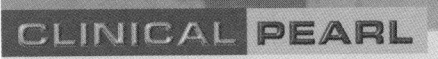

Remember that all ST elevations should be evaluated thoroughly for pathological causes. A young man having an AMI because of cocaine-induced arterial spasm can be misdiagnosed as early repolarization.

ECG 14-56 This ECG is also from a young patient, but this one was symptomatic. The changes are consistent with early repolarization. The patient had been doing some cocaine and was complaining of chest pain. Because he was young, there were no old ECGs to compare. What should you do with this patient? Send him home? Arrange outpatient follow-up?

The answer is that all chest pain in patients doing illicit drugs should be taken very seriously. We think they need to have a myocardial infarction ruled out prior to discharge. Why? Because they will fool you. The infarcts associated with many drugs are caused by spasm, not atherogenesis (plaque formation). In addition, many patients who chronically abuse drugs will develop advanced atherogenesis and heart disease.

Q U I C K REVIEW

1. Any ST elevation in a patient who is complaining of chest pain and has done cocaine or another illicit drug is benign. True or False.

2. Any ST elevation in a patient who has taken an illicit drug and who is complaining of chest pain should be taken very seriously. True or False.

3. Notching is always present in early repolarization. True or False.

1. False 2. True 3. False

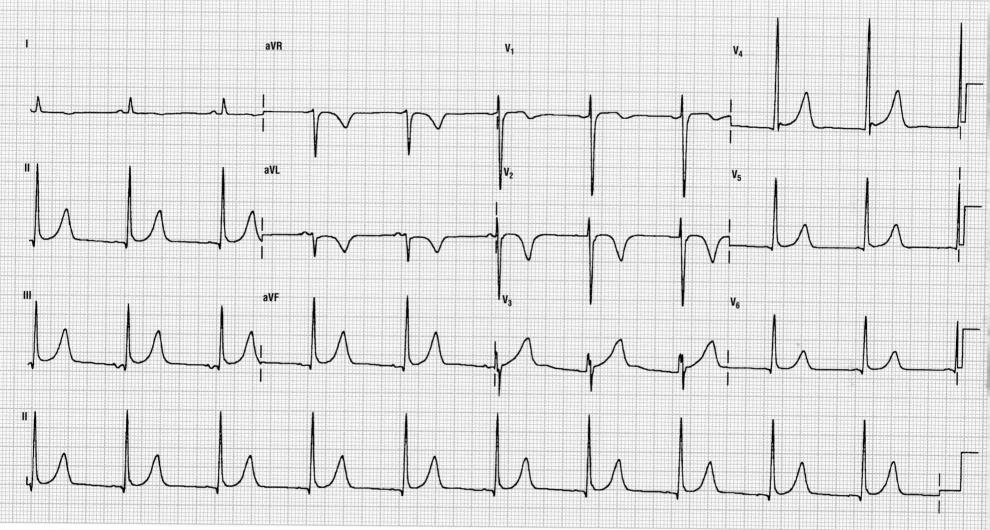

ECG 14-55

ECG CASE STUDIES: CONTINUED

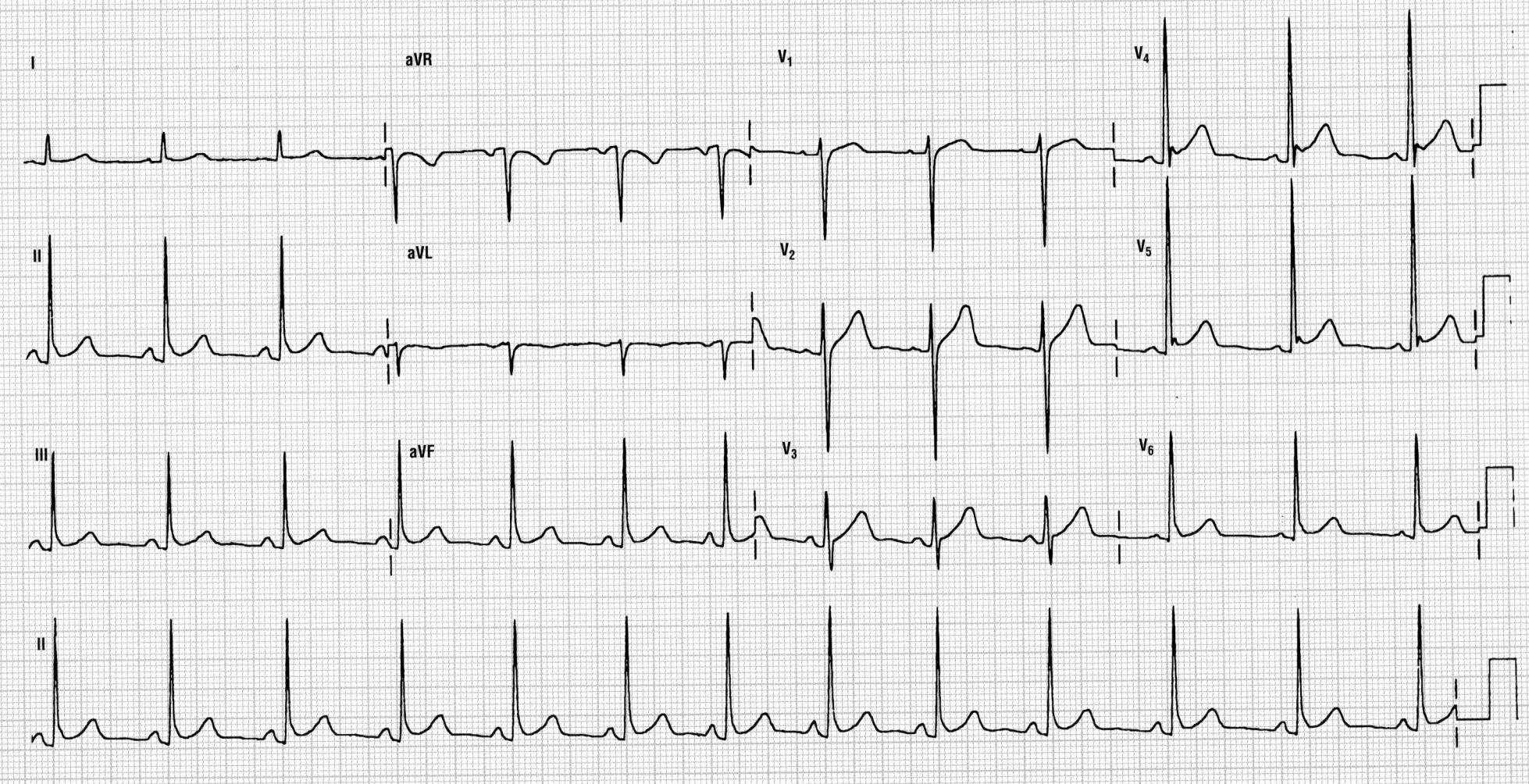

ECG 14-56

STs and T Waves in Blocks

When we look at an LBBB or RBBB pattern, we are struck by the complexity of the shapes. In order to make some sense of the complexes, we need to look at how a normal heart depolarizes and repolarizes, and how a heart with a block (or any other aberrancy) does the same thing. We covered a bit of this in Chapter 6 (The T wave), so you can go back there to review.

Under normal circumstances, the heart depolarizes from the endocardium to the epicardium (*yellow arrows*, Figure 14-28). Logic would dictate that the first cell to depolarize would also be the first wave to repolarize, but that would make this too easy. What really happens is that the epicardium is the first to repolarize, and the repol wave spreads inward toward the endocardium (*blue arrows*, Figure 14-28). This is because the pressure on the inside part of the ventricular wall is greater than the pressure on the outside.

The depolarization is a positive wave traveling toward the electrode in Figure 14-28. This creates a positive deflection of the QRS complex. The repolarization wave travels away from the epicardium, and from the electrode. Because this negative wave traveling away from the electrode is the same electrically as a positive wave traveling toward it, it results in a positive T wave (Figure 14-28).

The circumstance of a BBB or a VPC is one of pathological transmission of the action potential by cell-to-cell transmission (represented by the *diagonal arrows*). This will slow down the depolarization and repolarization of the cells. In turn, this produces a state in which the pressure gradient of the heart no longer alters the repolarization wave front. In these circumstances, the repolarization wave will follow the depolarization wave as you would originally expect. The result: The electrode now sees a positive wave coming toward it with depolarization (positive QRS), and a negative wave approaching it during repolarization (negative T wave; see Figure 14-29).

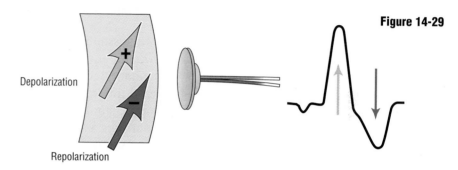

Figure 14-29

The final word is this: *in a bundle branch block, the T wave is always in the opposite direction of the terminal portion of the QRS complex.* This is called *discordance.* If the T wave travels in the same direction as the last part of the QRS, it is known as *concordance* (Figure 14-30). Concordance is bad, a sign of ischemia in a bundle branch block unless chronically present in old ECGs. In these chronic cases it represents an abnormal route of repolarization.

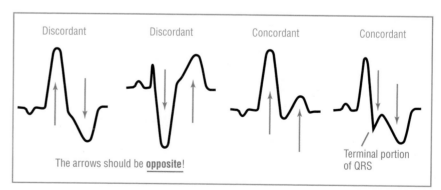

Figure 14-30: Discordant and concordant waves.

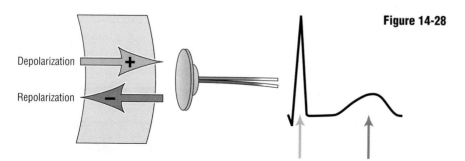

Figure 14-28

ECG CASE STUDIES: *STs and Ts in Blocks*

ECG 14-57 The first thing to decide is whether this is a BBB. Is it wider than 0.12 seconds? Yes. Does it match either an LBBB or RBBB pattern? Yes, it matches an LBBB pattern except in V₆. Before you label it an IVCD, let's think about this for a minute. Remember, we mentioned to you that leads I and V₆ should look identical or very nearly so, because they both represent the same area of the heart — the area both of them look at (remember the camera analogy). Then why do they look so different on this ECG? Whoever placed the precordial electrodes on the chest did not do a good job of putting them in the right places. The electrode for V₆ was either too high or too anterior. The result is a very different angle than should be seen in V₆. It is extremely important to place the precordial leads over exactly the right spots.

Now, imagine that V₆ looks like lead I. Would that be consistent with an LBBB? The answer is yes. If you look at V₃ to V₆, you'll see that the T waves are in the same direction as the last part of the QRS complex — in this case, an S wave. This makes the T waves concordant with the S wave, a sign of ischemic pathology unless it was present on an old ECG. Notice how, in the other leads, the T wave is opposite to the last part of the QRS complex (discordant). This is normal in a BBB.

ECG 14-58 This ECG shows an RBBB pattern; as a matter of fact, there is a bifascicular block. This is due to the left anterior hemiblock (LAH), which is evident from the limb leads. Which leads are concordant, and which are discordant? Well, the concordant leads are II, aVF, and V₂ to V₃. The rest are all discordant.

ECG 14-59 This, once again, is an LBBB pattern. Which are the concordant leads? Leads V₃ to V₅ and II are definitely concordant. Leads III and aVF both have T waves that start off negative and end up positive. The negative start makes them both discordant. Notice that there is some additional ST depression in II, III, and aVF. ST depression is normal in LBBB, but because it is not found anywhere else, it is highly suspicious of ischemia. The concordance in the leads mentioned above, along with the inferior ST depressions, makes inferolateral ischemia a very strong possibility.

 It has been a very long chapter, and the next one will also be long. The reasons are worth repeating. Most of the confusion about ECGs relates to ST segments, T waves, and infarct criteria. We have therefore concentrated on these sections. We hope this has been rewarding for you and has clarified some of your questions. It is crucial that you clearly understand the concepts put forth in these chapters. A little extra effort now will pay off in the future for both you and your patients.

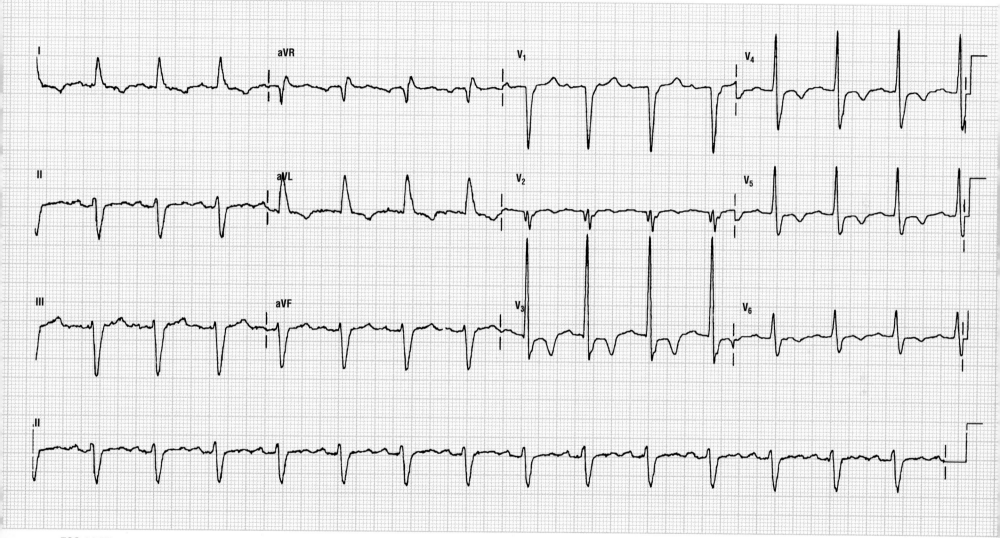

ECG 14-57

ECG CASE STUDIES: **CONTINUED**

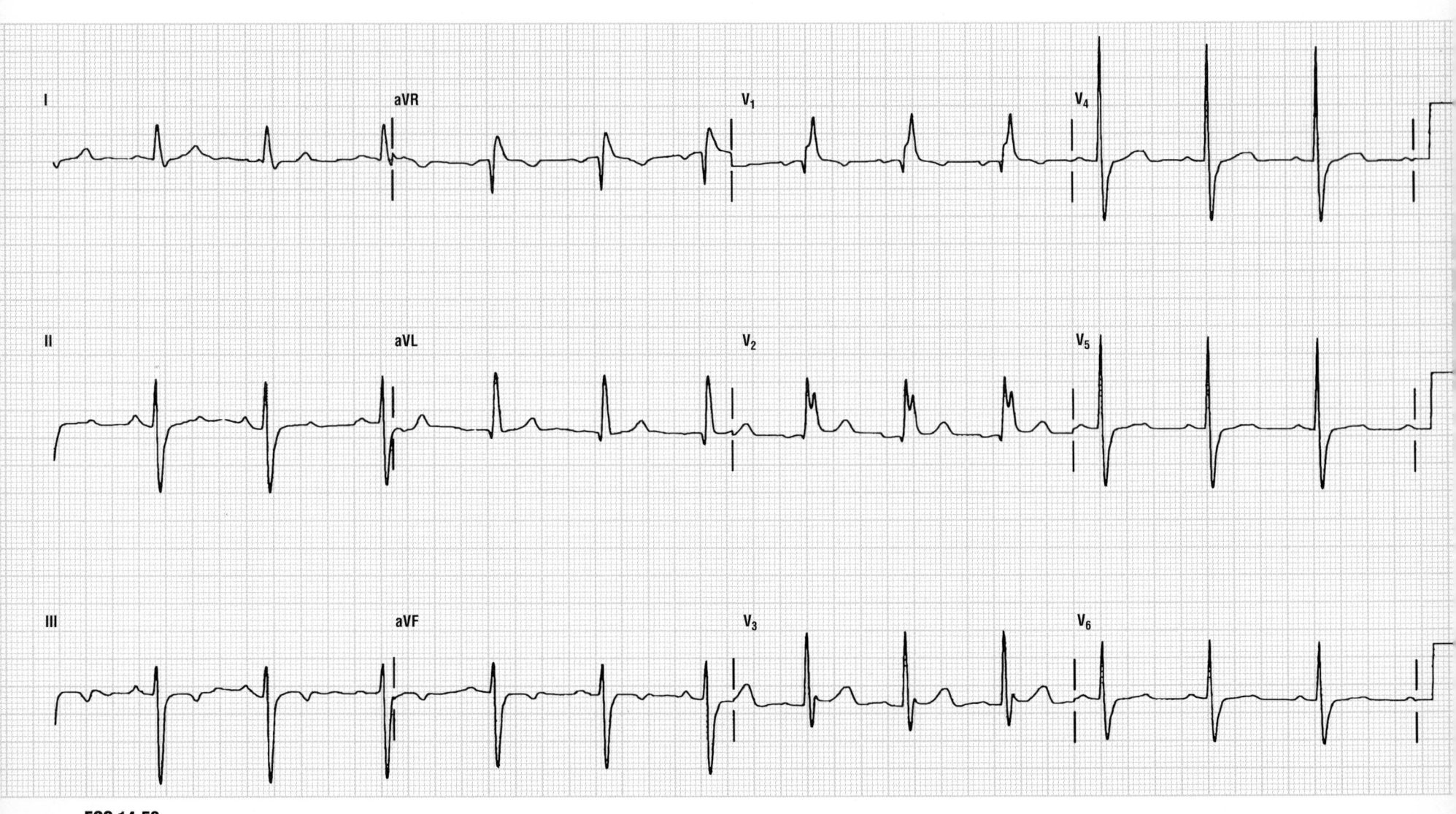

ECG 14-58

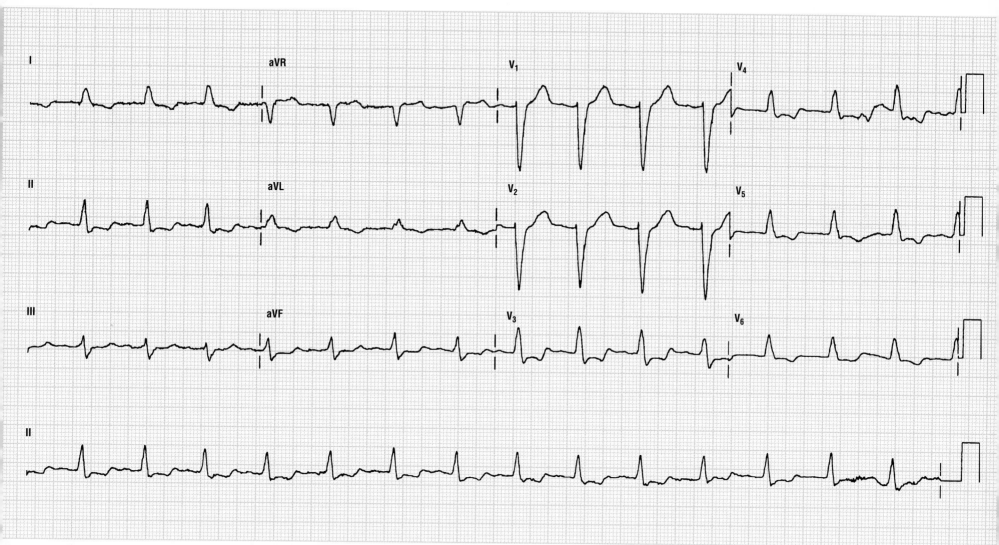

ECG 14-59

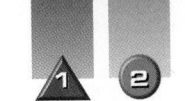

CHAPTER IN **REVIEW**

1. The J point is the point where the QRS complex and the ST segment meet. True or False.

2. T waves are normally positive in which leads?
   A. I
   B. II
   C. V_3 to V_6
   D. All of the above
   E. None of the above

3. The baseline is a straight line from TP segment to TP segment of adjoining complexes. Any ST elevation can be significant and should be evaluated thoroughly. True or False.

4. T waves are normally symmetrical. True or False.

5. If the T wave is more than _____ the height of the R wave, it is considered abnormal.
   A. $^1/_4$
   B. $^1/_3$
   C. $^1/_2$
   D. $^2/_3$
   E. $^3/_4$

1. True 2. D 3. True 4. False 5. D

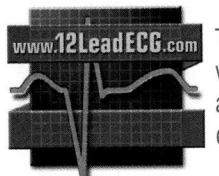

To enhance the knowledge you gain in this book, access this text's website at www.12leadECG.com! This valuable resource provides an online glossary and related web links. To learn more about the chapter topics, simply click on the chapter and view the link.

CHAPTER IN **REVIEW**

6. Tall, peaked, symmetrical T waves are usually found in:
   A. Myocardial infarction
   B. Ischemia
   C. Hypokalemia
   D. Hyperkalemia
   E. CNS events

7. Very broad, symmetrical T waves are classic for:
   A. Myocardial infarction
   B. Ischemia
   C. Hypokalemia
   D. Hyperkalemia
   E. CNS events

8. ST segment depression is classically found in:
   A. Q-wave AMI
   B. Ischemia
   C. Non-Q-wave AMI
   D. Both A and B
   E. Both B and C

9. Which of the following is **not** a criterion for RVH:
   A. P-pulmonale or RAE
   B. Right axis deviation
   C. Increased R:S ratio in V_1 to V_2
   D. Presence of RVH with strain pattern
   E. ST segment elevation in V_1 to V_2

10. Choose the **incorrect** answer. The differential diagnosis of increased R:S ratio in V_1 to V_2 includes:
    A. RVH
    B. LPH
    C. Posterior wall AMI
    D. WPW type A
    E. Young children and adolescents

11. Strain pattern is the greatest in the lead with the tallest or deepest QRS complexes. True or False

12. ST segment elevation or depression that is ischemic in nature is usually flat and is associated with symmetrical T waves. True or False.

13. You can see ST segment elevation consistent with LVH with strain even if the criteria for LVH are not met. True or False

14. LAE is always found in a patient with LVH with strain. True or False.

15. In a BBB, the T wave always deflects in the opposite direction from the terminal portion of the QRS complex. True or False.

6. D 7. E 8. E 9. E 10. B 11. True 12. True 13. False 14. False 15. True

CHAPTER **15**

This is the chapter you have been waiting for: the AMI. There is a tremendous thrill in making the diagnosis of an AMI and instituting treatment that will potentially save the patient's life, or at least lifestyle. We want to temper that enthusiasm, though, by stating that this topic is broad and covers many areas of the heart: the anterior wall, inferior wall, posterior wall, right ventricle, and apex. It also covers combinations of AMIs that occur — inferolateral, anterolateral, and infero-posterior, to list a few examples. Now, add the BBBs and atypical AMI presentations and there is some serious material to cover. Appropriate coverage of this topic would require an entire separate book. This chapter presents a broad overview. We will discuss some of the pathophysiological changes occurring in the heart as a result of an AMI and how the patterns of the ECG are altered.

Introduction

All cells need oxygen to survive, including myocardial cells. When the cell is oxygen-deprived, its function will begin to alter. It initiates anaerobic metabolism — the production of energy without oxygen — in order to survive. This creates acidosis and is generally a very ineffectual way for the cell to function. Eventually, the cell will begin to suffer injury from the buildup of these harmful metabolites, and this will proceed to cell death unless normal circulation and oxygenation are restored. As Figure 15-1 shows, the process occurs gradually along a continuum. For an analogy, think of a drowning man. He does not die the minute he goes under water. First, he uses up his reserves, then slowly becomes light-headed, panics, passes out, and eventually dies. We want you to think of ischemia, injury, and infarction as a similar continuum (panic is manifested as arrhythmia and hemodynamic

changes). The ECG proceeds in parallel through some quite well-defined presentations that we will cover shortly.

A short note on nomenclature. Ischemia and injury are reversible. The symptomatic manifestation of ischemia and/or injury is chest pain. Ischemia and/or injury develop because the demands of the heart are *transiently* overcome or not met by the blood supply to the area, for whatever reason. *Note that either an increase in demand or a decrease in supply can cause the ischemia and/or injury to develop.* Unfortunately, infarct (cell death) is irreversible.

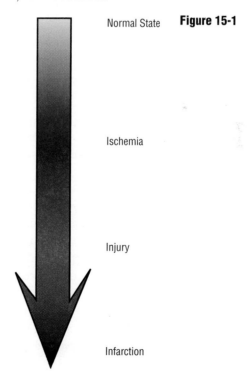

Figure 15-1

Normal State

Ischemia

Injury

Infarction

In order to understand the shapes of infarcts and their presentation on an ECG, we need to look at how blood circulates throughout the myocardium. Let's begin by thinking of cardiac circulation as a basic tree structure. The main trunk gives rise to the main branches. These, in turn, divide to form the large branches, then medium branches, and so on until you arrive at the terminal twigs and leaves. The main coronary arteries travel along the epicardium and penetrate into the myocardium at various points as seen in Figure 15-2. As these arteries approach the endocardium, they give off smaller and smaller branches until they form the capillary beds of the myocardium. Now, if we look specifically at a single big branch, we see that it supplies blood to a wedge-shaped section of tissue that grows fatter as we follow it distally, away from the artery's point of origin, as shown in Figure 15-3.

Now, remember the spectrum of ischemia we discussed above? Ischemia leads to injury and eventually infarction. When the cells die, they die along the pattern of distribution of the branch perfusing that section of myocardium, so the infarcted area will be wedge-shaped with the fatter side along the endocardium.

Then why are the wedges of the ischemic and injured areas (Figure 15-2) thinner along the endocardium? To answer this question, we need to look at three protective mechanisms of the heart:

1. The overlap of the areas of perfusion supplied by different arteries along the endocardium, called *collateral circulation*, allows some areas of the endocardium to be supplied by two different branch systems (Figure 15-3).
2. Oxygen from the ventricles can move directly, or *diffuse*, into the cells of nearby tissue.
3. There may be some small vessels, the *thebesian veins*, arising directly from the ventricles.

These mechanisms work to provide extra oxygen to the cells near the endocardium, making them less susceptible to ischemia and injury. There is, therefore, more ischemia and injury of the cells along the epicardial surface.

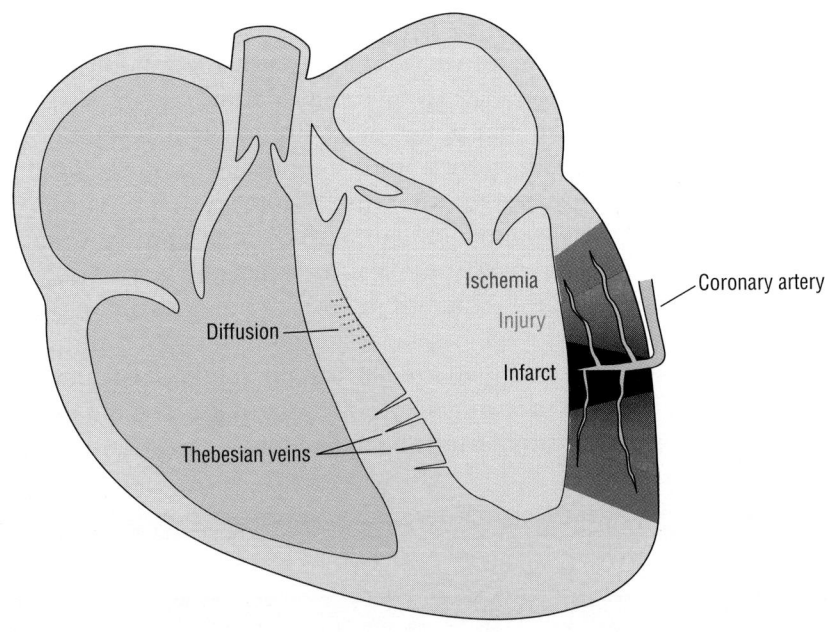

Figure 15-2

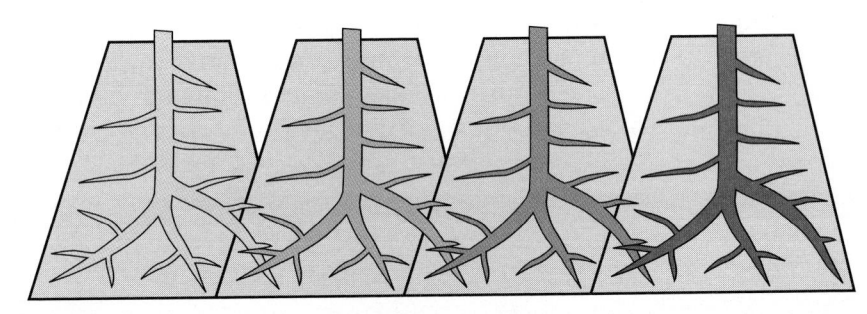

Figure 15-3: Overlapping wedges of perfusion from the coronary arteries.

Zones of Ischemia, Injury, and Infarction

Ischemia affects a wedge-shaped section of the heart. The wedge is thinner in the endocardium and wider along the epicardium, as depicted in Figure 15-4. This area of ischemia is more negative than the surrounding normal tissue, causing a pattern of ST depression. The T wave is flipped because ischemia causes repolarization to occur along an abnormal pathway.

Injury also influences a wedge-shaped section of tissue similar to that seen in ischemia, as shown in Figure 15-5. However, the zone of injury does not repolarize completely; it thus remains more positive than the surrounding tissue, leading to ST elevation. The T remains flipped because of the abnormal repolarization pathways along the injured and ischemic areas of the myocardium.

Infarction is dead tissue. It does not generate any action potentials and so is electrically neutral. This infarcted area acts like an electrical "window" in the wall of the myocardium. Looking through that win-

dow, an electrode can see the opposite wall. The unopposed, positive vector of the other wall, heading away from the electrode, produces the Q wave shown in Figure 15-6. The appearance of the rest of the complex results from the surrounding zones of infarct and injury.

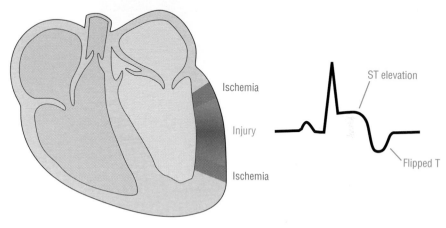

Figure 15-5: Ischemia and injury.

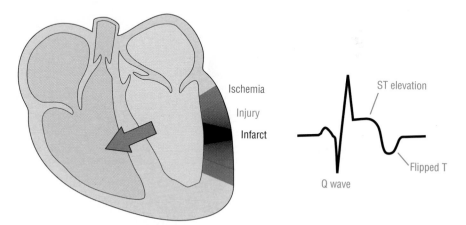

Figure 15-6: Ischemia, injury, and infarct.

Figure 15-4: Ischemia.

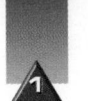
Infarct and Q Waves

Q Wave Infarct

There are two main electrocardiographic classifications of infarcts: Q wave and non–Q wave. We used to refer to the Q wave infarct as one caused by a transmural infarct — one involving the entire myocardium. Because there is dead tissue throughout the wall, we see the "window" effect and the development of a Q wave as seen in Figure 15-7.

That traditional thinking ended when autopsy studies showed that nontransmural infarcts could also give rise to Q waves. To understand how a nontransmural infarct can do that, we need to think in terms of vectors. As an example (and this is not the only possible explanation), suppose there were an area of infarct encompassing only the proximal one third of the ventricular wall. The infarcted area would also include an area of the Purkinje network. Because the Purkinje system transmits the electrical potential very quickly throughout the myocardium, if that system is not working in the infarcted area, the injured myocardium overlying the infarct could only be depolarized by slow, cell-to-cell impulse transmission as depicted in Figure 15-9. This slowing creates a brief interval during which the vector of the opposite wall appears to be unopposed. An electrode overlying the

infarct then reads the fast, unopposed vector of the opposite wall as a Q wave — and the vectors of the slow, injured area begin to appear.

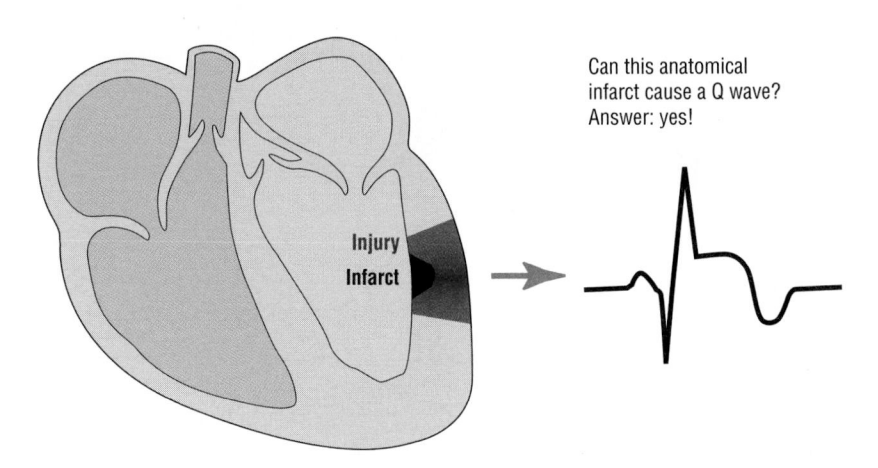

Can this anatomical infarct cause a Q wave? Answer: yes!

Figure 15-8

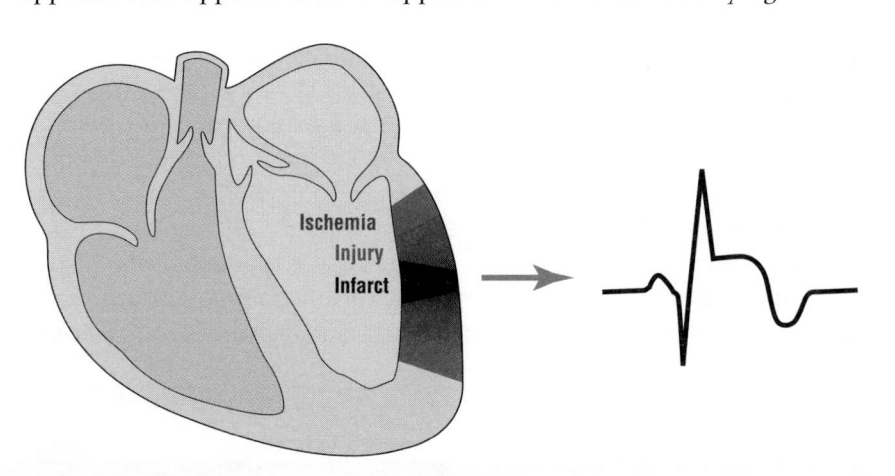

Figure 15-7: Q wave infarct.

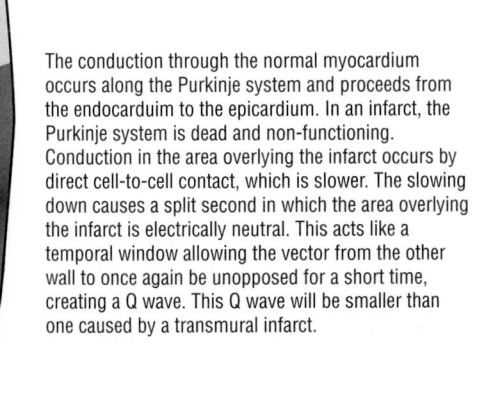

The conduction through the normal myocardium occurs along the Purkinje system and proceeds from the endocarduim to the epicardium. In an infarct, the Purkinje system is dead and non-functioning. Conduction in the area overlying the infarct occurs by direct cell-to-cell contact, which is slower. The slowing down causes a split second in which the area overlying the infarct is electrically neutral. This acts like a temporal window allowing the vector from the other wall to once again be unopposed for a short time, creating a Q wave. This Q wave will be smaller than one caused by a transmural infarct.

Figure 15-9

Non–Q Wave Infarct

Now, suppose that an infarct is small enough that it does not produce a visible Q wave, but big enough to cause an area of ST depression or T wave abnormalities, as in Figure 15-10. This ECG would not look like an AMI; we would initially think of it as ischemia or injury. However, we can confirm infarction by documenting an elevation in the biochemical markers used to diagnose AMI. This type of infarct, one that leaves no residual Q wave, is known as a non–Q Wave infarct.

Medical mythology used to state that this type of infarct was always along the endocardium, but this is false. This small infarct could occur in the endocardium or anywhere along the myocardium. It may be caused by the infarction of noncontiguous areas of myocardium. It may even be a small transmural infarct that for some reason is not giving rise to a Q wave. In addition, in this age of thrombolytic therapy and revascularization procedures, you can turn a transmural infarct into a nontransmural one very quickly by reversing the process causing the infarct — the clot. To clarify, you cannot use the presence of a Q wave to identify a transmural or nontransmural infarct, so we should put this fallacy to rest.

Then why bother with all of this Q wave and non–Q wave stuff to begin with? The main purpose of making the distinction lies in its prognostic significance to the patient.

Q wave infarcts are associated with higher incidences of acute mortality, increased tissue damage, and the development of congestive heart failure. Non–Q wave infarcts have higher long-term mortality if aggressive treatment strategies are not undertaken. Why? Look at Figure 15-11. Suppose there is an initial infarct at area #1 of the artery shown. This would infarct a small area of myocardium hardly worth noting, right? Wrong! With every infarct, there is a high chance — about 40% — of an arrhythmia that leads to sudden cardiac death.

Aggressive treatment could prevent the infarct zone from extending into subsequent events at areas #2, 3, and 4 in Figure 15-11. The cumulative effect would be the loss of much more myocardium, but the biggest danger is that 40% chance of sudden death that accompanies each of these events.

Statistics say that every time you toss a coin in the air, you have a 50% chance of calling it correctly — heads or tails — and 40% is close to 50%. Do you feel lucky enough to call four heads in a row?

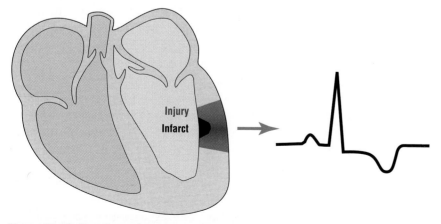

Figure 15-10: Non–Q wave infarct.

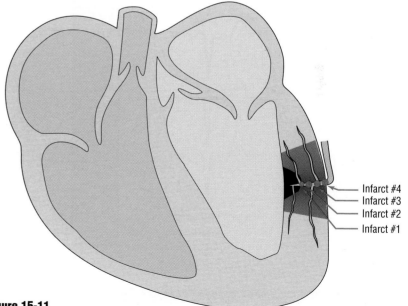

Infarct #4
Infarct #3
Infarct #2
Infarct #1

Figure 15-11

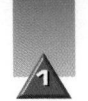
ECG Progression in Infarct

The ECG patterns in an AMI are not a static picture, but rather a continuum that extends from the normal state to a full infarct. This progression is shown in Figure 15-12. As you can see, the first thing that happens is that the T wave flips in early ischemia. Next, we see ST elevation that is either flat or tombstoning in character. The flipped T wave may disappear for a short time during this stage. Finally, we start to see Q waves.

Once the acute infarct is over, the chronic pattern of an old infarct begins to develop. The first thing to disappear is the ST segment elevation, with return of the segment to baseline. The T wave then reverts to upright. The Q wave remains permanently because of scar formation, however. The infarct pattern may take weeks to resolve to this level.

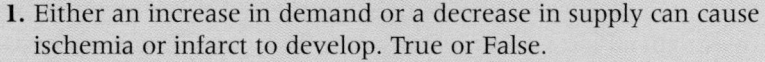

QUICK REVIEW

1. Either an increase in demand or a decrease in supply can cause ischemia or infarct to develop. True or False.

2. Myocardial cell death is reversible. True or False.

3. Infarcts are wedge-shaped with the broader end touching the endocardium. True or False.

4. Collateral circulation increases the chance of infarction. True or False.

5. Ischemia and injury are reversible. True or False.

1. True 2. False 3. True 4. False 5. True

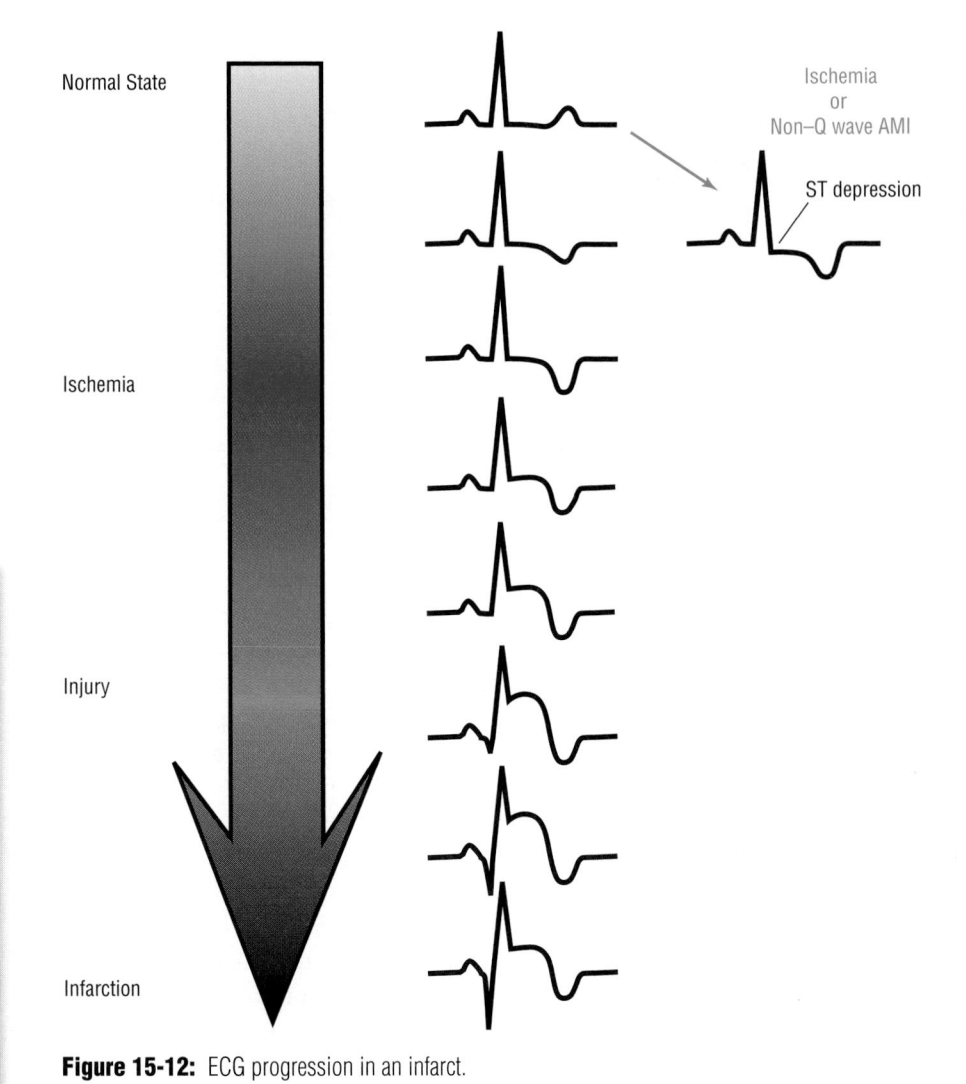

Figure 15-12: ECG progression in an infarct.

Reciprocal Changes

Reciprocal changes is a term that is bantered around by ECG interpreters on a regular basis. It refers to the "mirror image" that occurs when you have two electrodes viewing the same AMI from opposite angles. For example, take electrodes A and B in Figure 15-13. They are both viewing the same events at exactly the same time. However, they are recording complexes that are quite different from each other. Can you figure out why?

Let's start out by looking at electrode A. When the electrode looks through the window of the electrically neutral infarct zone, it registers only the unopposed vector heading away from it. This gives rise to

a Q wave, because the vector is heading away from it. Next, it registers the other vectors contributing to the QRS, and the more positive zone of injury that causes ST elevation. The T wave is flipped because of repolarization abnormalities generated by the areas of ischemia and injury.

Electrode B, on the other hand, originally sees an unopposed vector coming at it, giving rise to a high R wave. Then it registers the zones of injury and ischemia, respectively, as a pattern of ST depression and an upright T wave. It has, in essence, seen the "mirror image" of what electrode A is seeing. *The recording made by* **the lead on the wall exactly opposite** *an AMI is registering the reciprocal change of that AMI.*

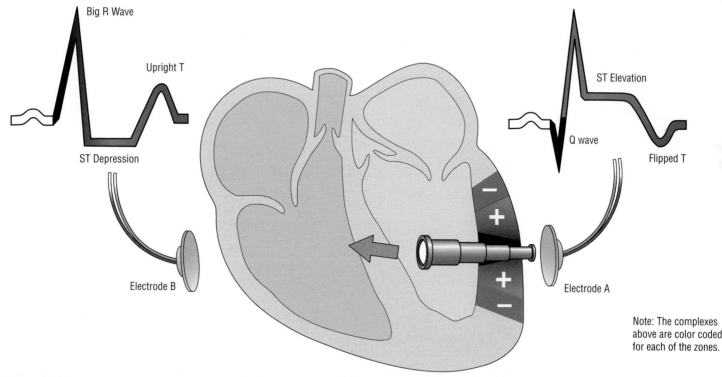

Big R Wave

Upright T

ST Depression

ST Elevation

Q wave

Flipped T

Electrode B

Electrode A

Note: The complexes above are color coded for each of the zones.

Figure 15-13

So what are the areas on the ECG that represent the individual walls, and which leads are truly reciprocal? Figure 15-14 gives a graphical answer to this question.

Infarct Regions on the ECG

The color-specific areas in Figure 15-15 represent the regions of infarction found on the ECG. Note that these areas are the electrocardiographic equivalents of the regions shown in Figure 15-14 using the hexaxial and Z planes. You need to see the changes of AMI or ischemia in a regional distribution in order to be certain that they are true changes.

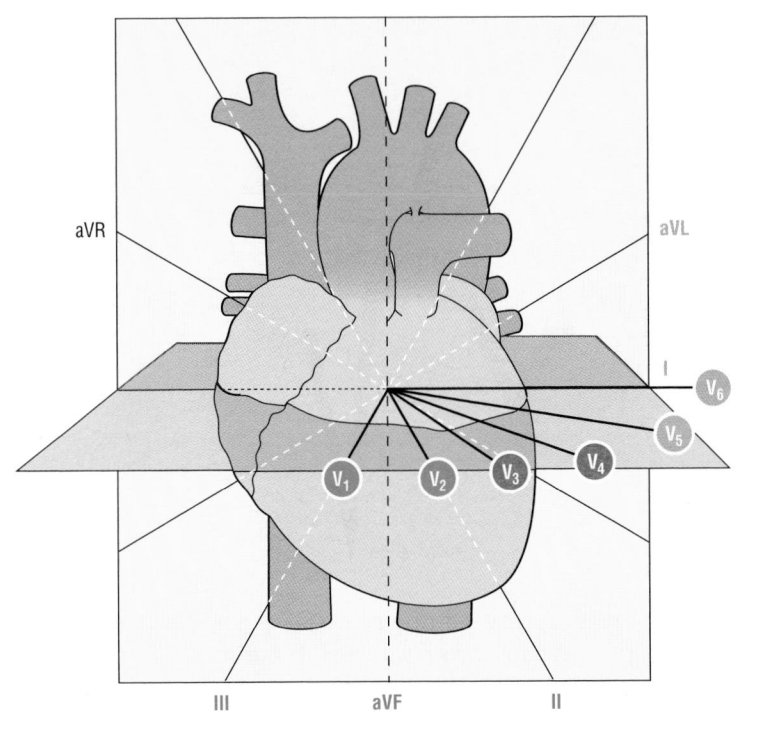

Anterior Wall = V_3 to V_4

Inferior Wall = II, III, aVF

Lateral Wall = I, aVL, V_5 to V_6

Septum = V_1 to V_2

Posterior Wall =
Reciprocal Changes
are found in V_1 to V_2

Reciprocal Changes occur in:

II, III, and aVF ⟷ I, aVL

V_1, V_2 ⟷ V_7, V_8, V_9

Note: V_7 to V_9 are posterior leads that will be discussed later in the chapter.

Figure 15-14

I	aVR	V_1	V_4
Lateral		Septal	Anterior
II	aVL	V_2	V_5
Inferior	High Lateral	Septal	Lateral
III	aVF	V_3	V_6
Inferior	Inferior	Anterior	Lateral

Figure 15-15

Infarct Regions in Combination

We have discussed the various regions in which AMIs occur in the preceding sections. We showed you the isolated regions involved and the leads that represent those infarcted areas. However, things do not occur that simply in real life. Real-life infarcts are caused by blocked arteries that usually involve more than one region of the heart and, therefore, of the ECG. (You can consult an anatomy textbook for a complete discussion of coronary artery anatomy.)

The amount of tissue infarcted depends on the size and location of the artery blocked, and the amount of area that it perfuses. When you look at an AMI at autopsy, you can physically see the amount of tissue infarcted and the arteries involved. Unfortunately, we can't be that accurate with the ECG. We can identify the regions affected and make an educated guess at the arteries that perfuse them, but we cannot state with any degree of certainty the extent of tissue involved.

This is because of other pattern-altering abnormalities that can affect the presentation on the ECG. The ECG is a representation of the vectors of the heart. Vectors representing LVH, RVH, conduction abnormalities, and so on can alter the appearance of the ECG in an acute AMI. In addition, there are many possible variations in the way that the arteries traverse the myocardium. The areas that they perfuse can, therefore, vary from individual to individual. This will alter the regions that are involved electrocardiographically, as well. We will begin by giving you some of the most established ECG patterns, but keep in mind that there can always be differences caused by factors such as other underlying pathology, dominant arterial systems, and the presence of collateral blood flow.

A larger artery usually affects more than one region. In addition, even though the infarct could be small, the zone of injury or the amount of myocardium at risk could be much greater. Hence, *acute* infarcts tend to involve more than one region: inferoposterior, anteroseptal with lateral extension, posterolateral, and so forth. This is especially true of infarcts involving the inferior and anterior walls. These infarcts result from obstruction of either the right coronary artery (RCA) or the left anterior descending (LAD) arteries, respectively. *Old* or *age-indeterminate* infarcts, represented by Q waves, are frequently found to affect the isolated inferior or anterior walls. Some acute infarcts, however, do involve only one region. These include high-laterals, true posteriors, and isolated RV infarcts; we will show you examples in their respective sections later in this chapter. We will concentrate here primarily on the acute infarcts. When you review some of the ECGs in the other chapters as an advanced reader, you will note many examples of old or age-indeterminate infarcts.

With that in mind, let's look at some of the main arteries and the areas that they perfuse. (RCA = right coronary artery; LAD = left anterior descending; LCx = left circumflex artery)

Inferior	RCA, LCx
Inferior-RV	Proximal RCA
Inferoposterior	RCA, LCx
Isolated RV	LCx
Isolated posterior	RCA, LCx
Anterior	LAD
Anteroseptal	LAD
Anteroseptal-lateral	Proximal LAD
Anterolateral, inferolateral, or posterolateral	LCx

Anterior Wall AMI

Anterior wall infarction rarely presents by itself. In fact, we were unable to provide a single example of isolated anterior infarct. It commonly occurs with infarcts of the septum, the lateral wall, or both. The leads that represent the anterior wall are V_3 and V_4, shown in Figures 15-16 and 15-17. When both the anterior wall and the septum are af-

fected (an anteroseptal AMI), the infarct changes will appear in leads V_1 to V_4. When the infarct occurs in the anterior and lateral walls (an anterolateral AMI), the changes will show in V_3 to V_6, and possibly I and aVL. When the anterior wall, septum, and lateral wall are all involved, the infarct is known as an antero-septal AMI with lateral extension. This will affect V_2 to V_5, and usually also V_1, V_6, I, and aVL.

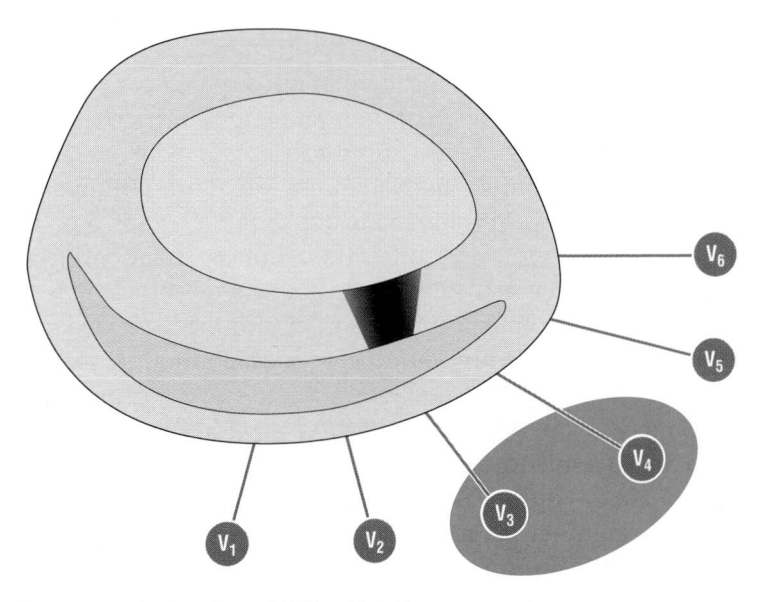

Figure 15-16: Anterior wall AMI = V_3 to V_4.

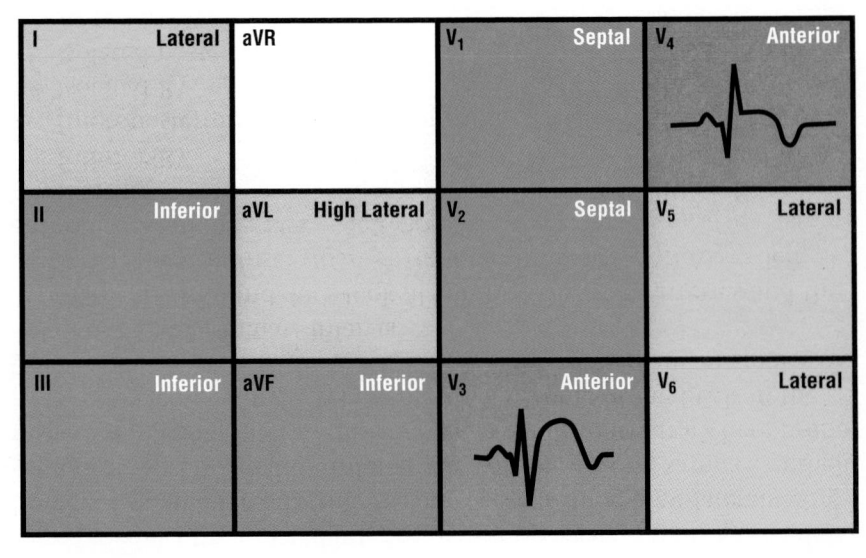

Figure 15-17

REMINDER:

Most infarcts of the heart involve more than one isolated area. Look for associated areas when an infarct is noted.

Anteroseptal MI

The anteroseptal AMI, an example of which is shown in Figures 15-18 and 15-19, is a common pattern and is frequently associated with hemodynamic compromise and cardiogenic shock, as are all the other anterior infarcts. It is critical to understand that this type of infarct does not cause any reciprocal changes in the limb leads, which are in a different plane. If you see changes in the limb leads, it is because of involvement of the additional walls of the heart represented by those leads, such as the high lateral wall.

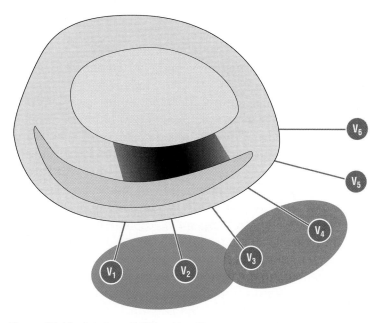

Figure 15-18: Anterior wall AMI = V$_3$ to V$_4$; septal wall AMI = V$_1$ to V$_2$.

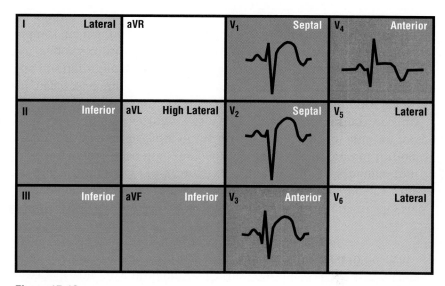

Figure 15-19

CLINICAL PEARL

If you see a reciprocal ST depression in leads II, III, and aVF, the infarct is probably affecting the lateral and high lateral areas of the heart as well.

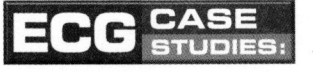 **Anteroseptal AMI**

ECG 15-1 This ECG is classic for an anteroseptal AMI. You see the rather large ST elevation with flat ST segments in V_1 to V_4, the hallmark of this type of infarct.

There is also minimal elevation in aVL, suggestive of some small involvement of the high lateral myocardium in the infarct. This elevation gives rise to reciprocal ST depression in II, III, and aVF. Note that reciprocal changes are usually the first electrocardiographic signs to appear. (In the sequence of this particular patient, leads I and aVL subsequently demonstrated clear ST elevation involving the lateral wall.) Leads I and V_6 eventually show some ST depression that could result from ischemia in those areas. Note that these leads are not reciprocal to the anteroseptal infarct. The leads that form reciprocal changes are 180° from the lead in question. In the case of an anteroseptal infarct, the reciprocal leads would be in the right posterior chest where we do not normally place any electrodes.

The concept of reciprocal leads is a critical one to understand. Study it carefully. Once again, leads that are reciprocal need to be 180° from the lead in question, and *lying in the same plane*. Limb leads and precordial leads cannot be reciprocal to each other because they rest on planes that lie at a 90° angle to one other. The negative zone of ischemia or secondary ischemia is the cause of ST segment depression in other, unassociated areas of an ECG.

ECG 15-2 The ST segment elevation in this ECG, noticeable in V_1 to V_3, makes this an anteroseptal infarct. There are Q waves starting to form in V_2 and V_3, and the T waves are markedly flipped in V_2 to V_4. This infarct had been going on for a few hours prior to the patient's arrival in the emergency department.

Note the appearance of the T waves in this patient and on the other ECGs in this chapter. You will notice that most, if not all, of the affected leads have symmetrical T waves. Symmetrical T waves, as mentioned in previous chapters, are a very bad thing. If you see them, you should begin to think of what kinds of pathology are involved and the clinical processes that the patient may have going on. Some Ts are just symmetrical by nature, however. An old ECG will help you with that distinction. All we ask is that you maintain a high level of suspicion when you approach an ECG with symmetrical T waves.

This is also a fine time to remind you about the ST segment. In infarcts, the ST segments are usually flat, upward sloping, or upwardly convex. If you have problems with this concept, go back and review Chapter 14 briefly before moving on. These points need to be clear when you are interpreting an ECG with a possible AMI.

ECG 15-3 This ECG also shows an anteroseptal AMI. There are elevated ST segments in V_1 to V_4, with Q waves in V_2 to V_4. The flipped, symmetrical T waves in V_5 to V_6 are a continuation of the ischemia from the acute infarct. Also note the poor R-R progression present throughout the precordium because of the infarct-related loss of anterior forces.

Is there an inferior infarct as well? No. Notice that there are tiny little R waves at the onset of the QRS complex in the inferior leads. The negative complexes are, therefore, not caused by an age indeterminate inferior infarct, but rather by a left anterior hemiblock. There are also changes consistent with an incomplete RBBB in V_1. Additional findings include LAE and nonspecific ST changes with flattening in the inferior and lateral areas.

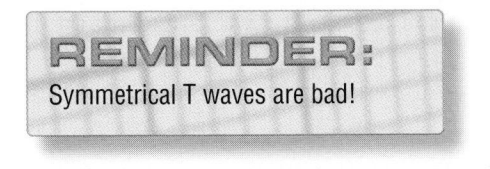
REMINDER:
Symmetrical T waves are bad!

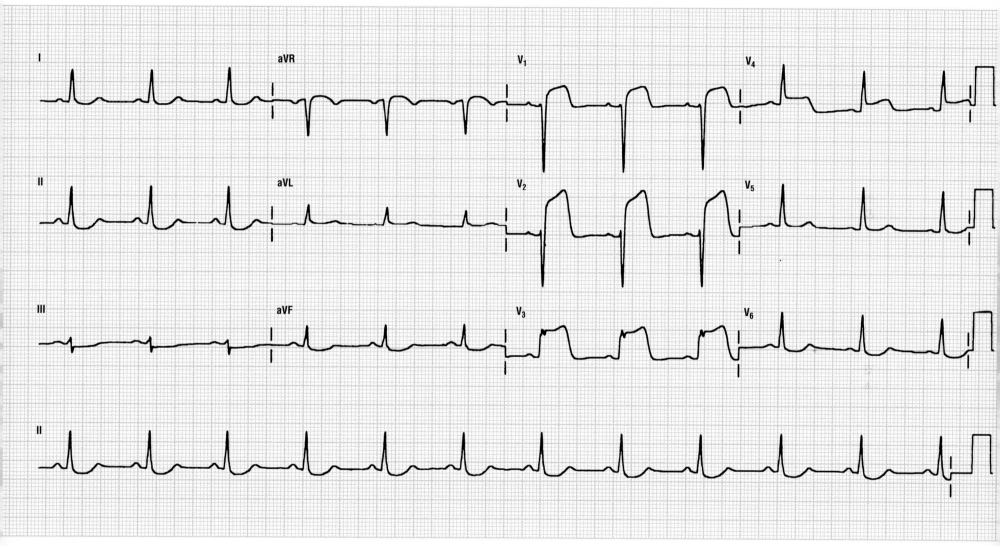

ECG 15-1

ECG CASE STUDIES: **CONTINUED**

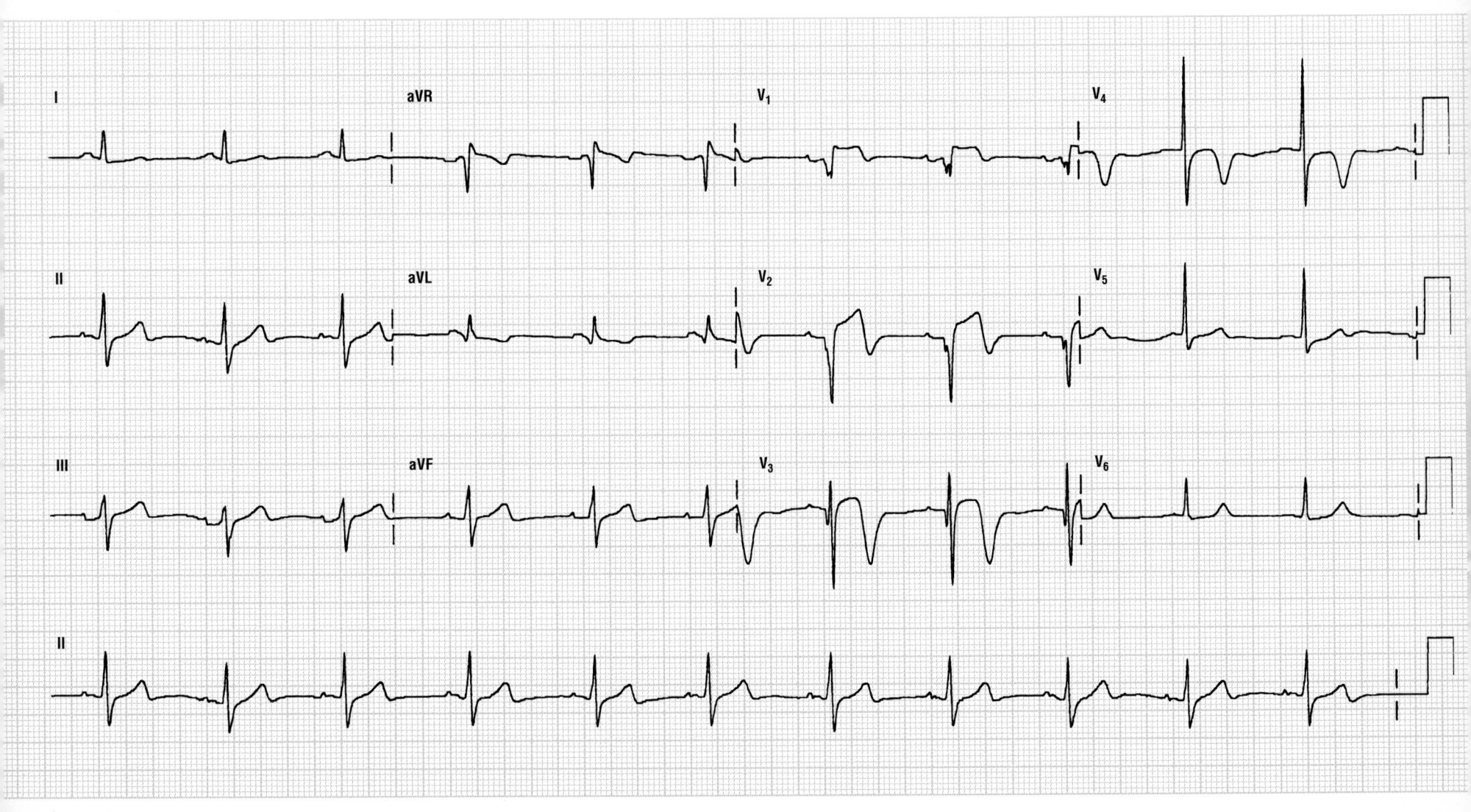

ECG 15-2

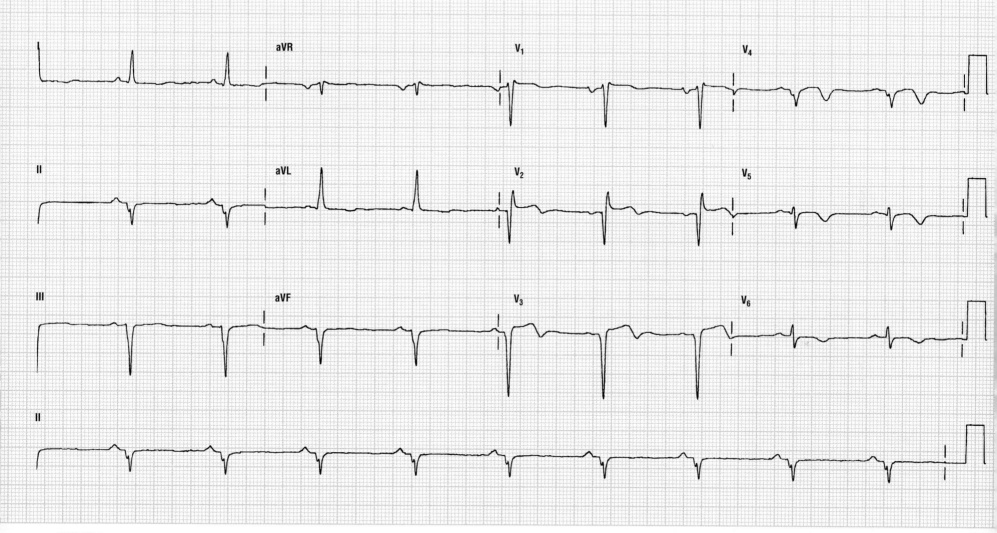

ECG 15-3

Anteroseptal AMI with Lateral Extension

The anteroseptal AMI with lateral extension occurs when there is extension of the infarct pattern to leads V_5 to V_6, I, and aVL. It is, once again, a common presentation for AMI and represents an infarct encompassing a large percentage of myocardial tissue. Reciprocal changes are commonly seen in leads II, III, and aVF.

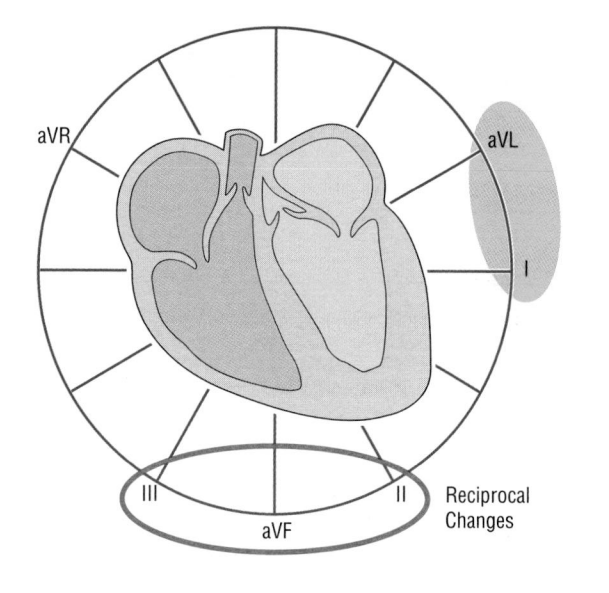

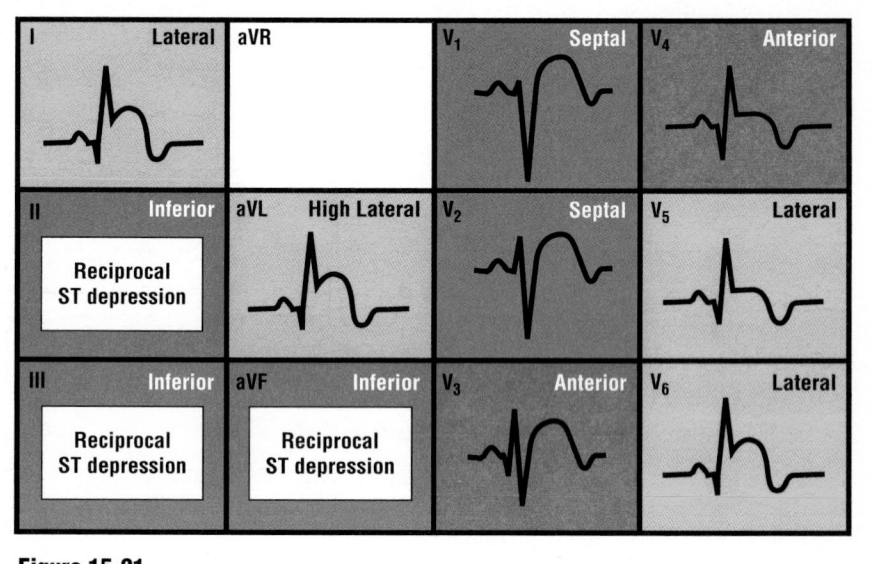

Figure 15-21

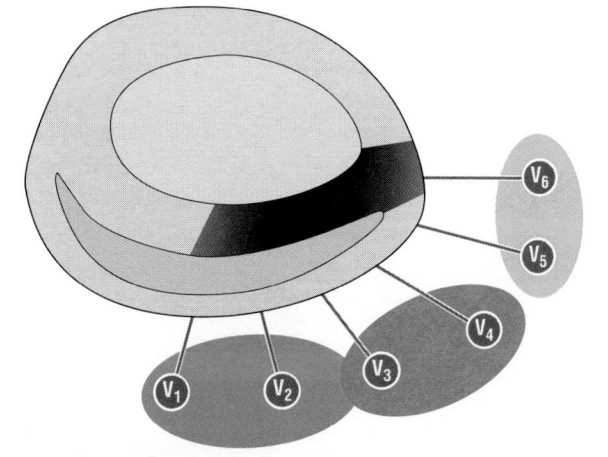

Figure 15-20: Anterior wall AMI = V_3 to V_4; septal wall AMI = V_1 to V_2; lateral wall AMI = V_5 to V_6 (I, aVL).

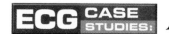

ECG 15-4 It is very difficult to confuse this ECG with anything but a big, ugly AMI. Anteroseptal AMIs with lateral extension are, unfortunately, a common form. Most anterolaterals also have some ST changes in V_2, making them truly anteroseptals with lateral extension. Some authors have called these ECGs "extensive anteriors," but we will simply call them anteroseptal AMIs with lateral extension.

This ECG shows ST elevation in V_2 to V_6 that extends to leads I and aVL. There are reciprocal changes in III and aVF. In addition, there are Q waves starting to form in V_3 to V_6, and in I and aVL.

Note the size of the ST segments and T waves. They are very elevated, consistent with what is known as the *hyperacute changes* of an early AMI. These changes occur during the first 15 to 30 minutes of an AMI, so this finding is usually missed because many patients do not present until 2 to 3 hours after the onset of chest pain — well past the hyperacute period. These patients are the ones that benefit the most from early revascularization because they have the most salvageable myocardium. Their stunned myocardium will also recover the fastest because the ischemic period has been relatively short. When you see these changes, be very aggressive.

ECG 15-5 This ECG also has the classic changes for an anteroseptal AMI with lateral extension. The ST changes occur in V_1 to V_5, and in I and aVL. The changes in V_2 are suggestive of the hyperacute changes we mentioned regarding ECG 15-4. However, because the hyperacute ST elevation is only found in V_2, these appear to be resolving into the more stable AMI pattern of tombstoning. There are reciprocal changes in II, III, and aVF, as expected.

 Anteroseptal AMIs with lateral extension are caused by obstruction of the proximal left main or the proximal left anterior descending (LAD) artery.

ECG 15-6 This is yet another anteroseptal AMI with lateral extension. The changes of a classic AMI are present in V_1 to V_6, and also in I and aVL. There are QS waves in V_2 and V_3. There are also Q waves in V_4 to V_6, I, and aVL, and reciprocal changes in II, III, and aVF.

Why didn't we say that V_1 has a QS wave? Because it doesn't! Note that there is a small *r* wave (we would say a ditzel of an *r*) before the S wave. This is just enough to make it an rS complex and not a QS.

 Poor R-R progression in the precordial leads frequently reflects a loss of the anterior forces (vectors) caused by a large, old anterior AMI.

ECG 15-7 This ECG also has some mildly elevated ST segments. Just kidding — they are *very* elevated. The leads involved point to an anteroseptal AMI with lateral extension: V_1 to V_5, I, and aVL. There are reciprocal changes in the inferior leads.

When they are faced with troublesome ECGs that they can't figure out, some people will give up on the interpretation and disregard the presence of abnormalities. We ask you to do the exact opposite. When you are faced with a troublesome ECG, spend the time to break it down into all of its components, look at each beat individually, and use the tools that you have available — rulers, calipers, and so on.

Additional points about this ECG include QT prolongation and LVH.

REMINDER:
Don't get hooked on the first thing you see on the ECG, no matter how impressive it is. Always break the whole thing down before making a definitive interpretation.

ECG CASE STUDIES: **CONTINUED**

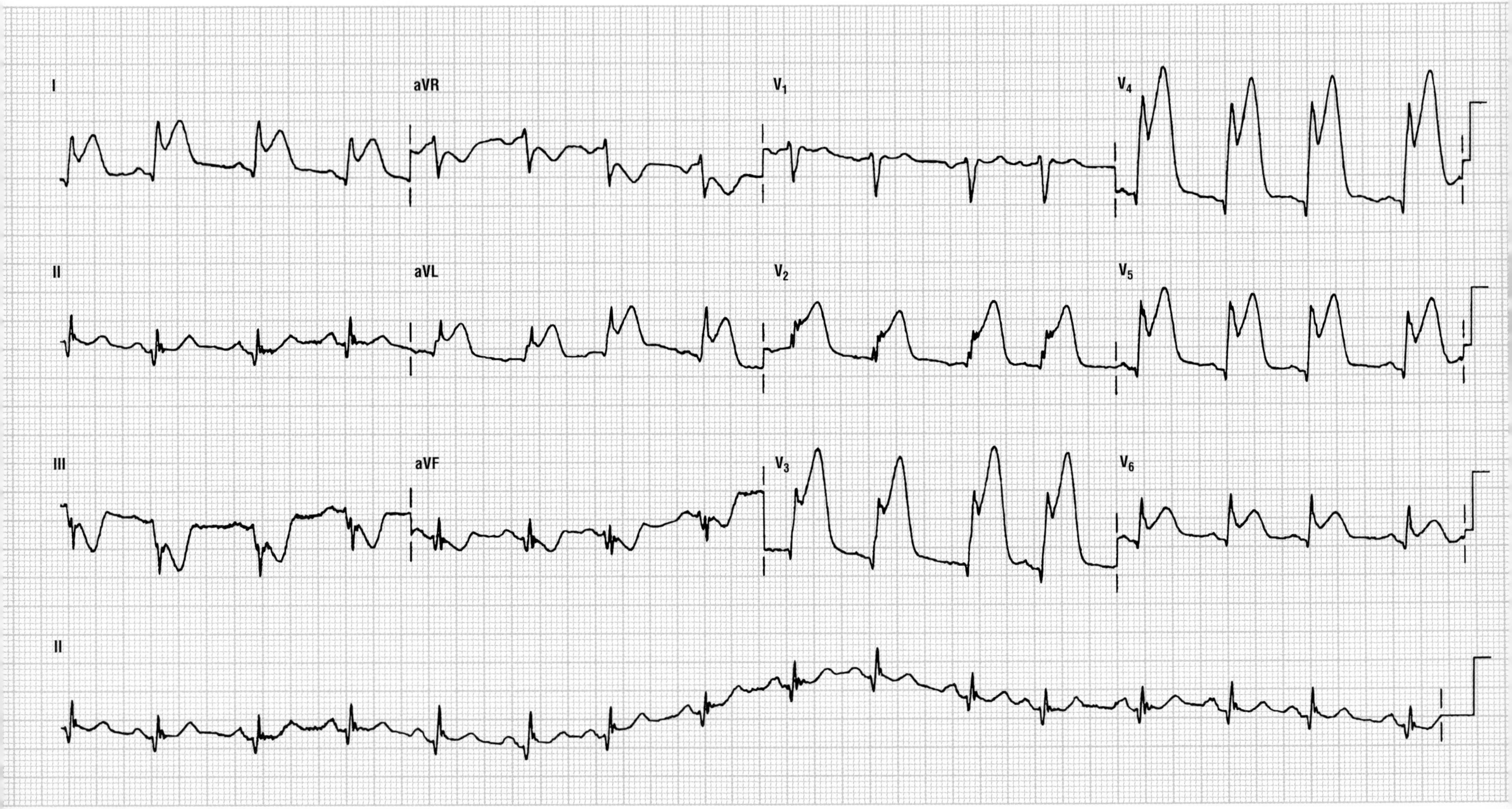

I   aVR   V₁   V₄

II   aVL   V₂   V₅

III   aVF   V₃   V₆

II

ECG 15-4

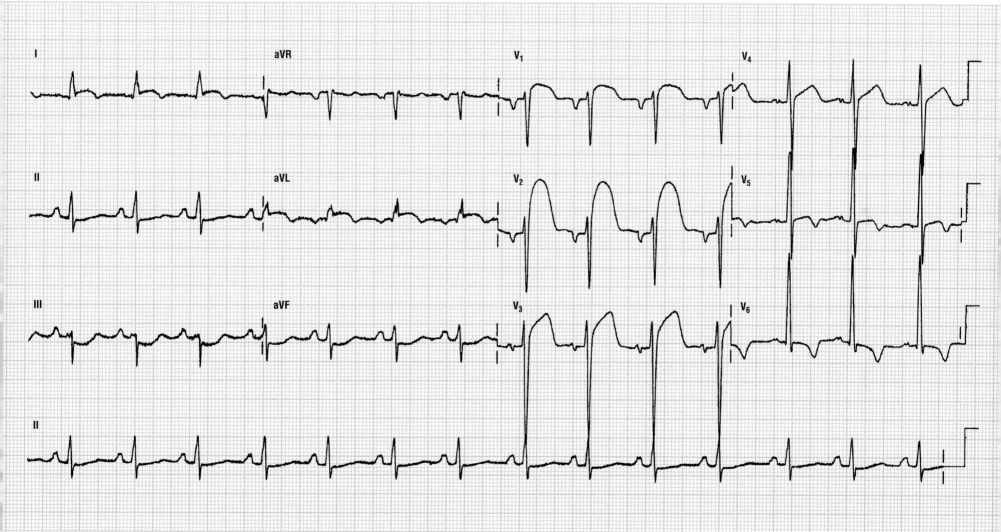

ECG 15-5

ECG CASE STUDIES: CONTINUED

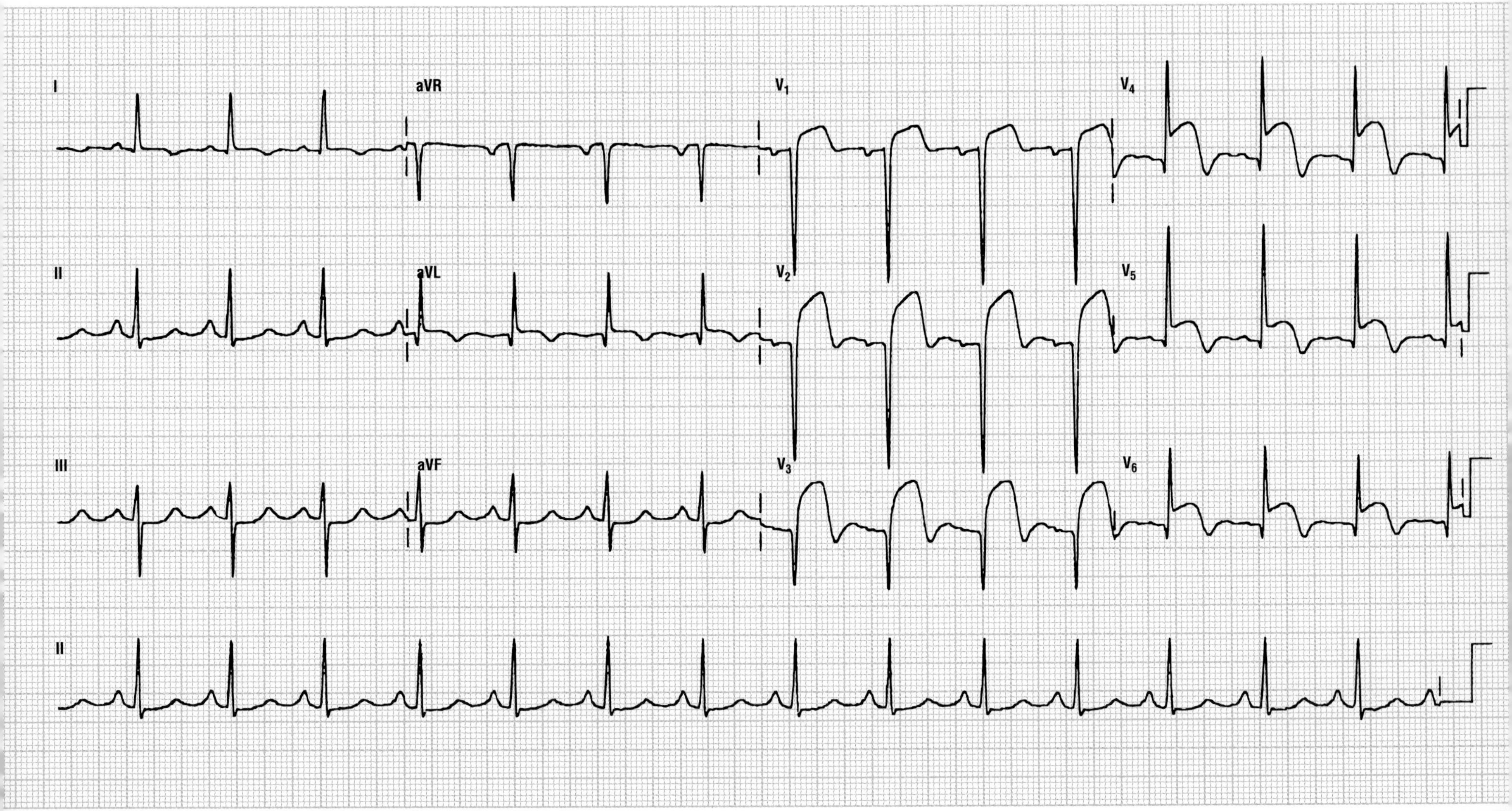

I aVR V₁ V₄

II aVL V₂ V₅

III aVF V₃ V₆

II

ECG 15-6

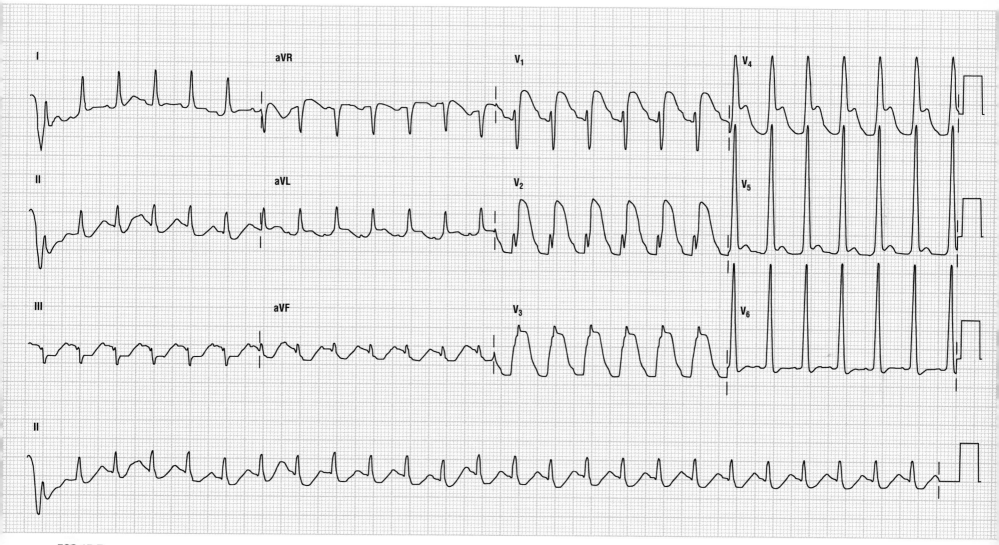

ECG 15-7

ECG CASE STUDIES: **CONTINUED**

ECG 15-8 The ST segment elevation in this ECG is classic for an anteroseptal AMI with lateral extension. Do you notice anything else unusual here? On ECG 15-7, we mentioned that it is critical to evaluate all aspects of an ECG in order to maximize your interpretation. The key thing to look at in this ECG, besides the obvious AMI, is the P waves. The inverted Ps beginning in II, III, and aVF are not normal (take a look at the rhythm strip for greater clarity). They are usually found in either a nodal or infranodal complexes with retrograde transmission of the P waves, or a low atrial ectopic pacemaker. Because the complexes are narrow and identical to the normal complex, they originate in the AV node. This makes it a junctional rhythm or a low atrial pacemaker. Because of the shortened PR interval, and the presence of the AMI, a junctional rhythm is the correct diagnosis.

REMINDER:
Always look for conduction or rhythm abnormalities on ECGs that show any kind of AMI.

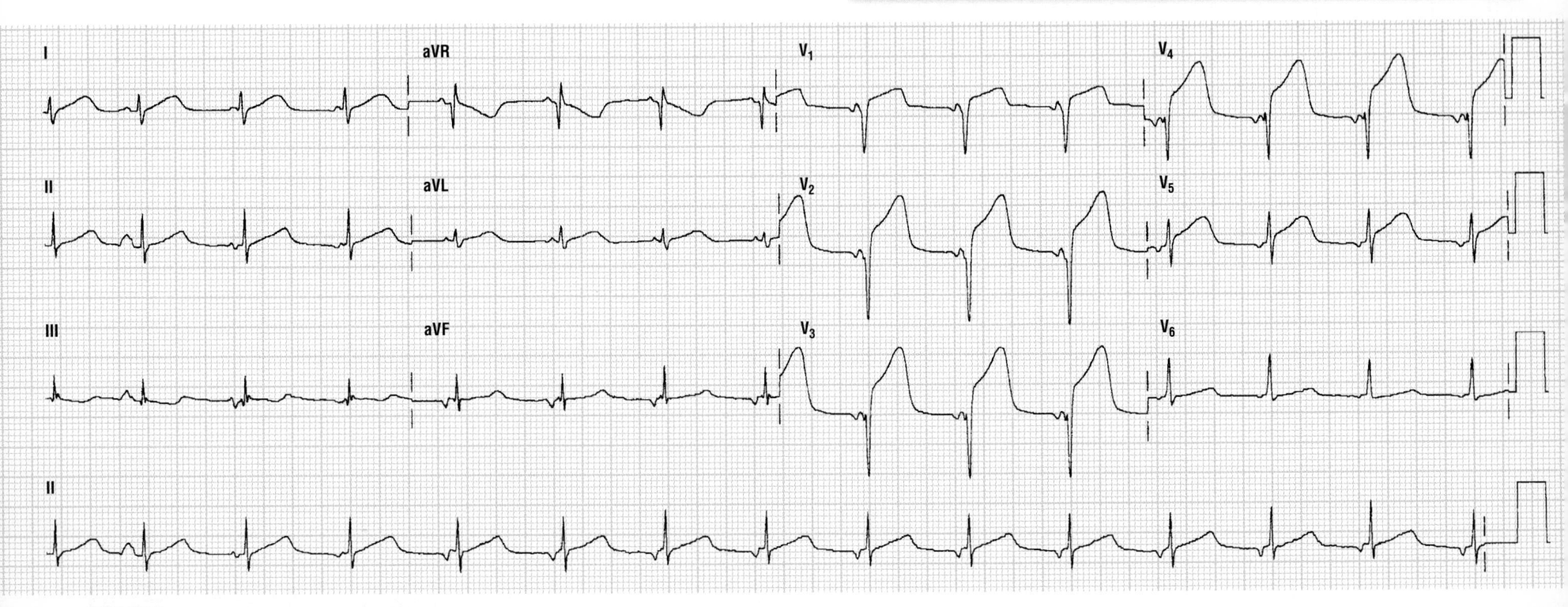

ECG 15-8

②

ECG 15-9 This ECG shows Q waves in V_1 to V_5, along with ST elevations in V_1 to V_5, I, and aVL. There are also the expected ST depressions consistent with reciprocal changes in the inferior leads. Once again, this is an anteroseptal AMI with lateral extension.

The PR prolongation is quite impressive. Whenever you have such prolonged PR intervals, consider the possibility that another P wave is buried in a complex at the halfway point between the two obvious P waves. If you take the distance between the obvious P waves in III, you arrive at approximately 22 mm, so the halfway point is at 11 mm.

Set your calipers at 11 mm and walk them along the ECG looking for any buried P waves. There are none in this ECG.

CLINICAL PEARL

When you see a very prolonged PR interval, consider the possibility of another P wave at the halfway point between the two visible Ps.

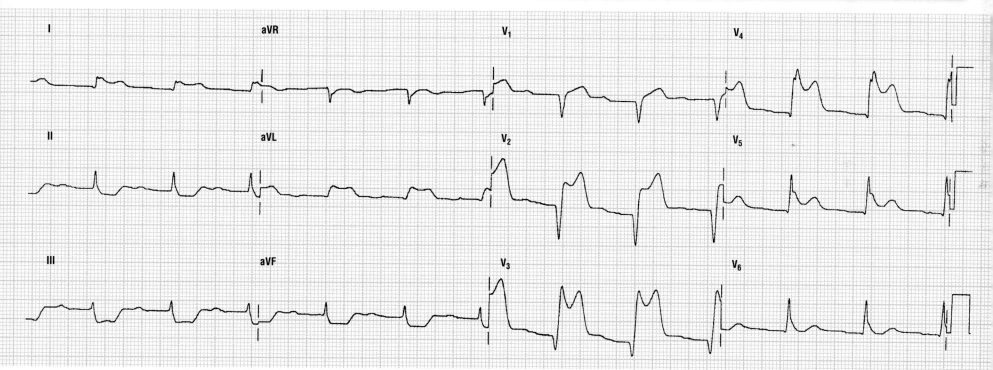

ECG 15-9

ECG CASE STUDIES: **C O N T I N U E D**

ECG 15-10 Yes, this is another anteroseptal AMI with lateral extension. We hope you're getting familiar with this pattern. We're giving you different looks at ECGs with the same underlying pathology. It is very difficult to see just one example of a pathological process and transfer that information to all existing ECGs. You'll find it much easier to do this when you have seen 5 to 10 examples of the varying presentations — some fast, some slow, with and without blocks, and so on. *Try to interpret as many ECGs as possible. Practice does make perfect.*

Compare this ECG to one with LVH with strain, such as ECG 14-41A, found on page 375. The ST segments are flatter and the T waves are more symmetrical. The clincher to the pathological process is the ST elevation in leads I and aVL, with reciprocal changes in the inferior leads. This can only be an AMI.

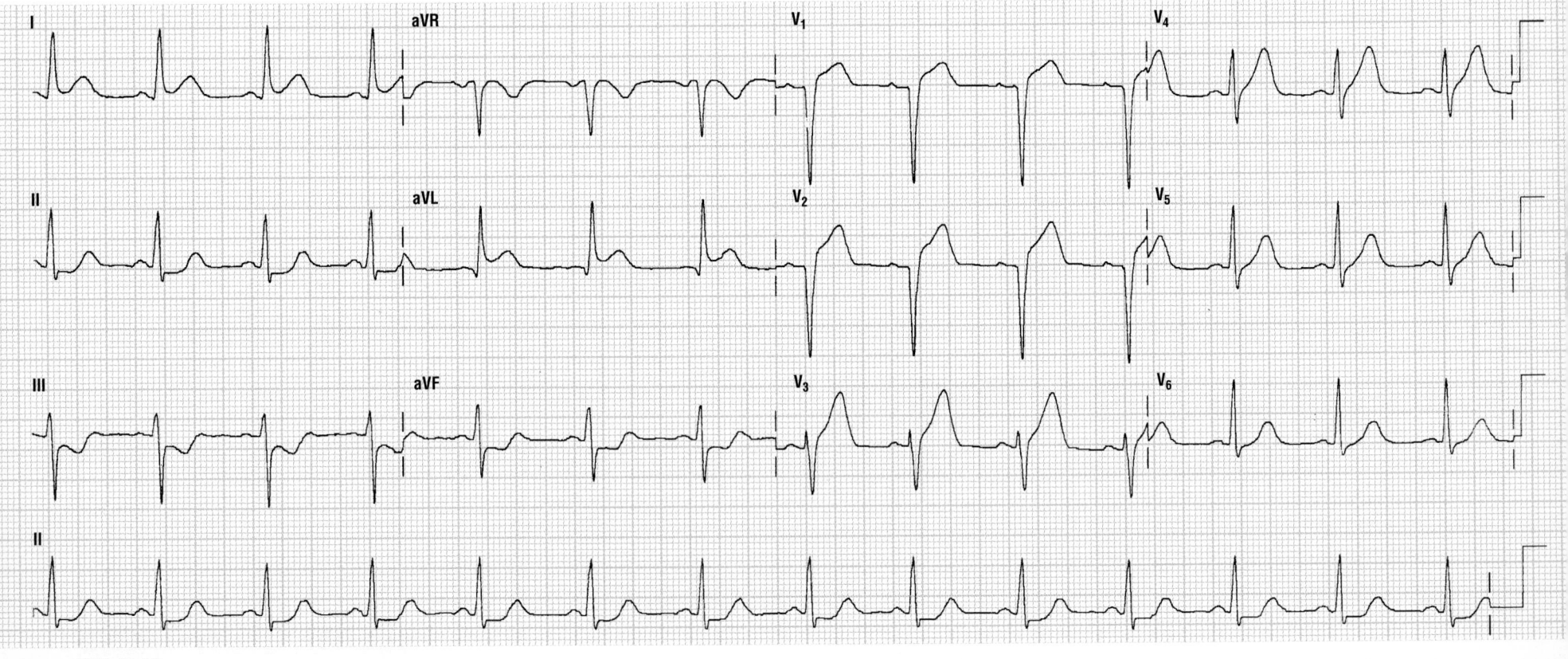

ECG 15-10

ECG 15-11 This ECG was obtained from a patient in obvious distress with significant hemodynamic compromise. It shows changes consistent with an anteroseptal AMI with lateral extension. Once again, notice the reciprocal changes in the inferior leads.

You need to obtain a new ECG whenever you see a change in the morphology of the complexes on the monitor, or when the patient's symptoms change at any point while having an AMI. Make this a habit. Don't think about it, just do it! Patients with AMIs have many rhythm abnormalities and blocks involving the AV node or the bundle branches. These will, in many cases, require the placement of a transcutaneous or transvenous pacemaker. Be prepared for any possible scenario.

> **REMINDER:**
> Obtaining serial ECGs is critical in an AMI patient to evaluate for new blocks or extension of the infarct.

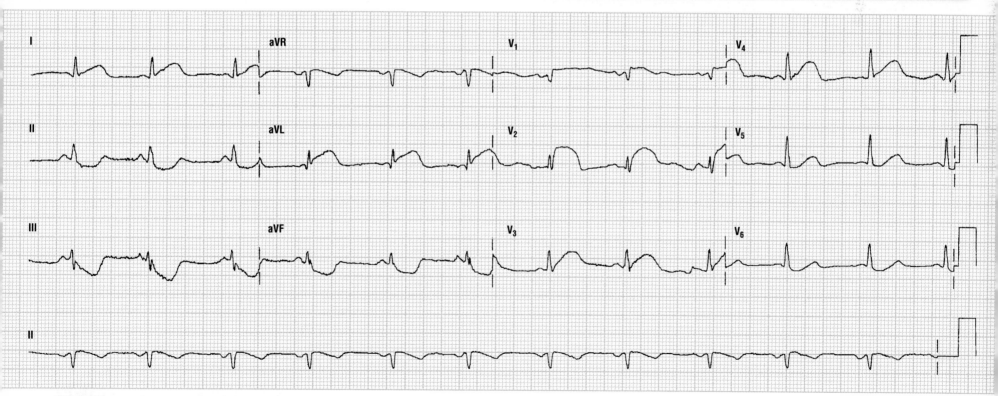

ECG 15-11

ECG CASE STUDIES: CONTINUED

ECG 15-12 This was obtained from the patient we saw in ECG 15-11, less than 10 minutes later. This looks like a totally different ECG, and it is. Why is it so different? Well, for starters, the QRS is wider than

> **REMINDER:**
> Understand the indications for pacemaker placement in an acute AMI. You always need to be prepared.

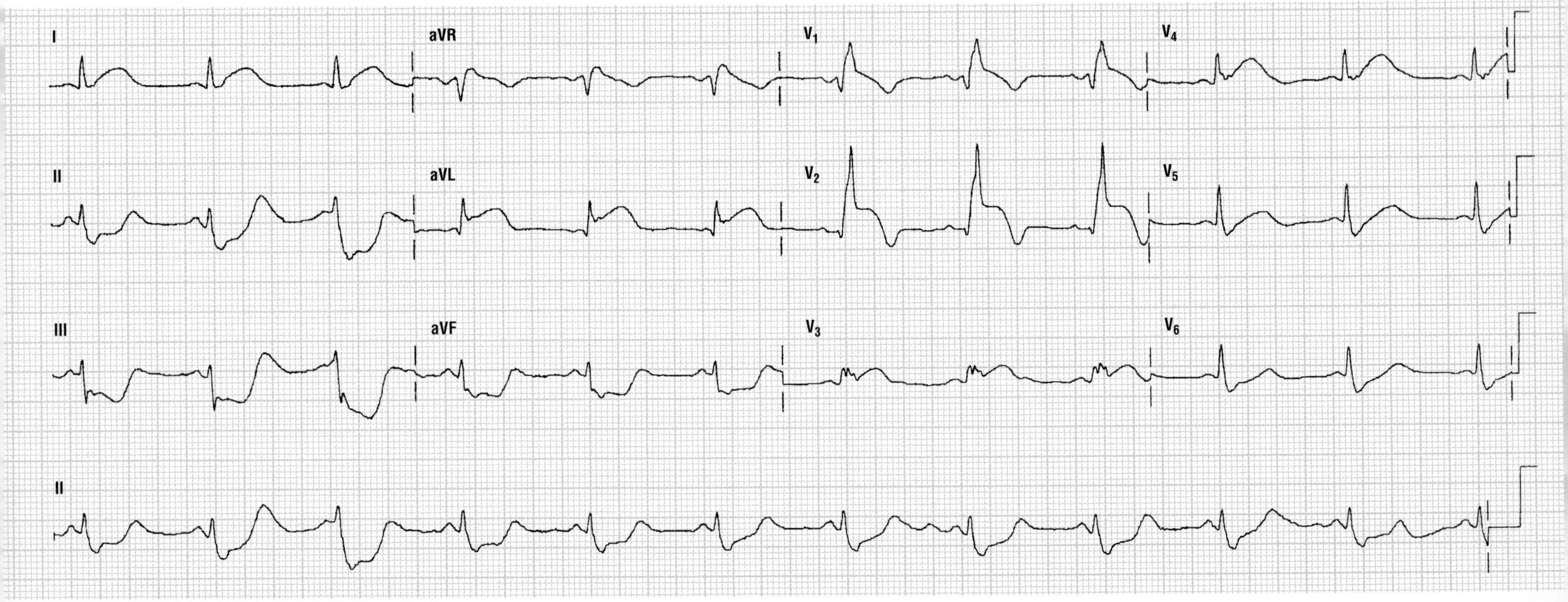

0.12 seconds. Think of the differential for this width. Are there slurred S waves in leads I and V_6? There definitely is in V_6. In lead I, the ST elevation is obliterating the slurred S. You can also see rabbit ears in V_1. These changes are consistent with an RBBB. Now look at the axis. It, too, has shifted because of a new LAH. A new bifascicular block, in the setting of an acute AMI, is an indication for pacemaker placement. You need to think and act quickly, because sometimes you only have seconds before significant hemodynamic compromise develops that could be life threatening.

ECG 15-12

ECG 15-13 Here is another example of a large anteroseptal AMI with lateral extension in a patient with a bifascicular block. The RBBB and LAH are old but the AMI pattern is new. The presence of a bifascicular block on an old ECG is comforting, but you should still take it seriously. Remember, there is only one fascicle transmitting the impulse to the ventricles. If anything happens to that fascicle, the patient is in serious trouble. We advocate placing a transcutaneous pacer as a preventive measure, in case it is needed. It is easier to turn on the machine when it is already hooked up than to turn your unit upside down looking for the machine or the pads in an emergency situation. Be prepared for the worst-case scenario. Don't gamble with the patient's life.

CLINICAL PEARL

An old bifascicular pattern is usually stable, but you should still be careful. An AMI with a new bifascicular block is very dangerous

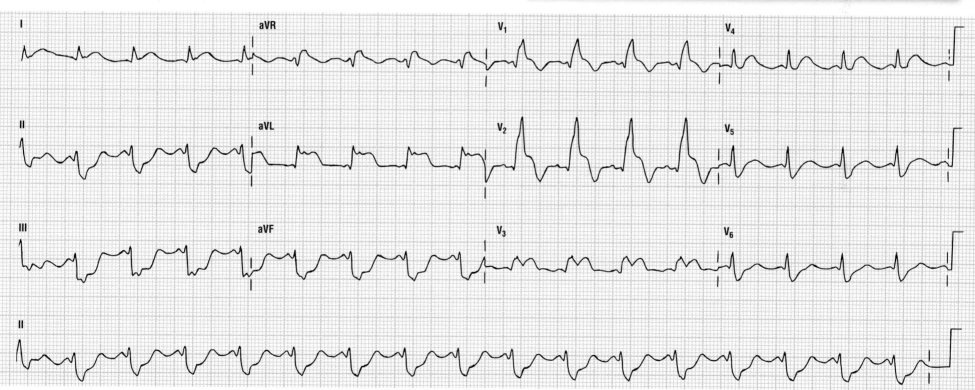

ECG 15-13

Lateral Wall AMI

Lateral wall AMIs can occur by themselves by showing changes in leads I, aVL, V$_5$, and V$_6$ or they can occur in combination with other infarct patterns. Most notable of the combination infarcts are inferolat-eral, anterolaterals, or anteroseptal with lateral extensions. They can also occur in combination with right ventricular and posterior infarcts as we shall see later in the chapter. Remember that high lateral AMIs do show reciprocal changes in the inferior leads.

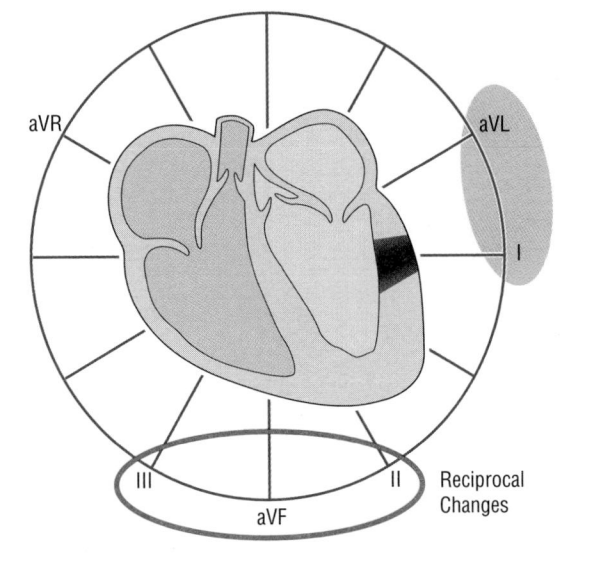

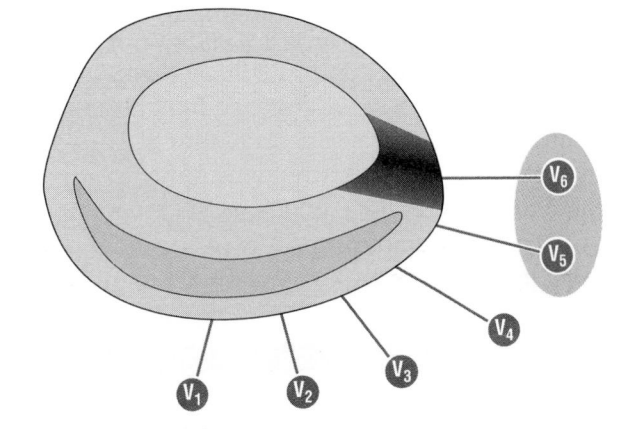

Figure 15-22: Lateral wall AMI = V$_5$, V$_6$; high lateral AMI = I, aVL.

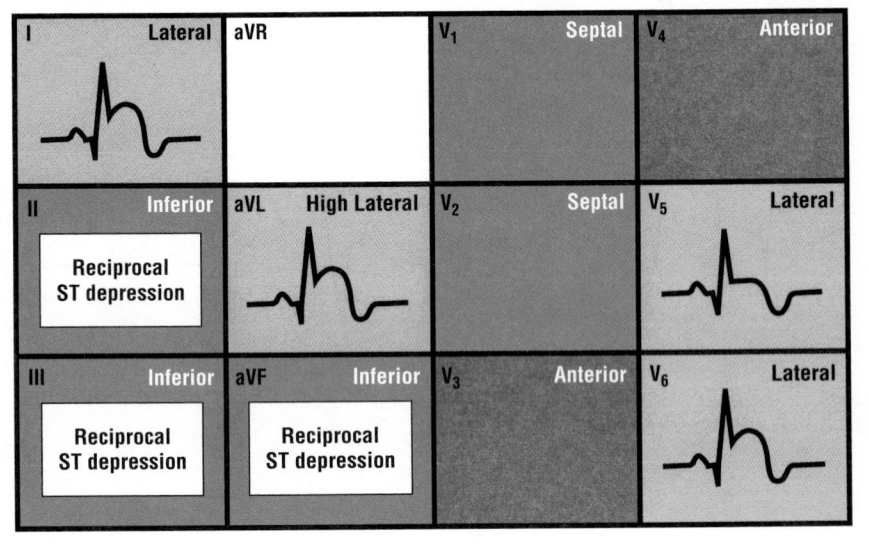

Figure 15-23

REMINDER:

Lateral infarcts can occur by themselves or in combination with anterior, anteroseptal, inferior, right ventricular, or posterior AMIs. Always look at all of the regions of the ECG and obtain additional leads to be sure.

ECG 15-14 This patient was suffering a high-lateral AMI. Notice that there is flat ST segment elevation in leads I and aVL. There are also reciprocal changes in the inferior leads, clinching the diagnosis.

There are changes caused by LVH with strain pattern, but notice that the T waves are symmetric in V_5 to V_6. LVH with strain is associated with asymmetric T waves in the lateral leads. The Ts in this ECG are secondary to ischemia until proven otherwise, especially in light of the high-lateral AMI. Also, remember that LVH with strain can be associated with ST depression and asymmetric T waves in leads I and aVL. In this ECG, the ST segments are elevated and the Ts are definitely symmetric, consistent with the AMI.

> **REMINDER:**
> Symmetric T waves are pathological until proven otherwise. Don't get fooled!

QUICK REVIEW

1. Lateral wall AMIs can occur by themselves or in combination with other regions. True or False.

2. Lateral wall AMIs show reciprocal changes in leads II, III, and aVF. True or False.

3. Lateral wall AMIs show reciprocal changes in leads V_1 and V_2. True or False.

4. Q waves in leads I and aVL are always due to a lateral infarct. True or False.

5. ST segment elevations in leads V_5 and V_6 are usually benign. True or False.

6. You should always look at *all* of the regions of the ECG whenever you find evidence of an infarct in any *one* region. True or False.

7. If you find evidence of a posterior infarct, you can discount any ST elevation in the lateral leads as insignificant. True or False.

8. Changes in V_4 are due to isolated lateral infarcts. True or False.

9. If you do not see any ST elevation in leads I and aVL, you will never see any ST depression in the inferior leads. True or False.

10. Lateral wall AMIs can be associated with infarcts in:
    a. Anterior wall
    b. Posterior wall
    c. Inferior wall
    d. Right Ventricular wall
    e. Anteroseptal areas
    f. All of the above are correct.
    g. None of the above are correct.

1. True 2. True 3. False 4. False. They can be benign Q waves, known as septal Qs. 5. False. Never assume any ST elevation is benign. Always evaluate the clinical scenario. 6. True! Whenever you find any evidence of infarct, look at all of the leads and regions very, very closely. In addition, always look closely at the rhythm. 7. False. They are evidence of anterior wall involvement in an anterolateral wall AMI. 9. False. Many times the ST elevation is minimal or developing. The ST depressions that represent reciprocal changes are the first visible signs occurring in AMIs in many cases. They commonly occur sooner than the ST elevations become apparent. 10. F.

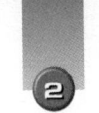

ECG CASE STUDY: **CONTINUED**

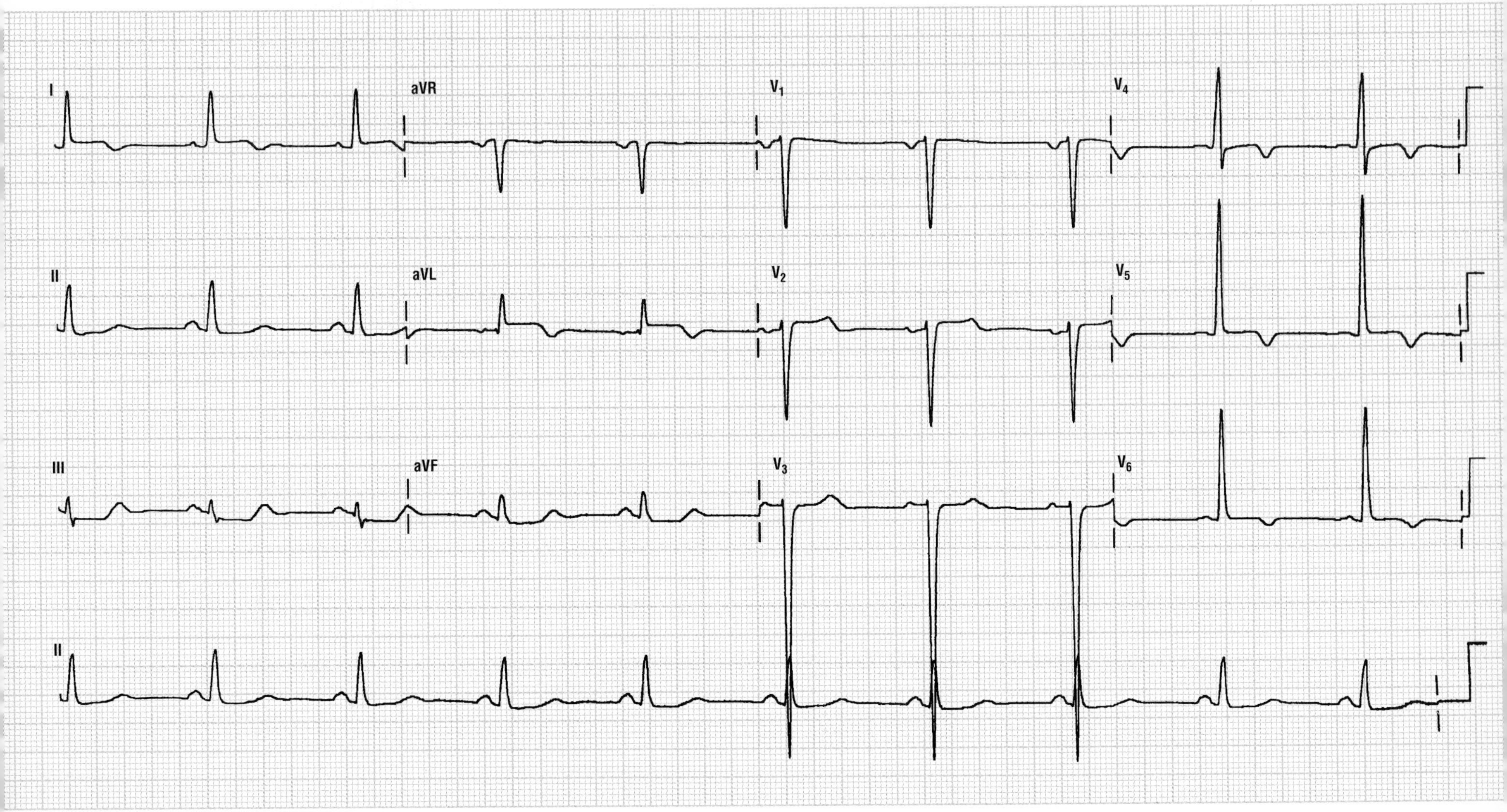

I aVR V₁ V₄

II aVL V₂ V₅

III aVF V₃ V₆

II

ECG 15-14

Inferior Wall AMI

Inferior wall AMIs, which produce changes in II, III, and aVF, depicted in Figure 15-24, are commonly associated with additional involvement of the lateral wall, the posterior wall, and the right ventricle. As you can imagine, inferolateral AMIs present with changes in II, III, aVF, and

V_5 to V_6, and may include I and aVL if the high lateral wall is involved, as shown in Figure 15-25. Reciprocal changes of an inferior AMI always present as ST depression in leads I and aVL unless the high lateral wall is also infarcting. Right ventricular infarcts and posterior infarcts (Level 2 material) will be covered later.

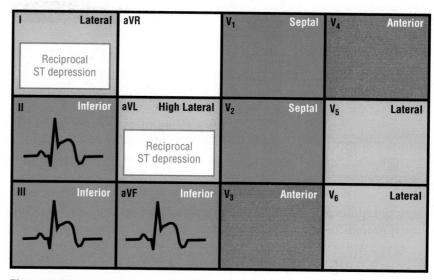

Figure 15-24: Inferior wall AMI = II, III, aVF.

Figure 15-25

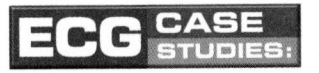 *Inferior Wall AMI*

ECG 15-15 Do you notice any ST elevation or depression on this ECG? Not really. There are some nonspecific ST-T wave changes with flattening of the T waves in aVF and V_5 to V_6. Then why would this ECG be in the infarct chapter? Well, notice the Q waves in III and aVF. These Qs are definitely pathological — wider than 0.03 seconds and deeper than $1/3$ the height of the associated R wave. They indicate an IWMI of indeterminate age. We use the term *age-indeterminate* when we are not sure when the AMI occurred, but know it is not an acute infarct occurring at this moment.

Isolated IWMIs occur mostly in age-indeterminate infarcts. This is because acute IWMIs usually involve the RCA, which perfuses parts of the posterior wall, right ventricle, and lateral wall. Therefore, acute infarcts will show changes in the leads representing those areas as well.

Notice the poor R-R progression. Many authors call this a sign of an old anteroseptal AMI that has caused a loss of anterior forces. This is something we should keep in mind as a possibility, but remember that there can be other causes of a poor R-R progression.

The eighth beat is a VPC. The last is an aberrantly conducted APC. Notice that there is a P wave before the complex, and that it starts in the same direction as the normal complexes.

ECG 15-16 The first thing that may strike you about this ECG is that the QRS complexes are wide and bizarre. This automatically raises the question of a BBB. Are there slurred S waves in leads I and V_6? Well, there sure are in lead I, but V_6 is another story. Why is there an RSR′ complex in that lead? You can sometimes see notched complexes in V_5 or V_6 in an LBBB, but this is not an LBBB. Could it be an IVCD? It could be, but there is a simpler explanation. Look at V_1 and V_2. They are very different from each other. Now, look at V_2 and V_6, which are very similar to each other. V_1 would look less out of place if it were in the V_6 slot, wouldn't it? What happened? The ECG tech placed the V_6 electrode in the V_1 location, and vice versa. These misplaced leads can alter your interpretation. Leads I and V_6 should be similar, if not identical. This is an RBBB.

Are there supposed to be Q waves in the inferior leads in RBBBs? No! Pathologic Q waves are pathologic Q waves, and they are a sign of infarct except in III and V_1 to V_2. In this case, the RBBB is accompanied by an age-indeterminate IWMI.

The first beat in the series is a pathologic beat, either a VPC or an aberrantly conducted complex. In order to make the call definitively, you would need to see what occurred prior to the start of this ECG.

CLINICAL PEARL

IWMIs usually occur in combination with other regions, namely the right ventricular, posterior, or lateral regions. Age indeterminate infarcts may only show changes in the inferior leads, but other regions were affected during the acute phase of the infarct.

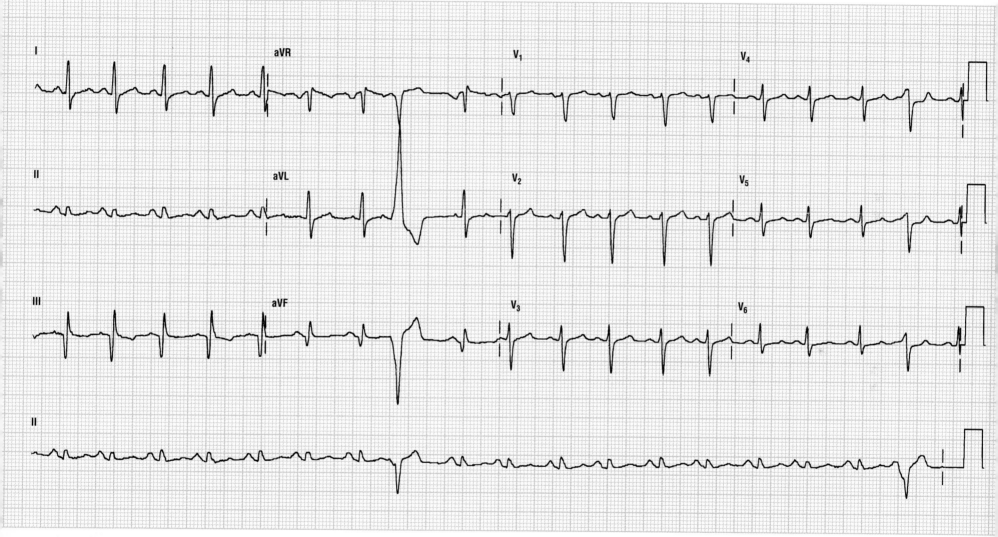

I   aVR   V₁   V₄

II   aVL   V₂   V₅

III   aVF   V₃   V₆

II

ECG 15-15

CHAPTER **15** • ACUTE MYOCARDIAL INFARCTION (AMI)

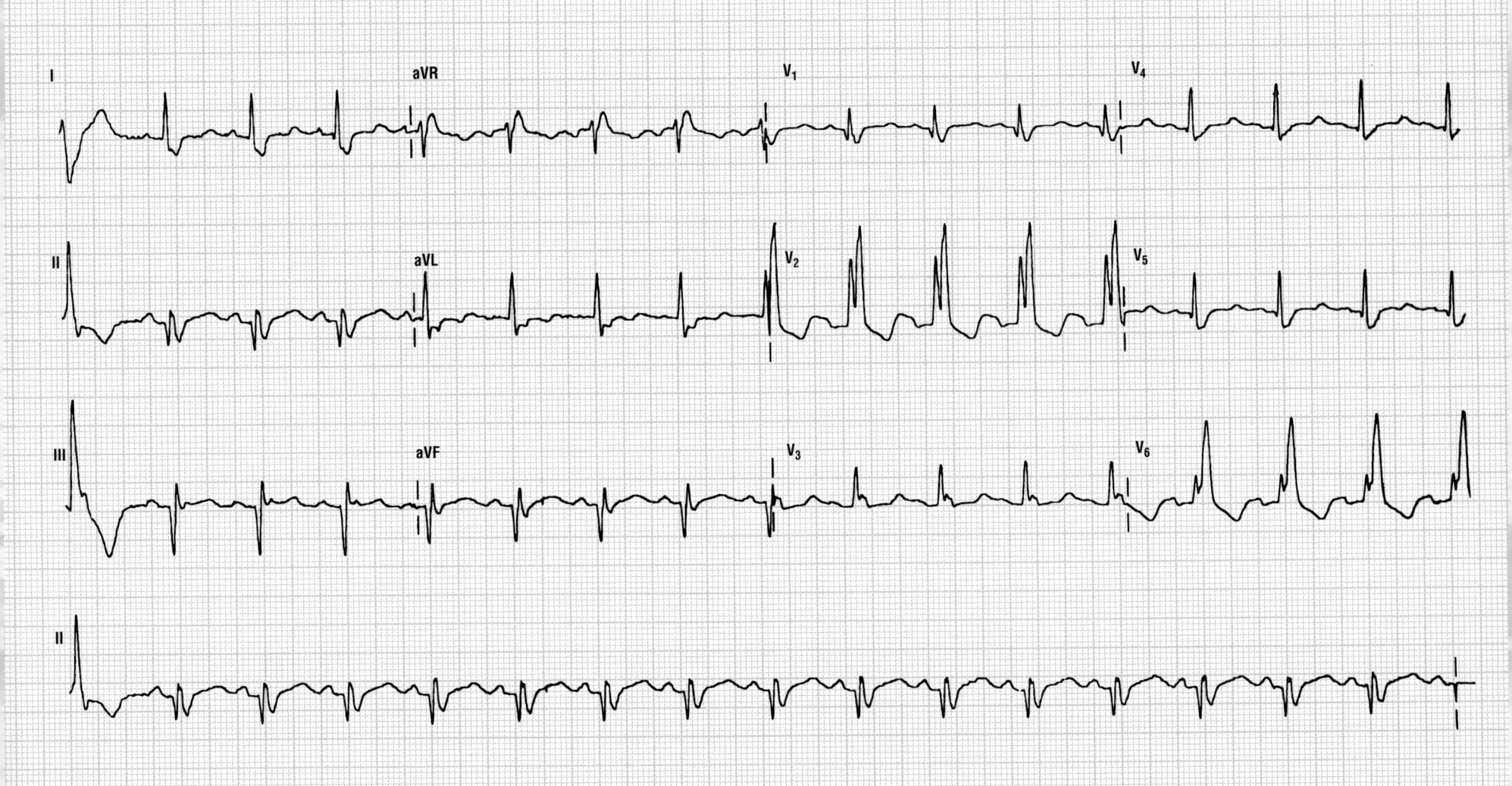

ECG 15-16

Inferolateral AMI

Inferolateral AMIs present with changes in leads II, III, aVF, V$_5$, V$_6$, I, and aVL. The changes in I and aVL will occur if the high lateral wall is involved. Also notice that the ST changes can occur in V$_2$ to V$_4$ as well

depending on how far anteriorly it extends. In these cases, however, you will always see the classic changes in V$_5$ and V$_6$ without exception and the extension to the anterior precordials will be contiguous with these leads.

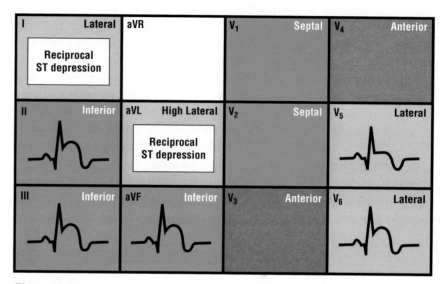

Figure 15-27

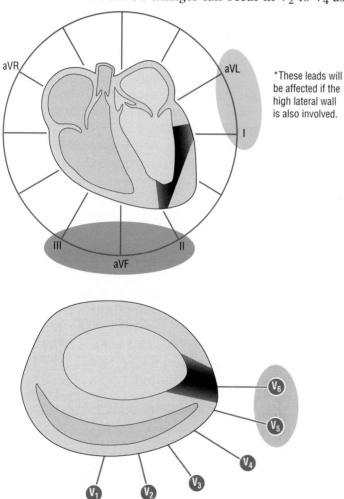

Figure 15-26: Inferior wall AMI = II, III, aVF; lateral wall AMI = V$_5$, V$_6$ (I, aVL*).

CHAPTER **15** • ACUTE MYOCARDIAL INFARCTION (AMI)

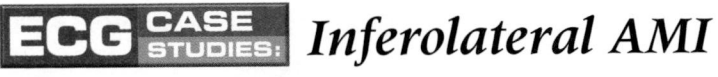 **Inferolateral AMI**

ECG 15-17 This is a great example of an inferolateral AMI (or, IWMI with lateral extension). You see the ST elevation in II, III, and aVF with reciprocal changes of ST depression in leads I and aVL. In addition, there is ST elevation in V_3 to V_6 consistent with the lateral infarct.

Take a good look at aVL. When you see a downward-sloping ST depression in that lead, think about an IWMI. This is the first sign of an IWMI, occurring before the ST elevation in the inferior leads. Other things can cause it, but always rule out the life-threatening problem before considering something benign.

ECG 15-17 The astute clinician will also notice that there is evidence of right ventricular infarction (RVI). The ST elevation in III is greater than the elevation in II, and there is ST elevation in V_1 that does not continue to V_2. This is a typical pattern for an inferolateral-RV infarct. The ST segment will be elevated in V_1 with a normal or depressed ST segment in V_2. Then in III, the ST segment again rises because of the lateral infarct. This patient had a positive V_4R as well, clinching the diagnosis. (*Additional ECG Leads* later in this chapter discusses V_4R.)

The rhythm is sinus arrhythmia.

> ## REMINDER:
> A downward sloping ST depression may be the first sign of an inferior infarct.

ECG 15-18 In this inferolateral AMI, there is obvious ST elevation in II, III, and aVF, as well as V_4 to V_6. Notice the Q waves beginning to form in the inferior leads, which could represent an old infarct in the area with some extension occurring acutely, or — more probably — an infarct that is a few hours old. There is reciprocal ST depression in aVL, but not in lead I.

Sinus arrhythmia is present with its trademark slowing and speeding pattern that shows a gradual change between each two beats. Note that all of the P waves and PR intervals are identical.

ECG 15-18 Lead V_2 is troubling because the *r* wave is broad and significant. In addition, there is minimal depression in the ST segment. This could suggest some early or resolving posterior injury and ischemia. Posterior and RV leads, discussed in *Additional ECG Leads* later in this chapter, are indicated in this patient.

You can use your knowledge to make an educated guess at times. Could you make a definitive call of posterior wall involvement in this case? Not without some additional information and leads (an echocardiogram would also be helpful). However, you always need to assume and prepare for the worst-case scenario. In this instance, the inferolateral AMI was very obvious, but the additional posterior involvement was not that clear. Does it make a difference? Yes, because an inferolateral-posterior AMI has more myocardium at risk than an inferolateral. In fact, it has one more entire wall of myocardium. Your interactions with your consultants need to reflect that additional level of concern so that the best management strategy can be instituted to salvage as much myocardium as possible.

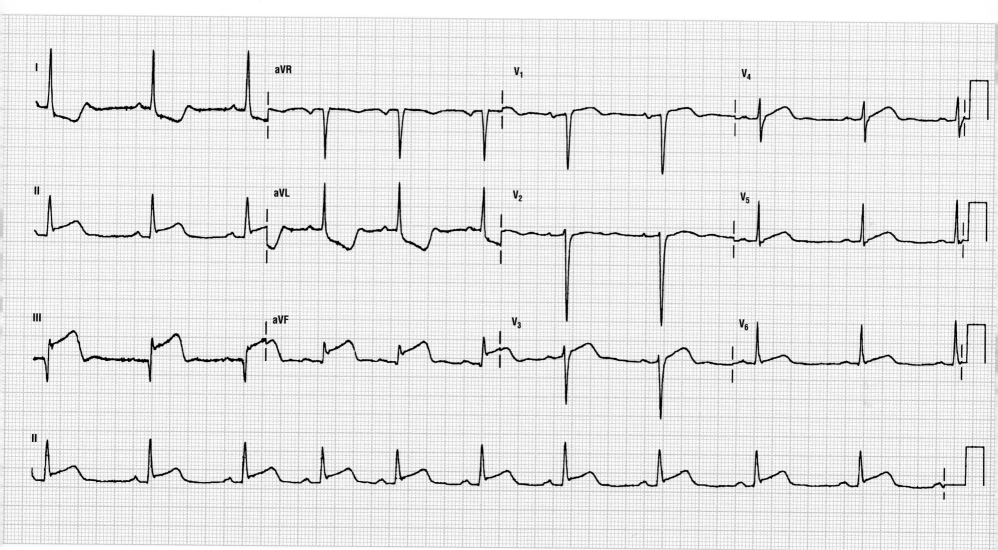

ECG 15-17

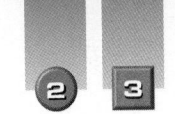

ECG CASE STUDIES: **CONTINUED**

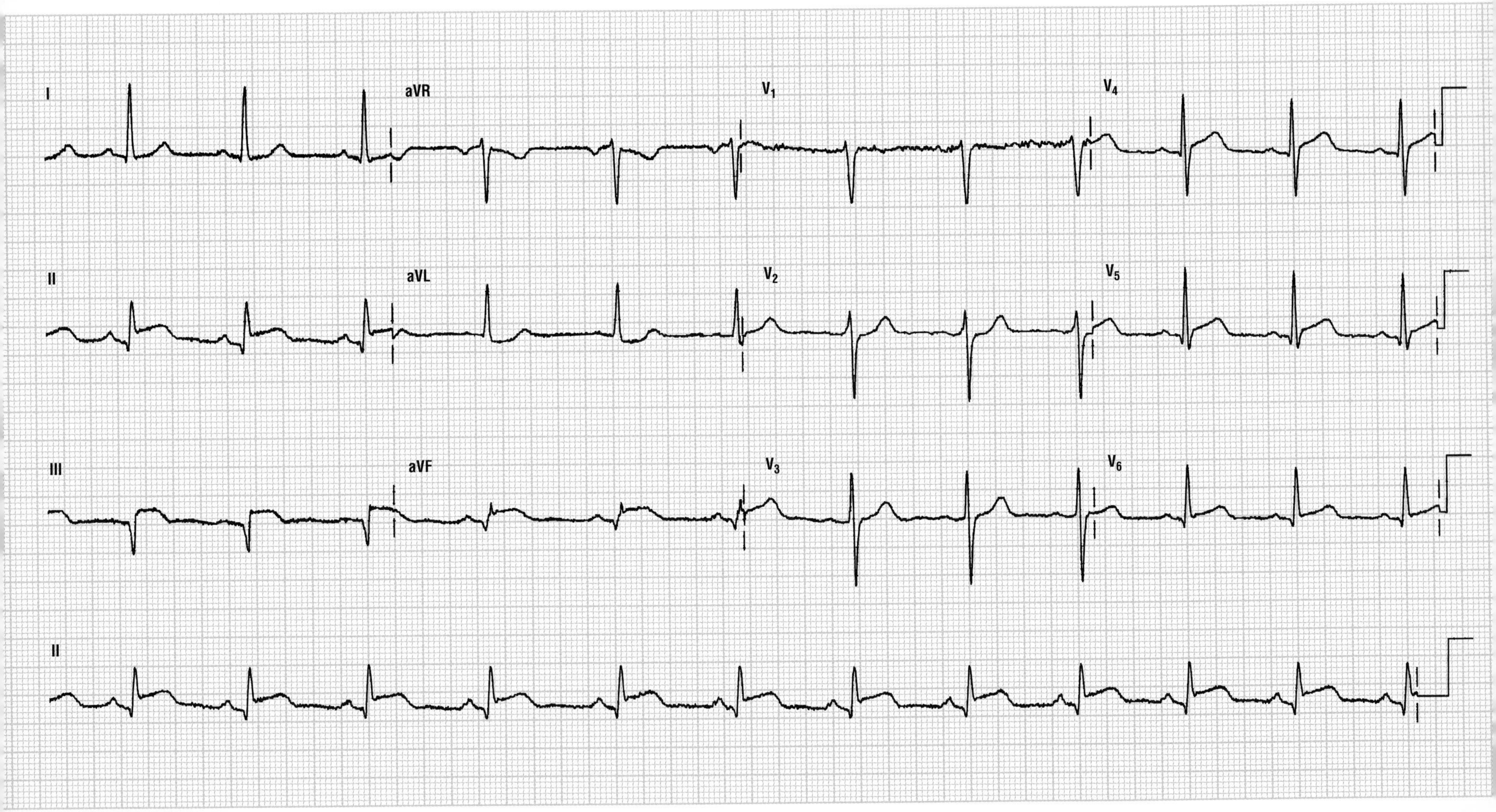

| I | aVR | V₁ | V₄ |

| II | aVL | V₂ | V₅ |

| III | aVF | V₃ | V₆ |

| II |

ECG 15-18

②

ECG 15-19 To start with, we just want you to look at aVL. This is the pathological ST depression we have mentioned a few times before. Note that lead I has some ST depression, but it is not overly impressive in its magnitude. If you were to have no ST elevation in the inferior leads at all, you should still be suspicious of an IWMI, especially if the clinical scenario includes a history consistent with ischemia. The ST segments in II, III, and aVF are elevated, however, making the diagnosis of an acute IWMI easier. ST elevation is also present in V_3 to V_6 consistent with lateral extension of the infarct/injury pattern.

③

ECG 15-19 The changes we mentioned in ECG 15-17 related to RVI are also present in this one, but in a much more subtle way. The ST elevation in III is greater than II. There is a small elevation in V_1 with a normal ST segment in V_2. Lead V_2 has another troublesome finding, the increased R:S ratio. This could be significant for a PWMI. Remember that inferiors, right ventriculars, posteriors, and laterals are frequently found in combination with one another. Once again, additional leads would be helpful. Clinical and echocardiographic correlation would also be useful in considering the diagnostic and therapeutic options available.

REMINDER:
In WPW, there can be Q waves in the inferior leads due to the pseudoinfarct pattern. Always look at "the company it keeps."

②

ECG 15-20 This ECG also has changes consistent with an inferolateral AMI. There are ST segment elevations in II, III, aVF, and V_3 to V_6, and reciprocal changes in leads I and aVL.

Some of you may be asking yourselves if this is a WPW pattern with slurring of the rise of the QRS complexes in the limb leads and V_1. Well, there are a few things that go against WPW in this ECG. First, the PR interval is normal. That can occur in approximately 12% of patients with WPW so this does not rule out the possibility. The other, more significant point is that the QRS complexes are not wide. WPW will cause a delta wave and that delta wave will cause a widening of the QRS complex. This is why WPW should be included in the differential diagnosis for wide complexes.

In WPW, a pseudoinfarct pattern occurs commonly in the inferior leads. This is caused by a negative delta in those leads, not by infarct. This is a true inferolateral infarct with an obvious intrinsicoid deflection, not WPW with a pseudoinfarct pattern.

We raised the possibility of WPW to challenge your thinking about ECGs. Think about the possibilities involved, and use the knowledge you have gained to make effective clinical interpretations. Another useful tool is the history. This patient presented with crushing substernal chest pain, which makes an inferolateral AMI very likely.

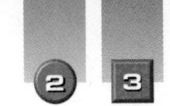

ECG CASE STUDIES: CONTINUED

I   aVR   V₁   V₄

II   aVL   V₂   V₅

III   aVF   V₃   V₆

II

ECG 15-19

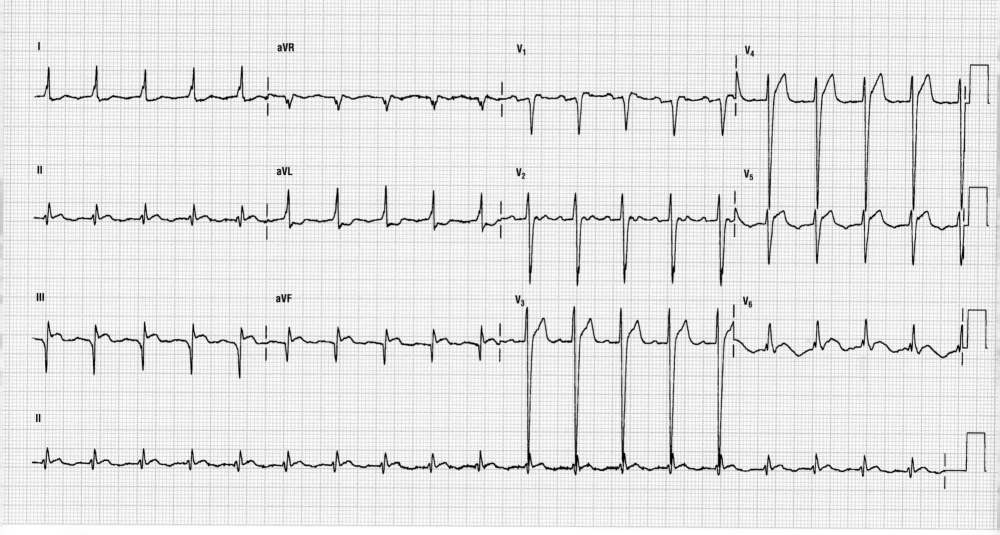

ECG 15-20

ECG CASE STUDIES: **CONTINUED**

ECG 15-21 This is a troubling ECG. We want you to take a good solid look at it and spend some time in arriving at an interpretation before you come back up for the discussion. (We suggest that you do that on all of the ECGs in order to derive maximum benefit from your studies.)

Let's start off with the rate. It's very fast. It goes from 150 to over 200 BPM. Is it regular? No. Is it regularly irregular? Again, no. Is it irregularly irregular? Yes. The differential diagnosis of an irregularly irregular rhythm includes wandering atrial pacemaker, multifocal atrial tachycardia, and atrial fibrillation. There are no discernible P waves in this ECG, so atrial fibrillation is the culprit. This is a patient with atrial fibrillation and a very rapid ventricular response.

Are the QRS complexes wide? No, the ST segment changes can fool you but the complexes themselves are not wide. There is no evidence of block. Where are the ST segments elevated? In II, III, aVF, and V_5. Where are the ST segments depressed? In leads I, aVL, and V_1 to V_3. The ST segment depressions in leads I and aVL are caused by reciprocal changes from the inferior AMI. The ST depressions in V_1 to V_3 indicate posterior wall ischemia or injury, which we will cover shortly. Which came first, the infarct or the arrhythmia? We can't tell that from the ECG, but we definitely need to control the rate in either case.

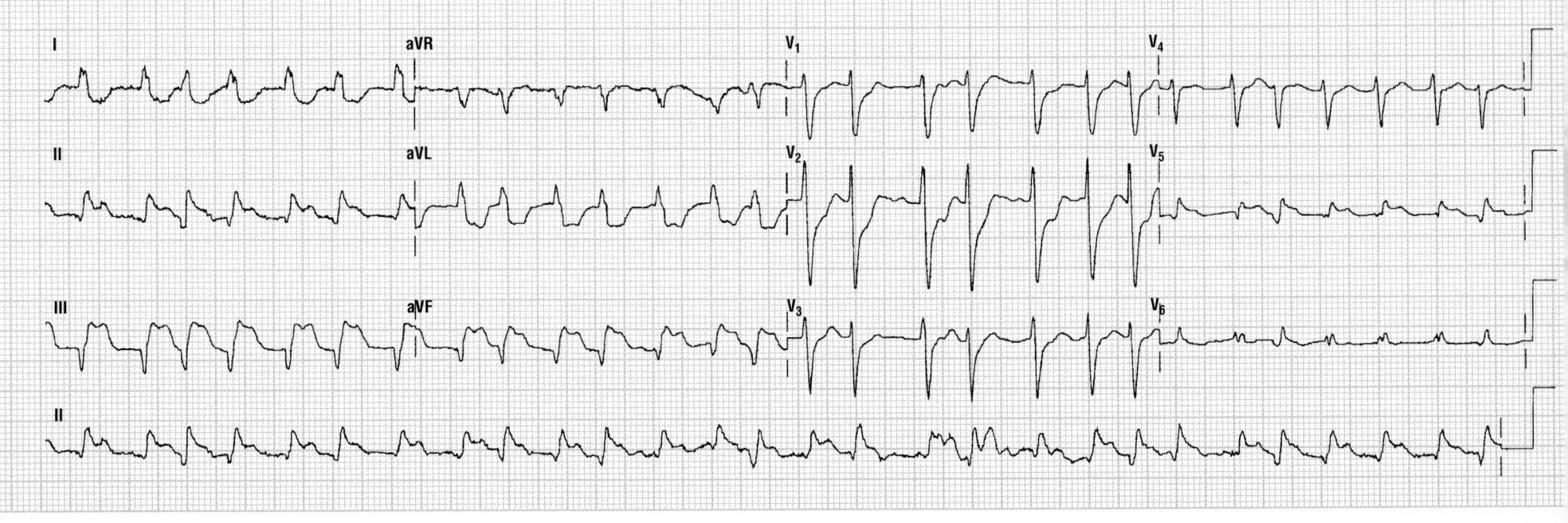

ECG 15-21

Apical AMI

An apical infarct occurs when a large right coronary dominant system infarcts. This causes direct changes in leads I, II, III, aVF, aVL, and V_2 to V_6.

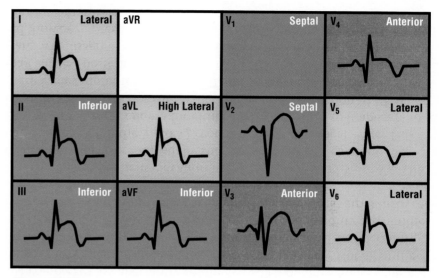

Figure 15-29

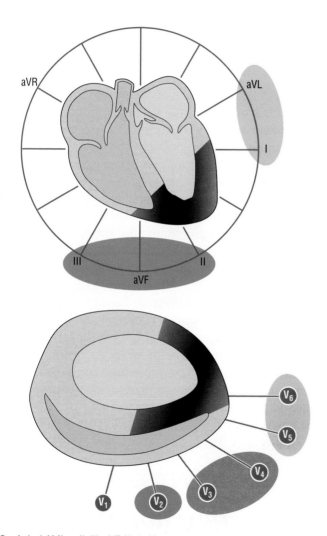

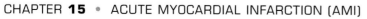

Figure 15-28: Apical AMI = II, III, aVF, V_2 to V_6.

ECG CASE STUDIES: *Apical AMI*

ECG 15-22 This ECG has ST elevation in I, II, III, aVF, and V_2 to V_6 consistent with an apical AMI. An apical infarct is really just a rather large inferolateral infarct with changes involving lead I and possibly aVL. We separate it out as an apical infarct because it is important to note the large area covered by this type of infarct. It also serves to differentiate it from a run-of-the-mill, inferolateral AMI because these ECGs are so commonly mistaken for pericarditis. As a rule, ST elevation in leads I and II indicates three possibilities: (1) pericarditis, (2) apical infarct, or (3) an aortic dissection causing occlusion of both coronary ostea and leading to a global infarct (very rare).

You will need to use your knowledge of electrocardiography and clinical medicine to differentiate between these three conditions. Look for associated PR depression, notching, tachycardia, and a history consistent with pericarditis to make that diagnosis. Check for unequal pulses, aortic regurgitation murmurs, CNS symptomatology, and radiographic findings to detect the possibility of an ascending aortic aneurysm or dissection. Finally, look for a history consistent with ischemia, progression of the electrocardiographic findings, and echocardiographic and catheterization results to make the diagnosis of apical infarct. The most important thing is to suspect the diagnosis and begin appropriate treatment promptly.

ECG 15-23 This ECG also has ST segment elevation in I, II, III, aVF, and V_2 to V_6 that is consistent with an apical infarct. There are Q waves in the inferior leads that confirm an AMI pattern.

Notice that there is minimal PR depression in the lateral leads. The amount of PR depression is not significant (deeper than 0.8 mm). This is an example of how easy it is to misdiagnose this problem as pericarditis. However, the treatment is very different: emergent revascularization for one, and for the other, nonsteroidal anti-inflammatory agents or surgical pericardotomy but definitely not any heparin, thrombolytics, or other anti-platelet agents.

What is the coronary artery pathology responsible for an apical infarct? Well, as you can imagine, it involves the RCA. There is a clot or obstruction of an extensively dominant RCA system occurring proximally. This leads to decreased perfusion of the inferior, anterior, lateral, and high-lateral walls, and possibly the septum, RV, and the posterior wall, as well.

Emergent revascularization is the treatment of choice because of the large extent of myocardium at risk in these patients. Aggressive management with hemodynamic control is essential.

ECG 15-24 This is a very difficult ECG to interpret. When you are faced with a tough ECG, break it down to its simplest components and then combine the results to arrive at your final interpretation. Let's start out by looking at the rhythm strip. We see that the third, sixth, ninth, and last complexes are aberrantly conducted APCs or JPCs. So let's mentally remove them from our ECG. Do we see P waves? Not all of the time, and their morphologies and PR intervals differ. There certainly are some R-R intervals that are the same, but the majority are of different lengths. Wandering atrial pacemaker and multifocal atrial tachycardia are definitely possibilities.

There is ST segment elevation in I, II, aVL, aVF, and V_2 to V_6. The complexes in aVF are unusually shaped. Why? If you examine the QRS complexes in the V_4 to V_6, you see that they appear wide. This ECG does not meet criteria for either RBBB or LBBB, so it appears to be an IVCD. We are not sure why there is no ST elevation in III, when there is elevation present in both II and aVF. The ST depression in V_1 may suggest posterior ischemia. This ECG is very difficult; many clinicians will disagree with our interpretation, and that is fine. The patient did, however, present clinically like an AMI and further studies verified the ECG interpretation above.

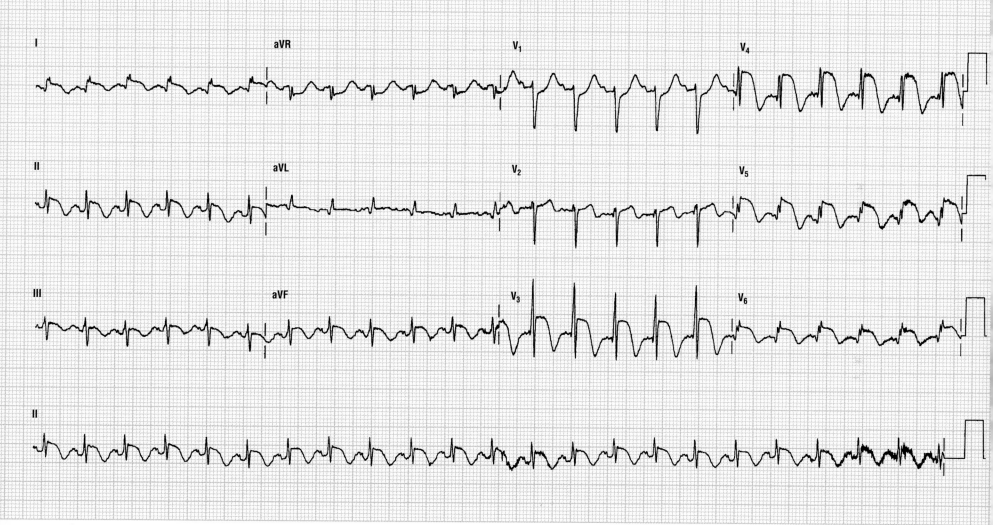

ECG 15-22

ECG CASE STUDIES: CONTINUED

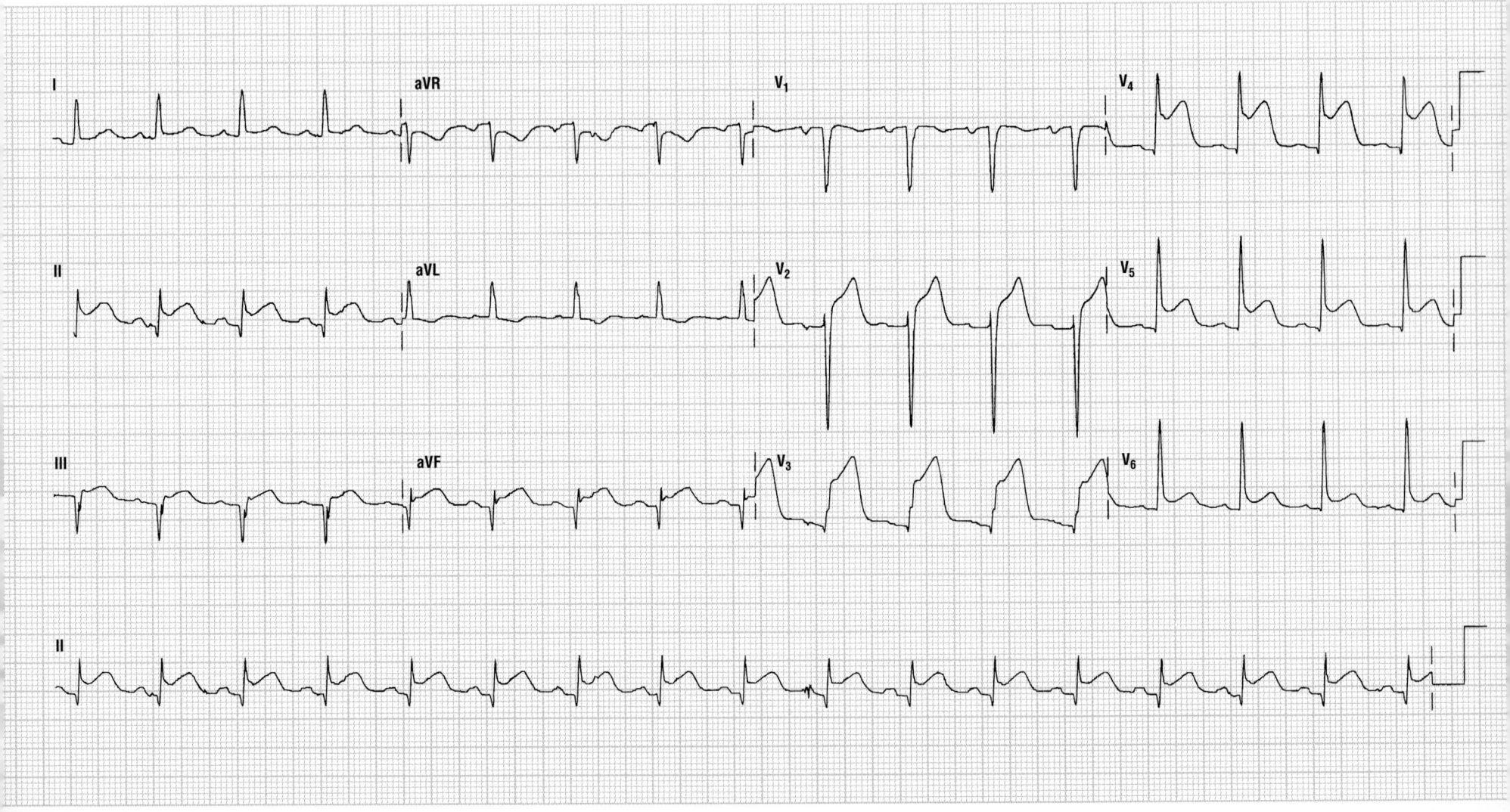

ECG 15-23

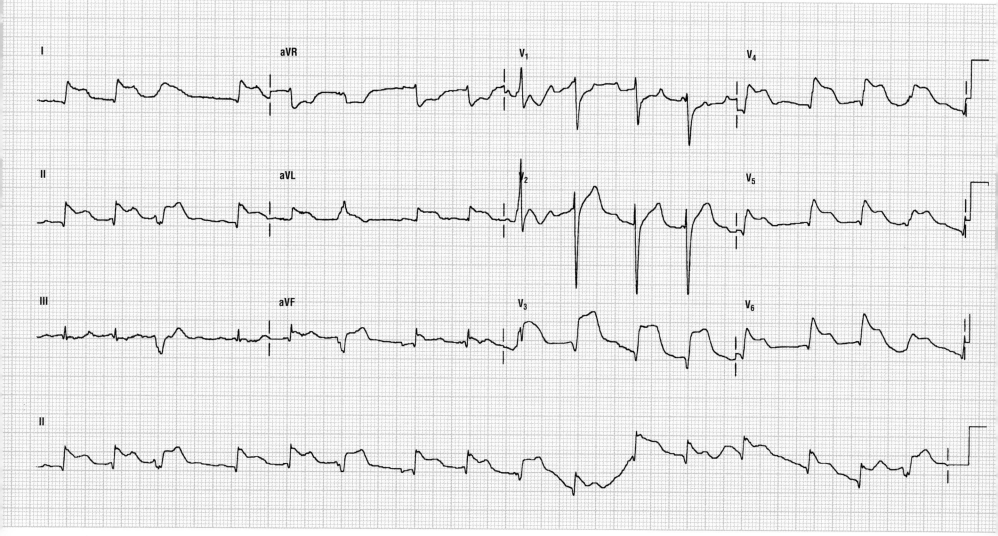

ECG 15-24

Additional ECG Leads

In addition to the standard leads, there are some extra precordial leads that come in very handy when we are evaluating AMIs. These leads help us diagnose both posterior and right ventricular infarcts, which occur quite frequently in combination with inferior infarcts. The posterior leads of V_7 to V_{10}, shown in Figure 15-30, are very helpful in diagnosing posterior wall AMIs. Normally, on a standard 12-lead ECG, we can only see the reciprocal changes of a posterior infarct. These reciprocal changes occur in V_1 and V_2. The use of the posterior leads lets us see the direct changes occurring in the posterior wall more clearly.

The right-sided leads similarly aid in the diagnosis of a right ventricular infarction, because the vector for the right ventricle points anteriorly and to the right. Direct changes occurring in the right ventricle are seen clearly in V_4R, V_5R, and V_6R.

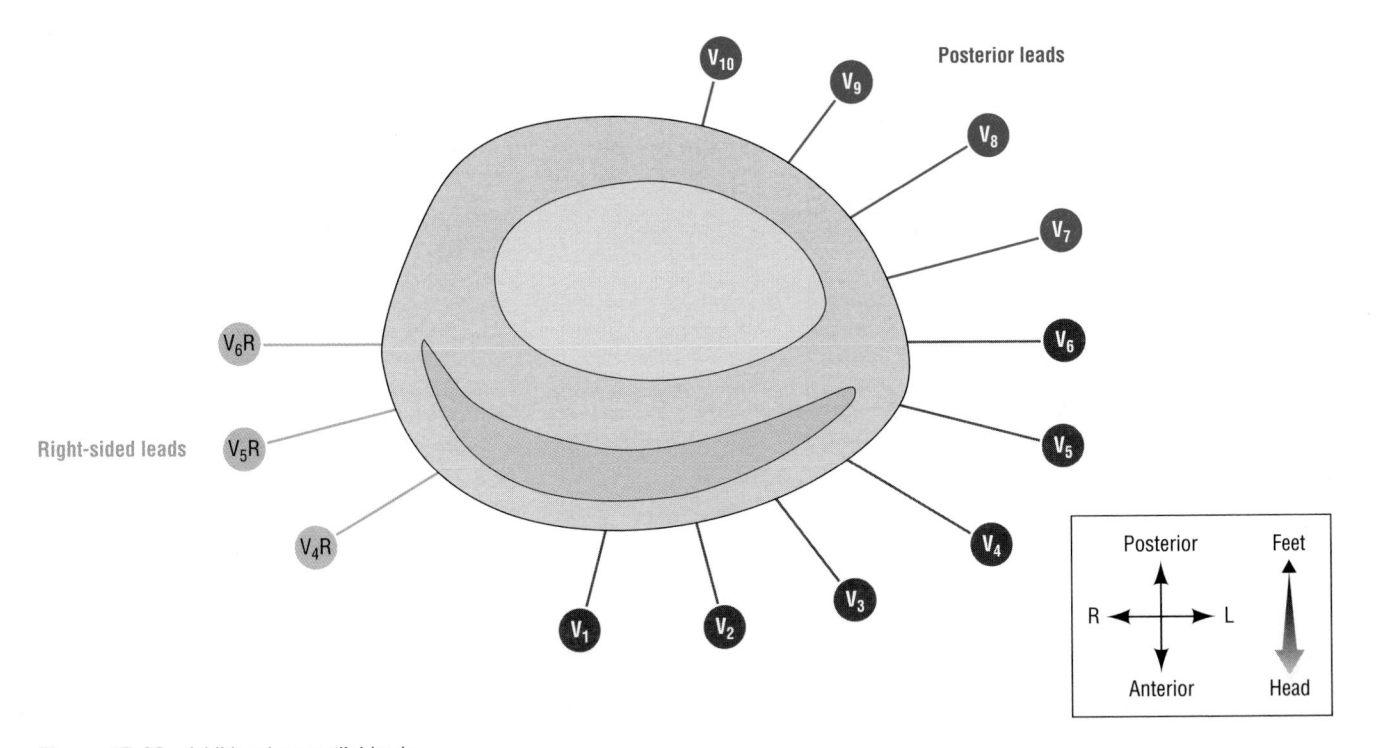

Figure 15-30: Additional precordial leads.

Placing Additional Right-Sided Leads

The right-sided leads, placed in a mirror image to V_4 to V_6, are known as V_4R, V_5R, and V_6R. Attach the patient to the ECG machine as you would ordinarily, then move V_4 to its mirror image on the right to obtain V_4R, as in Figure 15-31. Repeat the process for V_5 and V_6 to obtain V_5R and V_6R.

The right-sided leads show ST elevation in a right-side infarct. Key point: *Any time you see an inferior infarct, you should obtain right-sided leads.* Make it a habit. It will pay off for you tremendously and, needless to say, for your patients.

Placing Additional Posterior Leads

The posterior leads are used in the diagnosis of a posterior AMI. They will show the direct changes consistent with AMI — ST elevation, flipped T waves, and Q waves — rather than the reciprocal changes you'll see in V_1 and V_2. Obtain posterior leads in any patient with ST depression in V_1 to V_3 not associated with an RBBB.

Once again, you obtain the leads by moving V_4, V_5, and V_6, but this time to the spots for V_7, V_8, and V_9 (Figure 15-32).

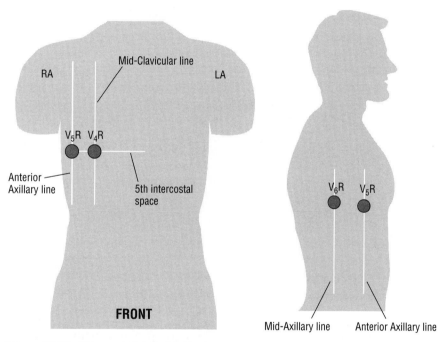

Figure 15-31: Placement of right-sided leads.

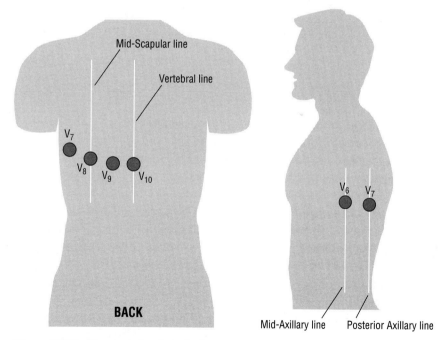

Figure 15-32: Placement of posterior leads.

Right Ventricular AMI

What makes a RVI special? Well, look at Figure 15-33. The RV is not working. Now, ask yourself how the blood is getting back to the left ventricle. Any ideas? The blood gets back almost exclusively by venous return. The atria pump with just enough pressure to push the blood into the ventricles and thereby assist the blood return slightly. How-ever, the main way that blood gets all the way around to the left ventricle is by venous return. Why is this important? If you increase venous capacitance, you decrease venous return. What are the medications we use to treat AMI, and what are their effects? We use nitrates, beta blockers, diuretics, and morphine, all of which cause decreased venous return. No return, no blood pressure.

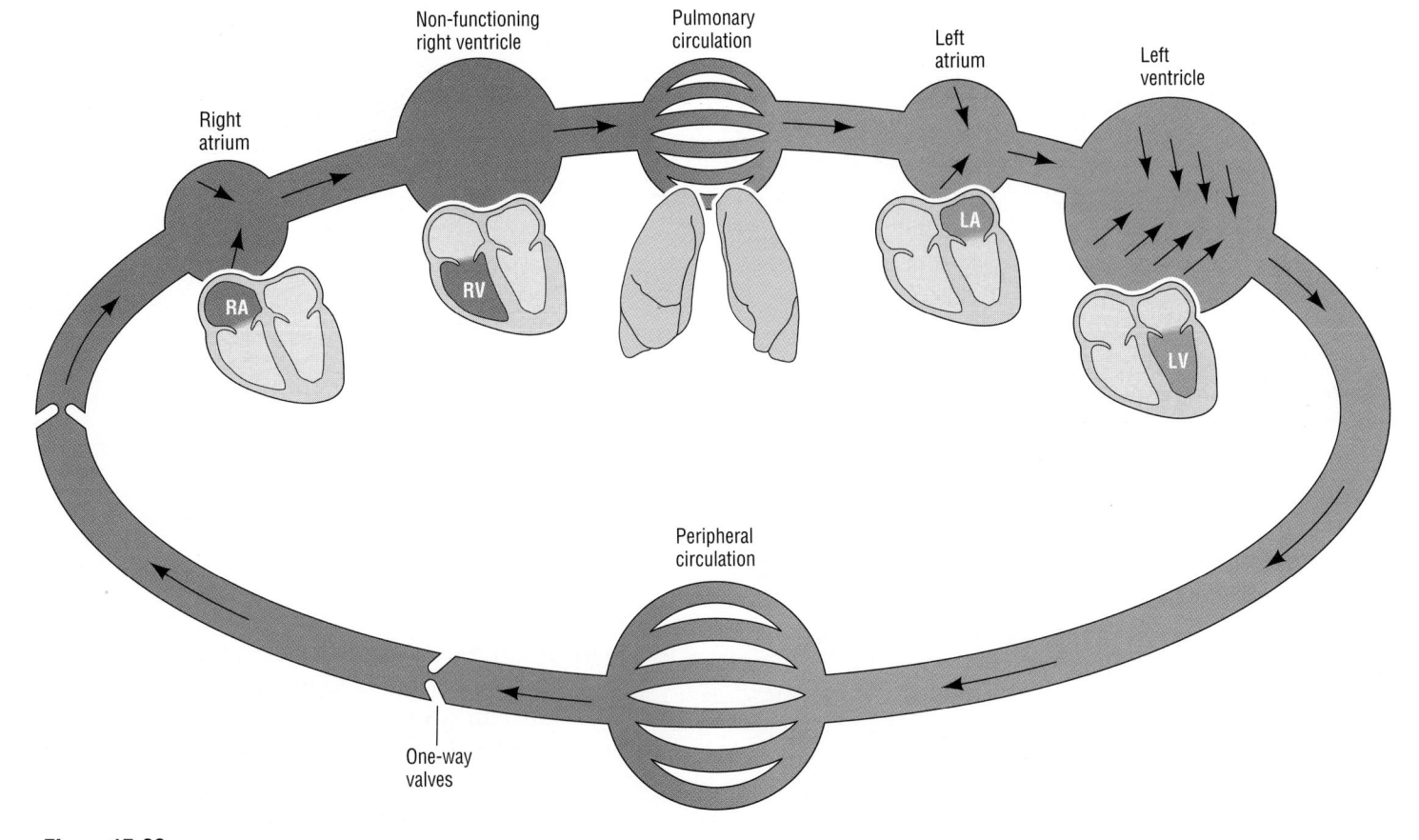

Figure 15-33

Criteria for Right Ventricular Infarction

As you can see from the material previously, the treatment of an RVI is very different from that of a left ventricular infarction. We refer you to a textbook of Cardiology for a review of the management and treatment principles for RVI patients. In this book, concentrate on the diagnostic criteria. The entire list of criteria is included below. Remember, as in most of electrocardiography, the presence of all of the criteria are not needed on one ECG to make a definitive diagnosis, and this usually does not occur. In other words, we will only see some of these criteria present on most ECGs with the diagnosis. We will discuss each item below:

1. IWMI
2. ST segment elevation greater in lead III than II
3. ST elevation in V_1 (possibly extending to V_5 to V_6)
4. ST depression in V_2 (unless elevation extends, as in #3 above)
5. ST depression in V_2 cannot be more than half the ST elevation in aVF
6. More than 1 mm of ST elevation in the right-sided leads (V_4R to V_6R)

Inferior wall MI

Most RVIs occur in conjunction with IWMIs — 97% of them to be exact. This is because they are usually caused by an obstruction in the right coronary artery, which also supplies the inferior wall. They can arise from a blocked left circumflex artery, but this is rare (3% of the time). Make it a habit to check for RVI when you see an IWMI.

ST segment elevation greater in III than in II

The infarct allows the vector from the interventricular septum to pass unopposed. This vector is directed anteriorly, inferiorly, and to the right. Lead III lies directly in its path, which causes the ST segment to be higher in this lead, as referenced in Figures 15-34, *top,* and 15-35.

ST elevation in V_1

The ST segment is elevated in lead V_1, also because of the unopposed vector and the direction of the injury current. This normally will elevate V_1 and depress V_2 as it passes by. This vector *can* cause ST segment elevation that extends through V_5 or V_6; however, this is uncommon. *Remember, if you see ST segment elevation in II, III, and aVF,* **as well as V_1,** *the most probable explanation is an RVI.* It would be very unusual to have an infarct of the right coronary artery (commonly supplies the inferior wall) and the left coronary artery (commonly supplies the anteroseptal area) at the same time. One possible exception is an aortic dissection blocking entry to both coronary arteries, but this is truly a rare occurrence.

ST depression in V_2

Classically, the direction of the vector will produce ST elevation in V_1 and depression in V_2. This is because the vector path points more towards V_1 and either away, or slightly away, from V_2.

ST depression in V_2 cannot be more than half the ST elevation in aVF

The amount of ST depression in V_2 is critical. If it is less than half the height of the ST elevation in aVF, then it is a simple inferior-RV infarct. If the ST depression is more than half the height of the ST elevation in aVF, it is consistent with an inferior-RV-posterior AMI. This means that there is a tremendous amount of myocardium at risk and infarcting, a critical point.

More than 1 mm ST elevation in the right-sided leads (V_4R to V_6R)

This is the most specific sign of an RVI. In the presence of an IWMI, if you find 1 mm or more of ST elevation in V_4R, you have made the diagnosis. Sometimes, you will find the elevation in V_6R, so make it a habit to obtain all three right-sided leads.

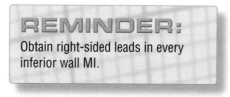

REMINDER:
Obtain right-sided leads in every inferior wall MI.

Right Ventricular AMI: Summary

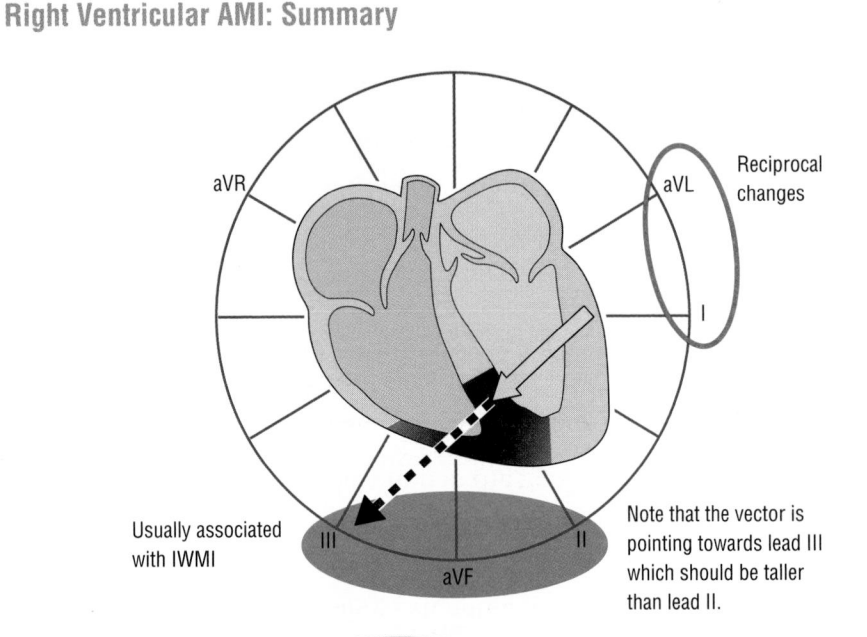

aVR

aVL

Reciprocal changes

I

Usually associated with IWMI

III

II

aVF

Note that the vector is pointing towards lead III which should be taller than lead II.

*ST elevation in lead V_1, but depending on how much of the RV is affected, it can extend up to V_6! In addition, the amount of ST depression has to be less than half of the ST elevation in aVF!

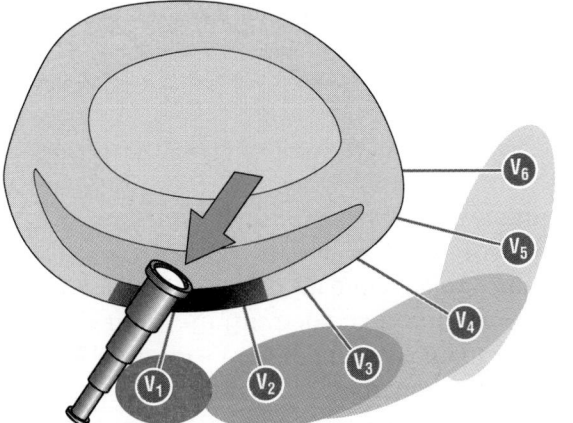

Figure 15-34: Right ventricular AMI = V_5, V_6, I, aVL.

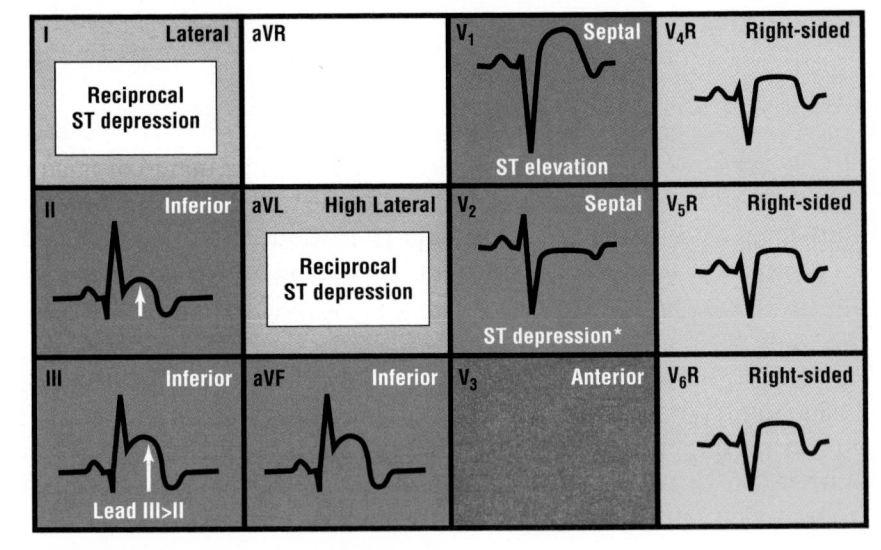

Figure 15-35

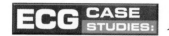 *Right Ventricular Infarction*

ECG 15-25 One of the reasons we did not offer too many examples of IWMIs earlier is that you will be covering many examples as we review RV and posterior infarcts. Here is such an example. This patient is definitely having an IWMI with ST elevations and Q waves in II, III, and aVF. There are reciprocal changes present in leads I and aVL. Note that the ST elevation is taller in III than II, and there is ST elevation in V_1 to V_3. These findings result from the right ventricular involvement of the AMI. We obtained right-sided leads; notice the elevations in V_4R, as well.

The P waves are only seen in V_3 to V_6, but the rhythm is NSR. The biphasic T waves in the lateral precordials are caused by LVH with strain; they are not reciprocal to the IWMI.

ECG 15-26 This ECG shows the classic findings of an RVI. There is an IWMI with ST elevation in II, III, and aVF with reciprocal changes in the inferior leads. Lead III has ST elevation greater than that found in II, consistent with an RVI. Also, note the ST elevation in V_1 with some small ST depression in V_2 that is less than half the ST elevation in aVF.

These are the criteria for RVI on a standard 12-lead ECG. We ordered right-sided leads, and the ST in V_4R was elevated, completing the criteria for diagnosis of RVI.

The ST elevation pattern seen in the precordials is very common in RVIs. The ST segments are elevated in V_1, then flat or depressed in V_2, and again elevated in V_3. It is unclear why this occurs. Always obtain right-sided leads in an inferior AMI.

ECG 15-27 This ECG also shows the criteria for an IWMI with RV involvement. It is critical that you understand the criteria for RV infarcts very clearly, both in the 12 standard leads and in the right-sided leads. This AMI is treated differently, and appropriate treatment cannot be instituted unless you first make the diagnosis. Get used to making the diagnosis from the standard 12-lead ECG, then use the right-sided leads to verify and confirm it. We cannot stress enough the importance of obtaining right-sided leads on any patient with elevation in II, III, and aVF. Make this standard protocol in your hospital or service if possible, so that they are recorded automatically.

ECG CASE STUDIES: **CONTINUED**

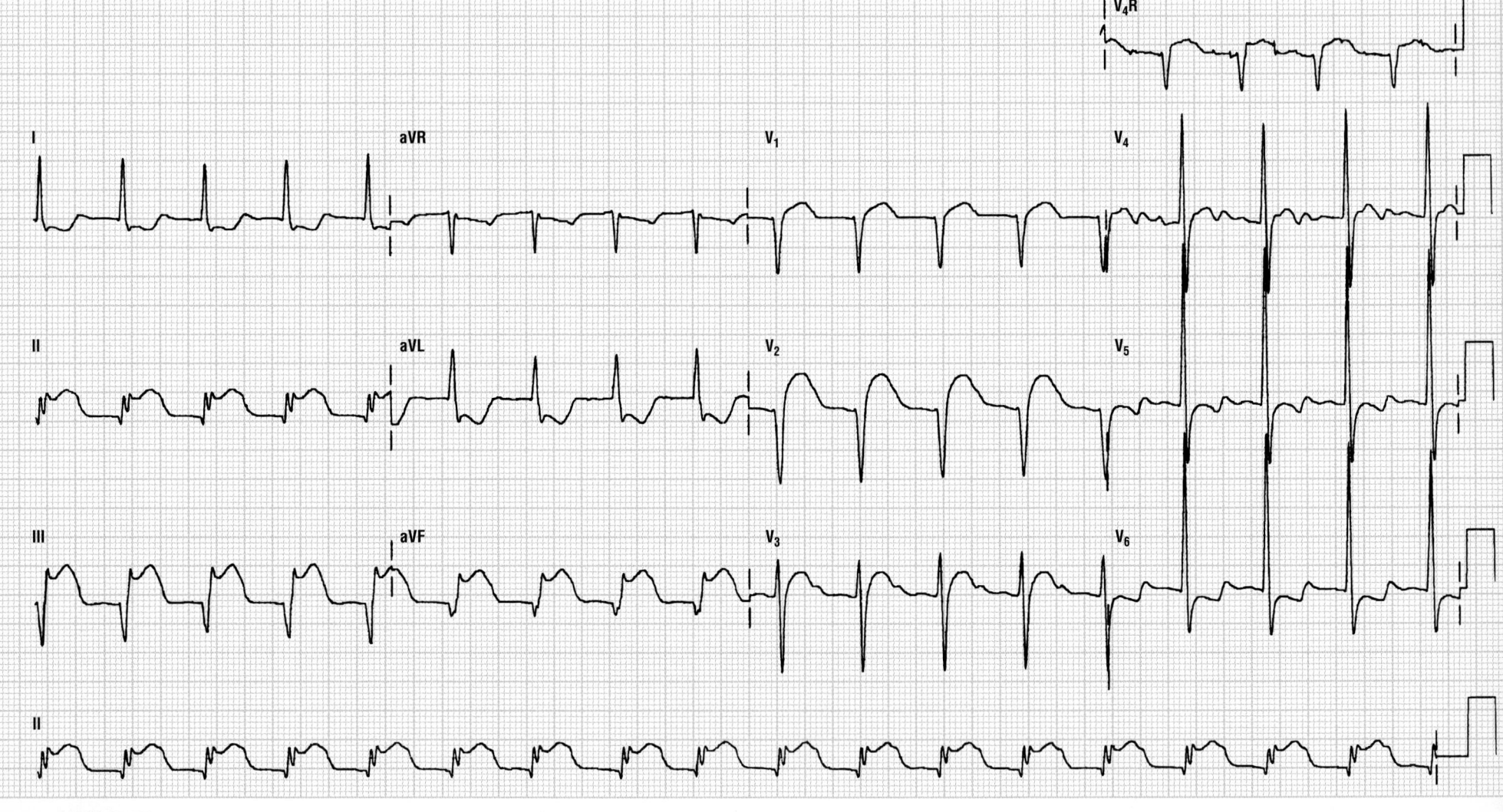

ECG 15-25

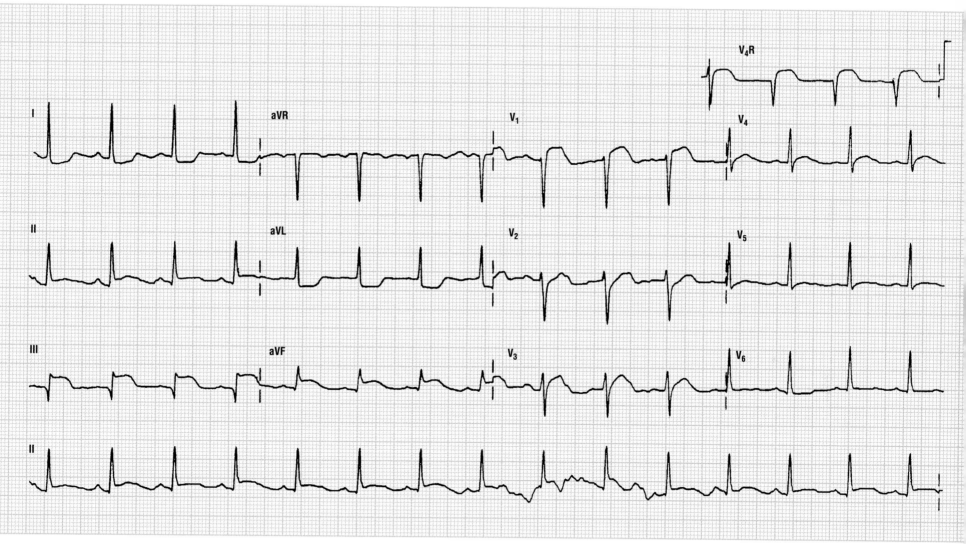

ECG 15-26

ECG CASE STUDIES: **CONTINUED**

I aVR V₁ V₄R

aVR V₁ V₄

II aVL V₂ V₅

III aVF V₃ V₆

II

ECG 15-27

2

Posterior Wall AMI

There are no direct leads that visualize the posterior wall on a regular 12-lead ECG. So how do you make the diagnosis? Well, the first thing you need to do is understand the concept of reciprocal leads. If you don't understand it clearly, go back now and review the Reciprocal Changes section earlier in this chapter. The diagnosis of PWMI is made on a regular ECG by seeing the reciprocal changes in V_1 and V_2. The reciprocal changes are almost a mirror image of the direct changes of AMI on the complex. You will see a tall and fat R wave, ST depression, and an upright T wave in leads V_1 and V_2 (Figure 15-36). There is a strong association between PWMIs and IWMIs.

Now, you may be faced with a diagnostic dilemma when you see ST depression in V_1 to V_2. Remember the old adage: the company it keeps. You will be able to make the correct diagnosis by looking at the rest of the complex and getting some posterior leads. If you have a normal R:S ratio, a thin R wave, and a flipped T with the ST depression, this is most probably anterior ischemia or a non–Q wave AMI. If there is a taller R wave that is fatter than usual (≥ 0.03 seconds) and an upright T wave, or if there is an associated IWMI, then it's likely a PWMI. The posterior leads are usually positive, but because of the distance of the electrodes from the heart, the ST elevation may not be impressive. Have a high index of suspicion.

REMINDER:

You need to have a high index of suspicion to diagnose a PWMI on an ECG. When you see any ST depression in V_1 or V_2, think of the possibility.

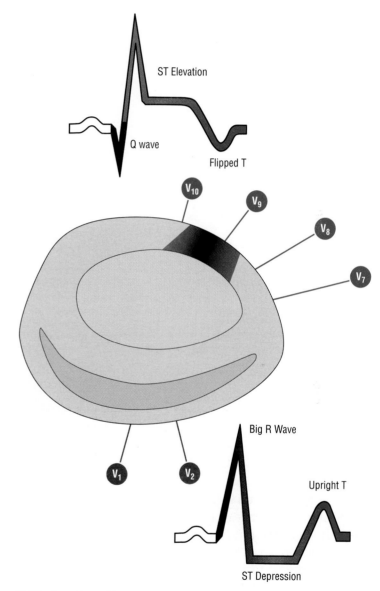

Figure 15-36: Posterior wall MI.

Carousel Ponies Are Bad on the ECG

Using your imagination, you can almost superimpose the figure of a carousel pony over the ECG complex shown in Figure 15-37. The ST depression makes a saddle, and the T wave is the back of the saddle that keeps you from sliding off. This upright T wave is a critical crite-rion in making the correct diagnosis. If you can picture someone sitting on the complex and holding on to the R wave, as the pole, you have a really good chance that it is a posterior AMI. RVH-with-strain, which also produces ST depression and a tall R wave, should have an asymmetric, flipped T rather than an upright, symmetric one.

Figure 15-37

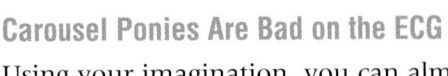

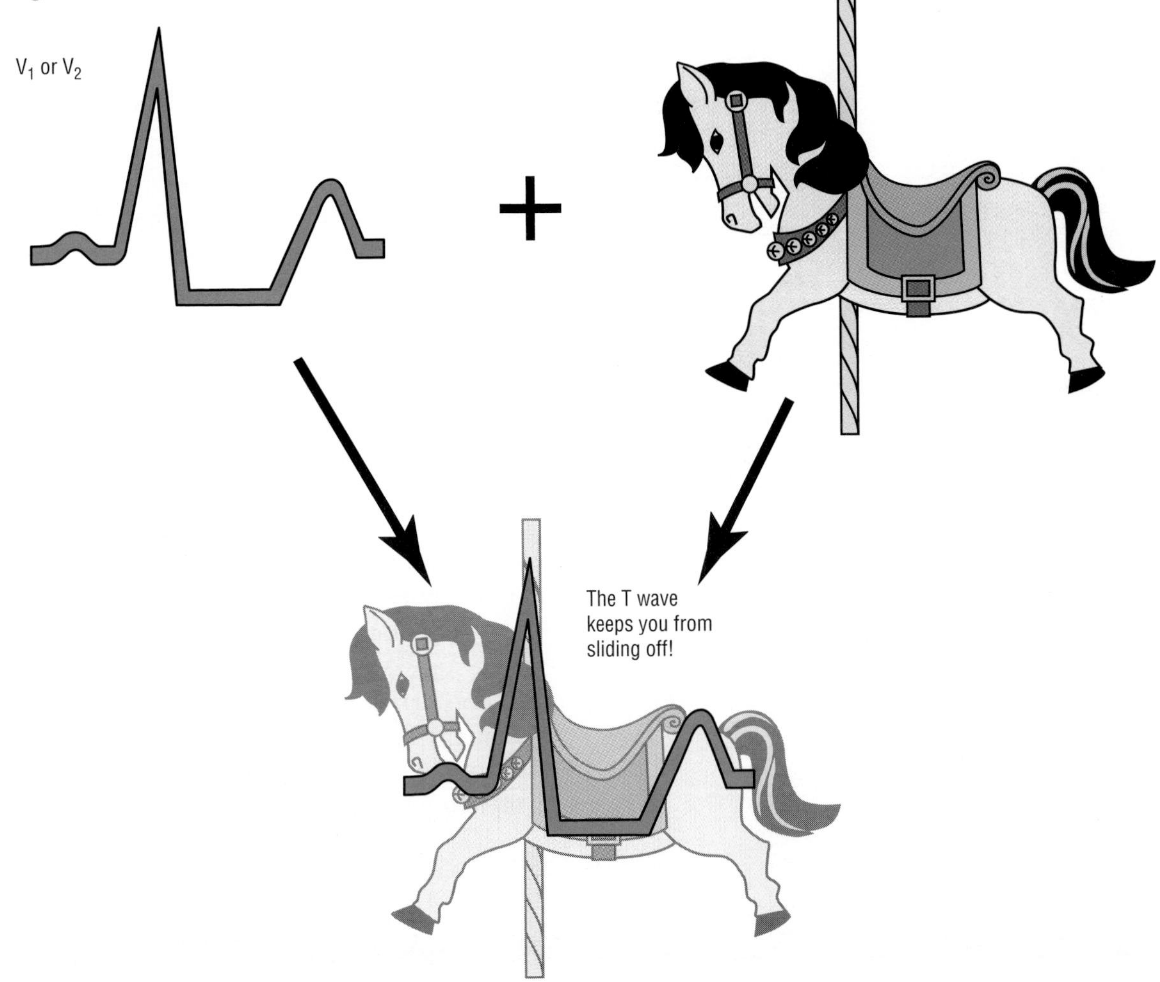

V₁ or V₂

The T wave keeps you from sliding off!

Posterior Wall MI: Summary

Remember that you're looking for reciprocal changes in the regular 12-lead ECG (Figure 15-38). If the AMI is occurring acutely, you will see ST depression as noted in Figure 15-39. If you do see it, order the additional posterior leads of V_7 to V_9. Age-indeterminate PWMIs present as just an isolated R:S ratio greater than 1 in V_1 or V_2. This is a diagnosis of exclusion; it can only be made after you have ruled out other causes of an increased R:S ratio that could occur in adult patients — RVH, WPW type A, and RBBB.

Most PWMIs are associated with IWMIs and RVIs, which we will review in subsequent sections.

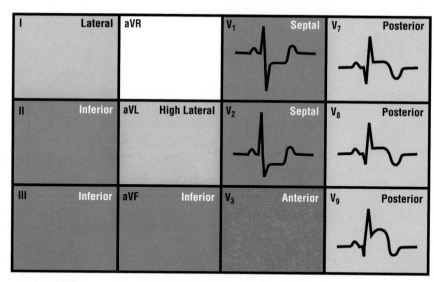

Figure 15-39

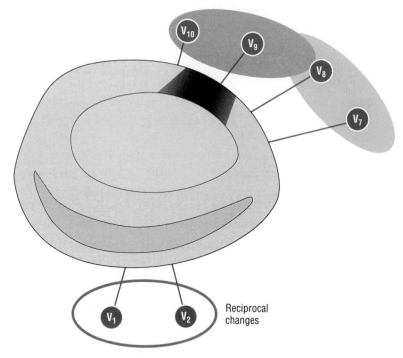

Figure 15-38: PWMI = V_7, V_8, V_9, reciprocal changes in V_1, V_2.

ECG CASE STUDIES: *Posterior Wall AMI*

ECG 15-28 This ECG shows the classic changes for an isolated or true posterior AMI. Note the increased R:S ratio in V_1 and V_2. Let's go through the differential diagnosis of increased R:S ratio one more time. Is the patient a child or adolescent? No, this patient was in his 50s. Is it an RBBB? No, there are no slurred S waves in leads I or V_6, and the complexes are not more than 0.12 seconds wide. Is it a WPW type A pattern? No, there are no delta waves present. What about RVH? Well, the axis is a bit vertical, but there is no evidence of RAE or $S_1Q_3T_3$ pattern. There are no clinical reasons for RVH, either. The last possibility is a PWMI. This is the diagnosis of exclusion in this case.

Let's look at some of the other findings that make a PWMI very probable here. The R wave is very wide in V_1 and V_2, consistent with a pathological R wave. According to some authors, you do not need to have a wide R wave, just a tall one, but it sure is nice when you do have one that is both tall and wide. The ST segment depression and the upright T wave are also very consistent with an acute or semi-acute posterior AMI. Is there any associated inferior or lateral infarct? No, not in this case. So this is an isolated posterior wall AMI.

Posterior leads would have been helpful in this case. Always ask for them to confirm the diagnosis.

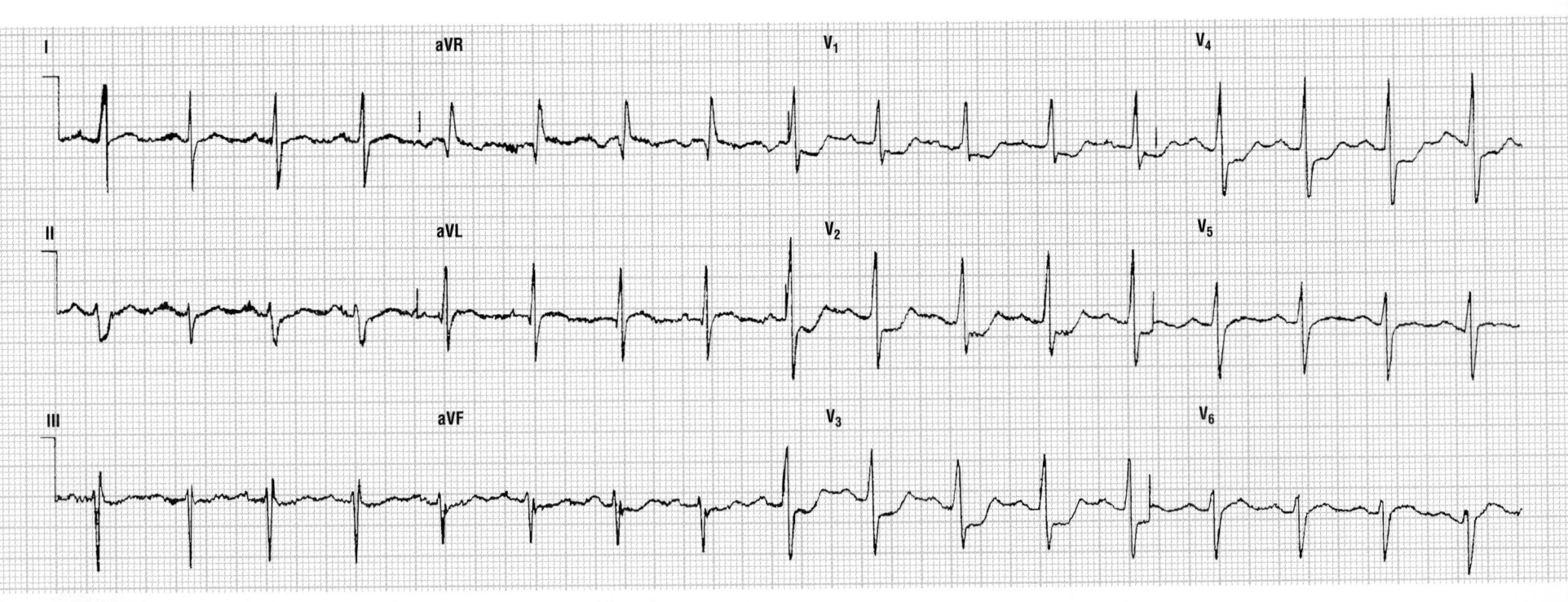

ECG 15-28

ECG 15-29 The R:S ratio in this ECG, also, is more than 1 in V_2. The R wave is wider than 0.03 seconds — pathologically wide. There is a flavor of ST depression, but this is not verified with a hairline ruler. It is an optical illusion of sorts.

What other infarct is evident on this ECG? Well, there are Q waves in the inferior and lateral leads consistent with an old or age-indeterminate, inferolateral infarct. As a matter of fact, the lack of ST segment changes and the presence of the old inferolateral AMI makes you think that the PWMI also occurred sometime in the past, probably at the same time the patient had the inferolateral AMI. Remember, PWMIs are commonly associated with IWMIs and RVIs. Can you figure out why this happens?

PWMIs, IWMIs, and RVIs are associated because the areas infarcted in these cases are perfused by the same arteries — the right coronary, the posterior descending, or the left circumflex. A blockage of one artery infarcts more than one area. You'll be spending more time on this in Level 3.

Finally, what is the rhythm on this ECG? Well, it is an irregularly irregular rhythm with no P waves. This makes the diagnosis atrial fibrillation with a slow ventricular response.

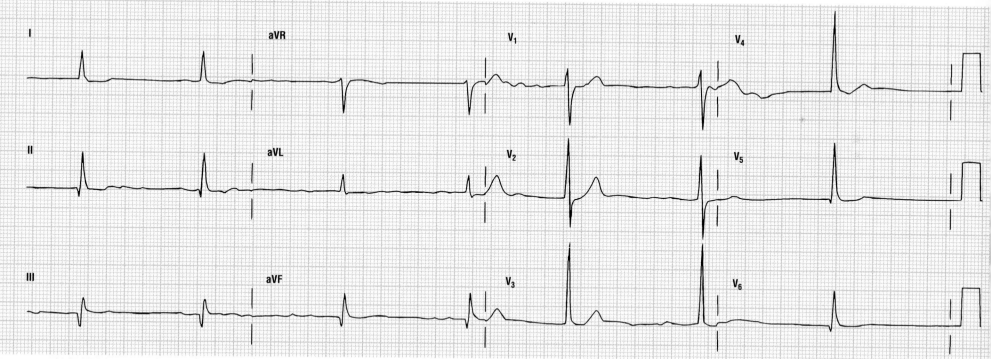

ECG 15-29

Inferoposterior AMI

We are now going to cover inferoposterior AMIs in greater detail. As mentioned previously, this is one of the possible combinations that commonly occurs with IWMIs. Remember, all of the criteria for both the IWMIs and PWMIs apply, but in combination.

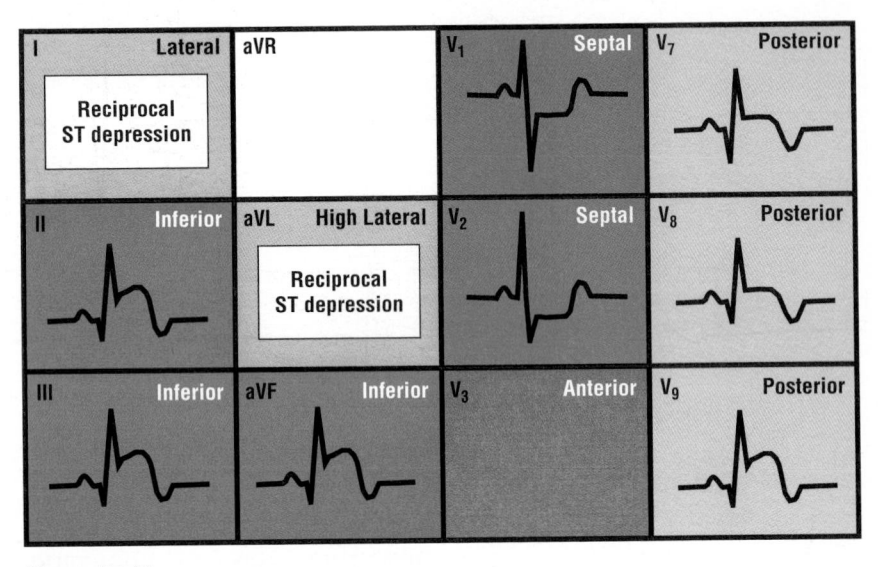

Figure 15-41

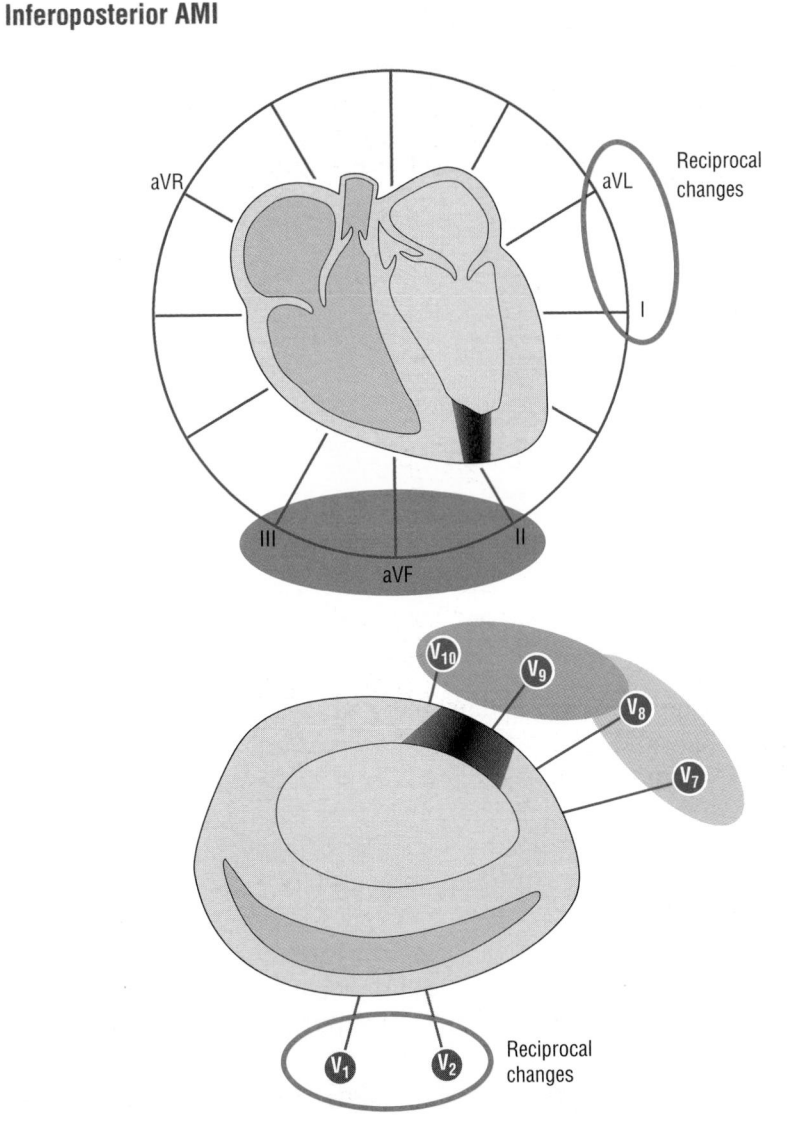

Figure 15-40: Inferior wall AMI = II, III, aVF; posterior wall AMI = V$_7$, V$_8$, V$_9$; reciprocal changes in V$_1$ and V$_2$.

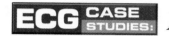

ECG 15-30 This is a great example of an inferoposterior AMI with lateral extension. Notice the ST segment elevations in II, III, and aVF. The amount of ST elevation in II and III is approximately the same, so right ventricular involvement is not suspected. However, you should still make it a point to obtain right-sided leads. There is reciprocal ST depression in aVL, consistent with the acute IWMI. Now, turning our attention to the precordial leads, we see an increased R:S ratio in V_1 and V_2. The R wave is wider than 0.03 seconds, and ST segment depression and an upright T wave are present — also see Figure 15-42. These findings are consistent with a PWMI. Finally, there are ST elevations in V_5 to V_6 to complete the infarct pattern by including the lateral leads.

ECG 15-31 This ECG also shows strong evidence of an inferior-posterior-lateral AMI. Take a look at the ST elevations in II, III, aVF, and V_4 to V_6, and the reciprocal ST depression in aVL consistent with an infero-lateral AMI. Note that the ST elevation in II and III is approximately the same, potentially excluding an RV infarct. (You should still obtain right-sided leads as an instinctual habit in any IWMI.) Now, look at V_1 and V_2. There are ST depressions in both leads, with upright T waves — also see Figure 15-43. In addition, there is a taller R wave that is wider than 0.03 seconds. These changes in V_1 and V_2 are consistent with a posterior wall AMI. Don't get fooled into thinking that the ST depression in V_1 and V_2 are reciprocal to the lateral changes; they are not reciprocal leads.

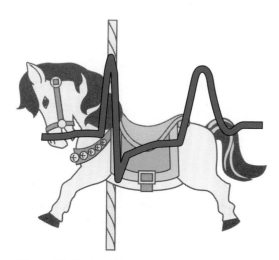

Figure 15-42: Lead V_2.

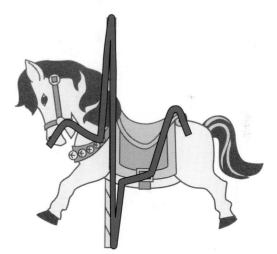

Figure 15-43: Lead V_2.

ECG CASE STUDIES: CONTINUED

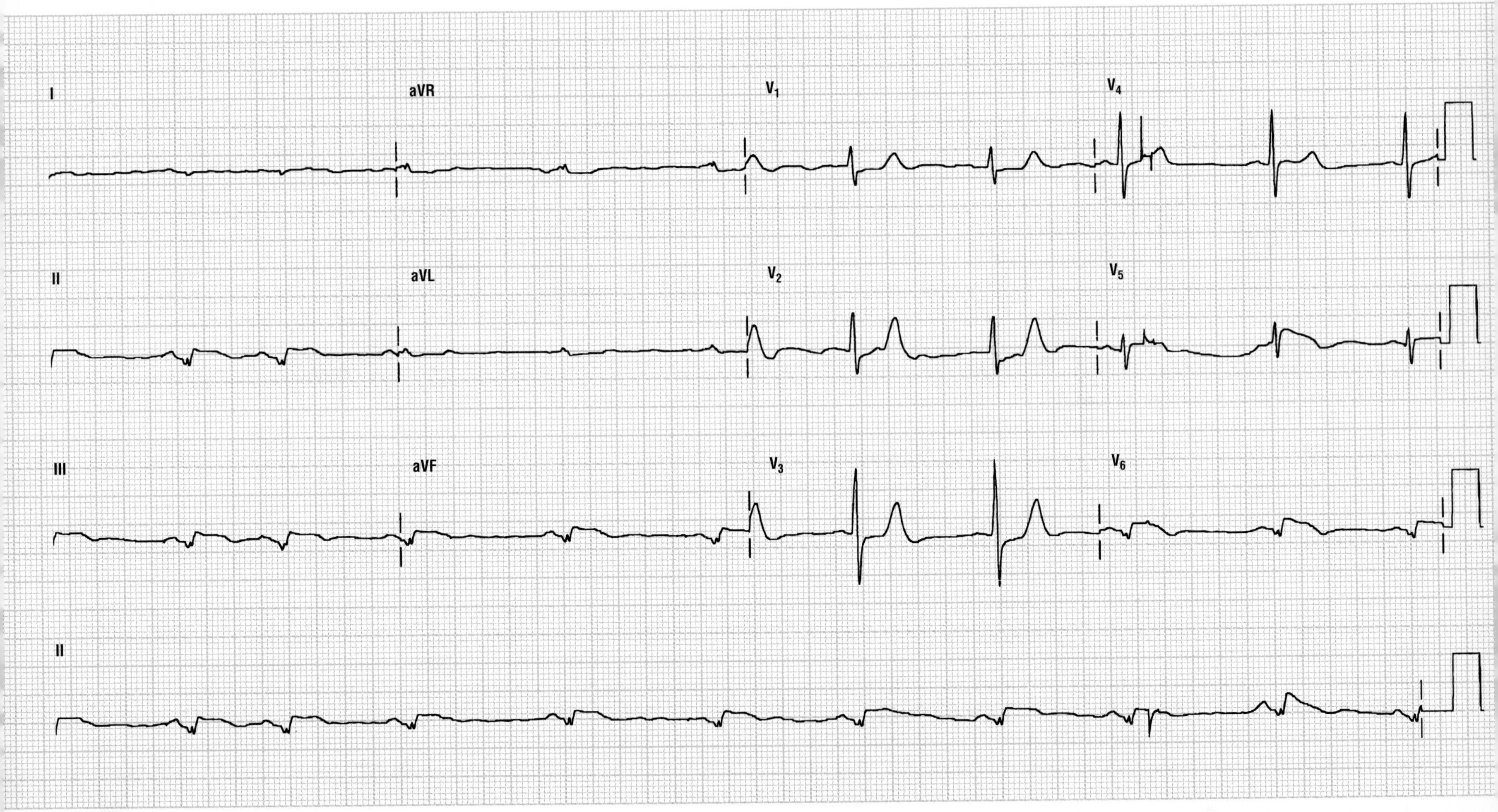

I

aVR

V₁

V₄

II

aVL

V₂

V₅

III

aVF

V₃

V₆

II

ECG 15-30

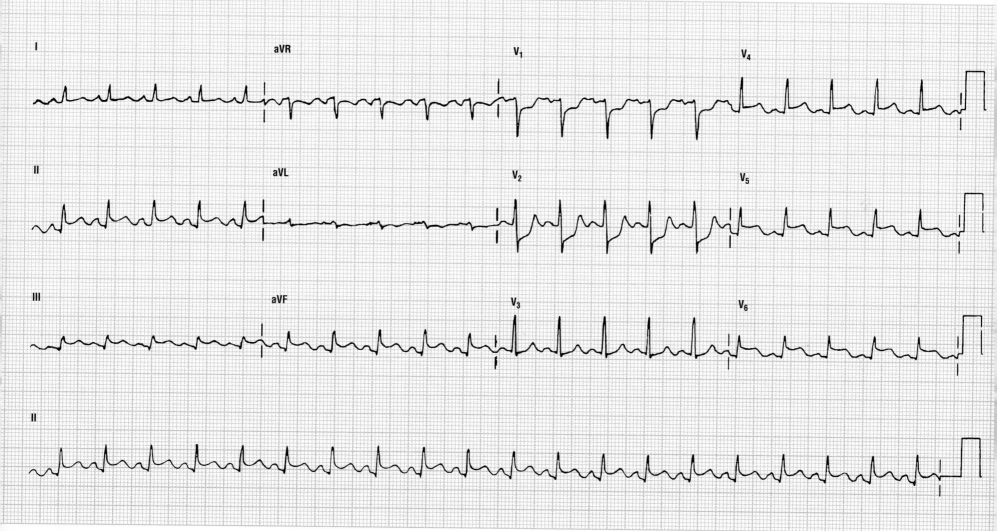

I   aVR   V₁   V₄

II   aVL   V₂   V₅

III   aVF   V₃   V₆

II

ECG 15-31

ECG CASE STUDIES: **CONTINUED**

3

ECG 15-32 This is a tough ECG! Take a good solid crack at interpreting this one before coming back up and going through the rest of this discussion.

Because this section is dedicated to inferoposterior AMIs, you probably have a good head start on the diagnosis. Indeed, this is an inferoposterior AMI, but what makes this ECG interesting is that it is occurring in a patient with an LBBB. Notice that the QRS interval is wider than 0.12 seconds consistent with the LBBB. There is a small R wave with a large S wave in V_1. Additionally, leads I and V_6 show monomorphic R waves. This is an LBBB pattern. Now, what do the ST segments look like normally in V_1 and V_2 with an LBBB? They are normally elevated in a discordant fashion.

The ST segments in V_1 and V_2 are depressed and the T waves are concordant. *Any ST depression in V_1 to V_3 in an LBBB is pathological and suggestive of a PWMI.* Now, look at the R waves in those same leads. They are wider than usual — wider than 0.03 seconds, in fact, which is also abnormal and consistent with the PWMI occurring in this patient.

Remember we mentioned earlier that pathologic Q waves are pathologic Q waves? This ECG has Q waves in the inferior leads consistent with an inferior infarct. Finally, V_6 shows ST elevation. Normally, LBBBs have ST depression in V_6, not elevation. These changes are consistent with a lateral injury pattern.

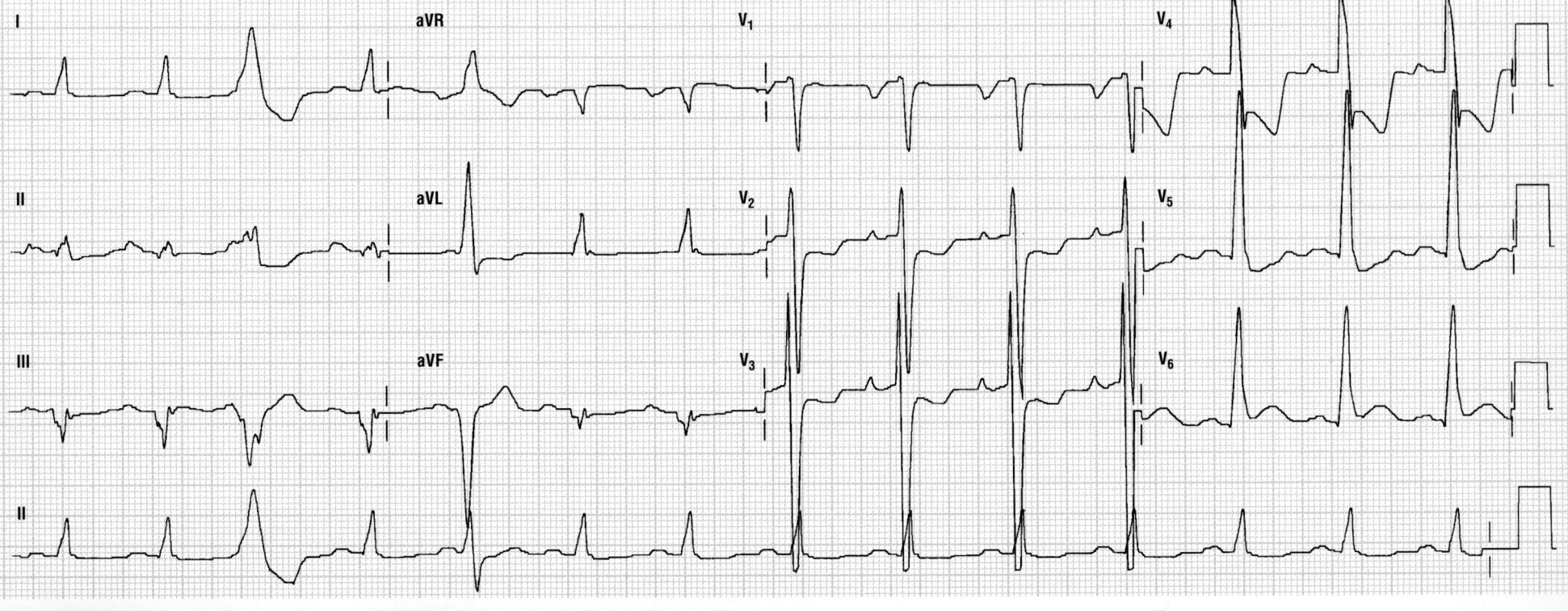

ECG 15-32

Inferior-RV-Posterior AMI

In this section, we are going to see the combination of inferior, right ventricular, and posterior wall AMIs. Note that these can still occur with lateral extension in many cases. These infarcts represent a large amount of myocardial tissue at risk and aggressive therapy. Consultation with a cardiologist is strongly encouraged as soon as possible.

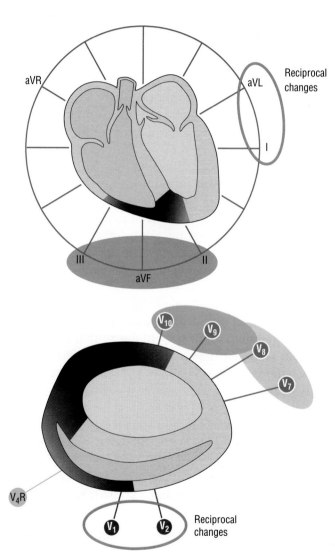

Figure 15-44: Combination of criteria for IWMI: ST elevation in III greater than II, and ST depression in V₂ greater than or equal to half the elevation in aVF.

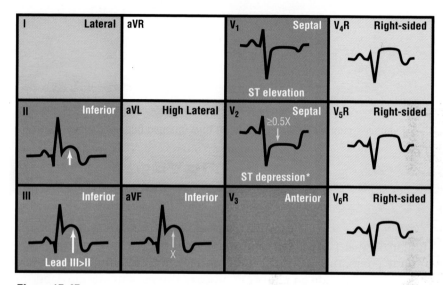

Figure 15-45

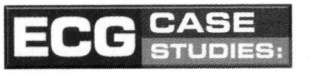 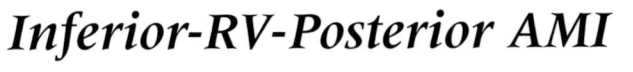 *Inferior-RV-Posterior AMI*

ECG 15-33 This ECG shows changes compatible with infarcts in three regions of the heart: the inferior wall, the right ventricle, and the posterior wall. The ST segment elevations in II, III, and aVF, and the reciprocal changes in aVL, are classic for an IWMI. The right ventricle shows involvement with the increased elevation of the ST segment in III compared with II. Right-sided leads verify the RVI. The posterior wall changes consist of the increased R:S ratio noted in V_1 and V_2 with ST segment depressions. The next ECG, done two minutes later, showed the T waves to be upright. The R wave is wider than 0.03 seconds. Finally, the ST segment depression in V_2 is more than half the elevation in aVF. As a matter of fact, the ST depression in V_2 and elevation in aVF are about the same.

ECG 15-34 This is another good example of an inferior-RV-posterior AMI. In the limb leads, the classic elevations in the inferior leads are present with reciprocal changes in the laterals. Also note that the ST elevation in III is taller than that in II, and the positive ST elevation in V_4R is consistent with an RV infarct. Finally, even though the R wave is not prominent in V_1 and V_2, the amount of ST depression is significant. Comparing the ST depression in V_2 with the ST elevation in aVF, we see that the depression in V_2 is much greater, suggesting a PWMI. Unfortunately, posterior leads were not obtained. As we keep saying, get used to obtaining right-sided and posterior leads on every patient with an IWMI. The additional information from those leads is very helpful.

ECG 15-35 The signs of infarct in this ECG are subtle and difficult to pick up. (Just kidding!) This is an inferior-RV-posterior MI with lateral extension. Go through the findings and spot the changes compatible with each of those four regions of the heart. This patient has a tremendous amount of myocardium at risk because of the blocked artery. We say *artery* because blockages usually occur in only one vessel at a time. (For advanced students: The only vessel that could potentially place this much myocardium at risk is the right coronary artery in a right-coronary-dominant system.) Treatment should be approached aggressively, but with the caution that the right ventricle is involved and preload should be maintained if at all possible. Reversing the obstruction to blood flow is the key to this patient's survival.

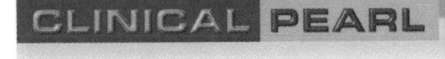

Be careful when treating patients with right ventricular infarctions. Maintaining preload is critical.

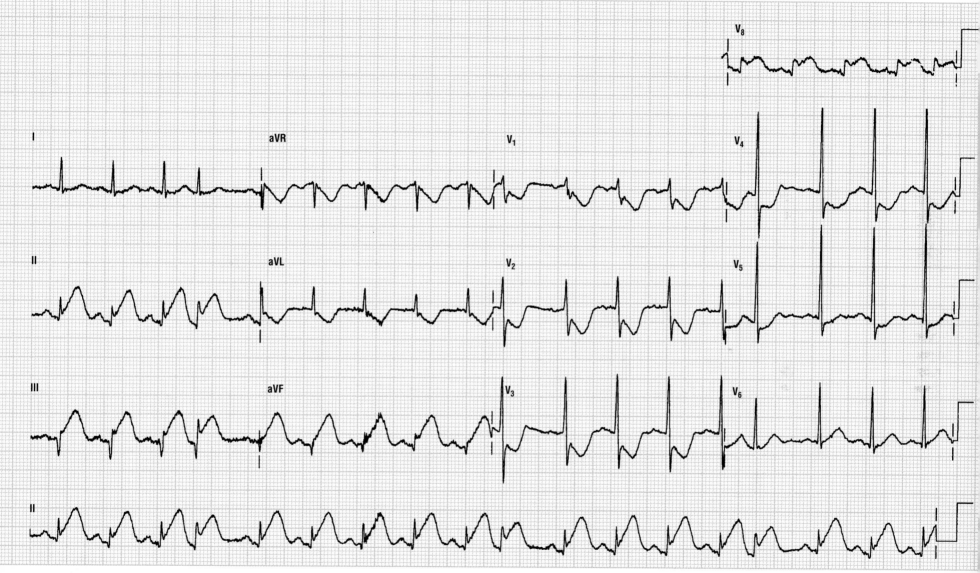

ECG 15-33

ECG CASE STUDIES: **CONTINUED**

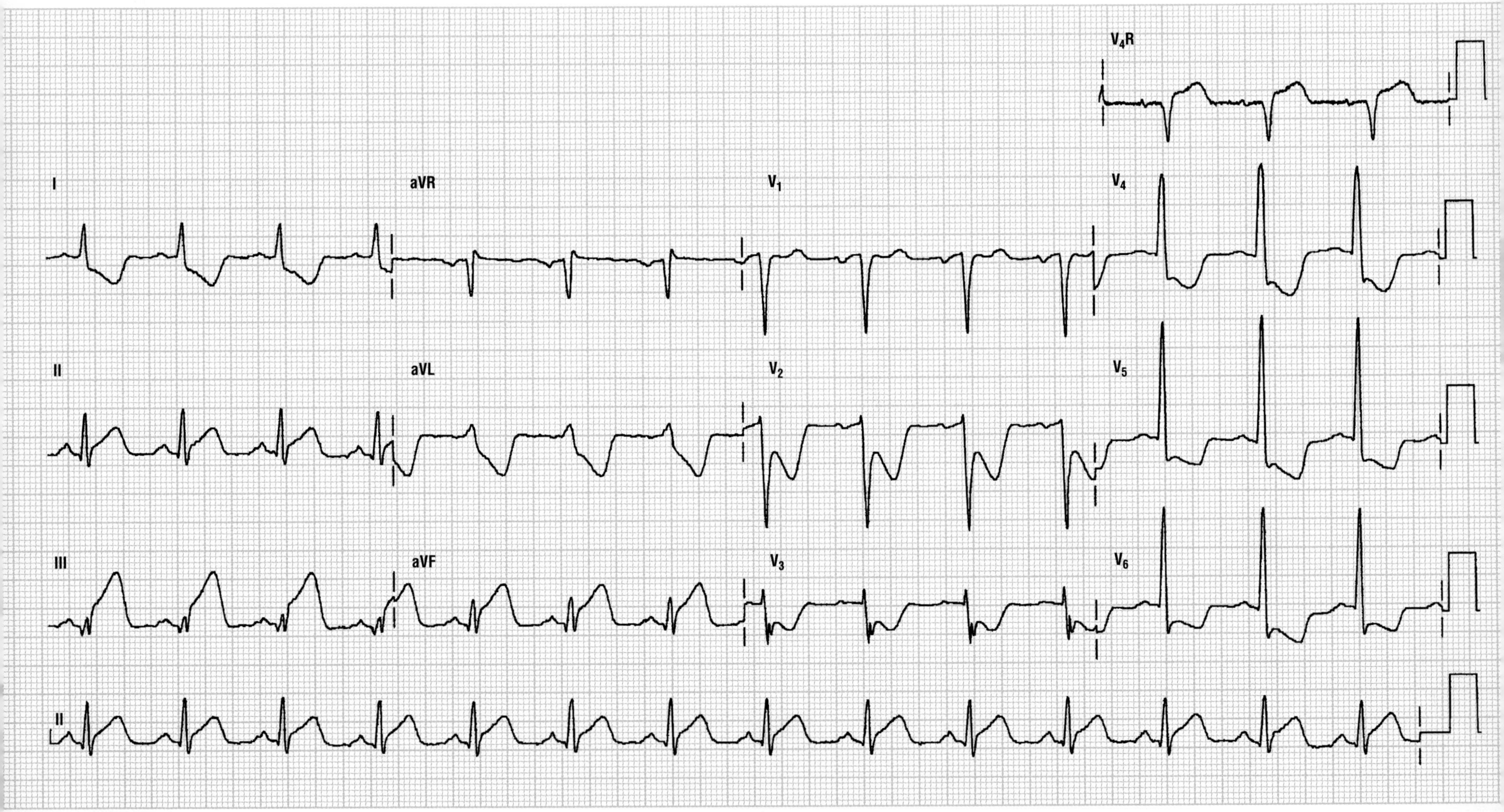

V₄R

I   aVR   V₁   V₄

II   aVL   V₂   V₅

III   aVF   V₃   V₆

II

ECG 15-34

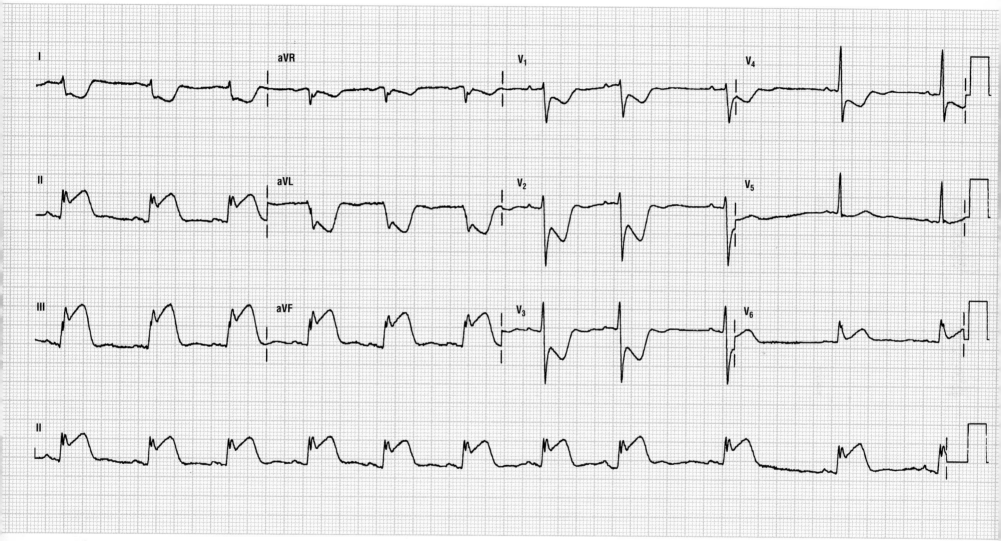

ECG 15-35

CHAPTER **15** • ACUTE MYOCARDIAL INFARCTION (AMI)

ECG CASE STUDIES: CONTINUED

ECG 15-36 Here is another inferior-RV-posterior MI with lateral extension. *Significant changes, for the purposes of thrombolytic protocols, involve elevation of 1 millimeter or more in two contiguous leads with a history compatible with an AMI.* Look at the amount of ST elevation in V_6. Is that pathologic ST elevation or just a variant of normal? In light of the infarct changes found throughout the ECG, that small amount of elevation is pathological. However, it is not significant enough to administer thrombolytics by itself, because it is not high enough and because it occurs in only one of the two lateral leads. The ST segment changes in the inferior leads, however, do match thrombolytic protocol standards. Remember, pathological changes do not always meet thrombolytic criteria, but they are still dangerous.

CLINICAL PEARL

Any ST elevation could be significant, needs to be explained, and may need to be treated. However, not all ST elevation is significant enough to justify administering thrombolytics.

ECG 15-37 Here, again, are changes consistent with an inferior-RV-posterior MI. These changes are a bit more subtle than the previous examples, though they are significant enough to treat, and they do meet the national standards for the administration of thrombolytics. Look at the ST segments in aVL. This is, as mentioned in an earlier chapter, the first sign of an IWMI.

Conclusion

We hope that this chapter has given you a good introduction into the electrocardiographic criteria for AMIs. We suggest that you review as many ECGs as possible, and, in particular, as many ECGs of AMI patients as you can. Keep a high index of suspicion in treating any patient with symptoms of the coronary ischemic syndromes. Also remember that RV infarcts behave differently and are treated differently than other AMIs. You will not know that the patient is having an RV infarct unless you think about the possibility to begin with. Only by making the thought process instinctual will you remember it when you are in the "heat of battle." Always think about RV and posterior wall infarcts when you diagnose an IWMI.

Finally, review this chapter and Chapter 14 as many times as you need to. They cover some of the most serious pathology that you will face. Any mistake could cost a patient's life, and will cause you extreme heartache and pain.

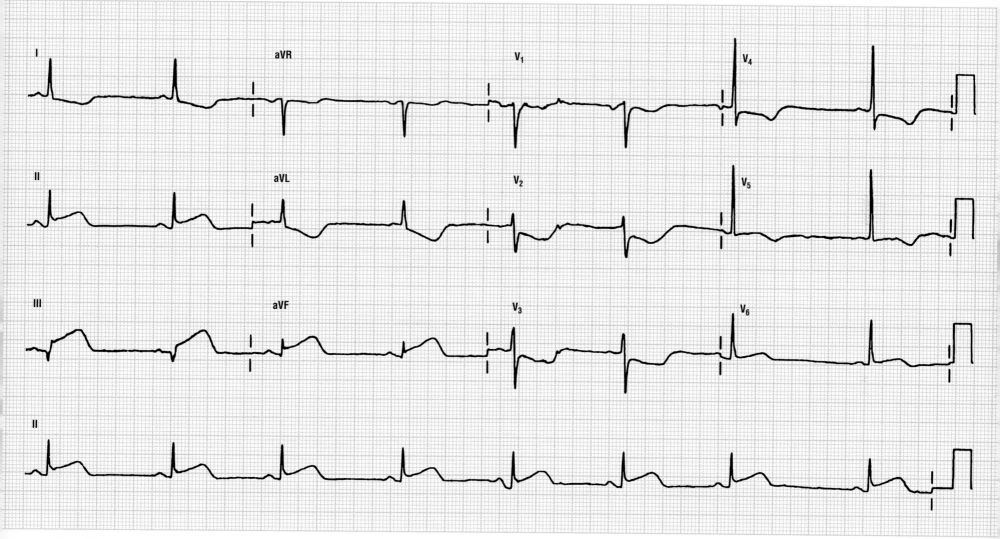

ECG 15-36

CHAPTER **15** • ACUTE MYOCARDIAL INFARCTION (AMI)

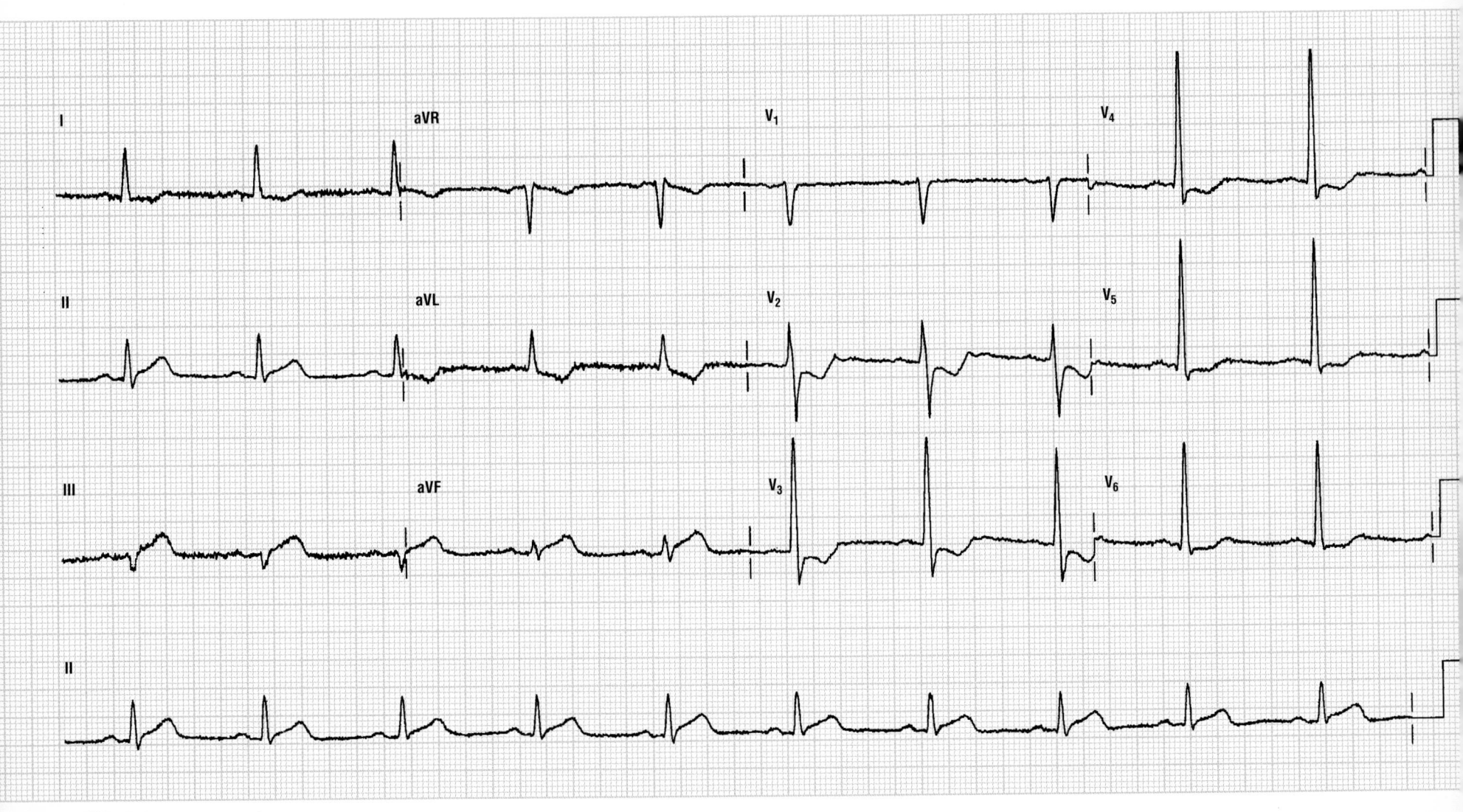

ECG 15-37

1. Ischemia, injury, and infarction are all reversible processes. True or False.

2. Infarcts are always broader along the endocardium. What are the protective mechanisms that cause zones of ischemia and injury to be narrower along the endocardium and broader along the pericardium?
   A. Collateral circulation
   B. Diffusion
   C. Thebesian veins
   D. All of the above
   E. None of the above

3. The zone of injury is more positive than the surrounding tissue, a factor represented electrocardiographically as ST elevation. True or False.

4. The area of infarction acts like an electrical "window." Q waves are the unopposed positive vector of the opposite wall heading away from an electrode overlying the infarcted area as it looks through the window. True or False.

5. Q wave infarcts are always transmural. True or False.

6. What is the chance of having an arrhythmia leading to sudden death in an AMI?
   A. 20%
   B. 40%
   C. 60%
   D. 80%
   E. 100%

7. Which is associated with a higher mortality rate?
   A. Q wave infarction
   B. Non–Q wave infarction
   C. Both are the same

8. The recording made by the electrode or lead on the wall exactly opposite an AMI is registering the reciprocal change of the AMI. True or False.

1. False 2. D 3. True 4. True 5. False 6. B 7. B 8. True

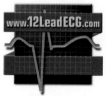

To enhance the knowledge you gain in this book, access this text's website at www.12leadECG.com! This valuable resource provides an online glossary and related web links. To learn more about the chapter topics, simply click on the chapter and view the link.

② CHAPTER IN **REVIEW**

9. A large coronary artery usually only perfuses one area of the heart. True or False.

10. Anteroseptal AMIs present with reciprocal changes in the inferior leads. True or False.

11. Anteroseptal AMIs with lateral extension represent a large amount of myocardium at risk. True or False.

12. Serial ECGs are critical to obtain in any AMI patient. True or False.

13. Inferior AMIs are usually benign, even when they are associated with right ventricular or posterior wall involvement. True or False.

14. The AV node is supplied by which artery?
  A. Right coronary
  B. Left anterior descending
  C. First obtuse marginal
  D. Left circumflex
  E. None of the above

15. The first electrocardiographic sign of an inferior AMI is:
  A. ST elevation in II, III, and aVF
  B. ST elevation in I and aVL
  C. Downward sloping ST depression in II, III, and aVF
  D. Downward sloping ST depression in aVL
  E. None of the above

16. Inferior wall AMIs are often confused with pericarditis. True or False.

17. Any time you have an IWMI you should obtain right-sided leads. True or False.

18. In a right ventricular infarct, blood returns to the left ventricle primarily because of:
  A. Pumping power of the right atria
  B. Pumping power of the left atria
  C. Venous return
  D. Gravity
  E. Peristalsis

19. Which is **not** a correct criterion for RVI:
  A. IWMI
  B. ST segment depression in III greater than that in II
  C. ST elevation in V$_1$
  D. ST depression in V$_2$
  E. ST depression in V$_2$ cannot be more than half of the ST elevation in aVF.
  F. 1 mm ST elevation in the right-sided leads V$_4$R to V$_6$R

20. Carousel ponies are bad on the ECG. True or False.

9. False **10.** False **11.** True **12.** True **13.** False **14.** A **15.** D **16.** False **17.** True **18.** C **19.** C **20.** True

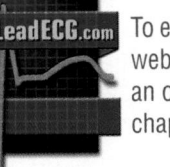

To enhance the knowledge you gain in this book, access this text's website at www.12leadECG.com! This valuable resource provides an online glossary and related web links. To learn more about the chapter topics, simply click on the chapter and view the link.

This chapter discusses two of the most important topics encountered in clinical practice. The material has been presented at Levels 1 and 2. By the time you reach Level 3, you should have a thorough understanding of these two topics. If you are a Level 3 reader, you may use this section for reference and to refresh your knowledge of these critical subjects.

Electrolytes are found in the extracellular and intracellular fluid of most cells (see Chapter 2). The most important electrolytes are sodium, potassium, calcium, and magnesium. Flow of these electrolytes into and out of the cells creates energy for depolarization and repolarization, and allows contractile mechanisms to function. As you can imagine, the levels of these electrolytes in the fluid bathing the cells will affect these currents and the appearance of the complexes on the ECG.

Drugs alter the electrolyte channels found on the cell membrane and thus cause changes in the flow of the electrolytes into and out of the cells. These drug effects also alter conduction patterns, and therefore the appearance, of the complexes on the ECG.

In this chapter, we are going to cover the two main electrolytes that cause diagnostic and recognizable changes on the ECG: potassium and calcium. Magnesium and some minor electrolytes will produce changes on the ECG that are both nonspecific and nondiagnostic. Because we would like you to concentrate on those aspects of electrocardiography that are useful clinically, we will not be covering those changes and refer you to the Additional Readings section.

It is also important to correlate ECG findings with possible drug effects. For instance, the patient has bradycardia and is taking beta blockers, so the beta blockers may be responsible for the bradycardia. The clinical correlation is the key to interpretation. We will not be offering examples of each drug effect because most are nondiagnostic for the drug. The exception is digoxin (dig). Because digoxin is associated with various changes and arrhythmias, we will cover it in greater detail.

Hyperkalemia and Its Effects

Of all the electrolyte changes that can occur, hyperkalemia is the most dangerous. Hyperkalemia can not only kill, but it can kill in seconds — and it prevents response to the drugs used in resuscitation. Hyperkalemia causes changes in the appearance of the QRS complex, symbolizing the changes in cell function, and can cause any and all arrhythmias. *Immediate recognition and action to stabilize the myocardial membrane and reverse the pathological processes are the keys to effectively combating the complications of hyperkalemia.* As we have said, if you don't think about the problem, you will never diagnose it!

Because the electrocardiographic changes in hyperkalemia take place along a spectrum that corresponds to blood potassium levels (Figure 16-1), the ECG can help you estimate the blood level. The main changes found in hyperkalemia include:

1. T wave abnormalities, especially tall and peaked Ts
2. Intraventricular conduction delays (IVCDs)
3. P waves missing or of decreased amplitude
4. ST segment changes simulating an injury pattern
5. Cardiac arrhythmias, any and all varieties

As a beginning student, concentrate on the T waves, remembering that any wide rhythm could be due to hyperkalemia. As an intermediate student, concentrate on the rest of the possible changes that can occur. We ask you to review the treatment of hyperkalemia in a text that covers treatment. Diagnosis is the most important aspect of treatment!

The Spectrum of Hyperkalemia

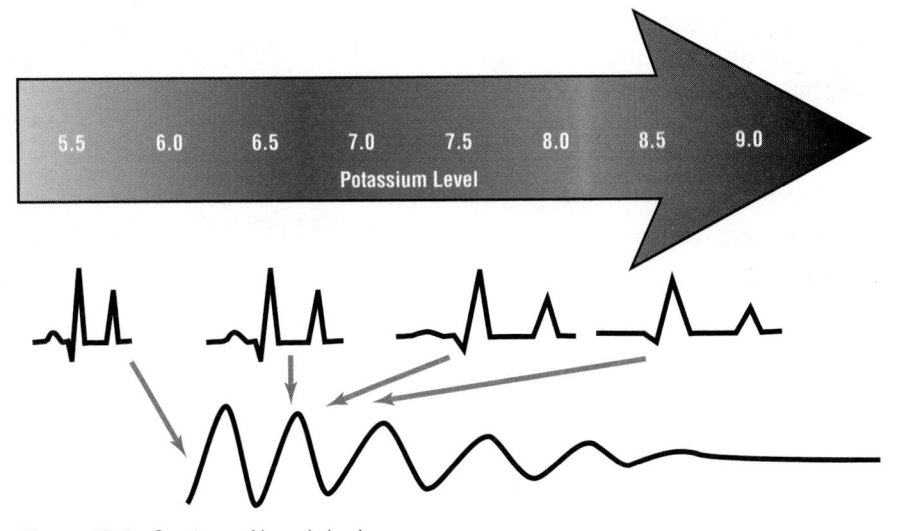

Figure 16-1: Spectrum of hyperkalemia.

Hyperkalemia occurs across a spectrum, both in actual blood levels and in the electrocardiographic representation of the pathology that occurs at those levels (Figure 16-1). Imagine those changes occurring smoothly on a continuous rhythm strip. As the level increases from normal, the T waves become tall and sharp. Next, all of the intervals begin to widen and decrease in amplitude. The P wave also loses amplitude until you can't see it any longer. As the potassium level continues to rise, the whole morphology of the complexes is lost and you arrive at a sine wave. Finally . . . straight line.

The rhythm can convert to a sine wave and asystole at any point after changes develop (*red arrows* in Figure 16-1). This can occur in seconds at any point along the spectrum. This and other arrhythmias are the main dangers of hyperkalemia.

T Wave Abnormalities in Hyperkalemia

Electrocardiographically, T wave abnormalities are the first changes noted in a patient developing hyperkalemia. The T wave changes begin to appear when the potassium level exceeds 5.5 mEq/L.

The most famous T wave change is the tall, peaked, and narrow T. There is an old medical adage that you wouldn't want to sit on a hyperkalemic T. When you look at some of the examples that follow, you'll see why. *However, these tall, peaked, and narrow T waves are found in only 22% of hyperkalemic patients.* The other 78% of the time, the T waves are any combination of tall, peaked, narrow, or wide. Examples include tall and wide, peaked but wide, and so on. The most common examples are tall and peaked but not narrow. All of the different combinations, however, show T waves that are symmetrical.

Another important point about T waves is that the morphology can change as the potassium level increases. Note in Figure 16-1 that the height of the T waves decreases as they widen. At a level of 5.5 mEq/L, the T waves are tall, peaked, and narrow, and there is a normal or slightly prolonged QT. However, as the level increases, the T waves and the PR, QRS, and QT intervals all widen, and the amplitudes become smaller. This will affect the appearance of the T waves.

Some clinicians believe that T waves have to be elevated in all leads to indicate hyperkalemia. We'd like to dispel this myth. *The T wave changes are usually first noted in V_2 to V_4.* Why, we cannot tell you. Perhaps because these are the leads in closest physical proximity to the heart itself. Don't be fooled into thinking that peaked, narrow T waves that only appear in V_2 to V_4 are not due to hyperkalemia!

CLINICAL PEARL

T Waves in Hyperkalemia

1. T wave changes are the earliest sign of hyperkalemia.
2. They are seen when the K+ exceeds 5.5 mEq/L.
3. Classic T waves that are tall, peaked, and narrow occur in only 22% of cases.
4. T wave morphology may be altered as a result of the IVCD that develops with severe hyperkalemia.
5. T wave changes may be localized to the anteroseptal leads, or the changes can be diffuse.

QUICK REVIEW

1. Hyperkalemia is many times very difficult to diagnose. True of False.

2. You should use calcium routinely in renal failure patients; it is a safe drug for minor problems. True of False.

3. With hyperkalemia, you only have seconds to minutes to intervene before possible life-threatening situations *could* develop. True or False.

4. IVCD presents like LBBB in leads I and V_6 and like RBBB in lead V_1. True or False.

1. True 2. False 3. True 4. False

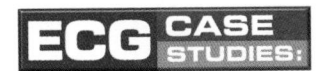 *T Wave Changes in Hyperkalemia*

ECG 16-1 It is kind of tough not to notice those massive T waves in leads V_2 to V_4 on this ECG. They are definitively tall, peaked, and narrow. This is the classic T wave change in hyperkalemia.

We want you to take a look at the T waves in the inferior leads as well. Note that they are not very impressive looking. However, they are still more than $^2/_3$ the height of the R wave in III and aVF. These are also pathological, and also caused by the hyperkalemic changes in this patient. You always need to be observant of changes that may not be too obvious because of other distractions on the ECG. Many times, those small findings are what will make the definitive diagnosis for you.

ECG 16-2 Are the T waves in this ECG consistent with hyperkalemia? Yes, they sure are! They are not as impressive as in ECG 16-1, but look at how tall they are in comparison to their respective R waves. These are some very tall, symmetrical T waves. They are pathological in leads I, II, III, aVF, and V_2 to V_6. These changes are quite global; they appear in most regions of the ECG.

Symmetrical T waves are generally due to some pathologic process. Whenever you see them on an ECG, rule out life-threatening causes of pathology before you label them "benign."

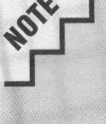

The String Theory of Hyperkalemia

The following analogy should help you visualize the T wave shape in hyperkalemia. Imagine an entire complex made of string. Now picture yourself grabbing the string just before the start of the P wave, and also at the top of the T wave. Slowly start to pull up on the string by the top of the T wave. The T wave begins to peak. If you continue to pull on the string from both sides, the intervals will widen and start to become smaller. The P waves disappear. Eventually, you would end up with a straight line. Sound familiar? These are the exact changes seen in hyperkalemia!

Hyperkalemia occurs commonly in patients with what underlying disorder?

End-stage renal disease

CLINICAL PEARL

Tall, peaked, and narrow T waves are found in only 22% of hyperkalemic patients. Beware of other possibilities!

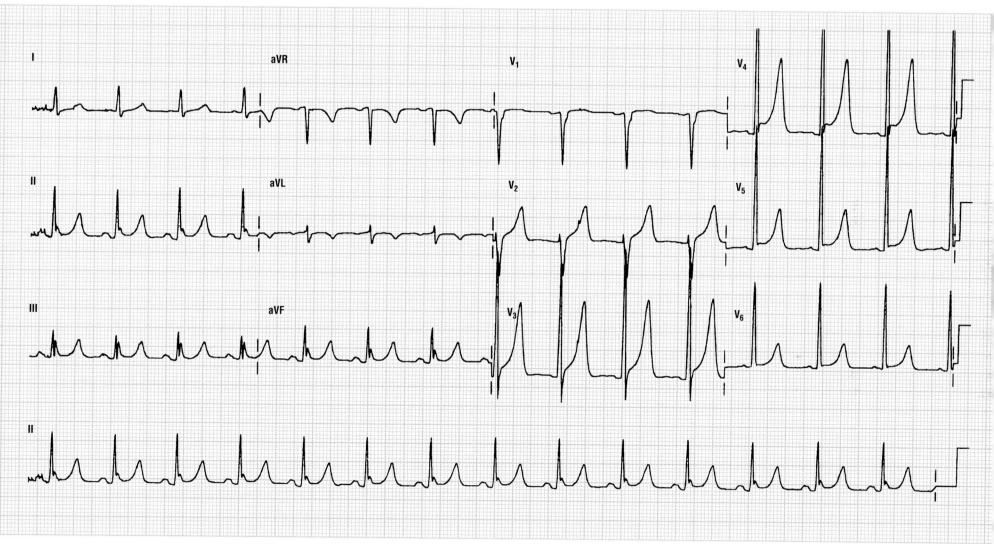

ECG 16-1

ECG CASE STUDIES: CONTINUED

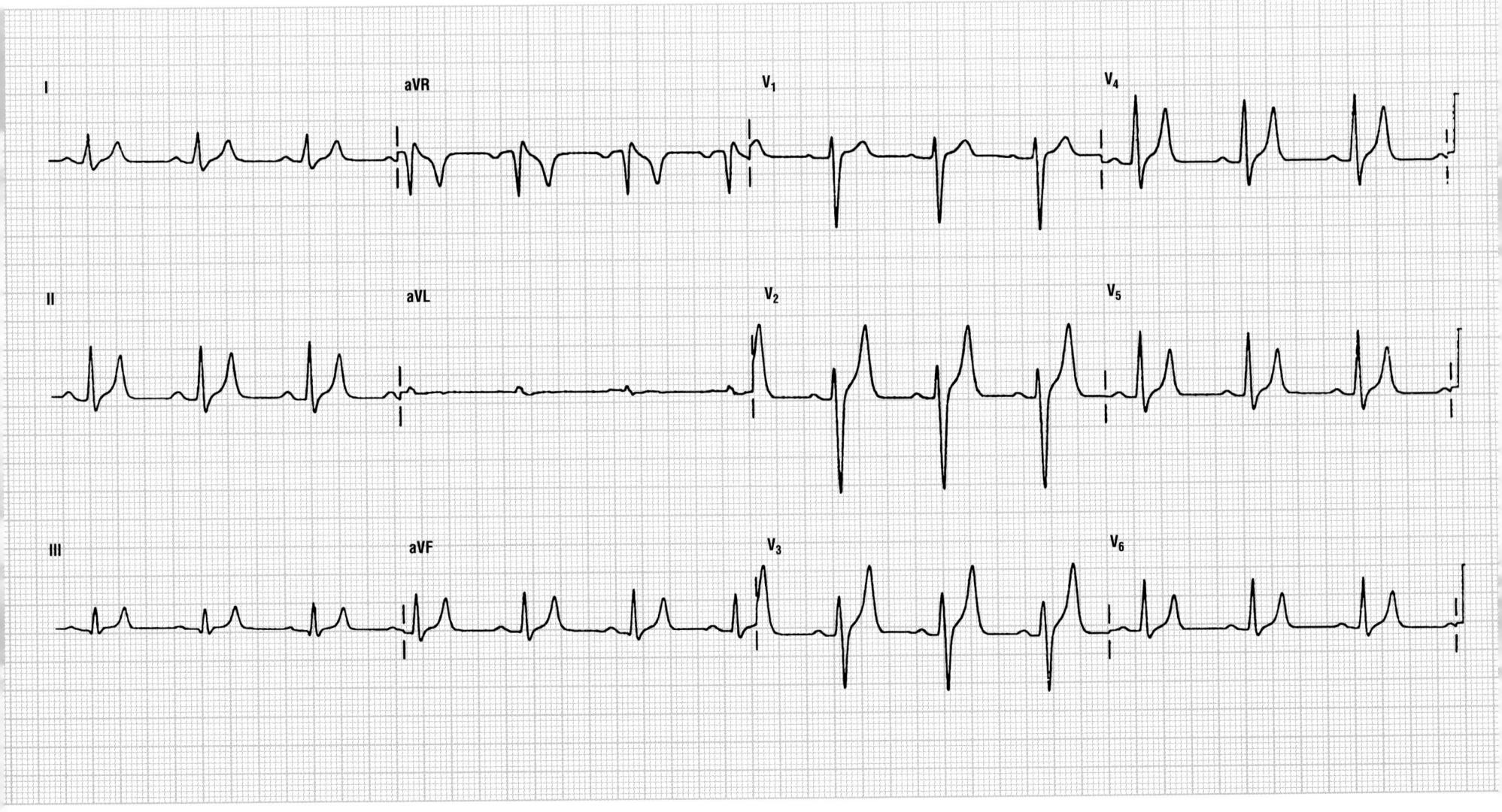

ECG 16-2

ECG 16-3 This ECG shows T wave changes in V$_2$ to V$_4$ that would be considered tall, narrow, and peaked. V$_5$ and V$_6$ are just a continuation of the changes of the anteroseptal leads. Note that the inferior leads show significant T wave changes, as well. There is prolongation of the QT interval that is out of proportion to the widening in the rest of the ECG. Why is this occurring? Well, renal failure — the most common cause of hyperkalemia — is also associated with hypocalcemia. And hypocalcemia, as we'll see later in this chapter, also causes QT prolongation. The prolongation in this ECG is the cumulative effect of widening caused both by high potassium and low calcium levels. Pericardial effusions with low voltage also occur commonly in these patients.

QUICK REVIEW

Besides hyperkalemia, what other changes of end-stage renal disease occur commonly?

.levretni eht nediw yltaerg ot dnet lliw lavretni TQ eht gnignolorp secrof eht fo noitammus sihT .noitagnolorp TQ sa ylnommoc stneserp ,txen ees llahs ew sa ,aimeclacopyH .snoisuffe laidracirep dna aimeclacopyH

ECG 16-4 Boy, these T waves would be painful to sit on, wouldn't they? In addition to the impressive T waves, we want you to look at how prolonged the QT intervals are. This is due, once again, to the combined hyperkalemia and hypocalcemia common to these patients. *In patients with mild hyperkalemia and end-stage renal disease, remember that you need to aggressively treat the potassium abnormalities, not the calcium imbalances!* Treatment with excessive calcium will cause crystallization

of the soft tissues, because *calcium + phosphate = calcium phosphate*. Renal failure patients typically have high phosphate levels; when calcium is added acutely, they form crystals.

CLINICAL PEARL

In dialysis patients, use calcium sparingly except when faced with life-threatening emergencies! However, calcium is the first-line drug in the treatment of life-threatening hyperkalemia. Use it in *any* patient with life-threatening arrhythmias or hemodynamic complications.

ECG 16-5 The T wave changes on this ECG are subtle, but they are present. The T waves are pathologic in V$_2$ to V$_5$, and the changes are highly suggestive of hyperkalemia. *Don't be fooled because the changes are subtle. You don't have more time before an arrhythmia develops just because the changes are subtle.* You may only have a few seconds or minutes before they turn deadly. You just don't know when it is going to happen. Don't gamble! This is one of those take-home points that we mention over and over because no one believes us. We'll show you some proof before the end of this chapter, but for now just keep repeating to yourself, "You only have seconds! You only have seconds! You only have seconds!" You'll thank us someday. Don't make us say, "We told you so" — we hate that.

REMINDER:

T wave changes do not have to be extreme to cause life-threatening rhythms or sine waves. They just have to be present to be dangerous!

ECG CASE STUDIES: CONTINUED

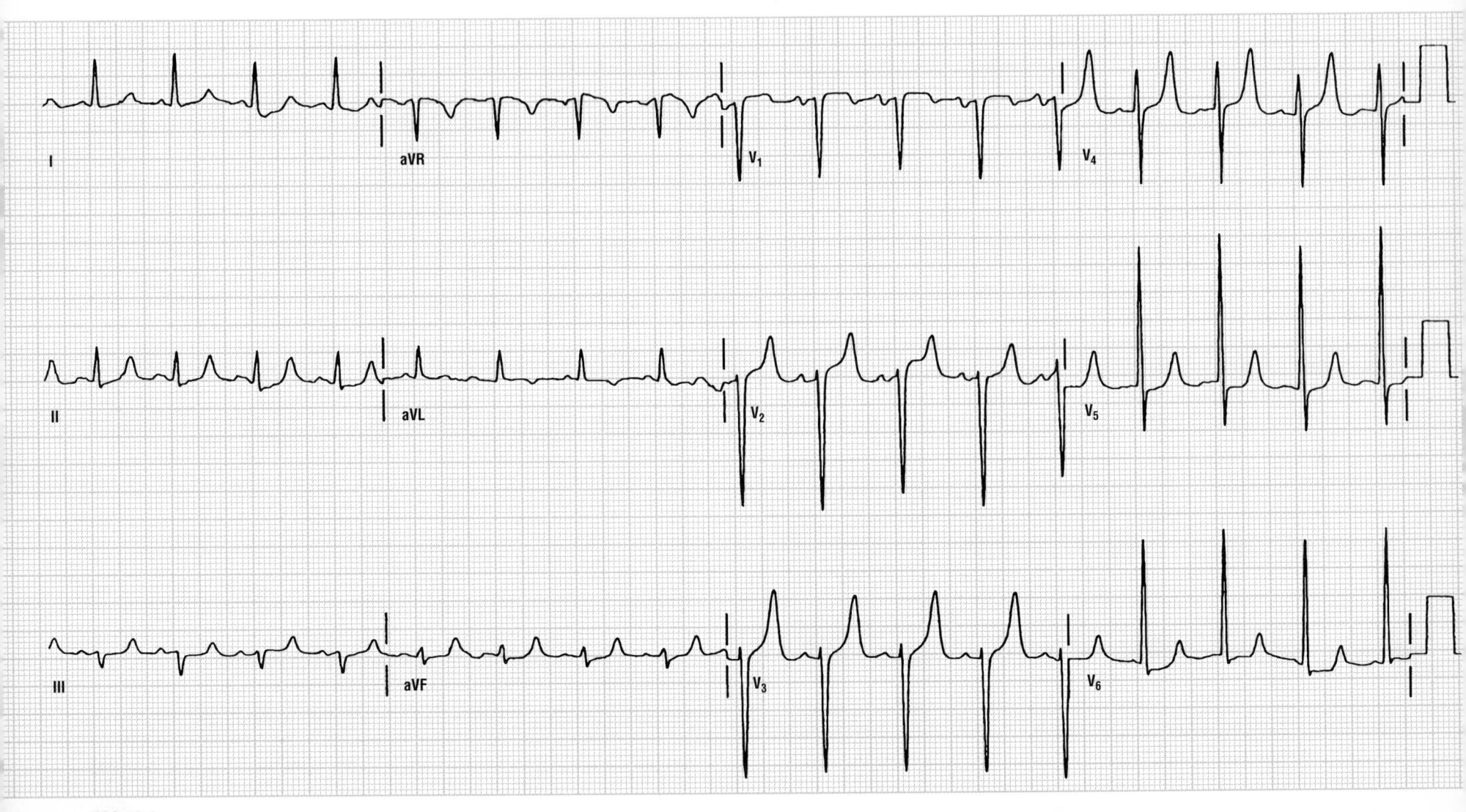

ECG 16-3

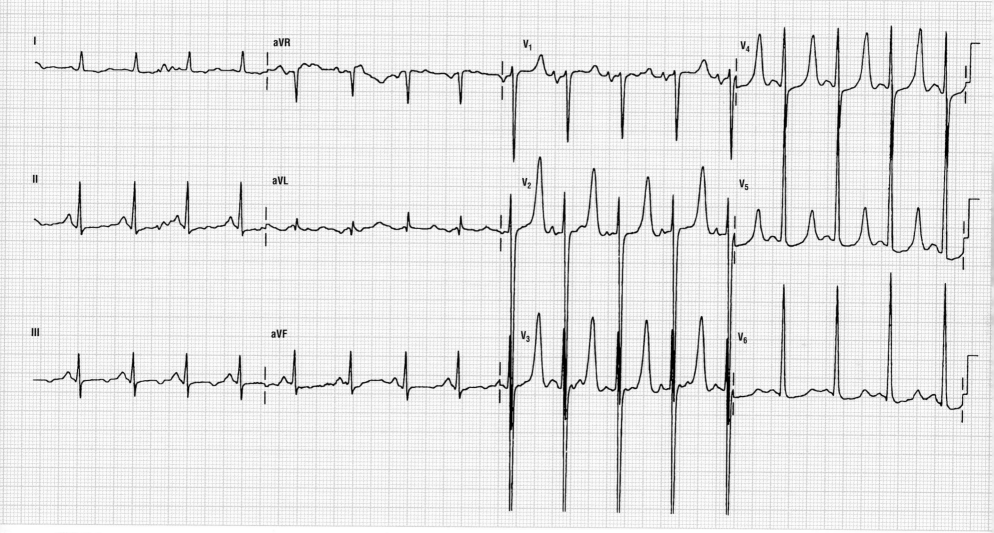

ECG 16-4

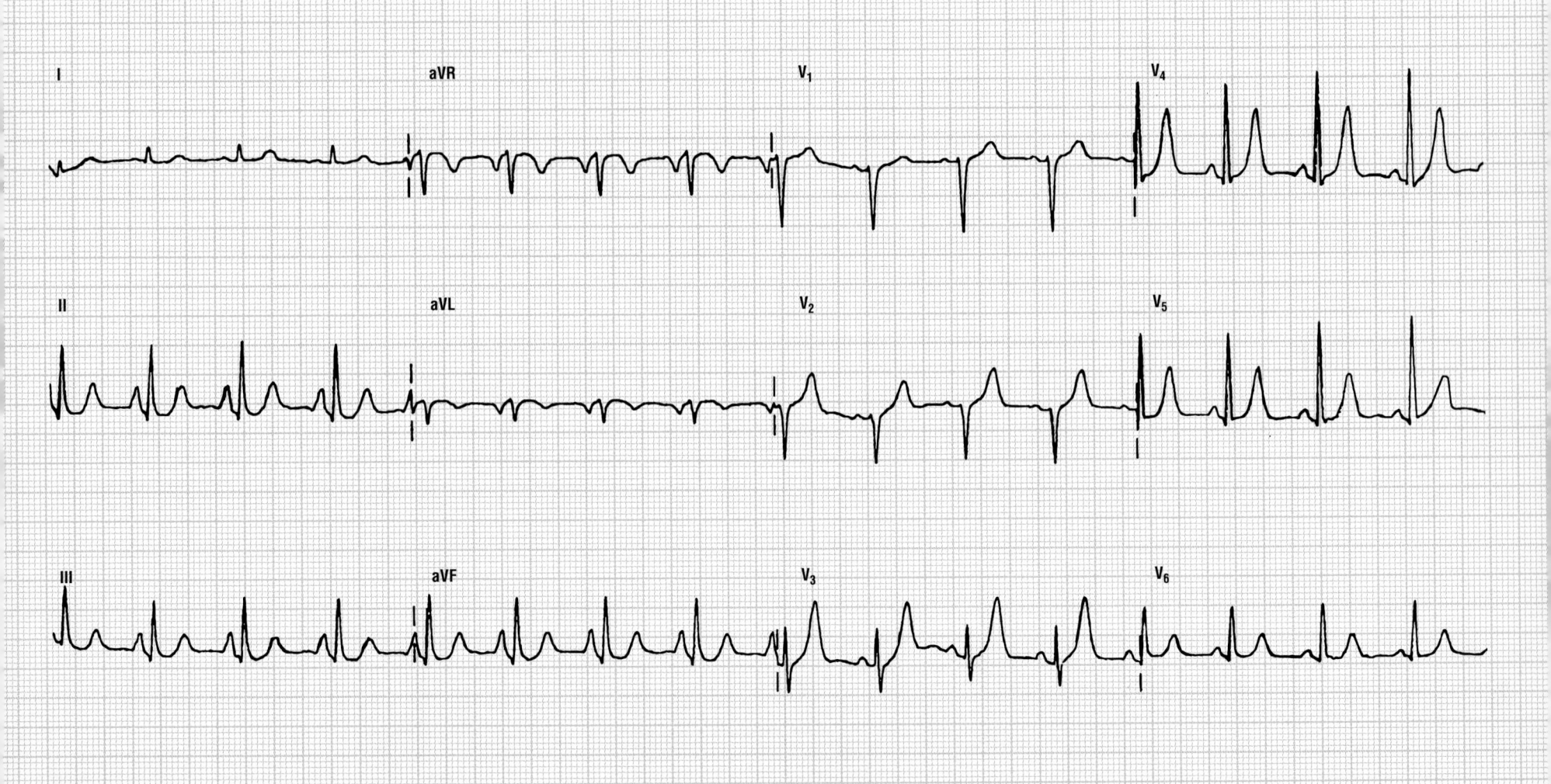

ECG 16-5

IVCD and Hyperkalemia

We covered IVCDs in Chapter 13, but here's a short review. An IVCD exists when the QRS width is more than 0.12 seconds and the ECG does not meet criteria for either LBBB or RBBB. In the most common presentation for an IVCD, V_1 looks like an LBBB with a monomorphic S wave or an rS complex, and leads I and V_6 look like an RBBB with the typical slurred S wave. *Whenever you see an IVCD, think of hyperkalemia first!* This is the most life-threatening cause of an IVCD, and it leaves you very little time to institute treatment. As always, clinical correlation and an old ECG are invaluable to the clinical diagnosis. If available, an arterial blood gas with a potassium level will give you a quick preliminary answer. You will probably not have time to wait for the regular potassium level to come back from the lab before you institute therapy, as this can take 30 to 90 minutes.

The widening of the complexes usually begins when the potassium concentration is at 6.5 mEq/L or greater. As the potassium level increases, the QRS complex will widen. The amplitude or height of the waves will slowly begin to decrease as the complexes continue to widen. Prominent S waves will start to form in leads I and V_6 as the IVCD progresses. The formation of a sine wave pattern can occur at any time.

The T waves in an IVCD will still be peaked, but will probably be a bit smaller than those found at lower potassium levels. They will usually be peaked, symmetrical, and wide. The axis of the ECG can change to an RAD or an LAD. You can also see a new LBBB or RBBB pattern instead of an IVCD. Finally, every conceivable arrhythmia can develop at this point.

> ## REMINDER:
> When you diagnose an IVCD, always think of hyperkalemia!

P Waves and Hyperkalemia

As the potassium level increases above 7.0 mEq/L, the PR interval increases, and the amplitude of the P waves decreases. Eventually, you will not be able to see the P waves. They will still be there — you just won't be able to see them. Why? As the potassium level increases, the atrial myocardial cells will stop depolarizing. The SA node and the special conduction system of the atria will continue to function but the myocardial cells will not. Because the atrial myocardium creates the atrial vectors that we pick up on the ECG as the P waves, we do not see any atrial activity on the ECG. Technically, this is still a sinus rhythm, because the complexes originate in the SA node; it just does not show up on the ECG. The problem is that you cannot distinguish this "P-less" sinus rhythm from an idioventricular rhythm. Treatment for hyperkalemia will cause a dramatic return of the P waves.

We have tried to stay away from treatment on purpose. However, keep in mind that when you are faced with an arrhythmia caused by hyperkalemia, response to the drugs you use will not be typical. The antiarrhythmics may not work appropriately, so you need to treat the hyperkalemia first. In addition, pressors and catecholamines, such as epinephrine, will not work normally on the hyperkalemic patient. *Treat the hyperkalemia first!* Give the patient calcium and sodium bicarbonate, then give the pressors if the patient is still in hemodynamic collapse. To top it all off, there is evidence that pacemakers will not work on hyperkalemic patients; that is, they will not capture.

You should always think about the possibility of hyperkalemia when a patient in cardiac arrest has an AVgraft. AV grafts are used for dialysis on end-stage renal failure patients, the group most likely to develop hyperkalemia.

> ## CLINICAL PEARL
> When you have a hyperkalemic idioventricular rhythm, reach for the calcium and sodium bicarbonate before you reach for the pacemakers or atropine!

ECG CASE STUDIES: *IVCD and P Waves in Hyperkalemia*

ECG 16-6 There are a few points that make this ECG just scream out, "Hyperkalemia!" The first is the PR interval prolongation, which is very marked — so prolonged that it falls on the preceding T wave. The QRS complexes are wide and they fall into the pattern of an IVCD. Look at V_1. It looks like a typical LBBB with a big, monomorphic S wave. V_6 is full of artifact; it's difficult to interpret, so look at lead I instead. It has the big, wide, slurred S wave you would expect in an RBBB. The QT interval is also very prolonged, and is more than $1/2$ the R-R interval. So we have an IVCD with prolonged intervals throughout. That should make you immediately think of hyperkalemia. Now, as if you needed more, look at the T waves. They are very wide and symmetrical. They are also pathologically tall in comparison with their respective R waves, greater than $2/3$ the height of the Rs in I, II, III, aVL, and V_3 to V_6. These T waves are the result of hyperkalemia.

Can you guess the potassium level? Well, you start to get T wave peaking at 5.5 mEq/L, and interval widening at 6.5 mEq/L. Prolongation of the PR interval and decreased P wave amplitude begin to appear at greater than 7.0 mEq/L. So we know the level is greater than 7.0 mEq/L. Finally, at levels greater than 8.8 mEq/L, we would get loss of the P waves altogether. A good guess would be between 7.0 and 8.8 mEq/L!

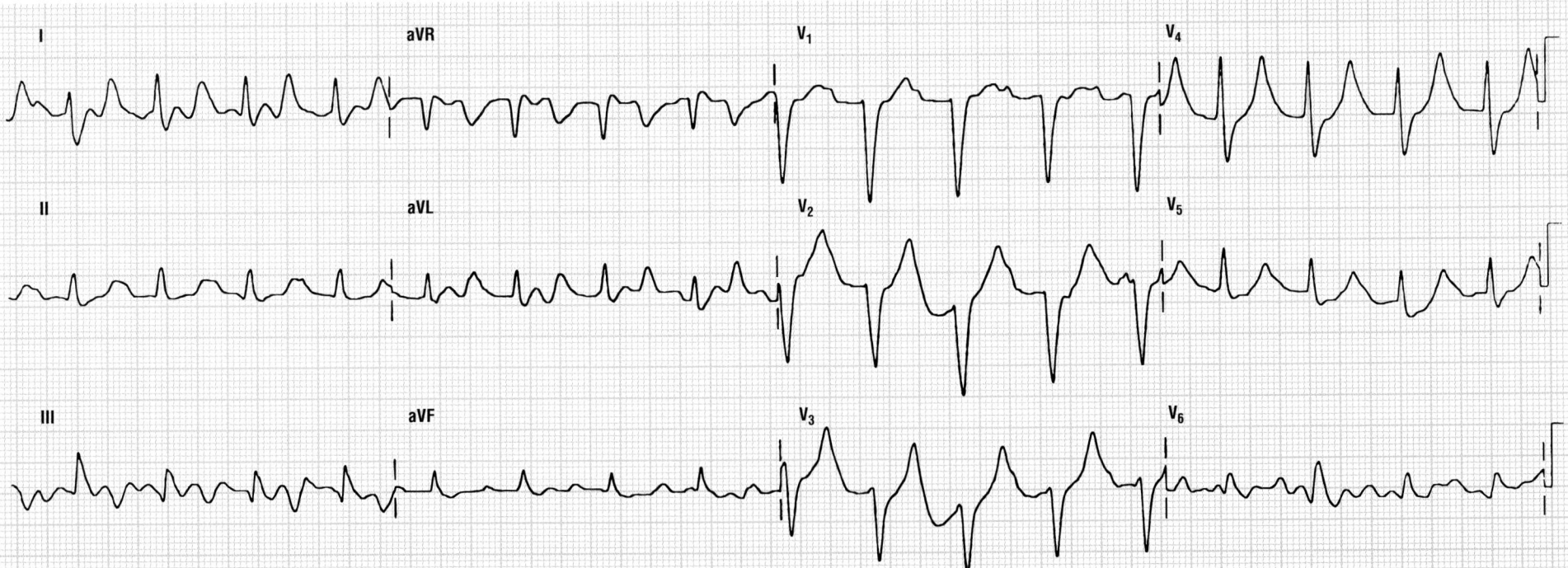

ECG 16-6

②

ECG 16-7 This ECG also shows changes characteristic of hyperkalemia. The things that jump out at you are the width of the QRS complexes and the IVCD pattern. Note that all of the intervals are widened throughout the ECG. The T waves do not have a tremendous amount of peaking but they are wide and symmetrical. What about the P waves — are there any? There is something that looks like a P wave right before the third complex in V₁, but that is the only place we see them, so the answer is no. What about the next-to-last complex? It is a premature complex with an associated compensatory pause, so it is either a JPC or an APC. Can you have an APC when you have no P waves? You can in hyperkalemia! Remember, in severe hyper-

kalemia, you will lose your P waves altogether. You can review the discussion several pages earlier (P Waves in Hyperkalemia) for further information.

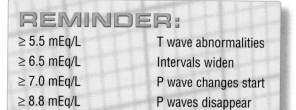

REMINDER:

≥ 5.5 mEq/L	T wave abnormalities
≥ 6.5 mEq/L	Intervals widen
≥ 7.0 mEq/L	P wave changes start
≥ 8.8 mEq/L	P waves disappear

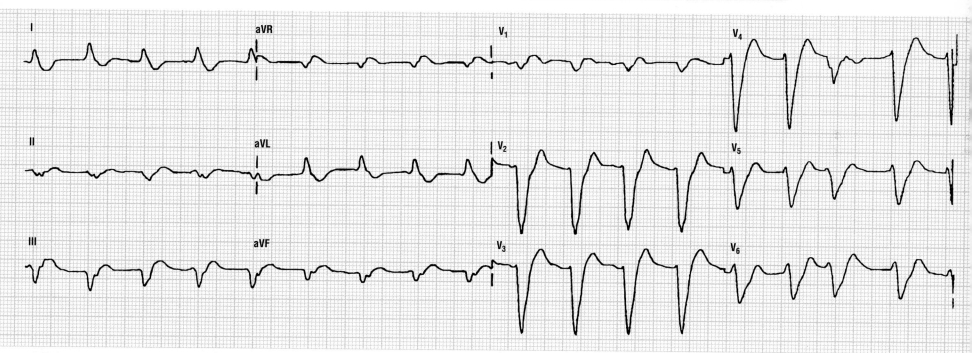

ECG 16-7

ECG CASE STUDIES: **CONTINUED**

②

ECG 16-8 This ECG shows a wide-complex rhythm. You would be hard pressed to state with any degree of certainty that it was not an idioventricular rhythm. However, one thing should raise a high level of suspicion that hyperkalemia is the cause. Most, if not all, idioventricular rhythms are either LBBB or RBBB patterns. This is an IVCD. Because the first thought that comes to mind in IVCD is hyperkalemia, we should do everything in our power to disprove it as the precipitating factor in this rhythm. In fact, this ECG was obtained from a dialysis patient with a potassium level of 10.4 mEq/L. The situation reversed quickly with aggressive treatment for hyperkalemia.

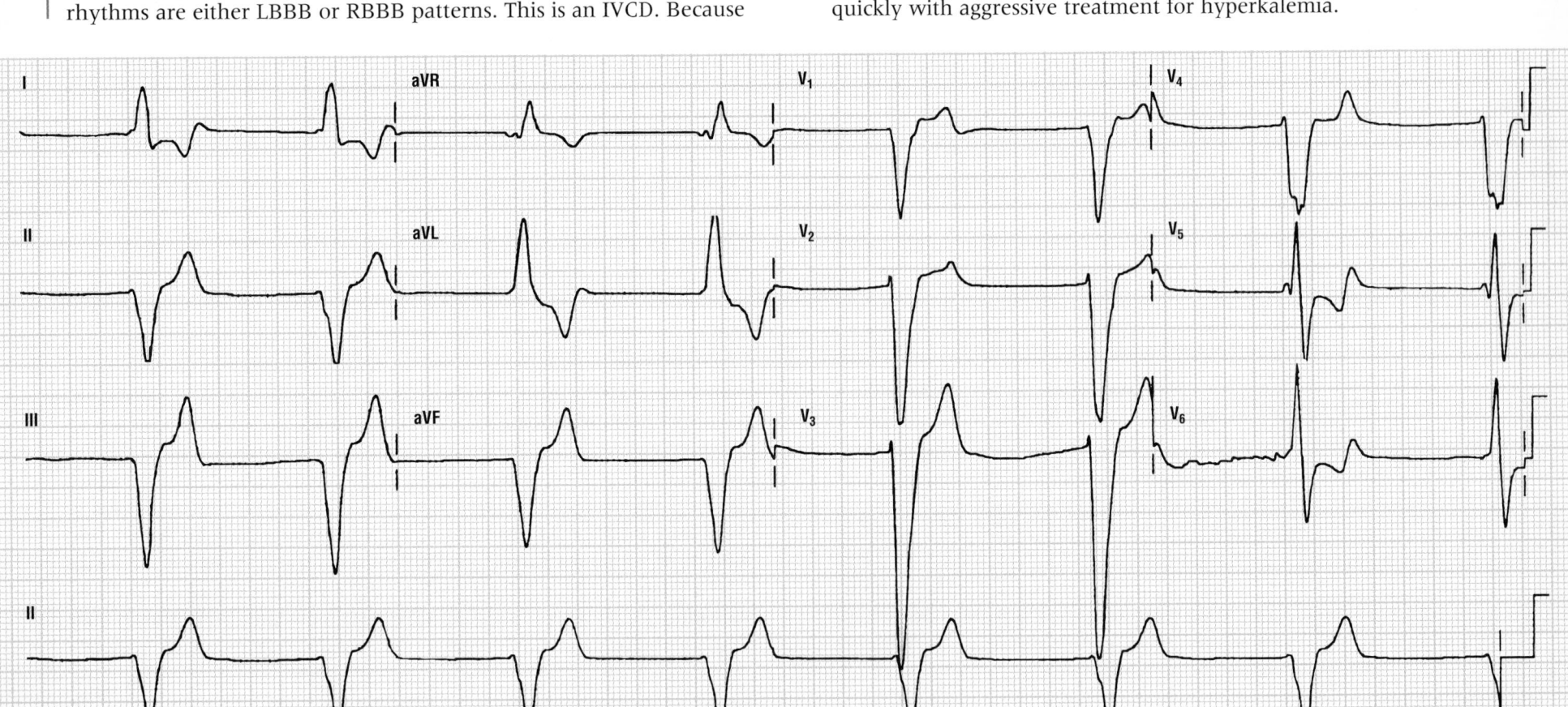

ECG 16-8

ECG 16-9 This ECG also shows a wide-complex rhythm with no discernible P waves, and once again the telltale signs of hyperkalemia are present: the IVCD, the widening of all of the intervals, the peaked T waves. All of those things should make you want to shout, "What is this patient's potassium level?!" *Remember, unless you think of it, you won't diagnose it!*

CLINICAL PEARL

Catecholamines (such as epinephrine), pressors (dopamine and others), and pacemakers will not work on hyperkalemic patients in cardiac arrest.

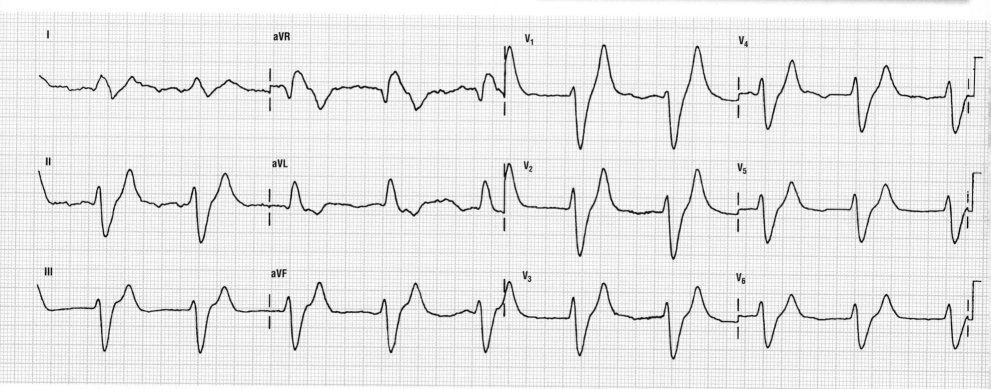

ECG 16-9

ECG CASE STUDIES: **CONTINUED**

ECG 16-10 This ECG shows a wide-complex rhythm with IVCD. This time the IVCD pattern has rabbit ears and a slurred S in V_6, but a monomorphic R wave in lead I. The QT interval is very prolonged, and the T waves are definitively peaked and wide. There are two more interesting points about this ECG. First, what is the rhythm? There are some P waves but they are different morphologies, and the PR intervals are different. The rhythm is also irregularly irregular. This is a wandering atrial pacemaker. Second, is the patient having a septal AMI? No, hyperkalemia can mimic the ST elevation of an AMI. When the potassium returns to normal, so will the ST segment. This is a very rare occurrence, and we mean *very* rare! Always correlate the ECG with the patient.

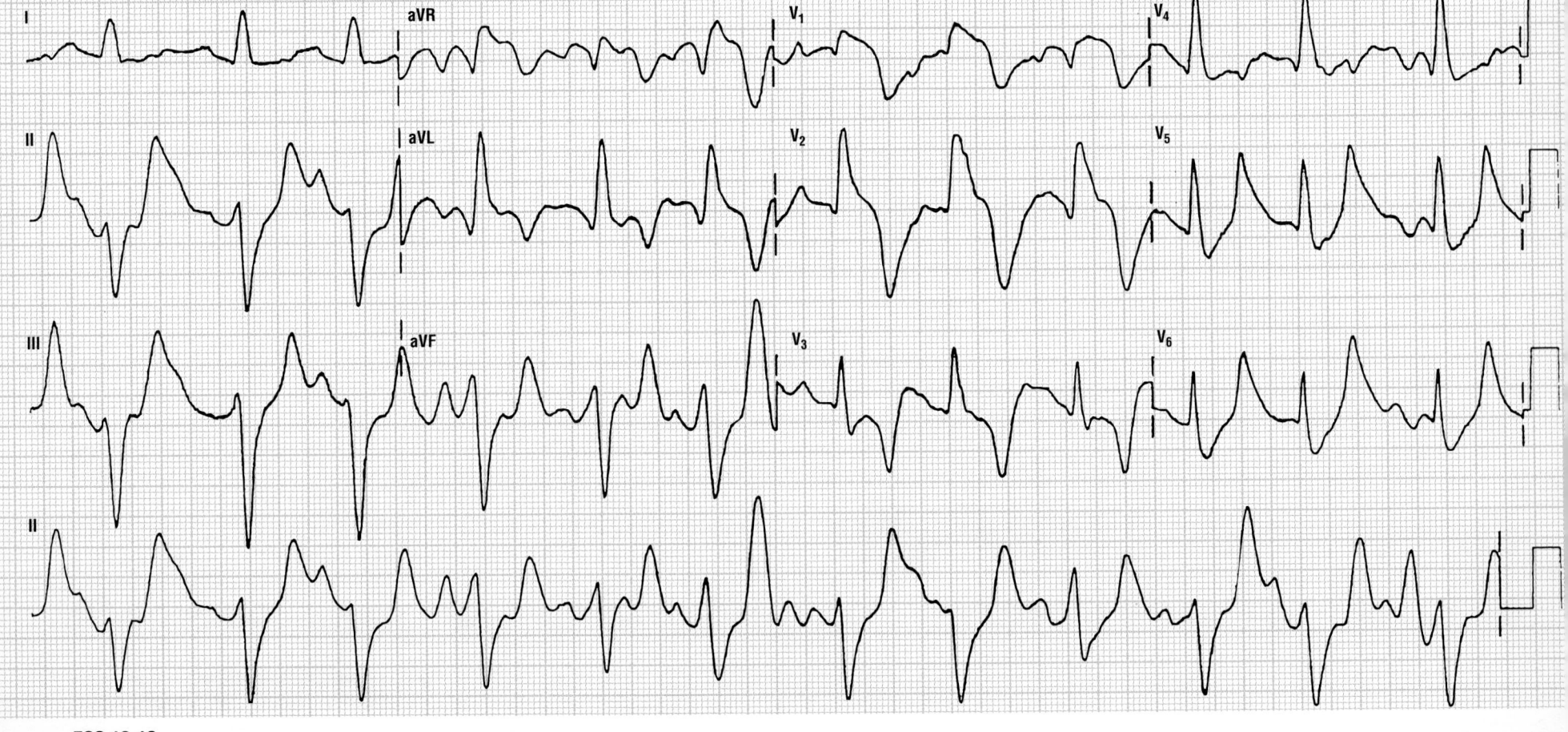

ECG 16-10

②

ECG 16-11 By now you should be starting to get familiar with the changes noted in hyperkalemia. This ECG should be saying, "Look at me! I'm hyperkalemic!" all over the place. You have peaked and wide T waves, an IVCD, QT prolongation, and PR prolongation. If you are not 100% comfortable with picking up these changes, go back and review the beginning of this chapter.

We don't know if you have noticed, but different authors emphasize what they consider important about the topics in their books. We have concentrated on three major points so far: (1) ST segments, (2) AMIs, especially the atypical regions, and (3) hyperkalemia.

ST segments cause the most confusion. There is tremendous clinical variation in what is considered pathological and what is benign. There is also a great deal of confusion about LVH with strain and infarcts. In Chapter 14, we tried to answer some of these questions for you. Chapter 15 covered not only the "easy" AMIs to pick up, but also the atypical regions involved, such as the posterior wall and the right ventricle. And, in this chapter we have discussed hyperkalemia. Hyperkalemia is a very lethal, very treatable entity. But first you need to make the diagnosis.

This ECG was obtained from a patient who arrived with some shortness of breath. The diagnosis was not made, and the patient waited. The ECG shows IVCD, interval prolongation, and abnormal T waves. The patient had no history of any renal problems. A short while after this ECG was obtained, the ECG pattern changed on the monitor and a repeat was obtained. Let's move on to ECG 16-12 for a continuation of this discussion. . . .

ECG 16-12 The patient was asymptomatic at this point, despite the horrible appearance of his rhythm strip. Lidocaine was immediately given, for treatment of the presumed diagnosis of hemodynamically stable ventricular tachycardia. Just when the ECG was completed and the leads were being removed, the patient arrested. The potassium level was later reported to have been 9.4 mEq/L. The take-home message: Know the changes of hyperkalemia and its treatment by heart. Think about the diagnosis, make it early, and institute treatment immediately. You don't have time to waste. You need to act, and act fast!

This is a sine wave pattern. You can still pick up the individual complexes on this ECG. Sometimes they will merge into one another. If the patient has progressed into this pattern, treat immediately for hyperkalemia. If the patient presents in this pattern, it is OK to start treatment for VTach and hyperkalemia at the same time. *You have only seconds. Use them wisely!*

ECG CASE STUDIES: **CONTINUED**

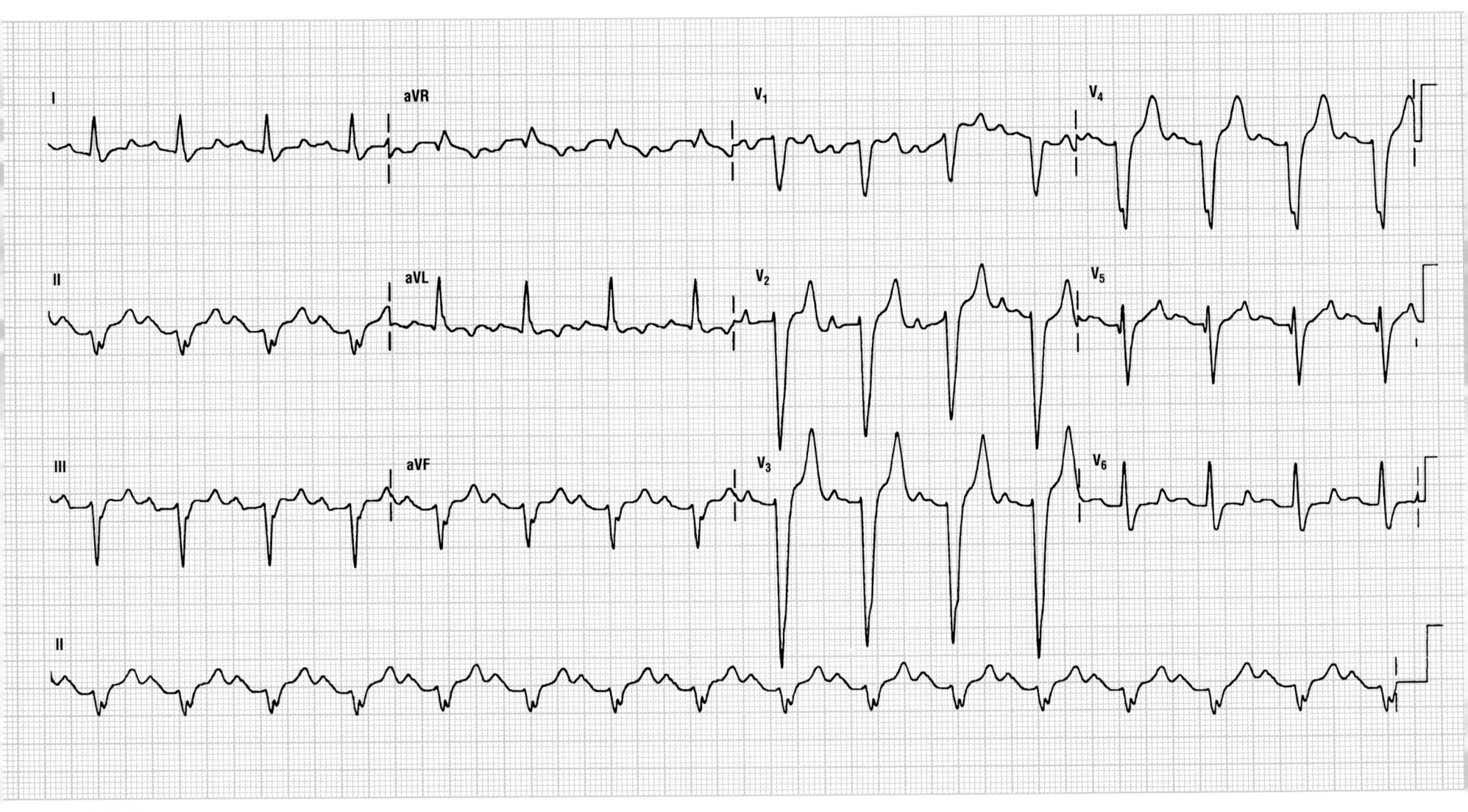

ECG 16-11

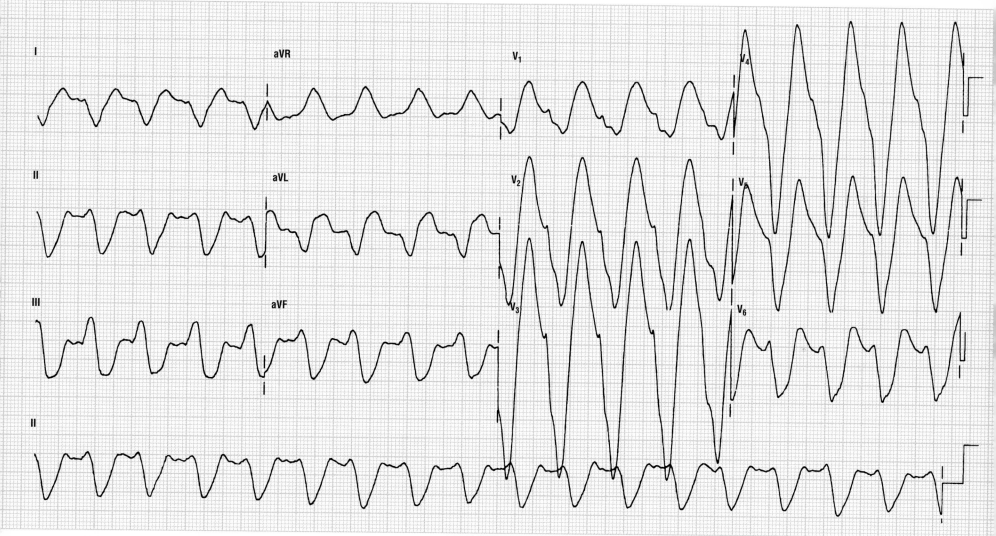

ECG 16-12

ECG CASE STUDIES: **CONTINUED**

ECG 16-13 So, if you are still skeptical about it only taking a few moments to go from bad to worse . . .

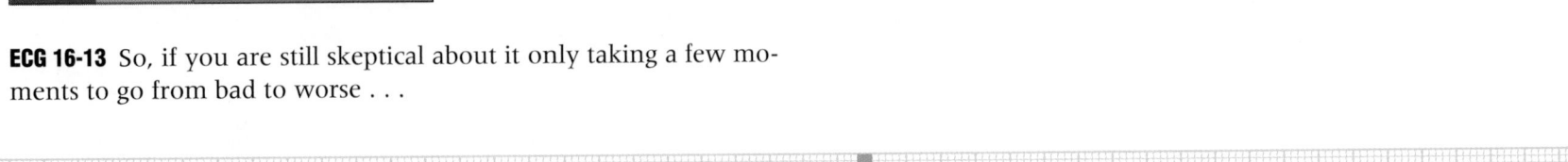

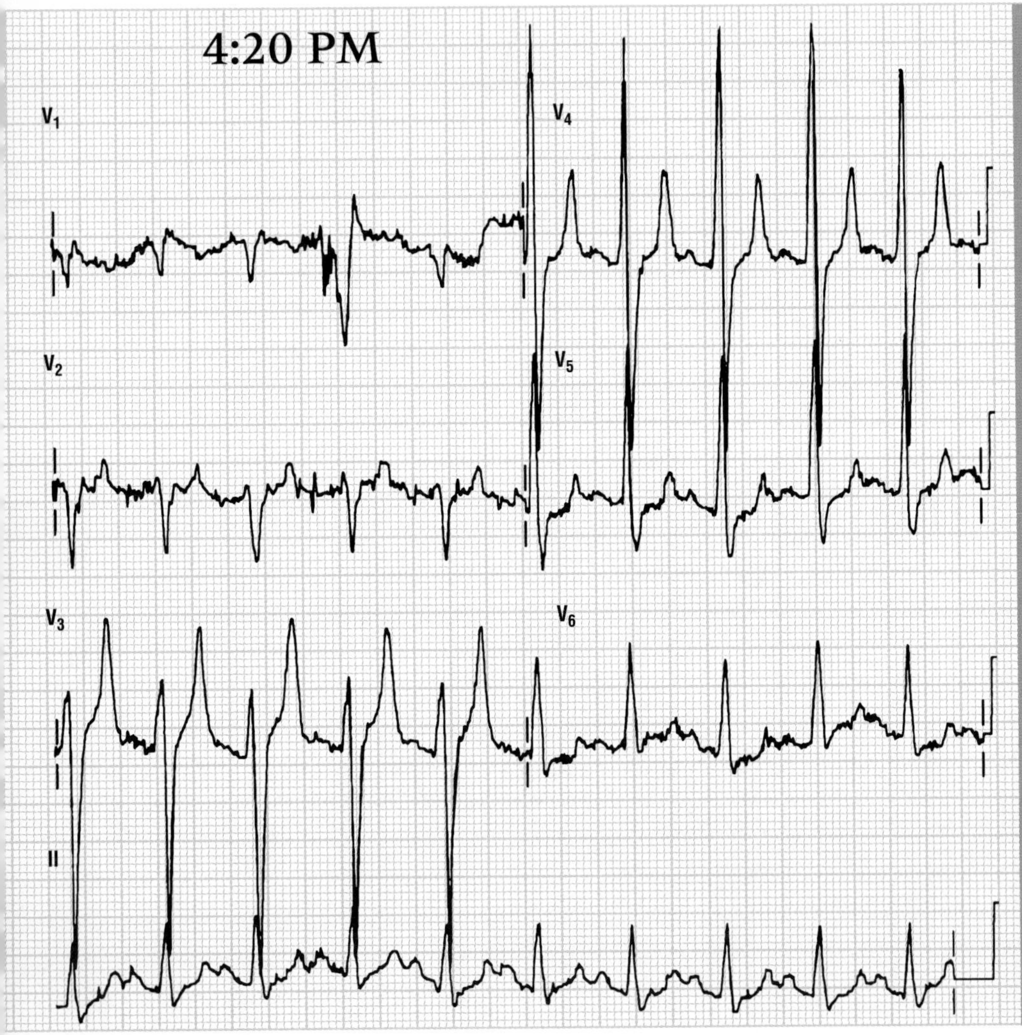

ECG 16-13A: 4:20 P.M.

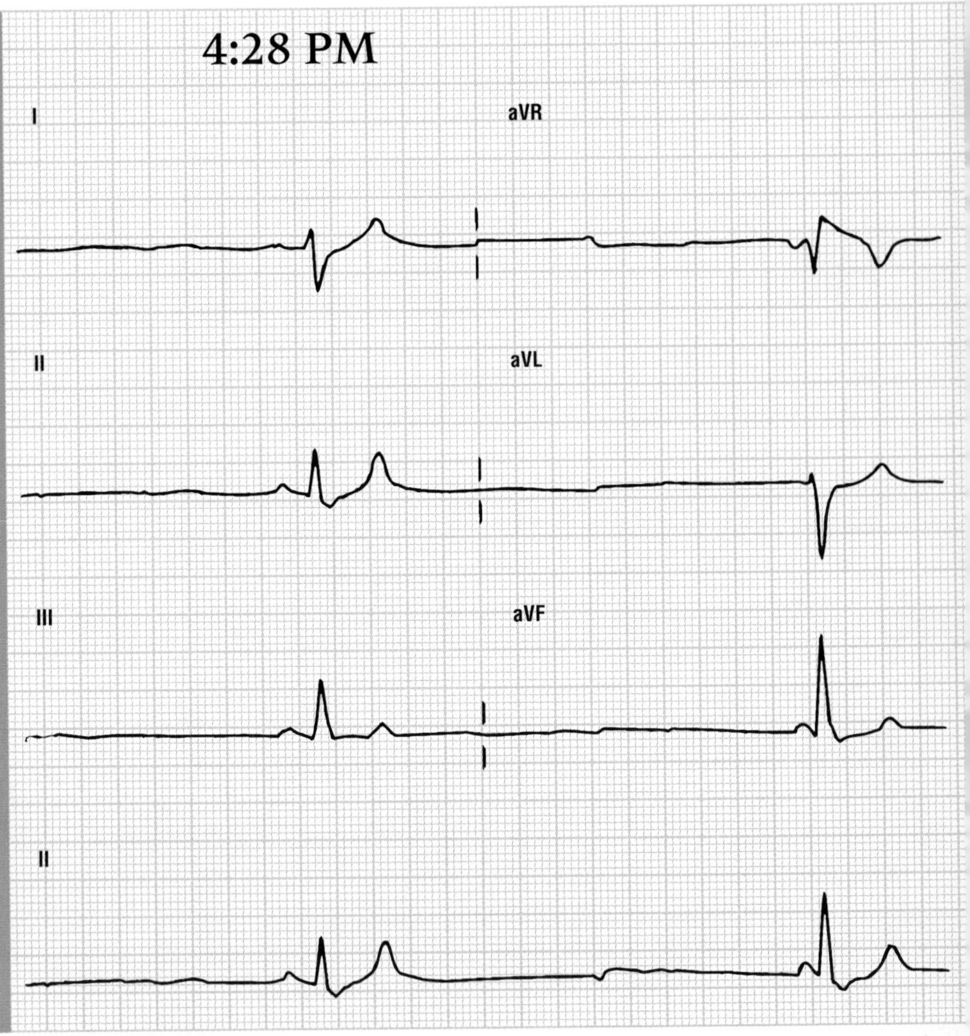

ECG 16-13B: 4:28 P.M.

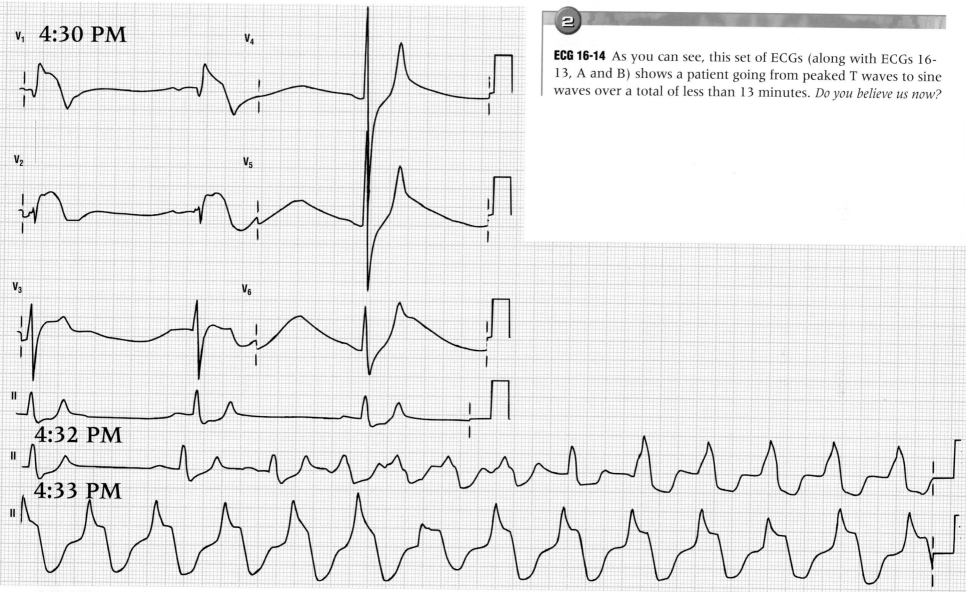

V_1 **4:30 PM**

V_4

V_2

V_5

V_3

V_6

II

4:32 PM

II

4:33 PM

II

ECG 16-14 As you can see, this set of ECGs (along with ECGs 16-13, A and B) shows a patient going from peaked T waves to sine waves over a total of less than 13 minutes. *Do you believe us now?*

ECG 16-14

CHAPTER **16** • ELECTROLYTE AND DRUG EFFECTS

Other Electrolyte Abnormalities

Hypokalemia

The hypokalemic changes on the ECG are not very dramatic. There are some nonspecific changes, such as mild ST segment depression, mild decreased amplitude of the T waves, and minimal prolongation of the QRS interval. However, the most common abnormality in hypokalemia is a prominent U wave. The U wave is a small wave that occurs immediately after the T wave, usually less than $^1/_{10}$ the height of the T wave (Figure 16-2). U waves can be caused by many different processes, however. (See differential diagnosis list below.)

By itself, the probability of developing an arrhythmia because of hypokalemia is extremely low. The real danger lies in a patient taking digoxin who is also hypokalemic. The combination causes an increased arrhythmic potential that can be life-threatening.

Differential diagnosis of U waves:

1. Hypokalemia
2. Bradycardia
3. Left ventricular hypertrophy
4. CNS events
5. Drug use: digoxin, Class I antiarrhythmics, phenothiazines

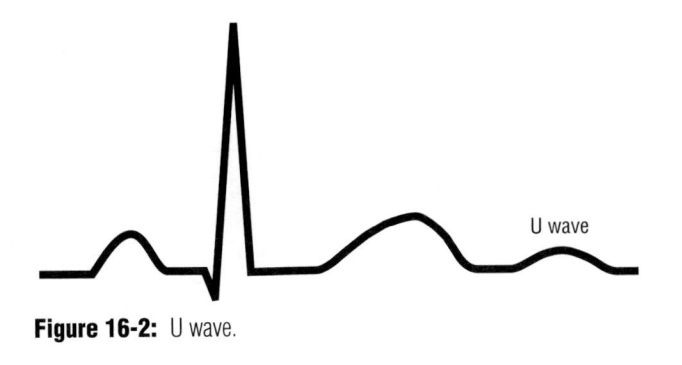
U wave

Figure 16-2: U wave.

Hypercalcemia

Hypercalcemic changes on the ECG are also minimal. The main change is a shortening of the ST segment, which in turn presents as a shortened QT interval (or shortened QTc. Remember, the QTc is the QT interval for heart rate). However, even this is difficult to correlate to the calcium level or the clinical presentation of the patient. Cardiac arrhythmias are rare.

Hypocalcemia

The main ECG change caused by a low calcium level is prolongation of the ST segment that produces an apparent lengthening of the QTc interval. Notice that this is the opposite effect of hypercalcemia. An easy way to keep the two in mind is to think that someone who is "hyper" moves quickly, so the movements appear shorter. A person who is "hypo," on the other hand, would take a long time to move, just as it takes a long time for the T wave to develop. Cardiac arrhythmias are rare.

The danger of QT prolongation, from any source, is the development of torsades de pointes, which can cause sudden death.

Differential diagnosis for a prolonged QT interval:

1. AMI and ischemia
2. Hypocalcemia
3. Drugs: Class Ia antiarrhythmics, amiodarone, phenothiazines, tricyclic antidepressants
4. CNS events
5. Hypothermia
6. Hypothyroidism
7. Congenital or idiopathic prolonged-QT syndromes
   a. Romano-Ward syndrome
   b. Jervell-Lange-Nielsen syndrome
   c. Sporadic long QT interval

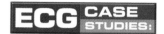

ECG 16-15 At first glance, this ECG doesn't look too pathological. It has a big P-pulmonale in lead II, it meets criteria for LVH, the axis is a little vertical, and there are some nonspecific ST-T wave (NSSTTW) changes throughout.

Then you look at V_2 and notice two distinct humps. The second hump does not align itself with the obvious P waves found in V_1 and V_3. So what is that hump? Is it part of the ST segment? If it is, then this ECG has some very prolonged QT intervals. T waves, however, are not usually shaped like roller coasters, going up and down and then up higher and down again. You start to notice that most of the other leads have the same small humps, but flatter.

What could possibly come between a T wave and the P of the next complex? The only thing that we can think of is a U wave. But what a U wave — it is taller than the T wave! Well, this is a U wave in an ECG obtained from a patient with a potassium level of 1.6 mEq/L — a very low number. As you would expect in hypokalemia this severe, there is flattening of the T waves and a definite U wave. The NSSTTW changes would also be expected. After correction of the hypokalemia, the changes resolved.

Remember, U waves can be found in various states. Go through the entire differential diagnosis list so you don't miss anything.

ECG 16-16 This patient presented to the emergency department with a complaint of a runny nose. She told the nurse that she also had some shortness of breath. Being new and very caring, the nurse ordered an ECG. The first thing we noticed was the markedly prolonged QT interval. In case you have never seen a prolonged QT interval, this is as prolonged as it gets! Anyway, the patient recounted that, since she was a young adult, she would suddenly faint for no reason. She had seen many doctors, and they had no reason or diagnosis for the fainting. She was labeled a crackpot and placed on many antidepressant and antipsychotic medications over time. She lost her job because of the meds and became homeless. Her only statement was, "I'm really not crazy, I just fall out."

Well, this doctor believed her, especially after looking at her ECG. Right after placing her on a monitor, the doctor started to examine her heart. He noticed that she slumped, and looked up to see her unresponsive. The monitor showed torsades de pointes. About 1 minute after she collapsed, during the chaos of gathering resuscitation equipment, she awoke and said, "See doc, I told you I pass out!" This poor patient's life was ruined because no one saw a prolonged QT interval. She had Romano-Ward syndrome and ended up doing fine.

ECG CASE STUDIES: CONTINUED

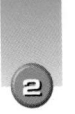

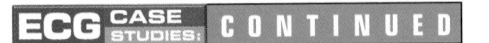

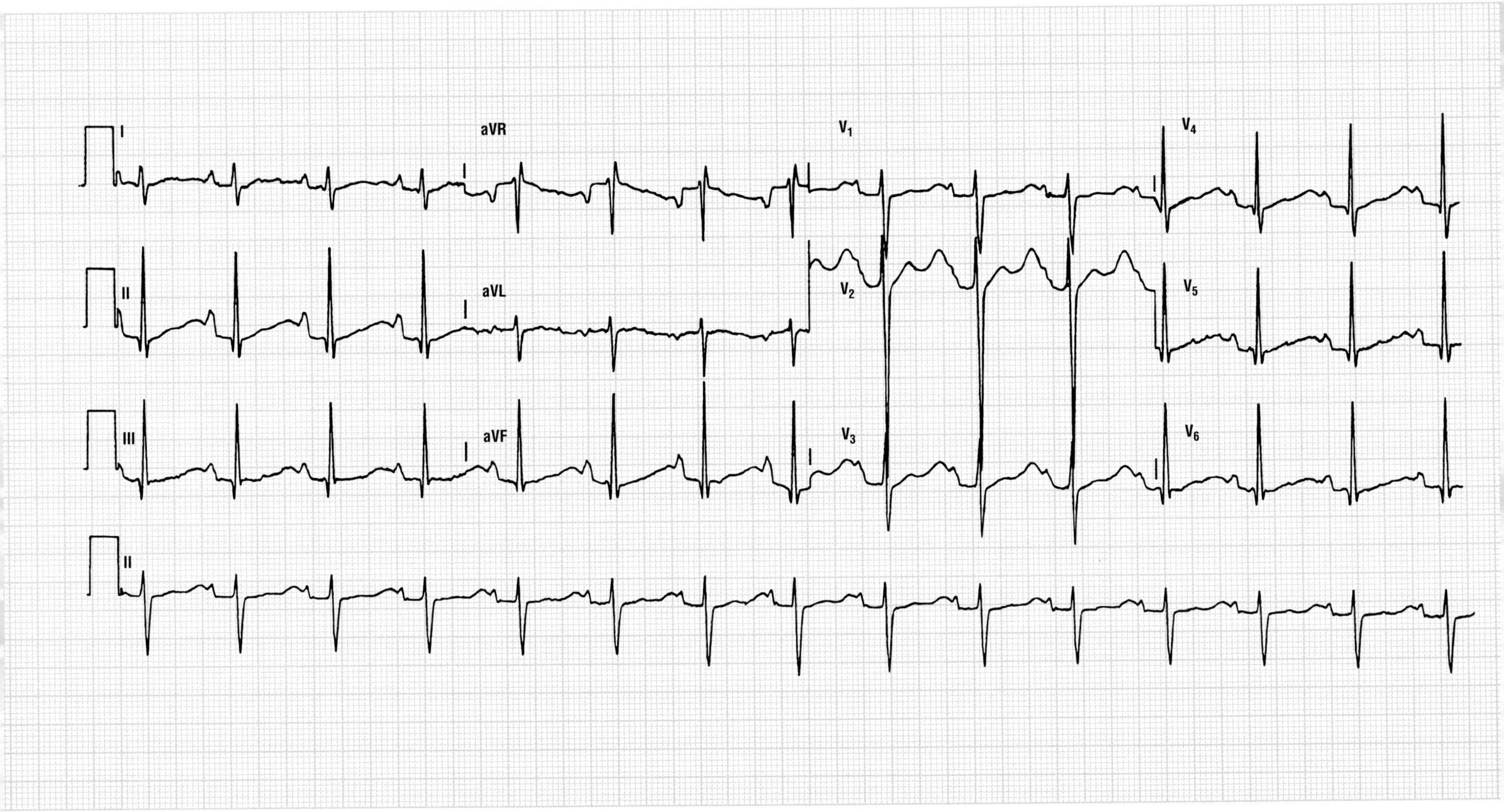
I
aVR
V1
V4
II
aVL
V2
V5
III
aVF
V3
V6
II

ECG 16-15

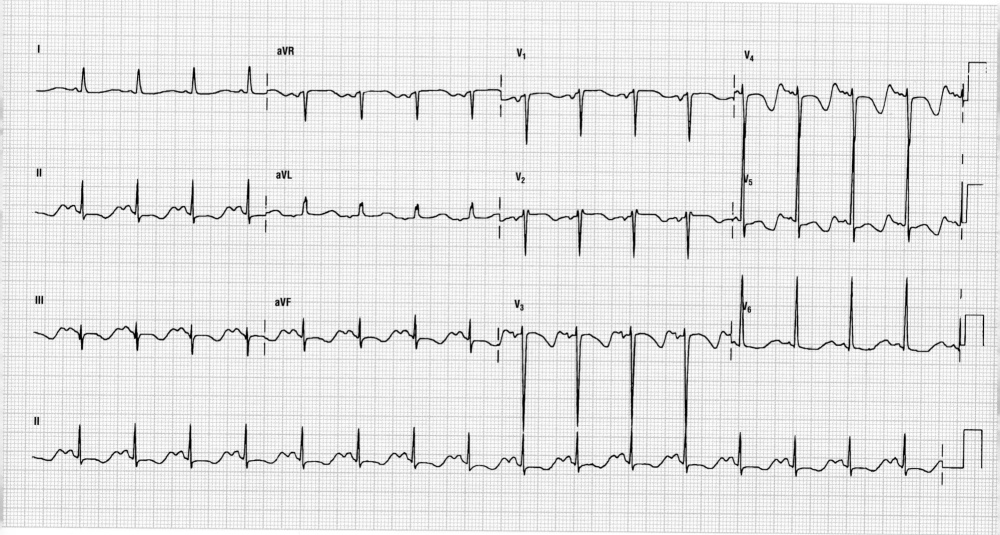

ECG 16-16

ECG CASE STUDIES: **CONTINUED**

ECG 16-17 This ECG shows a prolonged QT interval and, thus, a prolonged QTc. Generally, the ST segments and the T wave appear normal in cases of QT prolongation — the interval is simply more than $1/2$ the R-R interval. In this ECG, the ST segment is markedly prolonged and the T wave looks fairly normal. This is the usual presentation in hypocalcemia.

The ECG also shows changes consistent with LVH, possibly LVH with strain because of the flipped and asymmetric T waves in the lateral leads. There is also some ST segment depression in the inferior leads that could be due to ischemia. Clinical correlation, as always, is required because the most common causes of QT prolongation are ischemia and AMIs. In these cases, however, the ST segment and the T waves are usually equally prolonged.

NOTE

A quick test for QT prolongation is to use your calipers to measure the QT interval. If it is wider than half the R-R interval of the preceding complex, it is prolonged.

ECG 16-18 This ECG was obtained from a patient with a prolonged QTc interval. The patient began to have frequent aberrant beats and, during the ECG, decided to go into torsades. Needless to say, the tech was a little taken aback by the whole thing.

This is the biggest fear of a prolonged QTc interval. This usually occurs when the QTc is prolonged secondary to some precipitating factor such as AMI or drug overdose. We won't go into the treatment of this disorder other than to say that magnesium and overdrive pacing are the mainstays of therapy. Treat the underlying disorder to avoid this complication. If you see a prolonged QTc, ask yourself why it's there.

CLINICAL PEARL

Polymorphic ventricular tachycardia, a.k.a. torsades de pointes, is the most dangerous complication of a prolonged QT interval.

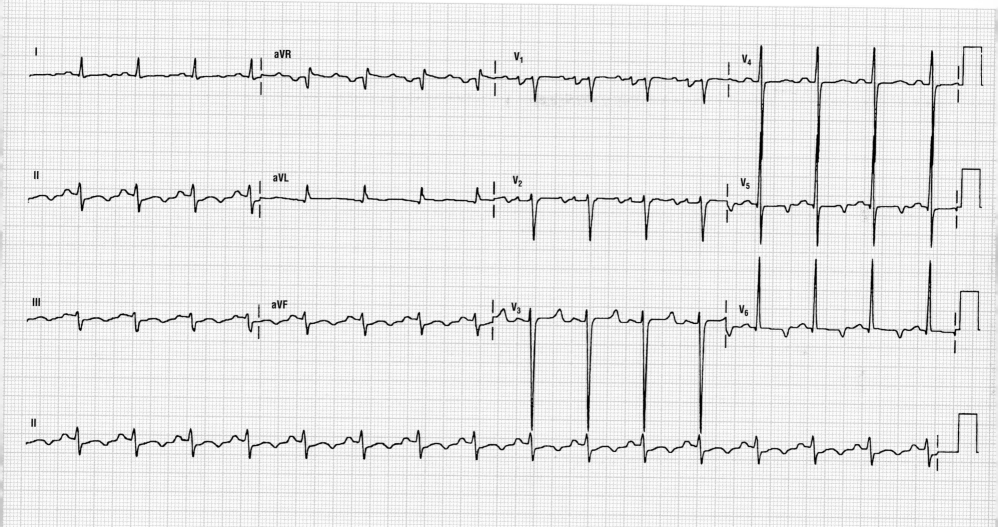

ECG 16-17

ECG CASE STUDIES: CONTINUED

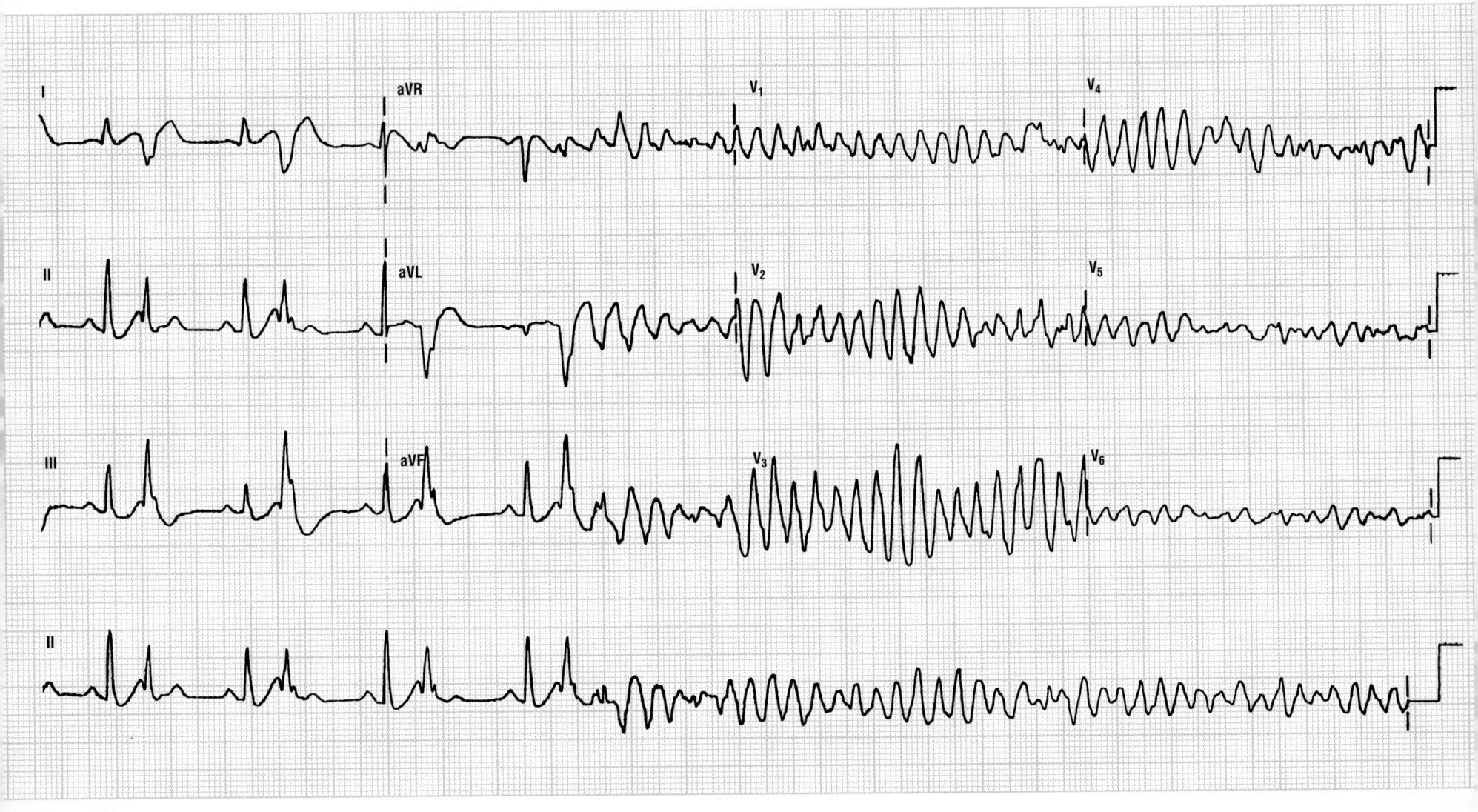

ECG 16-18

Drug Effects

Pharmaceutical agents also affect the function of the cells and the channels. This, in turn, alters the way the cells depolarize, repolarize, and innervate surrounding tissues. And this, in its own right, alters the vectors and — finally — the appearance of the ECG. We are going to focus primarily on digoxin, but we will give you a short table to discuss the toxicity associated with other drugs (Figure 16-3). For a complete discussion, consult a pharmacology textbook.

Drug	Possible Toxic Effects
Class I antiarrhythmics	• Lengthened QRS and QTc intervals • Possible AV blocks • Slowed or completely blocked SA node • Arrhythmias
Calcium channel blockers	• Blocked AV node primarily, but extent of block varies significantly within different drugs in this class.
Beta-blockers	• Slowed automaticity of the SA node and the Purkinje system • Blocked AV node
Amiodorone	• Slowed conduction everywhere: the SA node, atrium, AV node, Purkinje system, and ventricles
Phenothiazines and tricyclic antidepressants	• Widened QRS and QTc interval • T wave abnormalities • Arrhythmias are common in overdoses
Note ECG 16-21 shows how the ECG of a tricyclic overdose patient may look.	

Figure 16-3: Common toxic drug effects.

Digoxin

Digoxin and other members of the cardiac glycoside class are very useful in certain circumstances. However, because of a very low therapeutic-to-toxic index, they cause a tremendous volume of problems and deaths. In medical school our class was told that, over a career, every doctor will kill at least one person with digoxin. Having worked in the emergency departments of various academic institutions, we can say that this statement is probably correct or close to it. Thankfully, newer treatment strategies have narrowed the spectrum of use for this drug. Still, it is a common cause of severe or life-threatening complications, and you need to understand them. Once again, we refer you to the Additional Readings section for books that will completely cover the topic. We will be focusing on the ECG changes here.

The first thing to know is that digoxin overuse or overdose can cause any and all arrhythmias. The one most commonly discussed in relation to dig toxicity is paroxysmal atrial tachycardia (PAT) with block. PAT with block is diagnosed when there is a complete heart block with an underlying sinus tachycardia at a rate of 150 to 200 BPM. The escape rhythm can be either junctional or ventricular in origin.

On the ECG, digoxin causes a scooping of the ST segment that is rather unique. It is called a scooped-out appearance because it looks like someone took an ice cream scoop and dug a hole out of the baseline. (See Figure 10-11, page 132 for a graphic representation of this finding, and ECG 10-8 on page 133 for an example.) The T waves have a shorter amplitude and can be biphasic in nature. The QT interval is usually shorter than expected, and U waves are more prominent. Speaking of U waves, remember that hypokalemia will exacerbate the effects of the digitalis glycosides, and this increases the arrhythmogenic and toxic effects. *Any* dig level may be toxic in this case!

ECG CASE STUDIES: *Drug Effects*

ECG 16-19 Take a look at the ECG below. Note the scooped-out appearance of the ST segments in many of the leads. This is classic for digoxin and its glycoside relatives. The T waves are smaller than you would normally expect, as well. See ECG 10-8 for another example of scooped ST segments.

You will always find people talking about the scooped-out appearance, but we think the ladle analogy works as well or better. Take a look at Figure 16-4 and you'll see what we mean.

This ECG shows an APC and biatrial enlargement. Atrial enlargement is a big cause of atrial fibrillation (AFib), and digoxin is used to treat AFib in many patients.

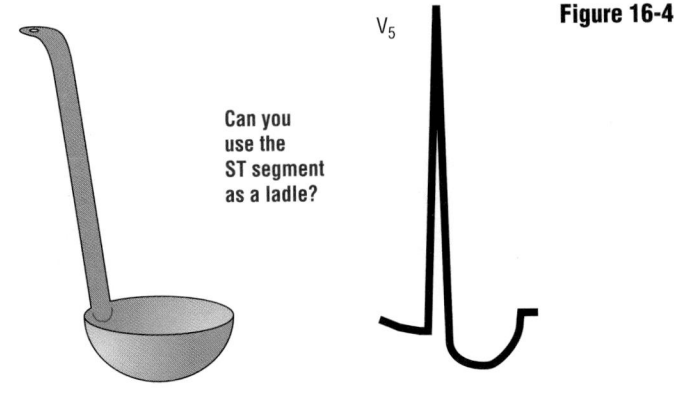

Figure 16-4

V_5

Can you use the ST segment as a ladle?

ECG 16-20 This ECG shows a complete heart block with a junctional escape rate of about 60 BPM. The underlying atrial rate is about 150 BPM. This is, therefore, PAT with block. The patient was taking digoxin and the level turned out to be 3.5 ng/ml, well into the toxic range.

PAT with block is commonly associated with dig toxicity. However, it is not pathognomonic of that toxicity by any means. It is found in other circumstances and can occur spontaneously. With all that said, when you see it, you had better order a dig level to be sure. If it is due to digoxin toxicity, how do you treat it? You treat the underlying problem. Antibodies against the compound are the mainstay of treatment for serious toxicity.

> **REMINDER:**
> PAT with block is present when there is a complete heart block with an underlying sinus tachycardia at 150 to 200 BPM.

ECG 16-21 This ECG shows an IVCD. There is no evidence of hyperkalemia, but at least we thought about it. There is also PR prolongation, a widened QRS interval, and a prolonged QTc. The patient came in for an overdose of tricyclic antidepressants. She subsequently died despite all aggressive therapy.

There is nothing about this ECG that makes it unique to tricyclics. The take-home message: If you have a lethargic patient who possibly overdosed on some medicine, think about tricyclics as the cause. They are real killers, and the faster therapy is instituted the better. These patients frequently develop life-threatening arrhythmias, so they need to be monitored closely.

> **CLINICAL PEARL**
> If you see an IVCD in an overdose patient, suspect tricyclic antidepressants.

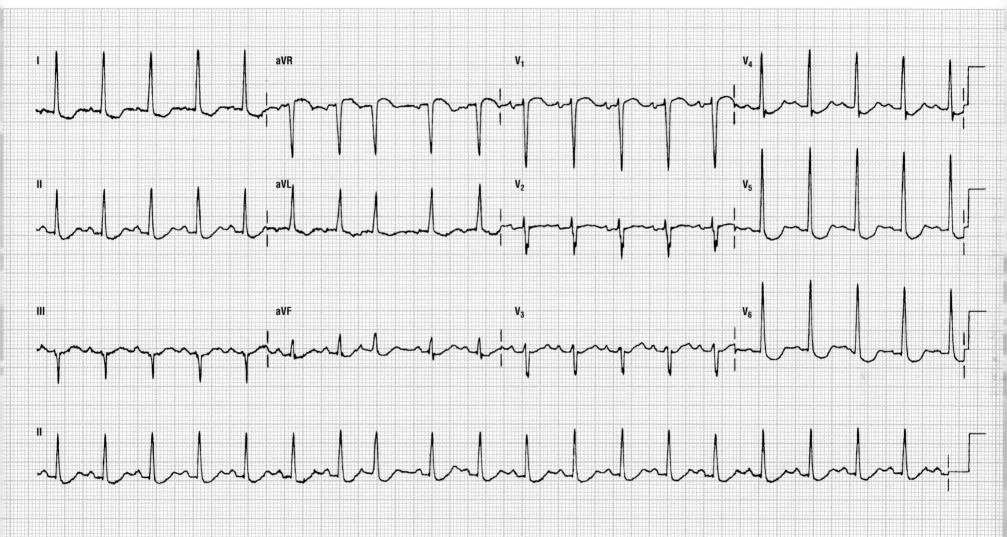

ECG 16-19

ECG CASE STUDIES: **CONTINUED**

ECG 16-20

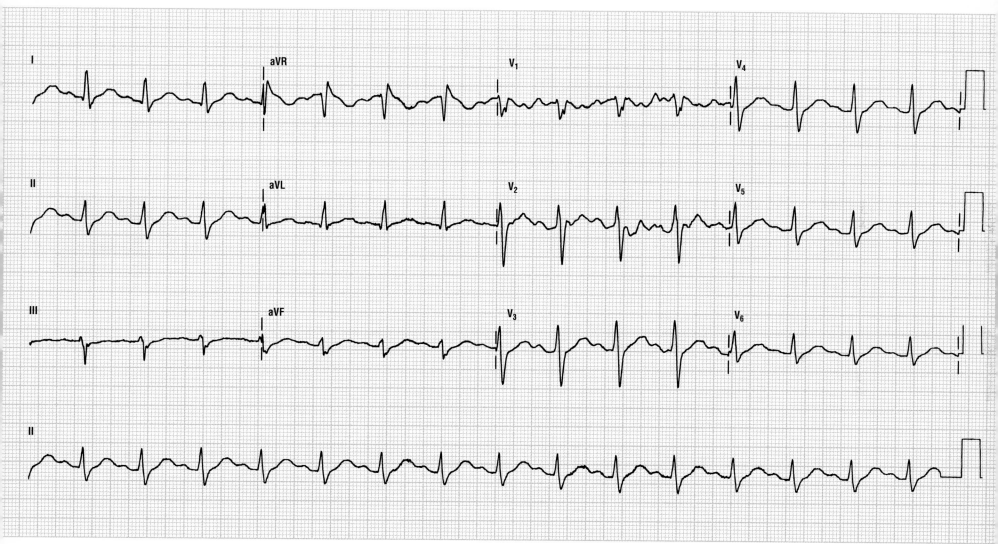

ECG 16-21

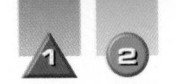
1 CHAPTER IN REVIEW

1. Hyperkalemia not only can kill, but it can kill in seconds and make the patient unresponsive to the drugs used in resuscitation. True or False.

2. Immediate recognition and action to stabilize the myocardial membrane and reverse the pathological processes are the keys to effectively combating the complications of hyperkalemia. True or False.

3. If you don't think about the problem, you will never diagnose it. True or False.

4. The ECG cannot be used to help estimate blood potassium levels. True or False.

1. True 2. True 3. True 4. False

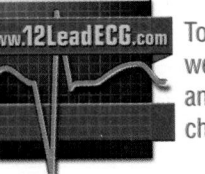

To enhance the knowledge you gain in this book, access this text's website at www.12leadECG.com! This valuable resource provides an online glossary and related web links. To learn more about the chapter topics, simply click on the chapter and view the link.

2 CHAPTER IN REVIEW

5. The main electrocardiographic changes found in hyperkalemia include:
   A. T wave abnormalities, especially tall and peaked Ts
   B. IVCDs
   C. P waves missing or of decreased amplitude
   D. ST segment changes simulating an injury pattern
   E. Cardiac arrhythmias, any and all varieties
   F. All of the above

6. Which of the following is **incorrect** with regard to T wave changes in hyperkalemia:
   A. They are the earliest sign of hyperkalemia.
   B. They are seen when the K+ level exceeds 5.5 mEq/L.
   C. The classic T waves that are tall, peaked, and narrow occur in only 22% of cases.
   D. T wave morphology may be altered as a result of the IVCD that develops with severe hyperkalemia.
   E. The changes are always diffuse and found in all leads.

7. Whenever you see an IVCD, you need to immediately think of hyperkalemia. True or False.

8. The differential diagnosis for the presence of U waves includes all **except**:
   A. Hypokalemia
   B. Bradycardia
   C. Left ventricular hypertrophy
   D. CNS events
   E. Medication use: digoxin, class I antiarrhythmics, phenothiazines
   F. All of the above are correct

9. Hypocalcemia is associated with:
   A. Shortened QT interval
   B. Prolonged QT interval
   C. None of the above

10. Hypokalemia will exacerbate the effects of the digitalis glycosides, which increases their arrhythmogenic and toxic effects. Any dig level may be toxic in this case. True or False.

5. F 6. E 7. True 8. F 9. B 10. True

New Ground

We are entering largely uncharted territory in this chapter. Only a few books try to demonstrate the thought process involved in reading an ECG. Most authors assume that you will use your innate instincts to interpret an ECG once you understand some of the basics. Unfortunately, ECG interpretation is not an instinctual ability imprinted on our RNA or DNA by mother nature to ensure survival of our species. It takes a lot of hard work to learn how to do it. Once you get the hang of it, though, you will wonder why you were never able to. It's kind of like riding a bike or reading.

Here is the secret of the electrocardiographic universe: Know what a normal ECG is supposed to look like. If the ECG you are looking at does not fit that pattern, then you have pathology present!

The 10 Questions of the Gram

You need a systematic approach to examining ECGs. In this block, we will be giving you a format to follow. It helps if you follow a stepwise approach to interpretation. Our system summarizes the basic steps of electrocardiography. We call it *The 10 Questions of the Gram.*

 1. What is my general impression?
 2. Is there anything that sticks out?
 3. What is the rate?
 4. What are the intervals?
 5. What is the rhythm?
 6. What is the axis?
 7. Is there any hypertrophy?
 8. Is there any ischemia or infarction?
 9. What is the differential diagnosis of the abnormality?
10. How can I put it all together with the patient?

Using this approach will simplify your life tremendously. If you answer each of the questions above, you have covered the essential points the ECG can offer.

When you first start using the system, write down all of the abnormalities that you come across. Don't rely on memory until you are comfortable with the process, because you will inevitably forget something important. When you are finished writing the answers to the questions above, synthesize the solution. The subtitle of this book, *The Art of Interpretation*, refers to the fact that this process is an art form, especially when you are putting it together with your patient. Keep this thought in mind: *The patient is the reason that you obtained the ECG in the first place!* This simple test, the ECG, can give you information about the anatomy, pathology, pathophysiology, and pharmacology of the heart. You just need to be able to tease the information out of the paper.

1. What Is My General Impression?

You start out by looking at an ECG and coming up with the main problem. Is the main problem an infarct? Is it hypertrophy? Is it an arrhythmia? Many times, you forget this general overview and you get caught up in the minutiae. This often leads to an incorrect diagnosis.

So how do we start making this initial overview? Well, we mentally compare the ECG in question to a normal example. *Know what a normal ECG is supposed to look like. If the one you're looking at does not fit that pattern, then you have pathology present!* Take a look back through the book and find a normal ECG (ECG 9-4, page 81), a normal RBBB (ECG 13-5, page 251), and a normal LBBB (ECG 13-18, page 273). (There are some "normal" variations to each of these types of ECGs, which have been mentioned at various points in the book.) What we want you to do now is study these normal ECGs in great detail. Look at each lead and the general patterns presented. When you are comfortable with the normals, look at abnormal examples of each. Mentally compare the two and pick out the major differences.

Let's start out by looking at the normal ECG. Note how the QRS complexes are nice and even. Are any of them exceptionally tall or short? Are they thin or wide? Note how the P waves interact with the QRS complexes. Look at the T waves. Are they slightly asymmetrical and not too prominent? They should all look alike. Are they upright in the leads where they should be? Look at the intervals. Do any of them seem longer or shorter than they should? Check the axis. Is it in the normal quadrant? What about the transition in the precordial leads — is it found somewhere in, or between, V_3 and V_4?

It may seem like a long time, but try to spend about five minutes looking at the normal ECG.

It is even more essential to understand the principles of the general impression in the bundle blocks because of their grossly abnormal appearance. Don't get flustered by the "ugliness" of the initial gram. Remember the tale of the ugly duckling — except in this case the ugliness will turn to beauty when you make the correct diagnosis.

Now, look at the normal RBBB. Are the QRS complexes 0.12 seconds or more? Is there a slurred S wave in leads I and V_6? Rabbit ears in V_1? Are all of the T waves opposite the last part of the QRS complexes? Note how the QRS complexes are thin at the onset and then they get wide. What about ST elevation — is there any? Are V_1 to V_2, and possibly V_3, normal? Are their ST segments depressed? Is there normally ST depression in these leads? Look at the complexes closely, and remember that all the intervals are the same. Is that ST segment elevation you are seeing in the inferior leads, or is part of the QRS complex causing it to *appear* to be ST elevation? Are there any Q waves? Are Q waves normally found in either bundle branch block?

Now, do the same for the ECG with LBBB. Are the ST segments elevated in V_1 to V_2? Are all the T waves discordant? Note which leads have elevation and which ones have depression. Is there ST segment elevation in V_1 or V_2, or is it depression? Is there ST segment depression in the left precordial leads of V_5 to V_6? Is that normal? What about the inferior leads — do they show ST depression? Are there prominent R waves in V_1 or V_2? Are Q waves anywhere except V normal in LBBB? Is this a new LBBB or was it there on a prior ECG? A new LBBB pattern signifies a possible AMI, aberrantly conducted complexes, or a ventricular rhythm. How does the patient look — stable or unstable?

Make sure you understand what we are getting at in this question. Don't let the details overwhelm you! Form a general impression. Sometimes you can get so wrapped up in the details that you forget the big picture. Don't make that mistake!

2. Is There Anything that Sticks Out?

We're talking about any *obvious* abnormality on the ECG. In Question 1, we were looking at the whole ECG. In answering this question, we are localizing it to smaller areas. It could be one complex or a group. It may be a couple of leads that just don't look right. Are they in a particular region of the heart, such as the inferior, lateral, or anterior wall? Are most of the complexes wide and bizarre with an occasional normal P-QRS-T cycle interspersed in the chaos? (If so, this is VTach until proven otherwise.)

If you can quickly diagnose the main pathology, it will help guide the rest of your evaluation of the ECG. Conversely, if you know the patient has some underlying pathology, you could look for related changes on the ECG. For example, if the patient came in having taken an overdose of digoxin, look for rhythm abnormalities associated with dig toxicity such as PAT with block.

Use your evaluation to guide your investigation. This confusing statement refers to the fact that an ECG may give you some clue to the patient's underlying pathology. Suppose someone shows you an ECG. You immediately notice that it is an IVCD with no P waves. It is wide and very, very ugly. The next question out of your mouth should be: "What is the patient's potassium level?" You then go and see the patient — who is in coma — and you look at both arms to check for a shunt. If one is present, end-stage renal disease is probably the culprit. Now, suppose you don't find a shunt, but instead notice that the patient's breathing is very fast and deep, and the mental status is altered. You examine the belly, and it is tender. You immediately ask for a fingerstick glucose and a set of blood gases. You have diagnosed

diabetic keto acidosis (DKA). The people around you will be amazed at your diagnostic acumen. You, however, repeat to yourself, "the company it keeps," and move on to your next case. Impressive!

3. What Is the Rate?

This is a simple question. We don't just want you to come up with a simple number, though. Tie the rate to the patient. For example, suppose you have a patient breathing rapidly who is also sweaty and in distress. The heart rate should be fast because of the obvious discomfort. However, the rate is 42 BPM. Following the principles you've learned in this book, you ask yourself, "Why is the rate so slow?" You notice that there is some ST depression, about 3/4 millimeter sloping down in aVL. Immediately, your razor sharp mind develops the following reasoning process. Could this be high lateral ischemia? Yes, but lateral ischemia is usually not associated with bradycardia. What type of ischemia/infarct is associated with bradycardia? Well, inferior wall IWMI increases vagal tone and causes bradycardia. Could the ST segment depression be a reciprocal change — the first sign of an inferior wall AMI? You'd better believe it! You immediately ask that a cardiologist be contacted to take this patient to the cath lab. You are a hero, and the patient thanks you. Maybe the story sounds a little corny. We understand. Our stories are meant both to teach and entertain. We hope you're picking up the concepts that they are trying to get across. Think! Put things together! It is not rocket science to come up with great diagnoses. Perhaps you don't know all the clinical medicine yet, but you will eventually. Use every bit of information that you have learned.

4. What Are the Intervals?

The intervals are crucial to the correct diagnosis. *Always measure the widest interval and use that measurement to gauge the other complexes and leads.* You need to measure the PR interval, the QRS complex, and the QT interval (Figures 17-1, 17-2, and 17-3, respectively).

The PR interval will either be normal, short, or prolonged. If it is normal, so much the better. If it is prolonged and regular, it is first-degree heart block. But don't stop there. If it is irregular but lengthening between subsequent beats, you've got to think about Mobitz I (Wenckebach) second-degree heart block. If it is irregularly irregular, there are various possible rhythm abnormalities.

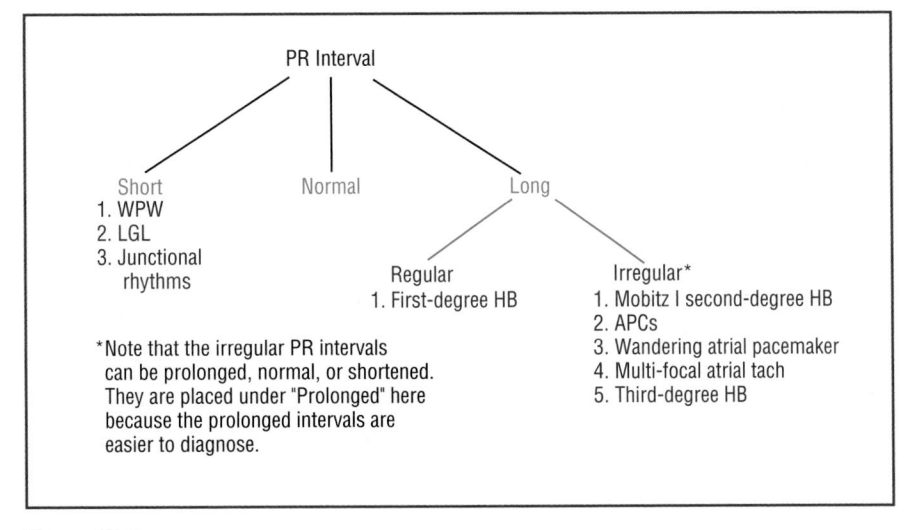

Figure 17-1

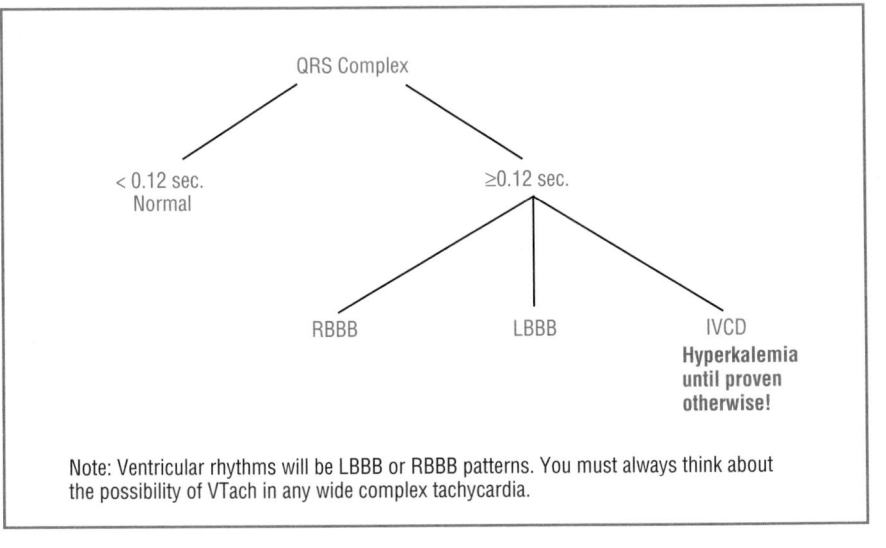

Note: Ventricular rhythms will be LBBB or RBBB patterns. You must always think about the possibility of VTach in any wide complex tachycardia.

Figure 17-2

Figure 17-3

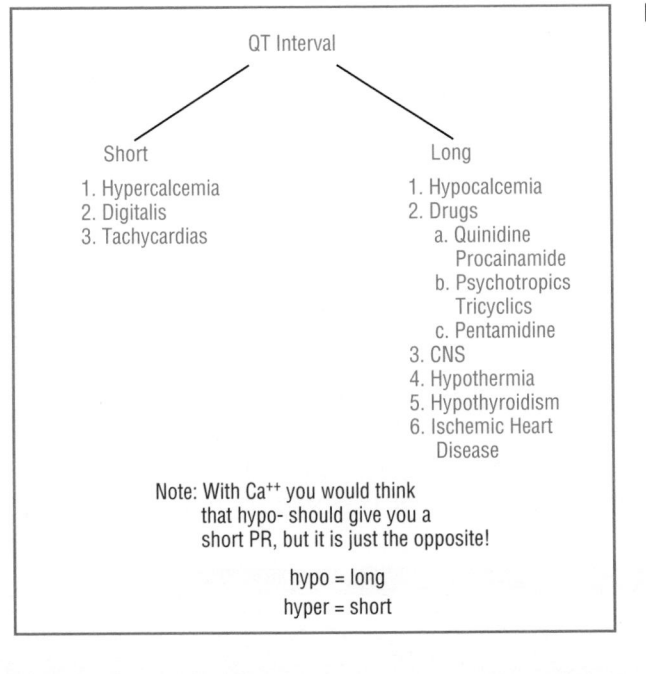

5. What Is the Rhythm?

In Chapter 8 we spent considerable time going over how to evaluate the rhythm. Here we highlight certain points that relate to the interpretation of the whole ECG. Always ask yourself the following questions when evaluating the rhythm:

General:

1. Is the rhythm fast or slow?

2. Is the rhythm regular or irregular? If irregular, is it *regularly* irregular or *irregularly* irregular?

P waves:

3. Do you see any P waves?

4. Are all of the P waves the same?

5. Does each QRS complex have a P wave?

6. Is the PR interval constant?

QRS complexes:

7. Are the P waves and QRS complexes associated with one another?

8. Are the QRS complexes narrow or wide?

9. Are the QRS complexes grouped or not grouped?

Is the rhythm fast, slow, or normal? Obviously, the differential diagnosis of a rapid rhythm is different from a slow one. We will give you some examples of each type of rhythm (Figure 17-4). You don't have to memorize them, and keep in mind that the list is not all-inclusive.

Do I see P waves? Are they all the same? The presence or absence of P waves really helps narrow the diagnosis of the rhythm. If there are no P waves, you know that the rhythm has to originate at or below the AV node. Retrograde P waves, however, can originate in the low atrium, or at or below the AV node.

The presence of different P waves will also assist you in making the diagnosis. If there are irregular beats with a differing P wave morpholo-

Slow	Normal	Fast	Can be fast, normal, or slow
Sinus Bradycardia	NSR	Sinus Tachycardia	Atrial Fibrillation
Junctional Escape	Accelerated	Accelerated	Atrial Flutter
Ventricular Escape	-Junctional	-Junctional	Third-degree HB
Idioventricular	-Idioventricular	-Idioventricular	Second-degree HB
Wandering Atrial	Wandering Atrial	Ventricular Tachycardia	First-degree HB
Pacemaker	Pacemaker	PSVT	APCs
		Multifocal Atrial Tach	JPCs
		Aberrantly Conducted	VPCs
		Supraventricular Tach	

Figure 17-4

gies, you are looking at either premature or escape complexes, depending on whether the different P wave comes early or late. If you have more than three different morphologies, with differing PR intervals, then you have either wandering atrial pacemaker (WAP) or multifocal atrial tachycardia (MAT).

In addition to seeing clear P waves, also think about *buried P waves* — those occurring at the same time as the previous complex's QRS complex or T wave. This buried P will give the previous T wave a different morphology than its siblings; the T wave with the buried P may have a hump or be taller than the other Ts around it. *Whenever you see a wave that is different than the others, stop and analyze why this is occurring!* This is a very critical point. Following this advice will save you a lot of heartache.

Speaking of buried P waves, here is another crucial point. *Whenever the heart rate is 150, give or take a beat, think about atrial flutter with 2:1 block.* This needs to become instinctual — you shouldn't even have to think about it. When you see a heart rate of 150 BPM, look at the lead with the smallest QRS complexes and try to find a buried P wave exactly midway between the two Ps you can see.

CLINICAL PEARL

150 BPM = Atrial flutter with 2:1 block until proven otherwise

Is the rhythm regular or irregular? This is another simple question whose answer will greatly assist your final interpretation. Regular beats have a pacemaker setting the pace. It could be atrial, junctional, or ventricular. Either the irregular beats have two or more pacemakers, or the irregularity is the result of irregular transmission through the AV node. The latter situation occurs in AFib, and AFlutter with variable block.

If the rhythm is irregular, evaluate it further by asking yourself if it is *regularly irregular* or *irregularly irregular*. In a regularly irregular rhythm, the irregularity occurs at a specified time or period, or in a predictable pattern. There is order in the irregularity. Examples of this type of rhythm include second-degree heart block and premature or escape beats. The latter may come irregularly, but the underlying baseline rhythm is regular.

There are only three true irregularly irregular rhythms: atrial fibrillation, wandering atrial pacemaker, and multifocal atrial tachycardia. This makes the decision easy once you have identified the rhythm as irregularly irregular. Look at the P waves; if you have some, it is either WAP or MAT, depending on whether the rhythm is tachycardic or not. If you don't see P waves, it's atrial fibrillation.

Are the complexes narrow or wide? This question demands an immediate answer. The main reason is that many of the possible sources of wide complex rhythms are life threatening. Just to name a few, possible sources include VTach, hyperkalemia, drug effects, idioventricular escape rhythms, CNS events, and so on. Right now a lot of you are thinking that stable bundle branch blocks appear as wide complex rhythms. However, even in these circumstances, the blocks could

hide serious underlying pathology. All in all, you need to be cautious when approaching an ECG with wide complexes.

Please, whatever you do, remember: *A wide-complex tachycardia is VTach until proven otherwise*. Ventricular tachycardia kills. An SVT with aberrancy is not as life-threatening. Always start the treatment as if the patient has VTach. If you find proof to the contrary, then you can change your management.

Narrow complexes, because they travel down the normal conduction pathway, must originate at or above the His bundles. Wide complexes may originate supraventricularly if they are aberrantly conducted or represent a BBB, but they can also originate in the ventricles. *With few exceptions, an atrial arrhythmia is of less clinical importance than a ventricular arrhythmia*. This is because the atria only pump blood to the ventricles, whereas the ventricles supply blood to the rest of the body. If you knock off the ventricular pumps, you die.

You can never rule out VTach. Several things can help you distinguish between aberrantly conducted supraventricular complexes and VTach:

1. The presence of P waves before each complex favors SVT
2. The abnormal beats begin in the same direction as the normal beats in an aberrantly conducted SVT
3. VTach is linked with AV dissociation
4. Capture and fusion beats are present in VTach

If you are lucky enough to catch the onset of the arrhythmia, you can sometimes follow the progression of an SVT or the origin of a VTach.

REMINDER:
Irregularly Irregular Rhythms:
• Atrial fibrillation • Wandering atrial pacemaker • Multifocal atrial tachycardia

---

REMINDER:
If you see a normal complex in the middle of a run of wide-complex beats, it is probably VTach.

Do I see any pauses? If you see a pause, ask yourself why it is occurring. It can be caused by premature complexes, which should have compensatory pauses. Pauses can also be caused by escape beats, with a prolonged P-P interval, or by AV blocks such as second-degree heart block Mobitz I (Wenckebach) or Mobitz II. Look at the company it keeps to make the diagnosis. If you see a progressively lengthening PR interval and then a dropped QRS complex with a pause, you've got Wenckebach.

> **REMINDER:**
> Always use your calipers to evaluate pauses and arrhythmias.

What is the relationship of the waves and complexes? The most common relationship of P waves to QRS complexes is 1:1. The P wave falls before each QRS complex at a specified distance, the PR interval. So what happens when you see two P waves for each QRS complex? Well, you have to look at the PR interval. If it varies completely and has no association with the QRS complex, then you are seeing AV dissociation and/or third-degree heart block. Now, suppose the PR interval is always the same. Your most likely culprit is second-degree 2:1 heart block. Are you starting to see how we put things together?

Let's suppose you have an ECG with very wide complexes and you notice some P waves that are not associated with the complexes. In addition, you see a change in the pattern of the complexes from wide to narrow for two beats. What is the diagnosis? That's right: VTach. It is sometimes easier to read a description of VTach than it is to see it in an ECG. That's why, in the beginning, we are asking you to write down your answers. When you review the things you wrote, they will make a bit more sense. Eventually you'll be able to interpret the same information in the middle of a cardiac arrest — without writing anything down.

How can I put it together? Write down all of the different things you found. Be a stickler about it! Don't let any abnormality get past you. The saying "God is in the details" holds true for ECG interpretation.

Many times, the diagnosis is found in one small area or even in one wave. If you don't know the answer, don't be afraid to ask someone else or look it up.

Remember the differential diagnoses of the various abnormalities. Use them and find the common thread. For example, tell us what the rhythm is:

1. Is the rhythm fast or slow? *Slow*

2. Do I see P waves? *Yes*

3. Are the complexes narrow or wide? *Wide*

4. Is the rhythm regular or irregular? *Regular*

5. Do I see any pauses? *No*

6. What is the relationship of the waves and complexes? *There are two P waves before some QRS complexes, but only one P before others. There is no apparent relationship between the Ps and QRSs.*

7. How can I put it together? *Your answer:*

   Your answer should be easy. The rhythm is slow and wide. If it is wider than 0.12 seconds, it is either going to be an LBBB, RBBB, IVCD, ventricular escape, or aberrantly conducted beat. Where is the money in the above seven questions? In the answer to F: the Ps and QRSs are not associated. Because we know that there is AV dissociation and it is slow, it is probably going to be an idioventricular escape rhythm. The final diagnosis: third-degree heart block with idioventricular escape. Let's go try some (e.g. ECG 10-22, page 155).

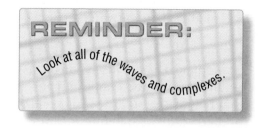

> **REMINDER:**
> Look at all of the waves and complexes.

6. What Is the Axis?

The axis is not really considered important by many practitioners. Boy are they wrong! The axis can be the only thing that shifted in an AMI. It gives you a mental picture of the main forces in play, and the areas of the heart with the most tissue. It is invaluable in diagnosis. Always calculate the axis as completely as possible. Your next review of this book will be as an advanced practitioner. (Congratulations!) When you get to the axis section, you will learn about the Z axis. Make sure you understand it completely. This will expand your axis horizon to a 3-D picture. It will be like adding a new 3-D game card to your computer. You'll be able to do and see much more with the added viewpoint.

When the axis is shifted, there are several things to think about. Did the patient lose myocardium in the area opposite that indicated by the axis? Is there a new block or hemiblock? Is the patient showing more signs of hypertrophy, and if so, why? When you answer these questions, you will be able to see the heart more clearly. You will start to form a mental picture of the actual heart, instead of just looking at lines on the paper.

CLINICAL PEARL

When you see a right axis, think about left posterior hemiblock.

Here is another very important point to remember about the axis. When you see an increased R:S ratio in V_1 or V_2 (Figure 17-5) — that is, the transition point is earlier in the precordial leads, the diagnosis will be one of these five conditions:

1. Right bundle branch block

2. Right ventricular hypertrophy

3. Posterior wall AMI

4. WPW type A

5. The patient is a child or adolescent.

V_1 or V_2 **Figure 17-5**

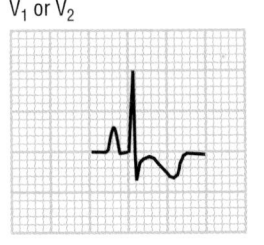

RBBB has the characteristic rabbit ear appearance, but it can be deceptive. Look for the slurred S wave in I and V_6. WPW has a delta wave and a short PR interval. RVH has a pattern similar to the one in Figure 17-5, with a flipped T. PWMI also has a pattern like the one in Figure 17-5, but the R wave is wide and the T is upright.

7. Is There Any Hypertrophy?

Look for hypertrophy in the atria and ventricles. If you don't remember the criteria, take a few minutes to go back and review them. Remember the company it keeps. The axis and the atria can both be affected in RVH, for instance.

We want you to visualize the heart when you think about hypertrophy. If you see an ECG with enlargement of the left and right atria and the right ventricle, it should paint a picture in your mind of a heart with a small left ventricle but enlargement of the other three chambers.

What causes this combination? Would hypertension give you this picture? No, because hypertension would increase the size of the left ventricle. You're looking for a problem that occurs before the left ventricle, in the sequence of blood flow. What structure lies before the left ventricle? The left atria — but that is also enlarged.

What is between the two chambers? The mitral valve! Would mitral regurgitation cause the three-chamber enlargement? No, because the blood is regurgitated back into the atrium after it enters the left ventricle. This would dilate the left ventricle, because it has to accommodate a larger volume of blood. Mitral stenosis perhaps? Right! Mitral stenosis causes an obstruction to blood flow before the left ventricle. The left atria would hypertrophy, and the increased pressure in the lungs would cause the right ventricle and subsequently the right atria to hypertrophy. An elegant diagnosis, isn't it? All because you artistically interpreted the ECG, rather than just read it.

Remember, there are two kinds of LVH: volume overload and pressure overload. This will help you visualize the heart and its pathology. Now, start adding all of the answers from the previous questions together, and you see where we're going. This is how you interpret an ECG. The ECG is a language, kind of like hieroglyphics, and you are interpreting the language so that everyone can understand. It takes time and perseverance, but have patience and you will get there.

8. Is There Any Ischemia or Infarction?

We spent a lot of time on this in Chapter 15. Hopefully, it will be rewarding to you. We are not going to rehash much of the information, but we will repeat this: look for regional changes. Regional changes are significant even when minimal. One thing that will greatly help you in assigning ischemia or infarction as a diagnosis is an old ECG. A previous ECG for comparison gives you a tremendous advantage. Many changes of early repolarization, depolarization-repolarization abnormalities, LVH-with-strain, ventricular aneurysm, and so on can be confused with myocardial infarction. When you are faced with these changes, an old ECG will be critical. If the changes were present six months ago, they are probably not related to a new event. However, remember that myocardial ischemia or infarction can present with no acute changes on an ECG; it is a clinical diagnosis. *Do not withhold treatment because the ECG is unchanged. Do not assume that the pain is benign because the ECG is unchanged.* Always assume the worst!

When looking at an ECG with a bundle branch block, remember what the normal block is supposed to look like. Anything abnormal or new is suspicious. Be careful with blocks.

The heart does not understand that it is only supposed to elevate certain leads in certain regions. Coronary anatomy will perfuse different regions in different people. Try to visualize the blocked artery that is causing the abnormalities you are seeing on the ECG. Remember that the treatment for a right ventricular infarction is different from any of the others. If you don't recall this, review it now. That fact is worth a patient's life!

9. What Is the Differential Diagnosis of the Abnormality?

This is our favorite section. The secret of medicine is the differential diagnosis. It is a lost art. This art is important to clinicians of all levels, whether it be physicians, nurses, paramedics, techs, or students. The principles are universal and can be applied to your particular needs and to your level of training. The following is a story told personally by Dr. Garcia, about his clinical thought process and how he acquired that process. Try not to over-focus on the medical facts; instead, concentrate on the process, which is the main point of this discussion . . . The greatest clinician I have ever met is Dr. Julio Ferreiro at the University of Miami. I once asked Dr. Ferreiro how he was able to formulate such unbelievable clinical diagnoses. His answer was modest and surprising. Can you guess what it was? Yes — the differential diagnosis.

All he did was ask the patient about her ailments by taking a history. He would then examine the patient and evaluate the signs of disease that were present. Next, he would figure out, in his mind, the differential diagnosis for each of the signs and symptoms. He found the one that was common to all and . . . bingo! That was the diagnosis.

Here is an example of the way we approached a particular patient using this simple system. A 50-year-old nun came to the emergency department. She was markedly short of breath, very pale, and had a swollen abdomen and diffuse edema throughout her body. Her heart rate was 135 BPM, and she was in sinus tachycardia; BP 100/50; RR 28, shallow, and labored. What do you think was going on? For brevity, we will only give you two to four differentials for each factor in the presentation (Figure 17-6).

What is the condition most commonly mentioned in the lists in Figure 17-6? Anemia. What else appears frequently? Well, two things: cancer and liver disease. Can cancer and liver disease cause anemia? Yes. Can they both cause hypoalbuminemia and anasarca? Yes. Can they both give you ascites? Yes. What is the most common cause of liver disease in the United States? Alcoholic liver disease. Do nuns have drinking problems? Usually not. Therefore, the diagnosis is most probably cancer with anemia causing a high-output failure. Now, what type of cancer? Possibilities include lung, intestinal, breast, ovarian, or a sarcoma. Any of these can cause this presentation. Because of the large amount of abdominal swelling, you should be highly suspicious of ovarian cancer. When we examined this patient, she had large, freely mobile masses in the abdomen. The diagnosis was correct. This was later verified by a CAT scan.

At first, you will not be fast. It takes quite a few years to develop this, but it is essentially a simple process. You could have come up with the same diagnosis by putting pencil to paper and thinking about it. Dr. Ferreiro's humble answer was correct.

In electrocardiography and in medicine generally, write your differentials down on a 3x5 card and carry them with you. When you have a few seconds of down-time, take one out and review it — between classes, on the bus, and so on. It will stick with you forever. Figure 17-7 shows an example of a differential diagnosis card we have carried. Notice the mnemonic in capital letters, to aid us in memorization.

Pale	SOB	Anasarca	Tachycardia	Ascites
Anemia	Anemia	Hypoalbumin	CHF	Hypoalbuminemia
Hypotensive	CHF	Anemia	Anemia	Liver disease
Vaso-vagal	Pneumonia	Liver disease	Sepsis	Cancer
		Cancer	Hypoxemia	

Figure 17-6: What is the common theme?

DDx for new onset AFib/Flutter:		
Myocardial infarction	**R**heumatic heart disease	**P**ulmonary embolus
Atherosclerotic heart disease	**A**lcoholic holiday heart	**P**neumonia
Drugs: digoxin	**T**hyrotoxicosis	**P**ericarditis
(MAD)	(RAT)	(PPP)

Figure 17-7: What is the common theme?

10. How Can I Put it All Together with the Patient?

We have already covered most of this topic in answering the other questions. The main point in making this into its own question is its importance. The reason you are there and the reason you have gone through all of this training is to provide the best care for your patient. The ECG is but one tool in your evaluation of the patient. However, there are very few things that you can obtain immediately, at the patient's bedside, and relatively inexpensively that can give as much information as an ECG. Some people say that electrocardiography is a lost art. It is a lost art because few people spend the time to learn about it. It seems easier to order an echocardiogram and obtain a real time picture of the heart — but it is *not* always easier. An ECG is a bedside test that can be easily obtained in any clinical setting in a fast and expeditious manner. The time spent waiting for specialized personnel and equipment could be disastrous for some patients!

Make a mental picture of the patient's heart as you read the ECG. Notice how the pathology that you are seeing relates to your patient, and you will quickly arrive at the appropriate treatment. How can you put it all together with the patient? Just by thinking about it!

Remember to use your differential diagnoses when you are evaluating the ECG. Be a bloodhound when you see an abnormality — sniff out the cause. *The little thing that you blow off will be the thing that is the most important.* This is the Murphy's law of electrocardiography.

The Big Picture

Let's recap how to read an ECG. First, get an impression of the whole gram. Then start your evaluation, writing down your findings. Look at what you have written down, and think about the differential diagnosis for each of the items. Miraculously, you will have the answer. Now, go on and try some of the practice ECGs we have included at the web site. After you're done, review the book quickly and try it again. Read as many ECGs as you can. That is how you'll become an expert in the art of electrocardiography.

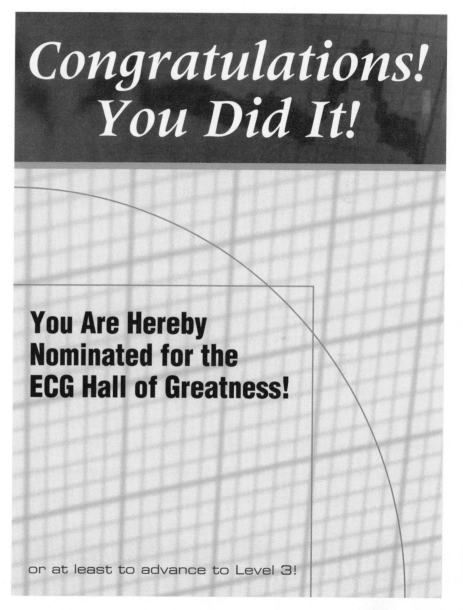

Congratulations!
You Did It!

You Are Hereby Nominated for the ECG Hall of Greatness!

or at least to advance to Level 3!

Acronyms

ACLS: advanced cardiac life support

AFib: atrial fibrillation

AMI: acute myocardial infarction

APC or PAC: atrial premature contraction

ASMI: anteroseptal myocardial infarction

BPM: beats per minute

CAD: coronary artery disease

CHF: congestive heart failure

CNS: central nervous system

COPD: chronic obstructive pulmonary disease

DDx: differential diagnosis

DKA: diabetic ketoacidosis

ED: emergency department

ESRD: End Stage Renal Disease

HB: heart block

IACD: intraatrial conduction delay

IRBBB: incomplete right bundle branch block

IVCD: intraventricular conduction delay

IWMI: inferior wall myocardial infarction

JPC or PJC: junctional premature contraction

LA: left arm (lead)

LAD: left axis deviation

LAE: left atrial enlargement

LAF: left anterior fascicle

LAH: left anterior hemiblock

LBBB: left bundle branch block

LCx: left circumflex artery

LGL: Lown-Ganong-Levine syndrome

LL: left leg (lead)

LPF: left posterior fascicle

LPFB: left posterior fascicular block

LPH: left posterior hemiblock

LVH: left ventricular hypertrophy

MAT: Multifocal Atrial Tachycardia

MI: myocardial infarction

NSR: normal sinus rhythm

NSSTWΔ: non-specific-ST-T wave change

PAT: paroxysmal atrial tachycardia

PSVT: paroxysmal superventricular tachycardia

PWMI: posterior wall myocardial infarction

RA: right arm (lead)

RAD: right axis deviation

RAE: right atrial enlargement

RBBB: right bundle branch block

RCA: right coronary artery

RL: right leg (lead)

RVH: right ventricular hypertrophy

RVI: right ventricular infarction

VPC or PVC: ventricular premature contraction

VTach: ventricular tachycardia

WAP: Wandering Atrial Pacemaker

WPW: Wolf-Parkinson-White syndrome

Additional Readings

Additional reading in electrocardiography is strongly recommended in order to strengthen your interpretive skills. There are quite a number of textbooks on the market and the search for a book that fulfills your particular needs can be quite daunting. We would like to make some suggestions on what we consider some excellent books on the subject. This list is intended as a reflection of the texts that appeal to us.

Electrocardiography in Clinical Practice, Fourth Edition, by Te-Chuan Chou, M.D., F.A.C.C., W.B. Saunders Company, 1996.

This is by far the most comprehensive and authoritative review of electrocardiography that has ever been written. It is an excellent text with all of the information you could ever possibly need. However, your knowledge of electrocardiography and medicine needs to be solid and extensive in order to fully comprehend the material. If you need the definitive reference on the subject, this is it.

Marriott's Practical Electrocardiography, Ninth Edition, by Galen S. Wagner, M.D., Lippincott, Williams and Wilkins, 1994.

This is the latest edition of Dr. Henry Marriott's excellent textbook on the subject. It is a classic that you should be able to understand easily if you are at an intermediate level. The eighth edition is the last one written directly by Dr. Marriott and is still worthwhile reading if you can obtain it.

Ventricular Electrocardiography, by J. Willis Hurst, M.D., J.B. Lippincott, Philadelphia, 1991.

This book is presently out of print to our knowledge. You can view an online copy of the 2nd edition at Medscape.com. This book has excellent historical information and extensive information on vectors and how they shape the ECG and your interpretation. The concepts are difficult to understand, but worth the effort.

The Complete Guide to ECGs: A Comprehensive Study Guide to Improve ECG Interpretation Skills, by James H. O'Keefe, Jr., M.D., Stephen C. Hammill, M.D., and Mark Freed, M.D., Physicians' Press, 1997.

This is a very good review of electrocardiography for intermediate and advanced students alike. You need a solid background in electrocardiography before you attempt to read this book, but the examples and the explanations are excellent.

Clinical Electrocardiographic Diagnosis: A Problem-Based Approach, by Noble O. Fowler, M.D., Lippincott Williams and Wilkins, 2000.

Once again, this is an extensive and excellent review of electrocardiography for the intermediate and advanced student. You need to have a solid background in electrocardiography to review this book as well. The examples are excellent and the clinical approach is refreshing.

Advanced ECG: Boards and Beyond, by Brendan P. Phibbs, M.D., Little Brown and Co., 1997.

This is not an extensive review, but what it does cover, it covers very well. It is written for the intermediate practitioner and is easy reading. There are many clinical pearls inside this book. This is a worthwhile read.

A

Aberrancy – The abnormal conduction of the electrical impulse through the heart. This aberrant conduction gives rise to wide complexes that are morphologically different from those that have gone through the normal pathways.

Accelerated idioventricular rhythm – A faster version of an idioventricular rhythm with a rate of 40 to 100 BPM.

Accelerated junctional rhythm – An escape rhythm with origins in the atrioventricular node or the surrounding tissue that is faster, or more accelerated, than expected. The rate is 60-100 BPM.

Accessory pathways – A pathway, other than the AV node, for the transmission of the impulse from the atria to the ventricles.

Action potential – The electrical firing of the myocyte, which leads to contraction. Consists of four phases.

Amplitude – The total height of a wave or complex.

Antegrade conduction – Normal conduction of the electrical impulse through the AV node from the atria to the ventricles.

Anterior wall – The vertical wall that lies along the anatomical front of the heart, that is, closest to the anterior chest wall.

Anteroseptal – Anatomically, the area of the heart that includes the anterior wall and the interventricular septum.

Antidromic conduction – A circus movement of the electrical impulse found in patients with Wolff-Parkinson-White syndrome in which the impulse travels down the Kent bundle and then reenters the atria via the AV node.

Arteries – Vessels of the circulatory system that carry blood away from the heart.

Atria – Small, thin-walled, chambers of the heart. They act as priming pumps for the ventricles. There are two: the left atrium and the right atrium.

Atrial fibrillation (AFib) – The chaotic firing of many atrial pacemakers in a totally haphazard fashion. There are no discernible P waves and the QRS complexes appear in an irregularly irregular pattern. The chaotic firing leads to a loss of the atrial mechanical contraction.

Atrial flutter (AFlutter) – A fast atrial rhythm (atrial rates are commonly 300 BPM), possibly caused by a reentrant mechanism, which gives the P waves a saw-toothed appearance on an ECG. Ventricular response rates can be variable.

Atrial premature contractions (APC) – An APC occurs when an ectopic pacemaker cell in the atria fires at a rate faster than that of the SA node. The result is a complex that occurs sooner than expected.

Atrioventricular (AV) node – Part of the electrical conduction system. It is responsible for slowing down conduction from the atria to the ventricles just long enough for atrial contraction to occur. This slowing allows the atria to "overfill" the ventricles and helps maintain the output of the heart at a maximum level.

Augmented limb leads – The limb leads aVR, aVL, and aVF.

AV blocks – Physiologic blocks of the AV node caused by disease, drugs, or vagal stimulation. They include first-degree heart block, Mobitz I second-degree heart block (Wenckebach), Mobitz II second-degree heart block, and third-degree heart block.

AV dissociation – An incomplete block of the AV node leading to the independent firing of the atria and the ventricles. The atrial impulse exerts some minimal control over the ventricular rate. In AV dissociation, the atrial rate is the same as or close to the ventricular rate.

AV node – see *atrioventricular node*.

Axis wheel – A tool used to calculate the electrical axis of the heart.

B

Bachman bundles – Part of the electrical conduction system that transmits the impulses through the interatrial septum.

Biatrial enlargement – Enlargement of both atria.

Bifascicular block – The combination of a right bundle branch block and a block of one of the fascicles of the left bundle, either the left anterior or left posterior fascicle.

Biphasic – A term used to describe a wave with both negative and positive components. Usually used in conjunction with P and T waves.

Bradycardia – A slow rhythm (< 60 BPM).

Brugada's sign – Brugada's sign, by definition, is the presence of an abnormally long interval from the R wave to the bottom of the S wave ≥ 0.10 seconds long. This is an abnormality that, if present, will help identify a wide complex tachycardia as VTach in comparison to an aberrantly conducted supraventricular tachycardia.

Bundle branch block (BBB) – A physiologic block of either the left or right bundle branch of the electrical conduction system.

Bundle branch – Part of the electrical conduction system. There are two: the left bundle branch and the right bundle branch. They originate in the bundle of His and end at the Purkinje system.

Bundle of His – Part of the electrical conduction system. It originates in the AV node and ends in the bundle branches.

C

Calibration box – A box or step-like displacement of the ECG baseline at the end of the ECG that is used to ensure that the ECG conforms to a standard format. The standard calibration box

The calibration box can also be set at half-standard or double-standard when evaluating height, or 25-mm or 50-mm standard in regard to width.

Calipers – A tool with two identical legs whose terminal points (pins) are used to evaluate distance. A measuring tool used in electrocardiography, architecture, and navigation.

Capture beats – Sometimes in AV dissociation a P wave falls during a period that enables it to innervate the ventricles. These complexes are narrower (identical to or close to the appearance of the normal complexes) than the ectopic ventricular beats due to the transmission of the electrical impulse down the normal conduction pathway.

Clockwise rotation – The term used to describe a late transition in the precordial leads.

Compensatory pause – A pause immediately following a premature complex that is longer than the interval between two normally conducted beats, allowing the rhythm to proceed, without any alteration of cycle length, around the premature complex. In essence, the pause compensates for the short interval preceding the premature complex and allows the rate to proceed on schedule.

Concordance – A state in which the T waves deflect in the same direction as the terminal portion of the QRS complex in bundle branch blocks. This likely represents an abnormal route of repolarization in most cases.

Coronal plane – An anatomical term used to describe a plane going from left to right, dividing the body or an organ into anterior and posterior segments.

Counter-clockwise rotation – The term used to describe an early transition in the precordial leads.

D

Delta wave – A slurring of the upstroke of the first part of the QRS complex that occurs in Wolff-Parkinson-White syndrome.

Depolarization – A state in which the cell becomes more positive, moving toward equilibrium with the extracellular fluid. Depolarization takes place during the latter part of resting state and is completed during activation by the action potential.

Discordance – The T waves are in the opposite direction of the terminal portion of the QRS complex in bundle branch blocks. This is the normal state in most cases.

Distal – Anatomically, describes the direction and relative distance away from midline. An object that is distal is further away from the midline than one that is proximal; the hand is distal to the elbow.

E

ECG ruler – A tool used to evaluate ECGs that contains various measuring systems and rulers.

Ectopic atrial tachycardia – A tachycardic rhythm of about 100 to 180 BPM that is due to the firing of an ectopic atrial pacemaker. The episodes of tachycardia are usually not sustained for an extended period.

Electrical alternans – A finding associated with a fluctuation of the electrical axis of the ventricles over two or more beats. It is usually associated with large pericardial effusions.

Electrical axis – The summation of the individualized vectors for all of the ventricular myocytes during activation.

Electrical conduction system – A specialized collection of cells that coordinate the bioelectrical activity of the heart. They are involved in initiating (pacemaking) and conducting the electrical impulse. They also coordinate the sequencing of the atrial and ventricular contractions to allow efficient pumping of blood.

Electrical potential – The difference between the charges on the outside and the inside of the cell wall. The electric potential of the resting myocyte is usually about -70 to -90 mV.

Electrodes – The electrical sensors placed on the chest to record the bioelectrical activity of the heart.

Endocardium – The internal lining of the atrial and ventricular walls.

Escape beat – A beat that occurs after a normal pacemaker fails to fire. The R-R interval is longer in these cases.

Extreme right quadrant – The quadrant of the hexaxial system represented by the area from $-90°$ to $-180°$.

F

First-degree heart block (1°AVB) – A prolonged PR interval (> 0.20 seconds) caused by a prolonged physiologic block in the AV node. The cause may be medications, vagal stimulation, disease, and so forth.

Fusion beats – Occur when two complexes with different inciting pacemakers fuse to form a complex unlike either the normal or the ectopic complex. Commonly seen in VTach.

H

Hemiblock – A block of one of the fascicles of the left bundle branch, either the left anterior or left posterior fascicle.

Hexaxial system – The system developed to describe the coronal plane that is created by the limb leads (I, II, III, aVR, aVL, and aVF).

Hyperacute infarct – An ECG pattern found during a very fresh acute myocardial infarction, usually only in the first 15 minutes. It is characterized by very tall, peaked T waves in the affected leads.

Hypercalcemia – An abnormally elevated level of calcium in the blood.

Hyperkalemia – An abnormally elevated level of potassium in the blood.

Hypokalemia – Abnormally depressed level of potassium in the blood.

Hypocalcemia – Abnormally depressed level of calcium in the blood.

I

Idioventricular rhythm – A rhythm occurring when a ventricular focus acts as the primary pacemaker for the heart. The complexes are wide and bizarre because of their ventricular origin.

Incomplete right bundle branch block (IRBBB) – The presence of RSR' complex in V_1, with a normal QRS interval, is considered an IRBBB. The only clinical significance is that it sometimes is a precursor to the development of a complete RBBB.

Inferior wall (IW) – Anatomically, the inferior wall of the heart, which lies on the diaphragm.

Innervation – Activation of the myocardial cells by an electrical impulse.

Intraatrial conduction delay (IACD) – A generic term to describe the presence of atrial enlargement, either left or right.

Intraventricular conduction delay (IVCD) – Either abnormal morphology of the QRS complex in one or two isolated leads, or an indeterminate widening of the QRS complex > 0.12 seconds that does not match LBBB or RBBB criteria.

Internodal pathways – Three pathways of the electrical conduction system found in the atria that transmit the impulse from the SA node to the AV node.

Intrinsicoid deflection – The amount of time it takes the electrical impulse to travel from the Purkinje system in the endocardium to the surface of the epicardium. It is measured from the beginning of the QRS complex to the beginning of the downslope of the R wave, and is usually measured in leads with no Q wave.

Ion – A positively or negatively charged particle in a solution. In the body, the main positively charged ions are sodium (Na+), potassium (K+), and calcium (Ca++). Chloride (Cl−) is the principal negatively charged ion.

Ischemia – Decreased perfusion of an area of myocardium, either relative or actual, that causes a decrease in the amount of oxygen and nutrients available.

Isoelectric lead – A lead that is exactly 90° from the electrical axis. It is usually the lead with the smallest amplitude and the one that is the closest to being neither positive nor negative.

J

J point – The transition point between the QRS complex and the ST segment.

J wave – A large terminal afterdepolarization (notching or hump) at the end of the QRS complex noted in patients with hypothermia. The J wave is also known as the Osborn wave.

James fibers – A bypass tract that connects the upper and central portions of the AV node, bypassing the physiologic block. This tract is found in Lown-Ganong-Levine syndrome.

Josephson's sign – A small notching near the low point of the S wave, seen in VTach.

Junctional escape beat – An escape beat with its origin in the AV node.

Junctional premature contraction (JPC) – A beat that originates prematurely in the AV node. Ventricular depolarization occurs along the normal conduction system distal to the AV node, so the QRS complexes are narrow and normal in appearance.

Junctional rhythm – An escape rhythm originating in the AV node, caused by failure of the proximal pacemakers to fire. The rate is 40 to 60 BPM.

Junctional tachycardia – A junctional rhythm with a rate > 100 BPM.

K

Kent bundle – An accessory pathway found in patients with Wolff-Parkinson-White syndrome.

L

Lateral wall – The lateral wall of the heart, along its left side.

Lead placement – The exact position on the body of the ECG electrodes.

Leads – 1. Any of the electrodes or conductors used to measure the biochemical activity of the heart. 2. The actual representation of the electrical activity of the heart based on the placement of the electrodes, analogous to camera angles.

Left anterior fascicle (LAF) – Part of the electrical conduction system. Responsible for innervating the anterior and superior areas of the left ventricle. It is a single-stranded cord terminating in the Purkinje cells.

Left anterior hemiblock (LAH) – A block of the left anterior fascicle. Causes an axis shift to the left quadrant.

Left atrial enlargement (LAE) – Enlargement of the left atrial wall caused by some underlying process.

Left axis deviation (LAD) – A displacement of the electrical axis of the ventricles toward the abnormal segment of the left quadrant (−30 to −90°).

Left bundle branch (LBB) – Part of the electrical conduction system that is responsible for innervating the left ventricle. It originates in the bundle of His and divides into the left anterior and left posterior fascicles.

Left bundle branch block (LBBB) – A physiologic block of the left bundle branch causing the characteristic ECG pattern of a QRS complex > 0.12 seconds, monomorphic S wave in V_1 and monomorphic R wave in leads I and V_6.

Left posterior fascicle (LPF) – Part of the electrical conduction system. Responsible for innervating the posterior and inferior areas of the left ventricle. It is a widely distributed, fan-like structure terminating in the Purkinje cells.

Left posterior hemiblock (LPH) – A block of the left posterior fascicle. Causes an axis shift to the right quadrant.

Left ventricular hypertrophy (LVH) – Enlargement of the left ventricular wall caused by some underlying process.

Limb leads – The leads that form the hexaxial system, dividing the heart along a coronal plane into anterior and posterior segments. These leads include I, II, III, aVR, aVL, and aVF.

Lown-Ganong-Levine (LGL) syndrome – A syndrome characterized by a short PR interval and a normal QRS complex.

M

Mahaim fibers – A short bypass tract that connects the lower AV node or the His bundles with the interventricular septum. They account for some of the delta waves seen in atypical Wolff-Parkinson-White syndrome.

Mobitz I second-degree heart block (Mobitz I 2°AVB) – Also known as Wenckebach. It is a grouped rhythm characterized by prolongation of the PR interval until a beat is completely dropped.

Mobitz II second-degree heart block (Mobitz II 2°AVB) – A grouped rhythm characterized by dropped beats with no prolongation of the PR intervals of the surrounding complexes. It is caused by a diseased AV node and is a harbinger of complete heart block.

Multifocal atrial tachycardia (MAT) – An irregularly irregular, tachycardic rhythm created by multiple atrial pacemakers, each firing at its own pace. By definition, there are at least three different P wave morphologies with varying PR intervals.

Myocardial infarction (MI) – A process, acute or chronic, that is characterized by the formation or presence of dead myocardial tissue.

Myocytes – The individual heart muscle cells.

N

Noncompensatory pause – A pause, immediately following a premature complex, that alters the rhythm, causing a resetting of the pacemaker and an alteration of cycle length, after the premature complex. In essence, this pause does not compensate for the short interval preceding the premature complex, and the rate is completely reset after the event.

Non-Q wave infarction – A small myocardial infarction acutely represented as ST depression or nonspecific changes. The diagnosis is made by enzymatic elevations noted in laboratory blood testing.

Normal quadrant – The quadrant of the hexaxial system represented by 0 to 90°.

Normal sinus rhythm (NSR) – The heart's normal state, with the SA node functioning as the lead pacer. The intervals should all be consistent and within normal ranges.

O

Osborn wave – A large terminal afterdepolarization (notching or hump) at the end of the QRS complex noted in patients with hypothermia. The Osborn wave is also known as the J wave.

Orthodromic conduction – A circus movement of the electrical impulse found in patients with Wolff-Parkinson-White syndrome, in which the impulse travels normally down the AV node and then reenters the atria via the Kent bundle.

P

P mitrale – A double-humped, M-shaped, P wave that is $\geq$ 0.12 seconds wide with the tops of the humps $\geq$ 0.04 seconds apart; found in the limb leads of I, II, and III. It represents left atrial enlargement.

P pulmonale – A tall P wave that is $\geq$ 2.5 mm high, found in the limb leads of I, II, and III. It represents right atrial enlargement.

P wave – The deflection used to identify atrial depolarization. It is the first wave of a complex or beat.

P-P interval – The interval represented by the space between the P waves of two consecutive complexes.

Pacemaker – The location that initiates cardiac depolarization and dictates the rate at which the heart will cycle. Pacemaking function is usually performed by the cells of the electrical conduction system, although any myocardial cell can perform this function.

Paroxysmal supraventricular tachycardia (PSVT) – A supraventricular tachycardia that starts and ends abruptly.

Pericarditis – An inflammatory process involving the pericardium.

Pericardium – The external lining or surface of the heart.

Polarization – The state in which the cell becomes more negative, moving toward disequilibrium with the extracellular fluid. Polarization occurs after the action potential and continues during the early part of the resting state.

Posterior wall (PW) – Anatomically in the heart, the vertical wall that lies closest to the posterior wall of the chest or thorax.

PR interval – That interval of time that occupies the space between the beginning of the P wave and the beginning of the QRS complex.

PR segment – The segment of the complex that occupies the space between the end of the P wave and the beginning of the QRS complex.

Precordial leads – Another term used to describe the chest leads. They are labeled from V_1 through V_6. They divide the heart along a sagittal plane.

Proximal – Anatomically, describes the direction and relative distance away from midline. An object that is proximal is closer to the midline than one that is distal; the elbow is proximal to the hand.

Pseudoinfarct – A pattern of Q waves found in the inferior leads of patients with Wolff-Parkinson-White syndrome type A. This pattern is not caused by a true infarct.

Purkinje system – Specialized cells that act as the final pathway of the electrical conduction system of the heart. They directly innervate the ventricular myocytes.

Q

Q wave – The first negative wave of the QRS complex.

Q wave infarct – An infarct that presents acutely or chronically with a significant Q wave. It usually represents a larger contiguous area of infarcted tissue.

QR′ wave – A complex seen in V_1 with RBBB and an anteroseptal infarct. The R wave, lost because of the infarct, is replaced by a Q wave.

QRS complex – The wave complex represented by ventricular depolarization. It may consist of individual or multiple waves in succession, which may appear in any combination: the Q wave, R wave, and S wave.

QRS interval – The interval of time occupied by the QRS complex.

QRS notching – A small hump or notch found at the end of the QRS complex. It is usually due to benign causes.

QS wave – By definition, a wave found in V_1 that is composed of only a negative component with no R wave.

QT interval – The interval of time represented by the space from the beginning of the QRS complex to the end of the T wave; may vary with heart rate.

QTc Interval – The QT interval, corrected mathematically for the heart rate.

Quadrants – The hexaxial system can be broken down into four quadrants: the normal, left, right, and extreme right quadrants. Each represents 90° of the hexaxial system.

R

R wave – The first positive wave of the QRS complex.

R-R interval – The interval represented by the space between the R waves of two consecutive complexes.

Rabbit ears – A slang term for the RSR′ pattern traditionally found in V_1 in an RBBB.

Rate – The number of beats per minute.

Refractory state – A short period of time, immediately after depolarization, in which the myocytes are not yet repolarized and are unable to fire or conduct an impulse.

Retrograde conduction – The conduction of the electrical impulse backward through the AV node, from the ventricles or AV node to the atria.

Right atrial enlargement (RAE) – Enlargement of the right atrial wall caused by some underlying process.

Right axis deviation (RAD) – A deviation of the electrical axis of the ventricles toward the right quadrant (90 to 180°).

Right bundle branch block (RBBB) – A physiologic block of the right bundle branch causing the characteristic ECG pattern of a QRS complex > 0.12 seconds, slurred S wave in leads I and V_6, and an RSR′ pattern in V_1.

Right ventricular hypertrophy (RVH) – Enlargement of the right ventricular wall caused by some underlying process.

S

S wave – The second negative wave of the QRS complex.

S₁Q₃T₃ pattern – A pattern of a small *s* in lead I, a small *q* in III, and a flipped T in III. This is usually a sign of acute or chronic right ventricular strain pattern. It is occasionally seen in cases involving pulmonary emboli.

Sagittal plane – Anatomically, a plane from anterior to posterior dividing the body or an organ into right and left segments.

SA node – see *sinoatrial node*.

Second marks – Small marks at the bottom of the ECG to represent an interval of time. They are usually found every three or six seconds depending on the system. At a 25-mm standard, five large boxes represent one second.

Septal Q waves – Small, nonsignificant Q waves that occur in leads I and aVL because of innervation of the interventricular septum.

Septum – Anatomically, the wall between the two atria and the two ventricles.

Sinoatrial block – A rhythm with interspersed dropped complexes. The P-P intervals are a multiple of the normal interval.

Sinoatrial node (SA) – The main pacemaker.

Sinus Arrest – A rhythm characterized by a discontinuation of the atrial pacemaker for an extended period of time. There are no strict criteria that state when a sinus pause becomes a sinus arrest.

Sinus arrhythmia – A variation of normal sinus rhythm involving a sequential acceleration and deceleration of the rhythm caused by the respiratory cycle. The rhythm becomes slower during exhalation and faster upon inhalation.

Sinus bradycardia – A slow rhythm (< 60 BPM) with its origin in the SA node.

Sinus pause – A time period during which there is no sinus pacemaker functioning. The time interval is not a multiple of the normal P-P interval.

Sinus tachycardia – A rapid rhythm (≥100 BPM) with its origin in the SA node.

Slurred S wave – A slow upstroke of the S wave noted in RBBB in leads I and V₆. Slurred S waves can have various morphologies.

ST segment – The section of the complex from the end of the QRS complex to the beginning of the T wave. Electrically, it represents the period of inactivity between ventricular depolarization and repolarization. Mechanically, it represents the time that the myocardium is maintaining contraction.

Strain pattern – Involves ST segment changes and flipped, asymmetrical T waves associated with right or left ventricular hypertrophy.

Supraventricular – Refers to an impulse or rhythm that originated above the ventricles.

T

T wave – The wave that represents ventricular repolarization.

Tachycardia – A rapid rhythm (≥100 BPM).

Threshold potential – The electrical value at which an action potential is triggered.

Third-degree heart block (3°AVB) – A complete block of the AV node leading to the independent firing of the atria and the ventricles. In third-degree heart block, the atrial rate is faster than the ventricular rate.

Torsade de pointes – An undulating sinusoidal rhythm in which the axis of the QRS complexes changes from positive to negative and back in a haphazard fashion.

TP segment – The area of baseline between the end of the T wave and the beginning of the next P wave. A line drawn from one TP segment to the TP segment of a consecutive complex is the true baseline of the ECG.

Tp wave – A wave representing the repolarization of the atria. It usually presents as PR depression or the ST segment depression seen in very fast tachycardias.

Transition zone – The area that represents the isoelectric point as the complexes transition from primarily negative to primarily positive in the precordial leads.

Transmural – Involving all aspects of the ventricular wall: the endocardium, myocardium, and pericardium; for example, a transmural AMI.

U

U wave – A small, flat wave sometimes seen after the T wave and before the next P wave. It could represent ventricular afterdepolarization and endocardial repolarization.

V

Vector – A diagrammatic term used to show the strength and direction of an electrical impulse.

Veins – Vessels of the circulatory system that carry blood toward the heart.

Ventricles – Large, thick-muscled chambers of the heart, the primary pumping chambers. There are two: the left and right ventricles.

Ventricular escape beats – An escape beat with its origin among the ventricular myocytes.

Ventricular fibrillation (Vfib) – The chaotic firing of many ventricular pacemakers in a totally haphazard fashion. There are no discernible QRS complexes. The chaotic firing leads to a loss of the ventricular mechanical contraction.

Ventricular flutter – A very rapid ventricular tachycardia occurring at 200 to 300 BPM. The complexes fuse into a sinusoidal pattern.

Ventricular premature contraction (VPC) – An aberrant complex caused by the premature firing of a ventricular cell.

Ventricular tachycardia (VTach) – A very fast ventricular pacemaker sets a pace of 100 to 200 BPM. The ventricles are always dissociated from the atria.

W

Wandering atrial pacemaker (WAP) – An irregularly irregular rhythm at a rate of < 100 BPM created by multiple atrial pacemakers, each firing at its own pace. By definition, there are at least three different P wave morphologies with varying PR intervals.

Wave – A deflection from the baseline in either a positive or negative direction, representing an electrical event of the cardiac cycle.

Wenckebach – Also known as Mobitz I second-degree heart block. It is a grouped rhythm characterized by prolongation of the PR interval until a beat is completely dropped.

Wide-complex tachycardia – A tachycardia with QRS widths > 0.12 sec. You should consider any wide-complex tachycardia to be ventricular tachycardia until proven otherwise.

Wolff-Parkinson-White (WPW) syndrome – A syndrome characterized by short PR intervals, delta waves, nonspecific ST-T wave changes, and paroxysmal episodes of tachycardia.

Z

Z axis – An axis system that adds a three-dimensional aspect to ECG interpretation because of its anterior and posterior orientation.

The abbreviation *f* refers to items shown in figures.

Internodal pathway, 8, *8f*
Interval; *see specific interval*
Interventricular conduction block, 108, *108f*
Intraatrial conduction delay, 94, *94f*
Intraventricular conduction delay, 277–280, *277f–280f*
  drug effects and, 508
  hyperkalemia and, 489–495, *490f–499f*
Inverted P wave, 73, 80
Ion movement, 16–17, *16f*
Ischemia, 521
  cell death from, 403
  inferior wall, 26
  in myocardial infarction, 405, *405f*
  right bundle branch block and, 246
  septal wall, 384, *384f*
  ST segment and, *311f*, 340–344, *340f–344f*
  subendocardial, *311f*, 372
Isolation of electrical axis, 227–228, *227f–233f*
IVCD; *see* Intraventricular conduction delay

J

J point, *310f*
J wave, 214–215, *214f–217f*
James fibers, 120, *120*
Junctional premature contraction, 268
Junctional rhythm, 80

K

Kent bundle, 132, 138

L

LAH; *see* Left anterior hemiblock
Large QRS complex, 164, *165f*
Lateral extension of anteroseptal myocardial infarction, 418, *418f*, 419, *420f–429f*, 424–429
Lateral wall myocardial infarction, 430, *430f*, 431, *432f*
Lead
  electrical axis calculation and, 227–228, *227f–229f*

manipulation of, 24, *24*
in myocardial infarction, 450, *450f*, 451, *451f*
placement of, 23, *23f*
representation of, 30
two-lead system, 24–25, *24f*, *25f*
Left anterior fascicle, 11, *11f*
Left anterior hemiblock, 282–284, *282f–288f*
  bifascicular block and, 297
  prolonged PR interval and, 151
  right bundle branch block and, 297, 299, *299f*, 300, 303
Left atrial enlargement, 74
  left ventricular hypertrophy and, 177
  left ventricular strain pattern and, 352
Left atrial hypertrophy, 101
Left axis deviation, 234
Left bundle branch, anatomy of, 10, *10f*
Left bundle branch block, 260–262, *260f*, *261f*, 262, *263f*, *264f*, 265, *266f*, *267f*, 268, *269f*, *270f*, 271, *272f*, *273f*, 274, *275f*, *276f*, 514
  bifascicular block and, 297
  criteria for, 261, *261*
  large QRS complex in, 164
  myocardial infarction and
    inferior wall, 434
    inferoposterior, 468
  ST segment and, 376, *376f*, 397–398, *397f–401f*
  T wave and, 397–398, *397f–401f*
  ventricular hypertrophy and, 277
Left posterior fascicle, 11, *11f*
Left posterior fascicular block, 73
Left posterior hemiblock, 255, 289, *289f*, 290, *291f*, *292f*, 293, *294f–296f*, 296
  bifascicular block and, 297
  P-pulmonale and, 88
  right bundle branch block and, 306–307, *306f*, *307f*
Left ventricular hypertrophy
  biatrial enlargement and, 107, *107f*
  bundle branch block and, 277
  large QRS complex in, 164, *165f*
  left bundle branch block and, 262, 265
  left ventricular strain pattern and, 352, 356, 359
  myocardial infarction and, 411

in P-mitrale, 83
P wave in, 80, *81f*
QRS complex and, 166–168, *166f–170f*, 171, *172f–173f*, 174, *175f–179f*, 177
right bundle branch block and, 252, 277
ST segment and, 342, 370, *370f*, 378, *378f*
strain pattern and, 352, 356, 359
Left ventricular strain pattern, 351–353, *354f–361f*, 356, 359
Localization, 26–27, *26f*, *27f*
Low atrial ectopic pacemaker, P wave and, 80
Lown-Ganong-Levine syndrome, 174

M

Measuring, calipers for, 33–36, *33f–36f*
Mechanics of contraction, 15–16
Membrane channel, 18–19
Mitral stenosis, 82
Mobitz I block, 142
Mobitz II block, 142
Monomorphic complex, 260
Multifocal atrial tachycardia
  P-pulmonale and, 89
  P wave in, 76
Myocardial cell, *15f*, 15–16
  death of, 403
Myocardial infarction, 403–478, 521
  additional leads in, 450, *450f*, 451, *451f*
  anatomy and, *404f*
  anterior wall, 412, *412f*
  anteroseptal, 413, *413f*, 414, *415f–418f*
    with lateral extension, 418, *418f*, 419, *420f–429f*, 424–429
  apical, 445, *445f*, 446, *447f–449f*
  ECG progression in, 408, *408f*
  flipped T wave and, 386
  infarct regions on ECG, 410–411, *410f*
  inferior wall, 25–26, 433–434, *433f*, *435f–436f*
  infero-RV-posterior, 469, *469f*, 470, *471f–473f*, 474, *475f*, 476
  inferolateral, 437, *437f*, 438, *439f*, 440f, 441, *442f–444f*, 444
  inferoposterior, 464, *464f–468f*, 465, 468
  large QRS complex in, 164, *165f*

lateral wall, 430, *430f*, 431, *432f*
non-Q wave, 407, *407f*
posterior wall, 459–463, *459f–463f*
prolonged PR interval in, 143
Q wave and, 205, *206f*, 343, 406, *406f*
QRS notching and, 214
QS waves and, 385, *385f*
reciprocal changes in, 409–410, *409–410f*
right ventricular, 452, *452f*, 453, *454f*, 455, *456f–458f*
ST segment and, *311f*, 342, 362, *363f–389f*, 364–368, 370–372, 372, 374, 376–380, 377, *377f*, *381f–384f*, 382–386, *387f*, 388
T waves and, 328
wide QRS complex and, 186
Wolff-Parkinson-White syndrome and, 125
zones of, 405, *405f*
Myocyte, atrial, 6
Myofibril, 16, *16f*
Myosin molecule, 15–16

N

Na+-K+-ATPase, 19
Node
  atrioventricular; *see* Atrioventricular node
  sinus, 77
Nomenclature, wave, 39–40
Non-Q wave myocardial infarction, 407, *407f*
Notching
  abnormal P wave and, 82, *82f*
  QRS, 214–215, *214f–217f*

O

Obstructive pulmonary disease, chronic, 92
Old infarct, 411
Orthodromic tachycardia, Wolff-Parkinson-White syndrome and, 122
Osborn wave, 214–215, *214f–217f*
Overload, volume, 168
Oxygen, 403